PEDIATRIC NURSE PRACTITIONER CERTIFICATION

REVIEW GUIDE

Sixth Edition

Primary Care

Edited by

JoAnne Silbert-Flagg, DNP, CPNP-PC, IBCLC
Assistant Professor
Johns Hopkins University School of Nursing
Baltimore, Maryland

Elizabeth D. Sloand, PhD, PNP-BC, FAAN
Associate Professor
Coordinator, Pediatric Nurse Practitioner Track
Johns Hopkins University School of Nursing
Baltimore, Maryland

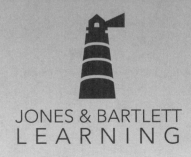

JONES & BARTLETT
LEARNING

World Headquarters
Jones & Bartlett Learning
5 Wall Street
Burlington, MA 01803
978-443-5000
info@jblearning.com
www.jblearning.com

Jones & Bartlett Learning books and products are available through most bookstores and online booksellers. To contact Jones & Bartlett Learning directly, call 800-832-0034, fax 978-443-8000, or visit our website, www.jblearning.com.

Substantial discounts on bulk quantities of Jones & Bartlett Learning publications are available to corporations, professional associations, and other qualified organizations. For details and specific discount information, contact the special sales department at Jones & Bartlett Learning via the above contact information or send an email to specialsales@jblearning.com.

07897-8

Production Credits

VP, Executive Publisher: David D. Cella
Executive Editor: Amanda Martin
Acquisitions Editor: Teresa Reilly
Editorial Assistant: Lauren Vaughn
Associate Production Editor: Alex Schab
Marketing Communications Manager: Katie Hennessy
Rights & Media Research Assistant: Wes DeShano
Media Development Editor: Shannon Sheehan

VP, Manufacturing and Inventory Control: Therese Connell
Composition: Cenveo Publisher Services
Cover Design: Kristin E. Parker
Cover Images: Top/bottom image: © flowerstock/Shutterstock;
    Middle image behind title: © Keo/Shutterstock
Printing and Binding: Edwards Brothers Malloy
Cover Printing: Edwards Brothers Malloy

Library of Congress Cataloging-in-Publication Data

Pediatric nurse practitioner certification review guide : primary care / [edited by] JoAnne Silbert-Flagg, Elizabeth D. Sloand. — Sixth edition.
    p. ; cm.
  Includes bibliographical references and index.
  ISBN 978-1-284-05834-5
  I. Silbert-Flagg, JoAnne, editor.   II. Sloand, Elizabeth D., editor.
  [DNLM: 1. Pediatric Nursing—Examination Questions.   2. Pediatric Nursing—Outlines.   3. Licensure, Nursing—standards—Examination Questions.   4. Licensure, Nursing—standards—Outlines.   5. Nurse Practitioners—Examination Questions.
6. Nurse Practitioners—Outlines. WY 18.2]
  RJ242
  618.92'00231—dc23
                    2015020529

6048

Printed in the United States of America
19 18 17 16 15   10 9 8 7 6 5 4 3 2 1

Contents

Chapter 4

Eye, Ear, Nose, Mouth, and Throat Disorders   81

Karen K. Buch

Chapter 5

Cardiovascular Disorders   117

Peggy Dorr

Chapter 6

Lower Respiratory Disorders   137

Shawna S. Mudd and Elizabeth D. Sloand

Chapter 7

Dermatologic Conditions   155

Brigit VanGraafeiland

Chapter 16

Advanced Practice, Role Development, Current Trends, and Health Policy   375
Janet S. Selway

Preface

Pediatric Nurse Practitioner Certification Review Guide presents the most up-to-date information and current standards of practice for the nurse practitioner (NP) in the pediatric primary care setting. It examines all the content areas required for the certification examinations for pediatric nurse practitioners (PNPs) in primary care. Each system chapter presents common pediatric disorders followed by a definition of the disorder and its etiology/incidence, signs and symptoms, differential diagnosis, physical findings, diagnostic tests, and management/treatment. Practice test questions follow content in each chapter. This format enables the reader to review essential information and to explore areas that may require further study. Bibliographies and relevant websites give the reader resources for further consideration and study.

All chapter authors are specialists in their areas. Clinical chapter authors are certified PNPs and expert clinicians who have practiced extensively in their specialty area. The editors are faculty members at the Johns Hopkins University School of Nursing who teach predominantly in the PNP primary care program.

We hope this review guide will assist PNP graduates to become certified and to provide competent and compassionate health care throughout their career to children, adolescents, and their families.

We are pleased to present the sixth edition of the *Pediatric Nurse Practitioner Certification Review Guide* from Jones & Bartlett Learning. It has a dual purpose. The book serves pediatric nurse practitioner (PNP) and family nurse practitioner (FNP) graduates who are doing self-study preparation for the PNP primary care certification exam. Students and graduates can be overwhelmed when faced with the vast body of knowledge required for certification. This book brings together the most current and essential information in an organized, concise, and comprehensive manner. This book also serves as a valuable clinical resource for practicing PNPs and FNPs in pediatric primary care.

The first chapter of the book reviews test-taking strategies to help students plan their certification preparation; it considers various approaches to test taking and to organizing one's study time. The second chapter reviews growth and development. The third chapter, which covers health promotion and well-child care for infants, children, and adolescents, includes expanded information on the promotion of breastfeeding in the first year of life. The subsequent chapters of the book review the following systems and disorders: HEENT, cardiovascular, lower respiratory, dermatology, gastrointestinal, infectious diseases, musculoskeletal, neurological, GU and GYN (including adolescent pregnancy), hematologic/oncologic and immunologic, endocrine, and multisystem and genetic. The book concludes with a chapter on advanced practice nursing, role development, current trends, and health policy.

Acknowledgments

We are pleased to have had the opportunity to revise the original work of Virginia Layng Millonig and Caryl Erhardt Mobley. We owe thanks to each chapter author for her diligence, knowledge, and expertise.

We are grateful to our professional colleagues who have mentored, supported, and taught us over the years, particularly those at the Johns Hopkins University School of Nursing.

JoAnne Silbert-Flagg and Elizabeth D. Sloand

As a practicing PNP for over 20 years at Columbia Medical Practice in Columbia, Maryland, I have had the opportunity to provide pediatric primary care to a generation of patients. I hope I have touched their lives as much as they have touched mine.

As books are revised and improved upon, so are our lives. I thank my husband, Jon (Kronheim), for his support and encouragement. I welcome my step-children, Sarah, Daniel, Anna, and Lauren, into my life. Last, I appreciate the love and support of my children, Chris and Jenn (Flagg), and my daughter-in-law, Melissa.

JoAnne Silbert-Flagg

I am personally indebted to my husband, Bob, who makes everything possible; my children, Daniel and his wife Kathryn, Christine, Rachel, and Rose, who are a continued source of wonder and pride; my grandchildren, James and Annette, who are pure joy; and my parents, Dorothy and Joseph, for their ever-present love.

Elizabeth D. Sloand

Contributors

Cheri Barber, DNP, CRNP
Clinical Assistant Professor
PNP Program Coordinator
School of Nursing and Health Studies
University of Missouri-Kansas City
Kansas City, Missouri

Karen K. Buch, MSN, CPNP
Gettysburg Pediatrics
Gettysburg, Pennsylvania

Peggy Dorr, DNP, CRNP
Pediatric Nurse Practitioner
Division of Pediatric Cardiology
University of Maryland Medical Center
Baltimore, Maryland

Marlo A. Eldridge, DNP, MSN, CPNP
Director, Pediatric Voiding Improvement Program
The Brady Urological Institute
Johns Hopkins Hospital
Baltimore, Maryland

Janice J. Hoffman, PhD, RN, ANEF
Associate Professor and Assistant Dean for
    the Bachelor of Science Nursing Program
University of Maryland School of Nursing
Baltimore, Maryland

Sheila Holdford, MS, RN, APRN-BC, CPNP-PC
Adjunct Clinical Instructor of Nursing
University of South Carolina College of Nursing
Columbia, South Carolina

Rita Marie John, EdD, DNP, CPNP, PMHS
Pediatric Nurse Practitioner Program Director
Associate Professor of Nursing at CUMC
Columbia University School of Nursing
New York, New York

Rachel Lyons, DNP, CPNP-PC/AC, DCC
Associate Clinical Professor
Pediatric Nurse Practitioner Specialty Director
Rutgers, The State University of New Jersey School
    of Nursing
Newark, New Jersey

Shawna S. Mudd, DNP, CPNP-AC, PNP-BC
Assistant Professor
Johns Hopkins University School of Nursing
Baltimore, Maryland

MaryLou C. Rosenblatt, RN, MS, CPNP
Lead Nurse Practitioner, Adolescent Medicine Clinic
Faculty, LEAH (Leadership Education
    in Adolescent Health)
Johns Hopkins Hospital
Baltimore, Maryland

Janet S. Selway, DNSc, CRNP, FAANP
Adult/Pediatric Nurse Practitioner
Assistant Professor
The Catholic University of America School of Nursing
Washington, D.C.

JoAnne Silbert-Flagg, DNP, CPNP-PC, IBCLC
Assistant Professor
Johns Hopkins University School of Nursing
Baltimore, Maryland

Elizabeth D. Sloand, PhD, PNP-BC, FAAN
Associate Professor
Coordinator, Pediatric Nurse Practitioner Track
Johns Hopkins University School of Nursing
Baltimore, Maryland

Brigit VanGraafeiland, DNP, CRNP
Assistant Professor
Johns Hopkins University School of Nursing
Baltimore, Maryland

Roseann Velez, DNP, CRNP, FNP-BC
Instructor
Johns Hopkins University School of Nursing
Baltimore, Maryland

Melissa Silva Wills, MS, PNP-BC
Pediatric Nurse Practitioner
Leukemia/Lymphoma Team
Department of Hematology/Oncology
Children's National Medical Center
Washington, D.C.

Lindsay Wilson, MSN, RN, CPNP
Lead Nurse Practitioner
Pediatric Gastroenterology and Nutrition
Johns Hopkins Children's Center
Johns Hopkins Hospital
Baltimore, Maryland

M. Elizabeth M. Younger, PhD, CPNP
Assistant Professor
Johns Hopkins University School of Medicine
Division of Pediatric Allergy and Immunology
Baltimore, Maryland

Test-Taking Strategies and Techniques

Janice J. Hoffman

CHAPTER 1

The decision has been made to take the certification examination, so it is now time to make plans. Based upon prior experiences with standardized testing situations, a candidate may have some anxiety and questions about the certification process. This chapter includes an overview of the test plans for primary care pediatric nurse practitioner certification, followed by study and test-taking strategies to assist in preparation for the examination.

☑ SELF-ASSESSMENT REGARDING SEEKING CERTIFICATION

The first question that only the nurse contemplating the certification process can answer is: "Why do I want to become certified as a pediatric nurse practitioner?" There are many benefits of professional certification, including demonstration of specialized knowledge and skills, recognition as an expert in the field, possible monetary benefits, possible career advancement, personal growth, and greater satisfaction as a professional nurse (Lamonte, 2007). Personal confidence in caring for patients is another benefit of professional certification. Perhaps most importantly, national board certification is required for NP practice in all states. Once the nurse decides to seek certification, questions may arise about how best to study and who and what can assist in the preparation. In addition, some nurses may have negative feelings about past testing experiences. In the following sections, specific content is provided about preparing for the examination and about ways to deal with the emotions associated with taking standardized examinations.

On the basis of past examination performance, most test takers consider themselves either strong or weak test takers. Nurses who have experienced success with formal or standardized tests in the past are wise to examine approaches used and to adapt these practices in preparing for this certification exam. For those who have not performed well on past tests, it is important to determine whether this past performance resulted from poor test-taking skills or lack of preparation, which may be related to lack of knowledge or insufficient review of the test plan. The area of pediatrics in which the nurse is currently working has an impact on performance as well as preparation. For example, nurses working in a specialized area such as pediatric cardiac surgery—although they are experts in cardiac surgery and care of the critically ill child—may need to focus on primary care, normal growth and development, and parent education.

Becoming familiar with areas of content to be reviewed is usually straightforward; examining and dealing with test anxiety is another issue. For those individuals with significant test anxiety, one approach is to become very familiar with the content and process of the certification examinations. Another strategy is to complete practice tests, even simulating testing circumstances like sitting in a quiet, monitored place and completing all questions prior to review. Online testing resources are available to further familiarize candidates with the examination process, which may decrease anxiety. Test taking is a skill, and as with any skill, it improves with consistent practice. Finally, the candidate needs to use personal strategies that have been successful in other high-anxiety circumstances, such as deep breathing, visualization, and exercise.

☑ KNOW THE TEST PLAN

Certification as a pediatric nurse practitioner (PNP) can be gained through the American Nurses Credentialing Center (ANCC) or the Pediatric Nursing Certification Board

(PNCB). One of the first priorities in certification examination preparation is to review the requirement for each organization. This information can be found at the following websites:

http://www.nursecredentialing.org/NurseSpecialties /PediatricNP.aspx (ANCC)

http://www.pncb.org/ptistore/control/exams/pnp /admin (PNCB)

Once eligibility for taking the examination has been determined, specific planning should begin. In preparing for the exam, make sure that sufficient time is planned for review of content and practice questions. Both of the above listed websites list specific resources to assist candidates in preparing for the certification examination. Other things to consider are work schedule and any other commitments or conflicts that might potentially compete with study time.

The next step is to review the test plan for each examination; the detailed plans for both the ANCC and PNCB examinations are available from the respective websites. Reviewing the content is important in guiding the individual plan of study and assists each individual candidate in estimating the time needed for review and study. In the next section, suggested guidelines for developing a specific study plan are described.

✓ DEVELOP A SPECIFIC PLAN

In reviewing the test plans, it is important to begin to prioritize the content areas where review is most needed. One strategy is to develop a rubric for self-assessment such as the following:

4 Very knowledgeable (little review needed)
3 Knowledgeable (some review needed)
2 Familiar (significant time needed for study and review)
1 Unknown (priority area for study and review)

In using this four-choice rubric, there is no middle or average choice, which forces a decision between an area needing significant study and review and one that requires less time.

Now that a self-assessment rubric has been developed, a review of the test plan is needed. **Table 1-1** provides an overview of the PNCB examination and **Table 1-2** provides the outline of the ANCC examination. It is important to schedule study time, with details about length of time allotted and content to be reviewed. One approach is to review your calendar for the next 3 months and to schedule specific study days and times, just as work and other appointments are scheduled. Based upon the self-assessment of baseline knowledge compared with the content outline and time frame until test day, an individualized plan of study can be developed. In addition to a review of content headings, Tables 1-1 and 1-2 provide percentages and numbers of test questions for the respective

examinations based upon the most recent practice analyses for PNPs. **Table 1-3** is a sample study plan for one week, based upon the PNCB test plan. While there are similarities in content, it is best to select study guides and review resources specific to the examination that is being taken.

A strategy to address potential content issues is to conscientiously review any new medication, term, diagnosis, and so forth that is encountered in practice or in a journal during the preparation time. Consider a small (2- by 3-inch) notebook or an electronic device to record this "new" data. Review this content to broaden your knowledge base. Both ANCC and PNCB suggest taking advantage of the review resources available, including books, audiovisual materials, and workshops.

This one-week calendar is used as an example in planning study time. It is important to plan study time in relation to work schedule. If a candidate works 12-hour shifts, it is probably not feasible to study on those days. To be more efficient with study time, it is beneficial to "schedule" the study time and the specific topic for study. Valuable time can be wasted "trying to decide what to study." With a plan, as in Table 1-3, not only are the times detailed but also the specific content is identified. The amount of time allotted for each category of the test plan should be based upon the individual self-assessment results.

✓ APPROACHES TO TEST TAKING

All items on the PNP certification examinations are multiple-choice questions. Each question includes the stem and four to five choices. The stem contains the content being tested and is sometimes stated as a question. The key to correctly answering these types of questions is to accurately determine what the question or stem is asking. Because questions may have distracting information that is not needed to answer the question correctly, one strategy is to reword the question into a short phrase that you can clearly understand and consider. For example, the question "A benign (Still's) murmur is most accurately described as" may be reworded to "Describe a Still's murmur."

Cognitive Levels of Questions

The PNP certification exam questions, as with most other professional nursing organization certification examinations (AACN, AORN, CEN, etc.), are based upon Bloom's taxonomy of cognition. The first levels, knowledge, comprehension, application, and analysis, are used in the development of multiple-choice examinations. As with other nursing examinations, the majority of questions are at the application and analysis levels. A short review of the different types of questions and examples are presented in this section.

In Bloom's taxonomy, knowledge-based questions are at the lowest cognitive level and test the ability to recognize

■ **Table 1-1** Primary Care Pediatric Nurse Certification Test Plan

Domains of Practice	Number of Questions	Knowledge Level	Percentage of Test	Hours for Study
Health Promotion	45		30%	
Counsel patients/caregivers about growth and development				
Counsel patients/caregivers with age/developmentally appropriate anticipatory guidance				
Provide patients/caregivers information about age/developmentally appropriate health promotion and illness prevention				
Counsel about age-appropriate injury prevention and safety				
Educate caregivers to recognize early warning signs of pediatric illness and emergencies				
Counsel about young adult concerns				
Counsel about age-appropriate transition to adult care				
Counsel child/family regarding age-appropriate response to death, dying, and loss				
Educate the community regarding pediatric health and wellness				
Assessment and Diagnosis	52		35%	
Growth and development				
History and physical examination				
Diagnostic testing and screening				
Analyzing information				
Diagnosis				
Management	45		30%	
Therapeutic interventions				
Procedures				
Counseling and education				
Collaboration and referral				
Case management				
Evaluation and follow-up				
Professional Issues	8		5%	
Leadership and professional development				
Research				
Business management				
Legal and ethical issues				

Data from PNCB Primary Care Pediatric Nurse Practitioner Detailed Content Outline (2013). available at http://www.pncb.org/ptistore/resource/content/exams/pnp/2012_CPNP_Content_Outline.pdf.

and recall information. An example of a knowledge-based question is as follows:

What is a common complication of a blood transfusion?

A. Fever
B. Elevated blood pressure
C. Hematuria
D. Change in level of consciousness

The correct answer is A. This question requires the test taker to remember only a fact in order to answer the question correctly. There are not large numbers of this

level of question on the exam, but basic knowledge is important to review.

The next level of question is comprehension, which requires the nurse to understand the meaning of the material. An example of this level of question is as follows:

The nurse understands that fever is a complication of a blood transfusion because antibodies in the patient's blood cause:

A. changes in the temperature set point in the hypothalamus
B. collapse of blood vessels

■ Table 1-2   ANCC Pediatric Primary Care Nurse Practitioner Board Certification

Domains of Practice	Number of Questions	Knowledge Level	Percentage of Test	Hours for Study
Foundations for Advanced Practice	56		32%	
Advanced Physiology and Pharmacology				
Advanced Pharmacology				
Advanced Health/Physical Assessment				
Care of Diverse Populations				
Clinical Prevention and Population Health				
Professional Practice	50		29%	
Quality Improvement and Safety				
Translational Science/Evidence-Based Care				
Informatics and Healthcare Technologies				
Healthcare Policy, Delivery, and Advocacy				
Interprofessional Collaboration				
Ethical and Legal Issues, Scope and Standards of Practice				
Independent Practice	69		39%	
Health Promotion and Maintenance				
Illness/Disease Management				
Advanced Diagnostic Reasoning and Critical Thinking				

Data from ANCC Web site, http://www.nursecredentialing.org

C.   an increase in the metabolic rate

D.   a reaction against donor proteins

The correct answer is D. The question is asking why fever occurs after a blood transfusion and requires the nurse to understand the physiologic etiology of the fever.

Application is the next level of question in Bloom's taxonomy, and these questions evaluate the nurse's ability to take information and apply it to a given situation.

The following question is an example of an application question:

The nurse is caring for a 15-year-old patient receiving a blood transfusion. Which findings would require the nurse to immediately stop the transfusion?

A.   Pain at the insertion site

B.   Coolness at the insertion site

■ Table 1-3   Sample One-Week Study Plan

	Sunday	Monday	Tuesday	Wednesday	Thursday	Friday	Saturday
6 a.m.	Work	Work				Work	
7 a.m.							
8 a.m.			Study Respiratory	Study Respiratory	Study GI Disorders		Study
9 a.m.							
10 a.m.							
11 a.m.							
12 p.m.							
1 p.m.			Study Respiratory	Study Respiratory			
2 p.m.							
3 p.m.							Study
4 p.m.							
5 p.m.							
6 p.m.							
7 p.m.					Study Infectious Diseases		
8 p.m.							
9 p.m.							
10 p.m.							

C.   Fever and chills

D.   Thirst

The correct answer is C. This question requires the nurse to know the side effects of a blood transfusion and which require an immediate intervention.

The highest cognitive level tested on the certification examination is at the analysis level. At this level, the nurse is often expected to take a familiar piece of information and apply it to an unfamiliar setting. An example of an analysis question is as follows:

Which dietary selections would be MOST effective for the patient with pernicious anemia?

A.   Peaches and cottage cheese

B.   Liver and onions

C.   Pasta with clam sauce

D.   Chicken breast and corn

The correct answer is B. This question requires the nurse to know that pernicious anemia is related to iron deficiency and to have knowledge of foods high in iron. Although some of the other food items contain some iron, liver and kidneys have large amounts of iron.

In review, the certification exam has questions from all four cognitive levels, but the majority of the questions are at the application and analysis levels.

Prioritization Issues

Prioritizing issues is a competency that is relevant to success on certification examinations. Many questions ask the nurse practitioner which intervention to complete first. There are two major approaches to prioritizing care: the "ABCs" (airway, breathing, and circulation) and Maslow's hierarchy of needs.

Consider the following question:

Four patients present to the emergency room. Which patient should the pediatric nurse practitioner see first?

A.   2-year-old with chest burns

B.   3-year-old with 2-day history of diarrhea

C.   4-year-old with suspected pneumonia

D.   5-year-old with cut to left thigh

The correct answer is A. Whereas all of these patients require an assessment, based upon the ABCs, the child with chest burns is the highest priority. All patients with burns to the face, chest, and abdomen require immediate evaluation for potential airway swelling secondary to heat near the airway. If airway swelling occurs, the patient may have a significantly compromised airway and require immediate intubation.

In using Maslow's hierarchy of needs, it is important to remember that physiologic needs always have priority over psychological needs. Another important concept from Maslow's hierarchy that guides prioritization relates to a focus on safety, food, and water as basic needs for all people. Refer to http://nursingcrib.com/abraham-maslows-hierarchy-of-needs for additional information on specific details of each category of needs.

Potential Test Item Traps

As described above, one of the key actions to increase the likelihood of correctly answering the questions is to clarify the meaning or intent of the question. Depending on the format of the question, several potential traps can lead to choosing an incorrect answer. Here are suggestions to help the test taker to correctly identify the topic of the question.

Many questions ask the PNP to prioritize or make a clinical judgment in order to select the correct answer. The stem of the question may ask the PNP to choose the "first" (indicating prioritization) or "most" or "best" (requiring discrimination and clinical judgment). It is really important to recognize these words and consider them carefully in selecting the correct answer.

Another potential trap is posed by "negative" questions. When was the last time the nurse reviewed the patient assignment and asked, "What will I not assess in this patient?" It is important to review the two negative formats used relatively frequently on standardized tests. Consider the following question:

The nurse practitioner is evaluating a 6-year-old admitted with a diagnosis of acute appendicitis. Which finding requires an immediate intervention?

A.   Nausea and vomiting

B.   Dry mucous membranes and scant urine output

C.   Abdominal pain and cramping

D.   Anorexia and constipation

The correct answer is B. The other options are expected clinical manifestations in patients with appendicitis. Option B indicates a complication; the patient is showing signs of dehydration secondary to the vomiting, anorexia, and decreased oral intake. This type of question asks the nurse practitioner to find something in the answer choices that requires an action or intervention.

The second potential trap involving a negatively formatted question is in the form of a patient teaching scenario. Teaching questions on a standardized nursing examination are typically asked in one of two ways:

"Which statement indicates that the patient/family member understands the information?"
"Which statement indicates the need for further teaching?"

The second question is an example of asking "what is wrong?" It is important with these types of questions that the nurse practitioner clarifies whether the question is asking for a correct or incorrect response by the patient. Consider the following example:

> Which statement, made by the parent of a 1-day-old child, indicates the need for further teaching?
>
> A. "I should bring the baby back for a checkup in two weeks."
> B. "The baby should have at least four wet diapers per day."
> C. "The baby will want to nurse every 2–3 hours."
> D. "The stool probably will be dark and sticky for the first couple of days."

The correct answer is B; all the other statements are correct about a newborn infant. A newborn with fewer than eight wet diapers per day is most likely not getting sufficient fluids. Consistently remembering to clarify the meaning of the stem with each question increases the likelihood of correctly answering these negatively formatted questions.

Maximizing Study Time

As discussed previously, it is very important to develop an individualized study plan based upon work schedule, personal commitments, and self-assessment of test plan content. Practice can improve test-taking skills. Most certification books include practice questions, and there are online resources available for both pediatric NP certification exams. Additionally, these practice items often familiarize the nurse with the types of questions to expect on the actual exams. Another consideration is whether to study in private or with a colleague who may also be taking the examination. Study groups may be very effective for the auditory learner who learns best through hearing and discussing content.

While practicing answering test questions is important, effective review of the correct answers is equally, if not more, important. After completing a practice examination, it is important for the candidate to review all questions to determine content areas in which further study is needed as well as those areas in which mastery of content is observed. During review, it is good to note not only that a question was answered correctly but more importantly that the question was answered correctly for the right reason. Examine the stated rationale for the correct answer as well as the rationale for the other incorrect choices. This strategy for reviewing exam questions familiarizes the nurse with the types of questions and reminds the nurse of relevant content that is available in the rationales for both correct and incorrect answers.

As the day for the exam draws near, consider simulating actual testing circumstances—quiet room, no interruptions, and no use of notes. Prepare a sample test, or plan on answering a set of 50 questions in 60 minutes as this closely reflects the approximate time given in the actual exams. Remember, both exams include 175 questions (150 scored and 25 experimental), and 3 hours are allotted to complete the exam.

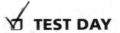

TEST DAY

Just as important as sufficient preparation for the examination is being attentive to preparation for the actual test day. Because last-minute cramming has not been shown to be effective, and because it may increase test anxiety, this is not a recommended strategy. On the schedule for the day before the exam, the "stop" time for studying needs to be clearly identified. Getting a good night's sleep and being well rested are more important at this stage of preparation than last-minute cram sessions. Also, at this late date, unfamiliar concepts, terminology, or diagnoses may undermine the confidence that has been growing over the weeks or months of preparation.

On the day of the exam, make sure you eat a healthy meal and take several healthy snacks and beverages with you to the testing site. Ensure that you are familiar with the location of the testing center, and make plans to arrive there 15–20 minutes early; many testing centers do not allow test takers to start the examination late. No study guides or books should be taken to the testing site as, again, coming across an unfamiliar concept may increase test anxiety. If you *must* have something with you, take flash cards or index cards with specific data to review—for example, development tasks that are expected at specific ages, normal laboratory values, or recommended immunization schedules and common side effects.

After completing the exam, consider some type of personal reward! You expended a lot of time and effort in preparing for the exam. Remember, although the ultimate goal is certification, a great deal of what you reviewed and learned in preparation for the examination contributes to professional growth and will benefit your patients. Once you receive your certification, make an effort to encourage a colleague to pursue this goal, and use your newly developed study habits and competence to mentor this potential candidate.

REFERENCES

American Nurses Credentialing Center. (2012). *Test content outline: Pediatric Primary Nurse Practitioner Board Certification Examination*. Retrieved from http://www.nursecredentialing.org/Documents/Certification/TestContentOutlines/PediatricNPTCO-Aug2013.aspx

Bloom, B. S. (1956). *Taxonomy of educational objectives: The classification of educational goals, by a committee of college and university examiners*. New York, NY: McKay.

Huitt, W. (2004). Maslow's hierarchy of needs. *Educational Psychology Interactive*. Valdosta, GA: Valdosta State University. Retrieved from http://chiron.valdosta.edu/whuitt/col/regsys/maslow.html

Keller, T. (2006). ICEA certification examination-taking: Strategies for test phobics. *International Journal of Childbirth Education, 21*(1), 14–16.

Lamonte, M. K. (2007). Test-taking strategies for CNOR certification. *AORN Journal, 85*(2), 315–332.

Nugent, P. M., & Vitale, B. A. (2011). *Test success: Test-taking techniques for beginning nursing students* (6th ed.). Philadelphia, PA: F. A. Davis.

Pediatric Nursing Certification Board. (2012). *Primary Care Pediatric Nurse Practitioner Certification Exam: Detailed content outline*. Retrieved from http://www.pncb.org /ptistore/resource/content/exams/pnp/2012_CPNP _Content_Outline.pdf

Quallich, S. (2013). Test taking strategies for the certification exam. *Uro-Gram, 41*(5), 13.

Straka, K. L., Ambrose, H. L., Burkett, M., Capan, M., Flook, D., Evangelista, T., . . . Thornton, M. (2014). The impact and perception of nursing certification in pediatric nursing. *Journal of Pediatric Nursing, 29*(3), 205–211.

Su, W. M., & Osisek, P. J. (2011). The revised Bloom's taxonomy: Implications for educating nurses. *Journal of Continuing Education in Nursing, 42*(7), 321–327.

Wilkerson, B. L. (2011). Specialty nurse certification affects patient outcomes. *Plastic Surgery Nursing, 31*(2), 57–59.

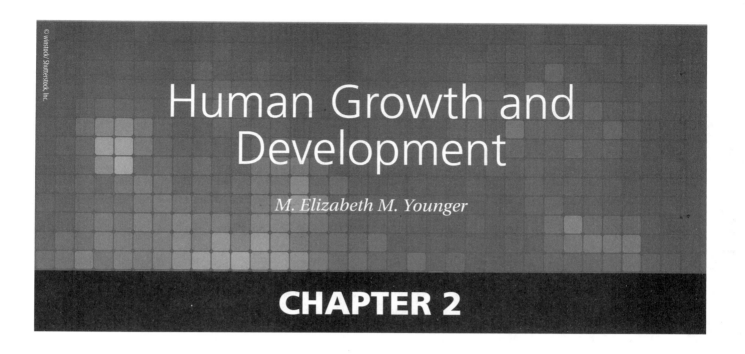

Human Growth and Development

M. Elizabeth M. Younger

CHAPTER 2

☐ HUMAN GROWTH AND DEVELOPMENT: UNDERLYING THEORY AND SCIENCE OF CHILD HEALTH

- Definition: How and why a person changes and/or stays the same over time
  1. Nature (heredity and genetic predisposition) vs. nurture (environmental influence)
  2. Continuity (continual process) vs. discontinuity (distinct stages)
- Three Fundamental Domains: Conceptual distinctions but overlapping processes in reality
  1. Physical domain
     a. Genetic factors
     b. Physical stature and appearance
     c. Nutritional status
     d. Physical health and well-being
     e. Fine and gross motor abilities
  2. Cognitive domain
     a. Perception, thinking, information processing, and memory
     b. Communication—receptive and expressive language
  3. Psychological and social domain
     a. Temperament and personality
     b. Interpersonal relationships
     c. Moral development
     d. Home environment and other social contexts

Classic Developmental Theories and Theorists

- Nature Positions: Emphasis on heredity and maturational process
  1. Jean-Jacques Rousseau (1712–1778)
     a. *Émile—Treatise on Education*

b. Child as an "untamed savage"
  2. Charles Darwin (1809–1882)
     a. *The Origin of Species*—human evolution (phylogeny) in order to adapt; "survival of the fittest"
     b. First use of "baby journal" as systematic method to document observed behavioral development
  3. Alfred Binet (1857–1911) and Theophile Simon (1873–1961)
     a. First standardized measurement of intelligence
     b. Intention was to identify "mentally defective" children needing specialized education
  4. G. Stanley Hall (1844–1924)
     a. *Adolescence* (1904)—classic work that first described adolescence as a critical developmental period of "Sturm und Drang" or "Storm and Stress"
     b. Development of questionnaires as method for the study of child development via adult retrospective recall
  5. Arnold Gesell (1880–1961)
     a. Maturational-organismic theory—biological basis of development; organizing principle of the theory is structure (closed system of transformational rules governing thought)
     b. *The Atlas of Infant Behavior* (1934)—developmental milestones
     c. Developed one of the earliest infant tests
  6. Sigmund Freud (1856–1939)
     a. *Three Contributions to the Sexual Theory* (1905)
     b. Stage theory of psychosexual development
        (1) Infancy: Oral stage
        (2) Toddler: Anal stage
        (3) Preschool: Phallic stage
        (4) School age: Latency stage
        (5) Adolescence: Genital stage
     c. Key principles

(1) Id: Principle of pleasure

(2) Ego: Principle of reality and/or self-interest

(3) Superego: Principle of morality or conscience

7. Neo-Freudian: Erik Erikson (1902–1994)—stage theory of psychosocial development across the life span

   a. Infancy: Trust vs. mistrust

   b. Toddler: Autonomy vs. shame and doubt

   c. Preschool: Initiative vs. guilt

   d. School age: Industry vs. inferiority

   e. Adolescence: Identity vs. role confusion

   f. Young adult: Intimacy vs. isolation

   g. Middle age: Generativity vs. stagnation

   h. Older adulthood: Integrity vs. despair

8. Neo-Freudian: Margaret Mahler (1897–1985)—psychological birth of the infant

   a. Psychological birth of the child with emerging sense of self as separate from mother

   b. Inadequate early mothering and "psychological birth" results in mental illness

   c. Phases of "psychological birth"

      (1) Autism from 0 to 2 months—no real social awareness or concept of self

      (2) Symbiosis from 2 to 5 months—mother–infant dependency

      (3) Separation–individuation from 6 to 36 months

         (a) Differentiation and practicing (6 to 12 months)—beginning awareness of self as separate from mother

         (b) Rapprochement (12 to 24 months)—exploration, emotional refueling, and ability to sustain brief separations

         (c) Consolidation (24 to 36 months)—increased ability to cope with separations through symbolic play

9. Jean Piaget (1896–1980)

   a. Interactionist—structuralist stage theory of cognitive development

   b. Sensorimotor stage: Birth to 2 years

   c. Preoperational thinking: 2 to 7 years

   d. Concrete operational thinking: 7 to 12 years

   e. Formal operational thinking: 12 years onward

• Nurture Positions: Emphasis on learning and environment

1. John Locke (1632–1704)

   a. *Essay Concerning Human Understanding and Some Thoughts Concerning Education*

   b. Child as "tabula rasa" or "blank slate"

2. John B. Watson (1878–1958)—behaviorism

   a. Classical conditioning—neutral stimulus associated with a meaningful one over time leading to a "conditioned" response that can be elicited by neutral stimulus alone as though it were the meaningful one

   b. *Psychological Care of the Infant and Child* (1928)

3. B. F. Skinner (1904–1990)—student of Watson

   a. Mechanistic-learning theory

b. Operant or instrumental conditioning—behavior is modified, reinforced, or extinguished by positively or negatively experienced consequences such as use of positive feedback for good behavior or "time-out" for misbehavior

4. Albert Bandura (1925–) and Walter Mischel (1930–)—Social learning theory

   a. Influenced by both behaviorism and psychodynamic theories

   b. Behavior results from interaction of individual characteristics, the environment, and the behavior itself

   c. Modeling—learning from direct observation and subsequent imitation of what is seen and done by significant others in the proximal environment

• Ethologic Theories

1. Konrad Lorenz (1903–1989)—*sensitive periods* as biologically programmed periods predisposed for particular learning, e.g., *imprinting*

2. Harry Harlow (1905–1981)—Wisconsin primate laboratory's classic rhesus monkey experiments on maternal deprivation (separation, isolation, and "terry cloth vs. wire surrogate mothers")

   a. Maternal separation and social isolation resulted in dramatic impairment of social-emotional development

   b. Physical contact and comfort as necessary for normal social and emotional development

3. John Bowlby (1907–1990): *Attachment and Loss* (1969)

   a. Attachment defined as "an affectional tie the infant forms to another specific person that binds the two together in space and endures over time"

   b. Importance of early mothering and consequences of "maternal deprivation" as observed in orphanages and asylums

4. Marshall Klaus (1927–) and John Kennel (1922–2013) *Maternal-Infant Bonding* (1976)

   a. Seminal studies on the impact of early contact vs. separation on maternal-infant bonding

   b. Influential in advocating change in hospital policies regarding rooming-in and father participation in the delivery room

5. Mary Ainsworth (1913–1999)—*Patterns of Attachment: A Study of the Strange Situation* (1978)—developed laboratory paradigm "strange situation" to assess security or insecurity of the attachment relationship

   a. Early maternal responsiveness to infant needs promotes secure attachment

   b. Secure maternal-infant attachment provides "safe base" from which the child can begin to actively explore the environment and a source of comfort when distressed

   c. Securely attached infants show more optimal cognitive gains and, later, school performance, illustrating the interconnectedness of psychosocial and cognitive domains

- Humanistic Theories
  1. Abraham Maslow (1908–1970)
     a. Theory of basic needs and human potential derived from study of healthy, creative individuals; few people achieve self-actualization
     b. Hierarchy of needs
        (1) Physiologic
        (2) Safety, security, and stability
        (3) Affiliation, acceptance, and love
        (4) Ego, self-worth, confidence, competence, and success
        (5) Self-actualization
  2. Carl Rogers (1902–1987)
     a. Client-centered approach from a phenomenologic perspective
     b. Key strategies for intervention
        (1) Unconditional positive regard, empathy, and genuineness
        (2) Empathy
        (3) Congruence or the ability to be genuine
- Moral Development
  1. Lawrence Kohlberg (1927–1987)—Stages of moral development
     a. Based on his original cross-sectional study of 84 school-aged boys (10 to 16 years) recruited from two suburban Chicago schools who were later followed longitudinally
     b. Responses to hypothetic moral dilemmas
     c. Preconventional or pre-moral level
        (1) Stage 1: Punishment-obedience—child behaves to avoid punishment
        (2) Stage 2: Instrumental-exchange—child behaves well for some gain or reward
     d. Conventional level
        (1) Stage 3: Good-boy/good-girl orientation—child behaves for approval
        (2) Stage 4: Law and order perspective—child behaves to avoid getting caught
     e. Postconventional level
        (1) Stage 5: Social contract—child/adolescent behaves in accordance with generally accepted social norms
        (2) Stage 6: Universal ethical principles—child/adolescent decides on moral standards of behavior through individual reflection and reasoning
  2. Carol Gilligan (1936–)—Gender differences in moral development
     a. Male social development orients to ethic of *principles*, with moral issues decided on the basis of fairness and justice
     b. Female social development orients to ethic of *interpersonal relationships*, with moral issues decided on the basis of compassion and caring
- Language Development: L. S. Vygotsky (1896–1934)
  1. Language as biologically programmed, but children learn language actively through direct experience and culture
  2. Zone of proximal development (ZPD): Zone between child's opportunity to observe/participate and ability to internalize the learned behavior

Transactional and Contextual Theories of Development

- Heredity–Environment Interactions
  1. Growth and developmental outcomes result from "main effects" and "interaction effects" of and between both heredity (nature) and environment (nurture)
  2. *Reaction range*—range of phenotypes that may emerge from similar genotypes developing under varied environmental contexts
- Transactional and Resiliency as Models of Development
  1. Transaction model first described in 1975 as a "continuum of reproductive risk and caretaking casualties" by Arnold Sameroff and Michael Chandler
  2. Research based on transactional model emerged in 1980s; describes risk and protective factors associated with vulnerability and resilience in the face of adversity
     a. Emmy Werner (1929–1982)—Kauai longitudinal study from birth to adulthood to explore perinatal risk and environmental factors on subsequent developmental outcomes, resiliency
     b. Michael Rutter (1933–1987)—epidemiological studies of children of mentally ill parents to examine risk and protective factors influencing subsequent psychopathology
     c. Alan Sroufe's longitudinal study of competence as a developmental construct
  3. Examples of clinical problems with multifactorial etiology better understood through a transactional perspective include failure to thrive, child abuse, attention deficit, hyperactivity, conduct, and eating disorders
- Ecological Model or "Development in Context"
  1. Developed and described by Urie Bronfenbrenner in 1979 publication—*Ecology of Human Development: Experiments by Nature and Design*
  2. Person–place–process model
     a. Microsystem—immediate settings within which a child spends time during development (e.g., home, school, hospital)
     b. Mesosystem—relationship or linkages between microsystems (e.g., service coordination)
     c. Exosystem—settings that may indirectly influence development (e.g., parent's workplace, school boards)
     d. Macrosystem—broad-based historical, cultural, demographic, and institutional context (e.g., managed care and welfare reform initiatives)
  3. Understanding how and why a child changes or stays the same over time requires examination not only of the child's emerging capabilities but also the quality

of the settings (places and processes) where children spend time; communication/linkages between these settings; influence of policy decisions; and overall social, cultural, and political context

4. Examples of clinical interventions better understood through an ecological perspective include early intervention services, home visiting services, and care coordination/case management strategies

5. Collaborative effort toward integration of scientific knowledge concerning childhood development and implications for policy and practice

☐ INFANT GROWTH AND DEVELOPMENT (BIRTH TO 2 YEARS)

- Physical Domain: Major tasks—physiologic regulation/ motor control
1. Definitions
   a. Preterm—newborn with gestational age estimated as less than 37 weeks. Late preterm is newborn born at 34 weeks to 36 weeks.
   b. Low birth weight (LBW) ≤ 2500 g
      (1) Very low birth weight (VLBW) ≤ 1500 g
      (2) Extremely low birth weight (ELBW) ≤ 1000 g
   c. Assessment of weight for gestational age
      (1) AGA—appropriate for gestational age
      (2) LGA—large for gestational age; weight is above the 90th percentile; often associated with diabetic pregnancies
      (3) SGA—small for gestational age
         (a) Symmetric intrauterine growth retardation (IUGR)—weight, length, and head circumference are SGA; reflects long-standing compromise and/or factors that are intrinsic to the infant such as a syndrome complex
         (b) Asymmetric intrauterine growth retardation (IUGR)—underweight for length and head circumference; reflects acute compromise extrinsic to fetus such as placental insufficiency
2. Average U.S. newborn is 20.16 inches (51.2 cm) long, weighs 7.63 pounds (3468 g) with head circumference of 14.2 inches (35 cm) and with chest circumference measuring approximately 0.8 inches (2 cm) less than head circumference
3. Initial 8–10% weight loss in average newborn in first 3 to 4 days of life is usually regained by 7 days if formula fed, 14 days if breastfed
4. Weight doubles by 6 months, triples by 1 year, and quadruples by 2 years
   a. 5–7 oz (150–210 g) weight gain per week during first 6 months
   b. 12–20 oz per month weight gain during months 6–12
   c. Average weight gain in second year is 8 to 9 oz (240–270 g) per month
   d. By 1 year, birth weight should be tripled
5. Length usually increases by 50% by 1 year, doubles by 4 years, and triples by 13 years—increases by 1 inch

(2.54 cm) per month during first 6 months, and then 0.5 inch (1.3 cm) per month through first year

6. Head circumference increases 0.5 inch (1.3 cm) per month during first 6 months, and then 0.3 inch (0.65 cm) per month through first year

7. Serial measurements and observation over time with use of standardized growth charts—http://cdc.gov/growthcharts/

8. Cranial sutures/fontanels
   a. Cranial sutures close during first year of life
   b. Posterior fontanel closes by 6–8 weeks of age
   c. Anterior fontanel closes by 12–18 months of age

9. Dental development
   a. Formation of teeth begins during the third fetal month and continues through adolescence
   b. Primary or deciduous teeth are first set of teeth that are later replaced by permanent teeth
   c. Eruption timing can vary greatly, but eruption sequence of deciduous teeth is generally consistent— see **Figure 2-1**

10. Motor development
    a. Early reflexive responses—involuntary responses to stimuli that may be viewed as precursors to late motor skills
       (1) Survival reflexes
          (a) Breathing, hiccups, sneezes, spitting up as infant tries to regulate breathing, sucking, and swallowing
          (b) Temperature control reflexes—cry, shivering, tucking legs close to body
          (c) Feeding reflexes—sucking, rooting, crying, and swallowing
       (2) Nonsurvival reflexes—Babinski, stepping, swimming, grasping, Moro or startle
       (3) Ontogeny of infant reflexes
          (a) Palmar grasp: strongest by 1–2 months, disappears by 3 months
          (b) Plantar grasp: disappears after 8 months
          (c) Moro reflex: disappears by 6 months
          (d) Stepping: disappears before voluntary walking
          (e) Asymmetric tonic neck (fencing) reflex: diminished by 3–4 months, disappears by 6 months
          (f) Gross and fine motor milestones—age of attainment varies, but sequence is generally consistent

- Cognitive Development: Major tasks—sensorimotor and early language development
1. Vision
   a. Presence of blink reflex and pupil constriction to light are indications of newborn vision
   b. Newborns can focus on objects between 4 and 30 inches away, including caretaker's face during feeding
   c. Binocular vision develops between 4 and 6 months
   d. Visual acuity is difficult to measure during infancy; distance acuity has been estimated between 20/150

1. Self-esteem—competence to think, learn, and make decisions as well as believe that one is worthy of love and respectful treatment from others
2. Peers and development of prosocial behavior through cooperative games, sports, and activities
3. The need for organized after-school activities has become critical with the increasing number of children who are regularly left unsupervised after school because of parental work schedules and variations in family structure in the United States

☑ ADOLESCENT DEVELOPMENT

- Physical Domain: Major tasks—puberty, sexual maturation
  1. Physical growth
     a. Average U.S. female gains about 38 pounds (17 kg) and 9 inches (24 cm) between 10 and 14 years
     b. Average U.S. male gains about 42 pounds (19 kg) and 9 inches (24 cm) between 12 and 16 years
  2. Puberty—period of rapid physical growth and sexual maturation resulting in adult size, shape, and reproductive potential
     a. Sequence of puberty—individual variation in onset, but sequence of somatic and physiologic changes is relatively set
        (1) Females
            (a) Puberty onset—9 to 10 years
            (b) Precocious puberty—before 8 years
            (c) Delayed puberty—after 13 years
            (d) First physical sign—breast buds
            (e) Peak height velocity—12.4 years
            (f) Menarche—12.5 years
            (g) Fertility—15 years
        (2) Males
            (a) Puberty onset—11 to 12 years
            (b) Precocious puberty— before 9 years
            (c) Delayed puberty—after 14 years
            (d) First physical sign—testicular growth
            (e) Peak height velocity—14.4 years
            (f) Spermarche—13 to 14 years
            (g) Fertility—15 years
     b. Anovulatory cycles are common during the first 2 years after menarche (50% of cycles vs. 20% after 5 years)
     c. Stages of genital maturity in males—takes approximately 4 years to move from stage 2 to 5 (Tanner staging)
        (1) Stage 1: Preadolescent testes, scrotum, and penis
        (2) Stage 2: Enlargement of scrotum and testes; scrotum reddens and roughens
        (3) Stage 3: Penis enlarges primarily in length
        (4) Stage 4: Penis enlarges in breadth and development of glans
        (5) Stage 5: Adult size and shape

     d. Stages of breast development in females (Tanner staging)
        (1) Stage 1: Preadolescent breast with nipple elevation
        (2) Stage 2: Breast buds with areolar enlargement
        (3) Stage 3: Breast enlargement without separate contour with nipple
        (4) Stage 4: Projection of areola and nipple as secondary mound to breast
        (5) Stage 5: Adult breast with areola receding and nipple projecting from breast
     e. Stages of pubic hair development in males and females (Tanner staging)
        (1) Stage 1: Preadolescent without pubic hair
        (2) Stage 2: Sparse, pale, fine pubic hair
        (3) Stage 3: Darker, more curled, increased amount of pubic hair
        (4) Stage 4: Hair is adult in character but doesn't cover entire pubic area
        (5) Stage 5: Adult distribution in quantity, quality, and pattern
- Cognitive Development: Major tasks—ability to abstract and make decisions
  1. Formal operational thought—ability to abstract (Piaget)
  2. Characteristic ways of thinking
     a. Egocentrism—difficulty an adolescent may have in thinking rationally about own personal experiences as completely unique
     b. Invincibility fable—sense of invincibility that can lead to risk-taking behaviors
     c. Personal fable—variation of adolescent egocentrism whereby adolescent feels personally gifted in some way
     d. Imaginary audience—exaggerated sense that everyone is watching and focused on the adolescent, resulting in feeling self-conscious
- Psychosocial Development: Major tasks—independence, intimacy, vocation or career goals
  1. Majority of adolescents cope well with their transition to adulthood and do not experience "storm and stress" as once assumed
  2. A second phase of "separation–individuation" occurs during adolescence that requires new approaches to parenting, communication, decision making, and independence
  3. Three psychosocial periods of adolescence
     a. Early adolescence—middle school (11 to 14 years)
        (1) Importance of peers and feeling "normal"
        (2) Moodiness
     b. Middle adolescence—high school (15 to 17 years)
        (1) Body image, sexuality, dating
        (2) Asserting independence
     c. Late adolescence—vocation and career choices (18 to 21 years)
        (1) Identity formation—achievement, moratorium, foreclosure, diffusion

    (2) Vocation and career choices, including college, military, and employment opportunities

    (3) Intimacy in relationships

☑ THE CHANGING AMERICAN FAMILY AS CONTEXT FOR GROWTH AND DEVELOPMENT

- Demographic Changes
  1. Increasing rates of divorce and remarriage
  2. Delays and declines in child bearing
  3. Rise in female participation in workforce—voluntary, dual-earner families, female head of household, and welfare reform work requirements
  4. Increasing incidence of single-parent families, childhood poverty, and homelessness
- Variations in Family Structure
  1. Decrease in "traditional" two-parent families
  2. Increase in single-parent households—divorce/separation, births to unmarried mothers, death of spouse, adoption
  3. Remarriage, blended families, and step-parenting
  4. Extended and/or "skip generation" families with grandparents as primary caregivers and/or with several generations living together
  5. Foster families—estimated 400,000 children in foster care at any given time; https://www.childwelfare.gov/pubPDFs/foster.pdf
  6. Group living, including homeless shelters—estimated 23% of the homeless population include families with children (National Coalition for the Homeless, 2009)
  7. Gay and lesbian families—sources vary regarding prevalence
- Family Functioning: Critical concepts
  1. Family functioning is more directly related to healthy growth and development than is family structure
  2. Components of family functioning include provision of a stable and safe physical environment as well as financial and emotional resources necessary to provide supportive and nurturing care with appropriate supervision and guidance
  3. Screening and assessment tools
     a. Family Inventory of Life Events (FILE)
     b. Family Coping Strategies (F-COPES)
     c. Adolescent-Family Inventory of Life Events and Changes (A-FILE)
     d. Parenting Stress Index (PSI)
  4. Family-centered care—Institute for Family-Centered Care
     a. Recognition that the family is the constant in a child's life
     b. Family–professional collaboration at all levels
     c. Respect for family diversity in structure, race, ethnicity, culture, and socioeconomic status
     d. Recognition of family strengths, uniqueness, and diversity in coping strategies
     e. Communication and sharing of information on an ongoing basis with families in a supportive and nonjudgmental manner
     f. Support and facilitation of family-to-family support
     g. Understand and incorporate strategies supportive of growth and developmental needs of children and their families into healthcare settings/systems
     h. Implementation of policies and programs to support emotional and financial well-being of families
     i. Accessible health care that is flexible, culturally competent, and responsive to family-centered needs
  5. Resources: Institute for Family-Centered Care: http://www.familycenteredcare.org

☑ DEVIATIONS IN PHYSICAL GROWTH AND BEHAVIORAL DEVELOPMENT

Failure to Thrive (FTT)

- Definition
  1. No consensus on definition
  2. Descriptive rather than diagnostic term
  3. Generally refers to infants and young children whose weight is below the 3rd percentile on National Center for Health Statistics (NCHS) growth standards and/or whose weight trajectory has decreased by two major growth percentiles
  4. Traditional categories include organic FTT, nonorganic FTT, and mixed etiology FTT
  5. Newer categories include neurodevelopmental FTT and socioemotional FTT
- Etiology/Incidence
  1. Multifactorial etiology, including underlying organic disease or predisposing medical condition, maladaptive parent–infant interaction, maternal depression, poverty, deficits in parenting information and skills, child abuse and neglect
  2. Accounts for between 3% and 5% of all pediatric admissions of infants younger than 1 year old, with as many as 50% of admissions without underlying medical condition
  3. Males and females are equally affected
- Clinical Findings
  1. Inadequate intake—inadequate maternal milk production, mechanical problems with suck/swallow coordination, systemic disease, errors in formula preparation, misunderstanding about infant needs and feeding practices
  2. Increased losses or decreased utilization—vomiting and/or malabsorption
  3. Increased caloric requirements—underlying disease process(es), including cardiac, respiratory, endocrine, cancer, and/or recurrent infection
  4. Altered growth potential—prenatal insult, genetic disorder, or endocrine dysfunction

- Differential Diagnosis
  1. Organic causes
     a. Gastrointestinal—gastroesophageal reflux disease (GERD), pyloric stenosis, cleft palate, lactose intolerance, Hirschsprung disease, milk-protein intolerance, hepatitis, malabsorption
     b. Cardiopulmonary—cardiac defects, bronchopulmonary dysplasia (BPD), asthma, cystic fibrosis (CF), tracheobronchial or tracheoesophageal malformations
     c. Endocrine—thyroid dysfunction, diabetes, adrenal insufficiency, pituitary disorders, growth hormone deficiency
     d. Infection from any organism
     e. Neurologic—mental retardation, fetal alcohol syndrome, lead poisoning, prematurity, neuroregulatory difficulties
     f. Genetic—mitochondrial diseases
  2. Social-emotional and environmental causes
     a. Maternal depression or other mental illness, isolation, marital/relationship difficulties
     b. Poverty/inadequate resources
     c. Inadequate parenting knowledge and skills
     d. Difficult temperament
     e. Child abuse and neglect
- Diagnostic Methods/Findings
  1. History—prenatal, perinatal, neonatal; complete diet history and feeding practices; environmental, social, and family history
  2. Identification of risk factors—prematurity, LBW, difficult temperament, regulation problems, social stresses
  3. Height, weight, head circumference; review longitudinal growth data, corrected for gestational age as appropriate; vital signs, including blood pressure
  4. Physical examination—signs of underlying organic disease; severity of malnutrition, evidence of abuse or neglect
  5. Developmental assessment and caregiver concerns
  6. Feeding observation to assess behavioral or interactional contributing factors
  7. Home visit or public health nurse referral to assess environmental factors
  8. Laboratory assessment should be judicious based on history and clinical findings; complete blood count (CBC), urine analysis (UA; if applicable); comprehensive metabolic panel; other labs as indicated by history, including blood lead levels, tuberculosis (TB) test; thyroid function; test for reflux/malabsorption; sweat test; stool specimen for parasites; bone age if height is poor
- Management/Treatment
  1. Address underlying organic cause if one is identified
  2. Importance of developing therapeutic alliance with caregiver
  3. Usually managed on an outpatient basis, if possible, with hospitalization indicated when there is evidence of abuse or severe neglect, severe malnutrition, medical instability, or when outpatient management has failed
  4. Interdisciplinary approach is optimal utilizing healthcare, nutritional, mental health, and social services
  5. Provide caregivers with necessary information regarding nutritional needs of child and appropriate feeding skills to promote optimal growth
  6. Close monitoring and follow-up on growth and development, social environment, and interdisciplinary/interagency communication

Stuttering

- Definition: Speech dysfluency with initial onset during the preschool years that is characterized by repetitions of sounds, syllables, and/or short words as well as pauses in timing of speech
  1. Mild or developmental stuttering—speech dysfluency most notable when a preschool-aged child is tired or excited that usually resolves spontaneously if not given excessive attention
  2. Moderate or severe stuttering (sometimes referred to as acquired stuttering)—persistent speech dysfluency that is inappropriate for age and usually has a neurologic and/or psychogenic etiology
- Etiology/Incidence
  1. Multifactorial etiology with a 3:1 male to female ratio of occurrence
  2. Prevalence estimated at 1% among prepubertal children with decrease to 0.8% postpuberty
  3. Mild developmental stuttering occurs in 4% to 5% of children between 2 and 5 years that spontaneously resolves; approximately 20% of early stuttering does not resolve without intervention
- Clinical Findings
  1. Repetition and/or prolongation of sounds, syllables, or short words
  2. Pauses within words or sentences
  3. Signs of physical tension and struggling with speech such as eye blinking and trembling lips
  4. Avoidance of words that cause particular problems
  5. Child and/or parents are frustrated and/or embarrassed by stuttering, posing difficulty at home, in school, or with peers
- Differential Diagnosis
  1. Normal developmental dysfluency
  2. Hearing impairment
  3. Speech-motor deficit
- Management/Treatment
  1. Assess frequency, type, and duration of dysfluency
  2. Encourage parents to avoid excessive attention to dysfluency and be patient in listening to child's speech
  3. Refer to speech and language pathologist for assessment if child is showing signs of embarrassment, speech dysfluency interferes with communication, and/or parent expresses significant concern regardless of severity

4. Stuttering Foundation of America
   3100 Walnut Grove Road, Suite 603
   P.O. Box 11749
   Memphis, TN 38111-0749
   (800) 992–9392
   http://www.stutteringhelp.org/

Autism

- Definition: Neurobiological disorders characterized by a spectrum of symptoms involving impairment in social interaction, impairment in interpersonal communication, and restricted and repetitive behaviors and interests. Symptoms range in severity but usually manifest themselves within the first 3 years of life
- Etiology/Incidence
  1. Unclear etiology
  2. In less than 10%, autism spectrum disorder (ASD) may be associated with another syndrome or disease, such as fragile X, tuberous sclerosis complex, Duchenne muscular dystrophy, Down syndrome
  3. Believed to have a primarily genetic cause, but environment may affect the expression of genetic material (e.g., advanced parental age, toxin exposure during early gestation)
  4. No association with vaccines
  5. Considered highly heritable (increased rate in siblings, and even higher in monozygotic twins)
  6. Affects 1 out of every 68 children in the United States; male:female ratio—4.3:1 (Centers for Disease Control and Prevention [CDC], 2015)
- Clinical Findings
  1. Normal growth and development usually reported until 2 to 2½ years when parents notice delays in language, symbolic or imaginative play, and/or other social interactions; onset of such delay or abnormal behavioral pattern before 3 years of age is considered part of diagnostic criteria
- *DSM-V* Classification:
  1. Autism Spectrum Disorder (ASD)
     a. Autistic disorder
     b. Asperger disorder
     c. Pervasive developmental disorder, not otherwise specified
  2. Other developmental disorders not considered ASD
     a. Rett's disorder
     b. Childhood disintegrative disorder
  3. Social (Pragmatic) Communication Disorder
- Diagnostic Criteria for Autism Spectrum Disorders
  A. Persistent deficits in social communication and social interaction across multiple contexts, as manifested by the following, currently or by history (examples are illustrative, not exhaustive):
     1. Deficits in social-emotional reciprocity, ranging, for example, from abnormal social approach and failure of normal back-and-forth conversation; to reduced sharing of interests, emotions, or affect; to failure to initiate or respond to social interactions
     2. Deficits in nonverbal communicative behaviors used for social interaction, ranging, for example, from poorly integrated verbal and nonverbal communication; to abnormalities in eye contact and body language or deficits in understanding and use of gestures; to a total lack of facial expressions and nonverbal communication
     3. Deficits in developing, maintaining, and understanding relationships, ranging, for example, from difficulties adjusting behavior to suit various social contexts; to difficulties in sharing imaginative play or in making friends; to absence of interest in peers
  B. Restricted, repetitive patterns of behavior, interests, or activities, as manifested by at least two of the following, currently or by history (examples are illustrative, not exhaustive):
     1. Stereotyped or repetitive motor movements, use of objects, or speech (e.g., simple motor stereotypies, lining up toys or flipping objects, echolalia, idiosyncratic phrases)
     2. Insistence on sameness, inflexible adherence to routines, or ritualized patterns or verbal nonverbal behavior (e.g., extreme distress at small changes, difficulties with transitions, rigid thinking patterns, greeting rituals, need to take same route or eat same food every day)
     3. Highly restricted, fixated interests that are abnormal in intensity or focus (e.g., strong attachment to or preoccupation with unusual objects, excessively circumscribed or perseverative interest)
     4. Hyper- or hyporeactivity to sensory input or unusual interests in sensory aspects of the environment (e.g., apparent indifference to pain/temperature, adverse response to specific sounds or textures, excessive smelling or touching of objects, visual fascination with lights or movement).
  C. Symptoms must be present in the early developmental period (but may not become fully manifest until social demands exceed limited capacities, or may be masked by learned strategies in later life)
  D. Symptoms cause clinically significant impairment in social, occupational, or other important areas of current functioning
  E. These disturbances are not better explained by intellectual disability (intellectual developmental disorder) or global developmental delay. Intellectual disability and autism spectrum disorder frequently co-occur; to make comorbid diagnoses of autism spectrum disorder and intellectual disability, social communication should

be below that expected for general developmental level

- Diagnostic Criteria for Social (Pragmatic) Communication Disorder
  A. Persistent difficulties in the social use of verbal and nonverbal communication as manifested by all of the following:
     1. Deficits in using communication for social purposes, such as greeting and sharing information, in a manner that is appropriate for the social context
     2. Impairment of the ability to change communication to match context or the needs of the listener, such as speaking differently in a classroom than on the playground, talking differently to a child than to an adult, and avoiding use of overly formal language
     3. Difficulties following rules for conversation and storytelling, such as taking turns in conversation, rephrasing when misunderstood, and knowing how to use verbal and nonverbal signals to regulate interaction
     4. Difficulties understanding what is not explicitly stated (e.g., making inferences) and nonliteral or ambiguous meanings of language (e.g., idioms, humor, metaphors, multiple meanings that depend on the context for interpretation)
  B. The deficits result in functional limitations in effective communication, social participation, social relationships, academic achievement, or occupational performance, individually or in combination
  C. The onset of the symptoms is in the early developmental period (but deficits may not become fully manifest until social communication demands exceed limited capacities)
  D. The symptoms are not attributable to another medical or neurological condition or to low abilities in the domains of word structure and grammar, and are not better explained by autism spectrum disorder, intellectual disability (intellectual developmental disorder), global developmental delay, or another mental disorder (*Diagnostic and Statistical Manual of Mental Disorders* [DSM-5], 2013)
  4. Associated problems may include other cognitive delays, problems learning, unusual responses to sensory stimuli, difficulties with sleeping and eating, differences in emotional responsiveness, and seizure activity
  5. Significant variation in clusters of symptoms and characteristics ranging from mild to severely affected
- Diagnostic Tests/Findings
  1. No specific medical diagnostic test for these disorders
  2. EEG indicated for associated problems, including seizures and language delay
  3. Laboratory studies to assess etiological factors
     a. Urine amino acids and organic acids; metabolic screen for metabolic disorders such as phenylketonuria (PKU)
     b. DNA probe for fragile X on blood plasma
  4. MRI or CT scan may show structural abnormalities in cerebellum, but otherwise not particularly helpful in absence of clinical signs such as asymmetries, focal tremors, or paralyses
- Differential Diagnosis
  1. Mental retardation
  2. Sensory impairment (hearing or vision)
  3. Severe abuse or neglect
  4. Rett's disorder
  5. Childhood psychosis or other mental illness
  6. Gifted child
  7. Tourette's syndrome
  8. Fragile X
  9. Childhood disintegrative disorder
- Management/Treatment
  1. No specific medical interventions currently available
  2. Screening: Early screening, diagnosis, and referral to early intervention is critical. American Psychological Association (APA) recommends:
     a. Ongoing developmental surveillance
     b. Targeted developmental screening at 9, 18, and 30 months
     c. ASD-specific screening at 18 and 24 months or at any time when there is a suspicion of problem
  3. Treatment is primarily psychoeducation requiring individualized plan
  4. Interdisciplinary team to coordinate care, including parents, teachers, primary care provider, psychologist, physical therapy, speech and language, and other early intervention staff as appropriate
  5. Address associated problems through specific therapies (sensory integration), counseling (family adjustment, behavioral management), medications (seizures and behavioral problems)
  6. Community education, resource identification, and parent-to-parent support
     a. Autism Society of America
        7910 Woodmont Avenue, Suite 300
        Bethesda, Maryland 20814-3067
        1-800-328-8476 (1.800.3AUTISM)
        http://www.autism-society.org
     b. CHAT—Checklist for Autism in Toddlers (Baron-Cohen et al., 2000)

Obesity

- Definition
  1. Excess accumulation of body fat relative to lean body mass that results from excessive caloric intake relative to energy expenditure
  2. Body mass index (BMI) > 95th percentile

- Etiology/Incidence
  1. Multifactorial etiology with interaction of genetic, environmental, developmental, and behavioral factors
     a. Genetic predisposition and/or parental obesity
     b. Dietary patterns
     c. Inactivity (television, video games)
     d. Cultural and familial food preferences
     e. Use of food as emotional buffer
     f. Physical disorders with decreased energy expenditure (spina bifida, Down syndrome, Prader-Willi syndrome)
     g. Endocrinopathy
  2. Most prevalent nutritional problem in United States
  3. According to CDC, 32% of children and adolescents in the United States are obese
  4. Ethnic differences: Non-Hispanic black girls and Mexican American girls are more likely to be obese than are non-Hispanic white girls; among boys, Mexican Americans are more likely to be obese than are non-Hispanic white boys
- Clinical Findings
  1. Parent and/or child concern regarding body weight
  2. Clinical observation of large size and/or excess fat on child
  3. Measurement of weight, height, and BMI
- Differential Diagnosis
  1. Endocrine dysfunction
  2. Congenital disorders/short stature
  3. Large frame
  4. Muscular hypertrophy
  5. Medication-induced obesity (including corticosteroids, psychotropic drugs)
- Diagnostic Tests/Findings
  1. History includes detailed dietary and activity level history (past and present); family history of obesity and related morbidities, including hypertension, cardiovascular disease, hyperlipidemia, diabetes, depression; review of systems for associated morbidity (glucose intolerance, orthopedic difficulties); developmental milestones; psychosocial concerns about weight
  2. Physical examination, vital signs, blood pressure
  3. Anthropometric measurements
     a. Weight for height ratio greater than 95th percentile on CDC growth charts is commonly used but doesn't account for large frame or increased muscle mass
     b. Percentage of ideal body weight greater or equal to 120%; calculated by dividing child's actual weight by ideal body weight (50th percentile for age and sex) and multiplied by 100
     c. Skin-fold thickness per calibrated caliper measurements at or above 85th percentile for age, sex, and race; triceps measurements are most common and reference charts are available
     d. BMI considered most useful index
        (1) Weight in kilograms/height in meters^2
        (2) Screening classifications using BMI in adolescents
           (a) Obesity—BMI equal or greater than 95th percentile for age and gender
           (b) At risk for obesity—between 85th and 95th percentile or with rapid weight gain of 2.0 BMI units in one year
  4. CBC, UA, thyroid function, lipid profile
- Management/Treatment
  1. Prevention in infancy through parent education regarding nutritional needs and feeding strategies
  2. Discuss moderate modification of diet and caloric content while increasing exercise program
  3. Goal for younger child is weight maintenance rather than weight reduction while linear growth catches up; goal for adolescent may include weight reduction if treated after growth spurt
  4. Behavior modification strategies directed at alternative coping measures to deal with stress, maintain motivation, and reinforce regimen
  5. Involvement of family in therapeutic program increases likelihood of success
  6. Refer to and collaborate with available community resources as appropriate
  7. Pharmacological and surgical treatment for severely obese adolescents

Child Abuse and Neglect

- Definition: *Abuse* usually refers to actual "acts of commission" and *neglect* refers to "acts of omission," although there remains no consensus on specific definitions
  1. First described as "battered child syndrome" by Dr. Henry Kempe in 1962
  2. Legal definitions and reporting requirements vary from state to state, but all 50 states have mandated reporting by healthcare providers of suspected abuse or neglect
  3. Categories include physical, sexual, and emotional abuse; negligent care; and Munchausen syndrome by proxy (MSP)
     a. Soft tissue injuries most common—bruises, abrasions, and lacerations
     b. Head injuries less frequent but cause majority of deaths—"shaken baby syndrome" (altered consciousness with or without signs of head injuries)
     c. Burns account for 10% of abuse injuries
     d. Abdominal injuries—usually blunt injuries from hitting or kicking; liver lacerations; kidney/pancreas contusions
     e. Fractures—rib, spiral, and multiple fractures at same or various ages should trigger suspicion
     f. Sexual abuse—probably least reported and underdiagnosed
     g. Munchausen syndrome by proxy (MSP)— disturbed parent-child relationship with

fabrication or actual harm to produce symptoms of illness requiring medical attention
- Etiology/Incidence
  1. Etiological factors associated with abuse and neglect
     a. Perpetrator—history of being maltreated as a child, cognitive or psychiatric impairment, socially isolated, inadequate parenting knowledge and skills, including unrealistic expectations of child
     b. Victim—unwanted pregnancy, difficult temperament, premature and/or disabled, no significant gender differences
     c. Social context—violence (family/community), poverty, unemployment, substance abuse
  2. National Child Abuse and Neglect Data System (NCANDS) data from 2012:
     a. 686,000 children per year reported to be victims of abuse or neglect (9.2 per 1000 children)
     b. 32% of victims were younger than age 4 years, 24% between 4 and 7 years of age
     c. Male:female ratio 48.7:50.9
     d. African American, American Indian, Alaskan Native, and mixed-race children have significantly higher rates of victimization than do Hispanic or white children. Asian children have the lowest rates of victimization
     e. Neglect (78.3%) is most common form of maltreatment followed by physical abuse (18.3%), sexual abuse (9.3%), and psychological maltreatment (8.3%)
     f. Most perpetrators (80%) are parents (39% mothers, 18% fathers, 17% both parents)
  3. Child abuse/neglect is a significant cause of pediatric mortality in infants (second to sudden infant death syndrome) and young children (second to accidents)
     a. 1640 deaths resulting from abuse or neglect were reported in 2012
     b. Most deaths (84.5%) were of children 6 years or younger
- Clinical Findings
  1. History is vague, inconsistent, and/or incompatible with child's developmental stage and severity of injury (e.g., bruises on legs if child is not yet cruising)
  2. History may change during course of interview
  3. Delay in seeking medical attention for injury
  4. History of recurrent injuries
  5. Soft tissue injuries with markings characteristic of source of abuse such as hand marks, curved mark of a belt, burn mark in shape of electric iron
  6. Bruises
  7. Burn markings characteristic of immersion
  8. Undernutrition, poor hygiene
  9. Developmental delays
  10. Inappropriate parent–child interaction
- Differential Diagnosis
  1. Unintentional injury
  2. Underlying disease process, e.g., hemophilia, leukemia, osteogenesis imperfecta

  3. Birth marks, Mongolian spots, and/or other variations in skin pigmentation
  4. Folk medicine and cultural practices, e.g., coin rubbing
  5. Sudden infant death syndrome (SIDS)
- Diagnostic Tests/Findings
  1. History to determine and precisely document type of injury, alleged circumstances, and action taken by caregiver
  2. Observation of parent and child for behavioral extremes or exaggerated responses
  3. Physical examination to assess location, type, and characteristic of any lesions or burns for characteristic pattern, shape, or outline
  4. Coagulation studies for severe bruising; radiographs of long bones, ribs, and/or skull series as indicated by history and physical examination; ultrasound for suspected visceral injury
- Management/Treatment
  1. Report of suspected neglect or abuse to child protective services is mandated
  2. Calling the police may also be immediately necessary
  3. Appropriate medical care for child, including immediate hospitalization if indicated by severity of injuries
  4. Ensure safety of child, utilizing foster care or relatives if necessary
  5. Assessment of siblings for maltreatment and assurance of safety
  6. Identify and make appropriate referrals to available community resources to facilitate interdisciplinary and interagency collaboration—child protective services, public health, parenting classes, child care/school programs
  7. Education and prevention
     a. Identify families with risk factors associated with child maltreatment and make referrals to appropriate community-based preventive resources before serious abuse occurs
     b. Close primary care supervision and acute care follow-up for at-risk families and children
     c. Mandated reporting of suspected abuse or neglect
     d. Support community-based child abuse prevention efforts

Attention Deficit Hyperactivity Disorder (ADHD)

- Definition
  1. A behavioral syndrome characterized by a persistent or ongoing pattern of inattention and/or hyperactivity-impulsivity that interferes with daily life or typical development. May have difficulties with maintaining attention, executive function, and working memory
     a. Onset is typically by the age of 3 years
  2. *DSM-V* presentations of ADHD
     a. Inattentive

    b. Hyperactive-impulsive

    c. Combined inattentive and hyperactive-impulsive

- Etiology/Incidence
1. Multifactorial etiology that remains poorly understood but may be associated with:

    a. Delayed CNS maturation

    b. Genetic factors

    c. Prenatal, perinatal, or postnatal trauma or illness

    d. Dysfunction of catecholamine neurotransmitters

    e. Male-to-female ratio ranges from 4:1 (general population) to 9:1 (clinic populations)

2. Controlled studies have not demonstrated evidence of additives, sugar, or salicylates as associated factors

3. Approximately 3% to 5% of school-aged children meet *DSM-V* criteria

4. *DSM-V* (American Psychiatric Association [APA], 2013) diagnostic criteria for ADHD include:

    1. Inattention: Six or more symptoms of inattention for children up to age 16, or five or more for adolescents 17 and older and adults; symptoms of inattention have been present for at least 6 months, and they are inappropriate for developmental level:

        o Often fails to give close attention to details or makes careless mistakes in schoolwork, at work, or with other activities.

        o Often has trouble holding attention on tasks or play activities.

        o Often does not seem to listen when spoken to directly.

        o Often does not follow through on instructions and fails to finish schoolwork, chores, or duties in the workplace (e.g., loses focus, side-tracked).

        o Often has trouble organizing tasks and activities.

        o Often avoids, dislikes, or is reluctant to do tasks that require mental effort over a long period of time (such as schoolwork or homework).

        o Often loses things necessary for tasks and activities (e.g. school materials, pencils, books, tools, wallets, keys, paperwork, eyeglasses, mobile telephones).

        o Is often easily distracted.

        o Is often forgetful in daily activities.

    2. Hyperactivity and Impulsivity: Six or more symptoms of hyperactivity-impulsivity for children up to age 16, or five or more for adolescents 17 and older and adults; symptoms of hyperactivity-impulsivity have been present for at least 6 months to an extent that is disruptive and inappropriate for the person's developmental level:

        o Often fidgets with or taps hands or feet, or squirms in seat.

        o Often leaves seat in situations when remaining seated is expected.

        o Often runs about or climbs in situations where it is not appropriate (adolescents or adults may be limited to feeling restless).

        o Often unable to play or take part in leisure activities quietly.

        o Is often "on the go" acting as if "driven by a motor."

        o Often talks excessively.

        o Often blurts out an answer before a question has been completed.

        o Often has trouble waiting his/her turn.

        o Often interrupts or intrudes on others (e.g., butts into conversations or games).

In addition, the following conditions must be met:

- Several inattentive or hyperactive-impulsive symptoms were present before age 12 years.
- Several symptoms are present in two or more settings (e.g., at home, school, or work; with friends or relatives; in other activities).
- There is clear evidence that the symptoms interfere with, or reduce the quality of, social, school, or work functioning.
- The symptoms do not happen only during the course of schizophrenia or another psychotic disorder. The symptoms are not better explained by another mental disorder (e.g., Mood Disorder, Anxiety Disorder, Dissociative Disorder, or a Personality Disorder).

Based on the types of symptoms, three kinds (presentations) of ADHD can occur:

Combined Presentation: if enough symptoms of both criteria, inattention and hyperactivity-impulsivity, were present for the past 6 months.

Predominantly Inattentive Presentation: if enough symptoms of inattention, but not hyperactivity-impulsivity, were present for the past six months.

Predominantly Hyperactive-Impulsive Presentation: if enough symptoms of hyperactivity-impulsivity, but not inattention, were present for the past six months.

Because symptoms can change over time, the presentation may change over time as well.

- Differential Diagnosis
1. Age appropriate for highly active child
2. Inadequate environments (understimulating or chaotic)
3. Learning disabilities/sensory impairment
4. Seizures or mental retardation
5. Situational anxiety and/or depressive reaction
6. Oppositional behavior and/or conduct disorder

- Diagnostic Tests/Findings
1. History—perinatal (maternal substance abuse); past (early health problems, including ear infections, lead poisoning, iron-deficiency anemia, frequent injuries due to activity); present (frequency, severity, and context of symptoms at home and school); social and developmental; parenting style; review of systems
2. Physical examination, screen for "neurological soft signs"; affective behavior; laboratory data of limited value; CBC, lead screen
3. Height, weight, blood pressure, vital signs
4. Vision and hearing screen

5. Sample behavioral assessment from multiple settings—(home, babysitter/child care, relatives, school) using rating scale of direct observation by different observers (e.g., parents, teachers, and babysitters/day care providers)
   a. Connor's Abbreviated Parent-Teacher Questionnaire
   b. ADHD Comprehensive Teacher Rating Scale
   c. Achenbach and Edelbrach's Child Behavior Checklist
   d. Edelbrach Child Attention Problem Scale
   e. DuPaul ADHD Rating Scale for Teachers
6. Psychological evaluation and cognitive testing
- Management/Treatment
   1. Provide structured environment—regular routine; clear and simple rules; firm limits; minimize distraction, overstimulation, and fatigue
   2. Behavioral management—formal operant conditioning techniques to reward/reinforce good behaviors; punishment strategies (time-out) or extinction techniques (systematic ignoring) to decrease unacceptable behaviors
   3. Evaluate need for mental health referral
      a. Child-based therapy for depression, anxiety, low self-esteem; cognitive-behavioral training to increase self-control
      b. Parenting classes or family therapy for relationship difficulties
   4. Pharmacotherapy—unacceptable side effects (including insomnia and growth retardation) and noncompliance are problematic; still no consensus that this is the gold standard for care
      a. Methylphenidate—effective in 75% to 80% with trial of at least 2 to 3 weeks; give 20 to 30 minutes before meals to maximize effectiveness; avoid p.m. doses to minimize insomnia
      b. Dextroamphetamine—effectiveness in 70% to 75% with rapid response
      c. Atomoxetine—nonstimulant, causes less insomnia
      d. If there is a psychiatric comorbidity such as depression or anxiety, treating the comorbidity may have a positive impact on the ADHD
   5. Close follow-up assessment and monitoring of growth and response to medication and behavioral management plan every 3 to 4 months
   6. Ongoing coordination and communication with family, school personnel, primary care provider, and mental health resources are critical to successful management
   7. Medication may be discontinued after 2- to 3-month trial if no change in behavior
   8. Nonconventional treatments (no documented evidence of effectiveness in controlled studies)
      a. Megavitamins, mineral therapy, fish oil, acetyl-l-carnitine
      b. Elimination of sugar, additives, coloring
      c. Neurophysiologic interventions (patterning, sensory integration, optometric training)

9. Community resources
   a. Children and Adults with Attention-Deficit/Hyperactivity Disorder (CHADD)—international nonprofit parent support organization
      8181 Professional Place—Suite 150
      Landover, MD 20785
      301-306-7070
      http://www.chadd.org
   b. Attention Deficit Disorder Association
      P.O. Box 7557
      Wilmington, DE 19803-9997
      1-800-939-1019
      http://www.add.org

Aggression, Defiance, and Disruptive Behavioral Disorders

- Normal behavior vs. dysfunctional patterns and clinical disorders
   1. Most children manifest some degree of developmentally normative aggressive, defiant, and disruptive behavior during infancy and early childhood, e.g., breath-holding, temper tantrums, lying, fighting, breaking things (i.e., some of this behavior is normal)
   2. Almost half of all parents consult with primary care providers regarding difficulty managing disruptive and defiant behaviors of their preschoolers
   3. Repetitive and persistent patterns of aggressive, defiant, and disruptive behaviors lasting longer than 6 months warrant detailed assessment and possible mental health referral
- Conduct Disorder: A repetitive and persistent dysfunctional pattern of aggressive behavior and/or violation of the law, social norms, and basic human rights
   1. Etiology/Incidence
      a. Multifactorial etiology—biological-genetic component suggested from twin/adoption studies
      b. Child onset (less than 10 years) has graver prognosis with increased risk of later substance abuse and antisocial personality disorder than adolescent-onset
      c. Incidence greater among males with estimates of 6% to 16%; female estimates of 2% to 9%
   2. Clinical Findings—*DSM-V* (2013) criteria include:
      a. Aggressive/threatening behavior to people or animals
      b. Deliberate, intentional destruction of property
      c. Lying, stealing
      d. Serious rule violations such as staying out all night, running away, truancy
   3. Differential Diagnosis
      a. Adjustment disorder
      b. ADHD
      c. Oppositional-defiant disorder
      d. Manic episode
      e. Other psychiatric diagnosis

4. Diagnostic Tests/Findings
   a. Separate interview with parent and child
   b. Assessment of parental anxiety regarding dependency/control issues; impact on family functioning
   c. Severity of behaviors with respect to intensity, frequency, duration, context, and developmental stage
   d. Identify contributing psychosocial risk factors—poverty, abuse, neglect, exposure to violence, parental mental illness, and/or substance abuse
5. Management/Treatment
   a. Identify and communicate concern for child and family well-being
   b. Refer for psychological/psychiatric evaluation and intervention
   c. Refer to social service and/or other community resources for parenting education, support, and to reduce family stress and potential for violence

- Oppositional-Defiant Disorder: A repetitive and persistent dysfunctional pattern characterized by negative, disobedient, defiant, and hostile behavior directed at authority figures
  1. Etiology/Incidence
     a. Multifactorial etiology associated with difficult temperament; disruption in early caregiving environment; harsh, inconsistent, and/or neglectful parenting; history of psychiatric disorder in at least one parent, including maternal depression
     b. Incidence among males is greater than among females until puberty, after which rates become more equal; overall estimates range from 2% to 16% depending on population
  2. Clinical Findings
     a. Loses temper easily
     b. Argumentative with adult authority figures
     c. Actively defiant of rules and adult requests
     d. Deliberately annoys other people
     e. Blames others for mistakes and misbehavior
     f. Edgy and easily annoyed
     g. Frequently resentful or angry
     h. Spiteful and vindictive behavior
  3. Differential Diagnosis
     a. Within normal range of oppositional behavior for age and developmental level
     b. Conduct disorder
     c. ADHD
     d. Mental retardation
  4. Management/Treatment
     a. Early identification and monitoring of defiant, aggressive, and oppositional behaviors
     b. Parenting education, support, and effective discipline
     c. Refer for family therapy/intervention if child manifests four or more of clinical behavioral features that have persisted for longer than 6 months

Learning Disabilities (LD)

- Definition
  1. Generic term referring to a heterogeneous cluster of disorders manifested by significant difficulties in the acquisition and use of language, listening, reading (dyslexia), writing (dysgraphia), reasoning, or mathematical abilities (dyscalculia)
  2. School performance in deficit areas significantly below that expected for age, grade, and level of intelligence
- Etiology/Incidence
  1. Multifactorial etiology of genetic and environmental factors
  2. Possible abnormal function in parietal and/or occipital lobes of brain
  3. Conditions associated with LD
     a. Developmental delay
     b. Lead poisoning
     c. Fetal alcohol syndrome
     d. Fragile X syndrome
     e. May be part of syndrome complex (e.g., Down syndrome, DiGeorge syndrome)
  4. General prevalence estimated at 6% to 11% of school-age children
  5. Dyslexia—most common LD, affects 5–15% of general population
- Clinical Findings
  1. Specific academic skill deficits
     a. Basic reading skills, reading comprehension, spelling
     b. Mathematical calculations and reasoning
     c. Disorders of written expression and writing skills
  2. Perceptual-motor impairments
     a. Distinguishing shapes and sizes
     b. Fine motor skills, e.g., writing, coloring, cutting
     c. May make letter and number reversals
  3. Memory and thinking impairment (integrative processing)
     a. Haphazard, ineffective study habits and strategies for memorization
     b. Sequencing of data
     c. Understanding abstract concepts, e.g., time, space, parts, whole
     d. Lacking skills for effective problem solving and task completion
  4. Speech and language deficits
     a. Language delay
     b. Difficulty with grammar (syntax), meaning (semantics), and/or social use of words (pragmatics)
  5. Attention deficits—difficulty concentrating and staying on task
  6. Hyperactivity—difficulty sitting still, constantly in motion
  7. Impulsiveness
     a. Often acting without thinking
     b. Poor planning skills
     c. Lack of self-regulation skills
  8. General deficits in coordination—clumsiness
  9. Emotional problems
     a. Lability and moodiness
     b. Often isolated or rejected by peers
     c. May exhibit inappropriate attention-getting behaviors
     d. Difficulty reading nonverbal social cues
     e. May be passive learners

- Differential Diagnosis
  1. Undiagnosed sensory impairment—vision or hearing deficits
  2. ADHD
  3. Seizure disorder
  4. Mental retardation
  5. Maladaptation to chronic disease
  6. Social and environmental factors
     a. Child abuse and neglect
     b. Situational anxiety or depressive reaction
     c. Ethnic or cultural minority
- Physical Findings
  1. Neurological soft signs commonly present
     a. Poor fine motor coordination and tactile discrimination
     b. Strabismus
     c. Poor hand–eye coordination
     d. Balance problems
  2. Phenotypic features of associated conditions—FAS, fragile X
  3. Other abnormal physical findings likely to be related to LD
- Diagnostic Studies/Findings: Diagnosis requires multi-dimensional assessment
  1. Complete medical and social history
  2. Developmental and behavioral history
  3. Educational history and school functioning
  4. Physical examination—soft neurological signs
  5. Laboratory studies—associated conditions
     a. Lead screening
     b. EEG if seizures suspected
  6. Psychoeducational testing
  7. Analysis of history, test results, and academic achievement leads to diagnosis
- Management/Treatment
  1. Developmental surveillance, early identification, and referral are critical
  2. Early intervention to optimize learning and minimize emotional sequelae
  3. Thorough psychoeducational evaluation to determine skills and deficits
  4. Interdisciplinary conference to evaluate findings
  5. Individualized education plan (IEP) developed based on multidimensional assessment
  6. Yearly reevaluation of IEP with revisions as needed
  7. Address other associated behavioral, social, and family issues through counseling and direct instruction
  8. Inform parents of legal rights under Individuals with Disabilities Education Act (IDEA) and availability of appropriate special services

Eating Disorders: Anorexia Nervosa and Bulimia Nervosa

- Definition: Chronic and often severe disturbances in eating behavior accompanied by distorted perception of body weight, size, and shape
  1. Anorexia nervosa—eating disturbance associated with weight loss and refusal to maintain body weight at minimally normal level (85% of expected body weight for age and sex; with subsequent amenorrhea in girls)
  2. Bulimia nervosa—eating disturbance associated with episodic binge eating followed by compensatory efforts to prevent weight gain (self-induced vomiting; dieting; fasting; excessive exercise or misuse of laxatives, enemas, and/or diuretics)
  3. Anorexia may occur with or without associated bingeing/purging (restricting vs. binge-eating/purging types); bulimia may occur with or without purging (purging vs. nonpurging types)
- Etiology/Incidence
  1. Family enmeshment hypothesis—rigid, overprotective families with difficulty with conflict resolution; separation–individuation
  2. Fear of sexual maturation; history of sexual abuse
  3. Social pressure to be thin
  4. Ballet dancers and gymnasts at particular risk
  5. Associated with psychological profile of low self-esteem in spite of outward successfulness
  6. Both disorders are more common among females
  7. Anorexia affects approximately 1% of white middle/upper-class females; 5% to 10% of cases are male, often associated with gender identity conflict
  8. Bimodal distribution with one peak at 14 years and second at 18 years
  9. Bulimia is more common than anorexia with later age onset
  10. Suicide rates of 2% to 5% of those with chronic anorexia with overall mortality rate as high as 10%
  11. Normal to high intelligence, overachievers, perfectionists
- Clinical Findings
  1. Self-imposed weight loss
  2. Anemia, jaundice, and secondary amenorrhea
  3. Vigorous exercise regimen to increase weight loss
  4. Constipation (chronic laxatives) and reflux esophagitis (self-induced vomiting)
  5. Dry skin, brittle nails
  6. Lower body temperature, blood pressure, and heart rate
  7. Lanugo
  8. Sore throat, calluses on dorsum of fingers, loss of tooth enamel (from induced vomiting)
- Differential Diagnosis
  1. General medical condition—gastrointestinal disease, diabetes, thyroid disorder, AIDS, systemic lupus erythematosus
  2. Pregnancy
  3. Depressive disorder or substance abuse
- Diagnostic Tests/Findings
  1. History—include nutritional patterns as well as effort to lose weight (dieting, exercise, vomiting); preoccupation with food and/or "feeling fat"; past medical, family, and social history; review of systems (amenorrhea)

2. Weight and height percentiles—degree of malnutrition determined as percentage below ideal body weight (IBW)
   a. Mild malnutrition—<20% below IBW
   b. Moderate malnutrition—20% to 30% below IBW
   c. Severe malnutrition—>30% below IBW
3. Physical examination—signs of malnutrition; dry skin, brittle nails, muscle weakness, flat affect, decreased blood pressure, pulse and body temperature; Tanner staging delays
4. CBC, serum albumin, glucose, electrolytes, thyroid function, ECG; others as appropriate based on history and clinical findings

- Management/Treatment
1. Interdisciplinary treatment plan, including nutritional intervention, behavior modification techniques, psychotherapy (individual, family, and/or group therapy); pharmacologic management with antidepressants if appropriate
2. Hospitalization for rehydration, refeeding, and/or psychiatric treatment if condition warrants. As the family is a contributing factor, hospitalization as a means to remove the child from the family is sometimes effective
3. Approximately one-half of patients show varying degrees of improvement, 25% show long-term improvement, 25% do poorly regardless of intervention
4. Refer to appropriate community resources for assessment tools, support, and education:
   a. Psychological Assessment Resources, Inc. (PAR, Inc.)
      16204 North Florida Avenue
      Lutz, FL 33549
      1-800-331-8378
      http://www4.parinc.com/Default.aspx
   b. National Eating Disorders Association
      603 Stewart Street, Suite 803
      Seattle, WA 98101
      1-800-931-2237
      http://www.nationaleatingdisorders.org
   c. National Association of Anorexia Nervosa and Associated Disorders
      P.O. Box 7
      Highland Park, IL 60035
      847-831-3438
      http://www.anad.org

Childhood Depression

- Definition: Behavioral pattern lasting at least 2 weeks that is characterized by affective and behavioral symptoms, including sad or tearful moods, irritability, and/or social withdrawal with associated decreased interest and pleasure in developmentally appropriate activities
- Etiology/Incidence: Multifactorial etiology with associated risk factors, including:

1. History of traumatic event(s) involving significant separation(s) or loss(es) of parent, caregiver, or significant other
2. Family history of depression, especially in mother; evidence of genetic component from twin and adoption studies
3. Chronic neglect and lack of nurturance due to family disruptions or dysfunction, including long-term effects of poverty and/or homelessness
4. Substance abuse, physical or sexual abuse in household
5. Chronic illness and/or disability may increase risk, especially with familial predisposition
6. Estimated incidence of 3% for overall pediatric population and as high as 9% for adolescents; no gender differences in early childhood depression, but increases among females in adolescence with ratio of 5:1

- Clinical Findings
1. Major depressive episode—significant distress and/or interference with normal daily functioning lasting at least 2 weeks associated with:
   a. Depressed or irritable mood and/or decreased interest and pleasure in developmentally appropriate activities and a minimum of four additional symptoms
   b. Appetite changes with associated weight gain or loss
   c. Insomnia or hypersomnia
   d. Difficulty concentrating; decline in school performance
   e. Feelings of worthlessness, guilt, fearfulness, isolation
   f. Social withdrawal from friends, family; school refusal and/or truancy
   g. General somatic complaints of aches and pains with nonspecific etiology, e.g., fatigue, headaches, stomachaches
   h. Agitation, irritability, and/or disruptive behavior
   i. Recurrent thoughts of death and/or suicidal ideation
2. Dysthymic disorder—long-standing depressed or irritable mood lasting 1 year or more, but symptoms of distress and interference with normal daily functioning not as pronounced as a major depressive episode
3. Adjustment disorder with depressed mood—depressed or irritable mood, sadness, tearfulness, and/or feelings of hopelessness causing some degree of impairment of daily functioning that occurs within 3 months of a significant and identifiable stressful life event

- Differential Diagnosis
1. Normal periods of sadness and/or mood swings
2. Acute depressive reactions/adjustment disorder with depressed mood in response to identifiable life stress
3. Masked depressive disorder—somatization and denial of feelings

4. Underlying physical disorder
5. Substance abuse
6. Psychiatric depressive disorder with suicidal risk
- Diagnostic Tests/Findings
  1. Behavioral symptoms according to *DSM-V* diagnostic criteria
  2. History—developmental, family, social, and school; current medications; chronic disease/disability
  3. Separate interview with child or adolescent is essential
  4. Physical examination—neurological screening
  5. Height, weight, vital signs, assess for recent weight loss or gain
  6. Laboratory tests—as indicated by history (drug screen, pregnancy test)
- Management/Treatment
  1. Early screening and identification of children and adolescents at risk for depression
     a. Center for Epidemiologic Studies Depression Scale for Children
     b. Children's Depression Rating Scale
     c. Children's Depression Inventory
     d. Child Behavior Checklist
     e. Rose Institute Adolescent Depression Scale
     f. Mood Questionnaire for Adolescents
  2. Evaluate severity of depression, including suicidal risk, and make appropriate referrals
  3. Psychiatric intervention is necessary for major depressive episode or dysthymic disorder
     a. Family and/or individual psychotherapy
     b. Pharmacotherapy—may be included as part of multimodal treatment plan
        (1) Selective serotonin reuptake inhibitors (SSRIs)—most effective medication for major depressive episodes (fluoxetine or sertraline)
        (2) Tricyclic antidepressants have limited clinical use with equivocal effectiveness demonstrated in controlled studies (monitor blood levels)
  4. Supportive counseling for adjustment disorder with depressed mood
  5. Resources
     a. Depression/Awareness, Recognition, and Treatment (D/ART)
        National Institutes of Mental Health
        Science Writing, Press, and Dissemination Branch
        6001 Executive Boulevard, Room 8184, MSC 9663
        Bethesda, MD 20892-9663
        1-866-615-6464
        http://www.nimh.nih.gov/index.shtml

Suicidal Behavior

- Definition: Passive or active thoughts/wishes about death and dying (suicidal ideation); talking and/or threatening to take one's life or self-injury without intent to die (suicidal gesture); deliberate self-injury with the intent to die, but not resulting in death (suicide attempt); and self-inflicted death (completed suicide)
- Etiology/Incidence (CDC, 2015)
  1. Accounts for 11% of teenage deaths, representing the third leading cause of adolescent mortality
  2. 15% to 40% of completed suicides were preceded by one or more suicide gestures/attempts
  3. Females have higher rates of suicide attempts; males have higher rates of completed suicides
  4. Higher rates among Native American, Asian, and chronically ill adolescents
  5. Ingestion of medication is most common method; violent methods (hanging and shooting) are more frequently used by males than females and are more often fatal
- Clinical Findings
  1. Severe and/or chronic depression
  2. Hopelessness
  3. Previous suicidal gestures
  4. History of suicide in family
  5. Existence of specific plan
- Differential Diagnosis
  1. Unintentional injuries due to carelessness and/or adolescent sense of "invincibility"
  2. Suicidal gesture as desperate call for help
  3. Imminent risk/acute suicidal intent
  4. Psychotic episode
- Diagnostic Tests/Findings
  1. History—past and present health, chronic depression, chronic illness, disability; school performance; family history of depression and/or suicide; current medications; substance abuse
  2. Suicidal risk—suicidal ideation, extent of premeditation and existence of plan, likelihood of rescue, suicide notes, previous suicidal gestures
  3. Observation and/or reports of suicidal behavior by family, teachers, or peers
- Management/Treatment
  1. Refer immediately for crisis intervention resources, e.g., 24-hour hotline
  2. Suicidal ideation and/or gestures with existence of plan requires immediate psychological evaluation
  3. Ensure safe environment for child/adolescent, including hospitalization if necessary
  4. Short-term hospitalization is recommended for all suicide attempts; attending to emergency treatment and/or surgical management is necessary but insufficient without additional follow-up intervention
  5. Treat underlying depression
  6. Inform child/adolescent of seriousness of concern and need to notify family and mobilize necessary community resources
     a. American Association of Suicidology
        5221 Wisconsin Avenue, NW
        Washington, DC 20015
        202-237-2280
        1-800-273-TALK (8255) – 24/7 Suicide prevention hotline
        http://www.suicidology.org/Resources/Crisis-Centers

Substance Abuse (Tobacco, Alcohol, and Other Drugs)

- Definition: Use of any drug or chemical for purposes of stimulation, pleasure, or in a way that interferes with normal functioning and/or threatens health; includes misuse of legal "recreational" drugs, prescribed or non-prescribed medications, as well as illegal substances; *DSM-V* distinguishes substance abuse from dependence
  1. Substance abuse—a maladaptive pattern of substance use associated with significant impairment or distress, including inability to meet expected daily obligations, use of substance in situations/context that may be hazardous to self or others and/or resulting in legal and/or other interpersonal conflicts
  2. Substance dependence—a pattern of repeated substance abuse that results in tolerance, withdrawal, and/or compulsive use that can be psychological and/or physiologic-based
  3. Categories of substances include—alcohol, marijuana (cannabis), nicotine, amphetamines, caffeine, cocaine, hallucinogens, inhalants, opioids, phencyclidine (PCP), sedatives and hypnotics, anabolic steroids
- Etiology/Incidence
  1. Multifactorial etiology, including some evidence of biological predisposition along with psychosocial and environmental risks such as impulsivity, nonconformity/rebellion, peer pressure, ineffective coping with stress, undiagnosed depression, family dysfunction, history of child abuse or neglect, parental substance abuse
  2. Majority of adolescents will engage in some form of drug use at some point
  3. More frequent use of all substances among males vs. females
  4. Highest overall incidence of substance abuse among Caucasian teenagers followed by Hispanic youth; lowest incidence among African American teenagers
  5. Most recent national drug use survey (2012) reported prevalence of current illicit drug use is 8.8% of teenagers from 12 to 17 years of age
  6. Trend is away from street drugs toward prescription drugs used illicitly
- Clinical Findings
  1. Nicotine—decreased exercise tolerance, fatigue, muscle weakness; pallor, tachycardia, staining of teeth, tobacco odor on breath and clothes
  2. Alcohol—initial euphoria and talkativeness; grogginess; impaired short-term memory; decreased reaction time; hypoglycemia
  3. Marijuana (THC, pot, cannabis, joint, reefer, weed, hash, grass)—euphoria, drowsiness, slowed reaction time and motor coordination, time distortions, tachycardia and transient hypertension, bloodshot eyes
  4. Amphetamines—dilated pupils, tachycardia, anorexia, insomnia, weight loss, anxiety, and suicidal behavior
  5. Cocaine (coke, freebase, crack, nose, flake)—agitation, hyperactivity, euphoria followed by depression, confused thinking, occasional paranoid ideation, tachycardia, habitual "snorting" induced nasal septum scabbing or necrosis
  6. Hallucinogens
     a. LSD—dilated pupils, visual and auditory hallucinations and flashbacks, disorganized and confused thinking, increased attention to stimuli; chronic use can lead to psychosis and major personality changes
     b. PCP—euphoria, motor incoordination, hallucinations; paranoia with aggressive/violent behavior
  7. Inhalants/volatile substances (glue, cleaning agents, hydrocarbons)—relaxation, hallucinations, light headedness, giddiness; seizures, coma, cardiac arrhythmias, and sudden death
  8. Anabolic steroids—used to increase muscle mass and strength; fluid retention, mood swings, menstrual abnormalities; male gynecomastia, female hirsutism, breast atrophy
  9. Opiates include naturally occurring (e.g., morphine, codeine), semisynthetic (e.g., heroin, hydromorphone), and synthetic (e.g., fentanyl, meperidine, methadone); constricted pupils; respiratory depression; euphoria; analgesia; dermatologic lesions, "tracks"; tattoos in unusual places to conceal track marks; chronic infections (skin, HIV, scarring, and cellulitis); constipation; decrease in libido; urinary retention
- Differential Diagnosis
  1. Social recreational use of legal substances
  2. Experimentation vs. abuse
  3. Chronic depression
  4. Neurological disorder
  5. Learning disabilities
- Diagnostic Tests/Findings
  1. History—past and present, environmental, family, social, and academic history; review of systems; current medications; specific drug history, including specific drugs, frequency of use, settings of use, impairment of daily functioning including suspensions or legal difficulties
  2. Interviews with and observations from child/adolescent, parents, school personnel, peers
  3. Physical examination with close assessment of skin integrity (nasal septum, skin lesions/track marks); neurological assessment; vital signs, weight, height, blood pressure
  4. Serum and urine toxicology, HIV testing, others as appropriate to specific history
- Management/Treatment
  1. Ensure appropriate privacy, confidentiality, and nonjudgmental atmosphere
  2. Referral to appropriate substance abuse treatment resources
  3. Identify and provide appropriate referrals for management of underlying psychosocial difficulties contributing to substance abuse

4. Educate and counsel regarding legal and physical risks of substance abuse
5. Support community-based prevention programs
6. Additional national resources
   a. National Institute on Drug Abuse (NIDA)
      (800) 662–HELP
      http://www.nida.nih.gov
   b. National Family Partnership
      (800) 705–8997
      http://www.nfp.org
   c. Substance Abuse and Mental Health Services Administration
      1-800-662-HELP (4357)
      http://www.samhsa.gov

☐ HEALTH SUPERVISION AS ONGOING SURVEILLANCE, SCREENING, AND ASSESSMENT OF PHYSICAL GROWTH AND BEHAVIORAL DEVELOPMENT

- Definitions
  1. Surveillance: A continuous process of periodic assessment and monitoring of growth and development over time through a variety of methods, including direct observation, health history, parent/child interviews, and physical examination
  2. Screening: Use of standardized or generally accepted methods with essentially well populations in order to identify individuals who may be at risk for physical, cognitive, or psychosocial abnormality and warrant further assessment; good screening tools are simple, inexpensive, acceptable, valid, and reliable
  3. Assessment: A more systematic evaluation using a standardized or generally accepted method leading to recommendations for intervention
  4. Sensitivity: Proportion of those with the abnormality who are correctly identified through screening (true positives)
  5. Specificity: Proportion of those without the abnormality who are correctly identified as negative through screening (true negatives)
  6. Positive predictive value (PPV): Proportion of those individuals correctly screened as positive of all those who actually have the abnormality
- Examples of Screening and Assessment Tests Used in Child Health Supervision
  1. Physical assessment and laboratory screening
  2. Developmental screening and assessment
     a. Global development
        (1) Newborn Behavioral Assessment Scale (NBAS)—assessment of newborn's behavioral capacities, including state control, autonomic reactivity, reflexes, habituation, and responsiveness to visual and auditory stimuli
        (2) Bayley Infant Neurodevelopmental Screener (BINS)—screens for basic neurological, receptive, expressive, and cognitive functions in infants between 3 and 24 months
        (3) Bayley Scales of Infant Development, Second Edition (BSID-II)—current "gold standard" for diagnosing developmental delays and recommending intervention for children birth through 42 months with separate mental, motor, and behavioral rating scales
        (4) Ages and Stages Questionnaires (ASQ)—parent-completed child monitoring system for children 4 to 48 months
        (5) Denver II—screens in personal-social, fine motor-adaptive, language, and gross motor domains in children birth to 6 years
        (6) Parents Evaluation of Developmental Status—Developmental Milestones (PEDS:dm) Tool that uses parent observations for behavioral and developmental screening (http://www.pedstest.com/default.aspx)
        (7) First Step—screening test for evaluating preschoolers
     b. Cognitive development—intelligence
        (1) McCarthy Scales of Children's Abilities
        (2) Weschler Preschool and Primary Scale of Intelligence Revised (WPPSIR)
        (3) Weschler Intelligence Scale for Children (WISC III)
     c. Language
        (1) Early Language Milestones Scale (ELM)—0 to 42 months
        (2) Receptive and Expressive Emergent Language Scale (REEL)—0 to 36 months
        (3) Clinical Linguistic and Auditory Milestone Test (CLAMS)—0 to 36 months
        (4) Language Development Survey—screening tool for toddlers using vocabulary checklist for enumeration of words
        (5) The MacArthur Communicative Development Inventory—words and gestures
        (6) The MacArthur Communicative Development Inventory—words and sentences
     d. Behaviors
        (1) Achenbach's Child Behavior Checklist (ACBCL)
        (2) Connor's Abbreviated Parent-Teacher Questionnaire
     e. Temperament
        (1) Infant Temperament Questionnaire—4 to 8 months
        (2) Toddler Temperament Scale—1 to 3 years
        (3) Behavioral Style Questionnaire—3 to 7 years
        (4) Middle Childhood Temperament Questionnaire—8 to 12 years
  3. Parent–child relationship and home environment
     a. Parenting Stress Index (PSI)
     b. Home Observation for Measurement of the Environment (HOME scale)—infant, preschool, and elementary school versions

c. Pediatric Review and Observation of Children's Environmental Support and Stimulation Inventory (PROCESS)

d. Nursing Child Assessment Feeding (NCAF) and Teaching (NCAT) scales

4. Mental health screening and diagnostic classifications
   a. *DSM-V*

❑ QUESTIONS

Select the best answer.

1. Most stage-based theories of development focus primarily on:
   a. The continuity of development
   b. The discontinuity of development
   c. Persistence of inherent personality characteristics
   d. The influence of context on development

2. The common practice of using "time-outs" with young children is a direct application of:
   a. Operant conditioning
   b. Classical conditioning
   c. Separation–individuation
   d. Maturational reinforcement

3. Good communication among families, schools, and primary care providers is an example of which ecological concept?
   a. Microsystem
   b. Mesosystem
   c. Exosystem
   d. Macrosystem

4. Which of the following findings would most likely be associated with asymmetric intrauterine growth retardation?
   a. Weight, length, and head circumference ranging from 3rd to 5th percentile
   b. Heavy maternal smoking throughout pregnancy
   c. Weight at 3rd percentile and length at 25th
   d. Gestational diabetes

5. Early reflexive responses that are not related to survival include all but:
   a. Babinski
   b. Moro
   c. Swimming
   d. Rooting

6. The most likely weight of a 1-year-old child whose weight at birth was 6 pounds would be:
   a. 19–20 pounds
   b. 13–14 pounds
   c. 25–26 pounds
   d. Impossible to estimate

7. One of the major psychosocial tasks of infancy is:
   a. Development of secure attachment
   b. Separation–individuation
   c. Symbiosis
   d. Regulation

8. Which developmental theory best explains the multifactorial etiology of failure to thrive?
   a. Organismic-maturational theory
   b. Social learning theory

c. Transactional theory
d. Psychoanalytic theory

9. Most healthy infants are able to reach, grasp, and hold on to a rattle or other small toy by about:
   a. 2 months
   b. 6 months
   c. 8 months
   d. 10 months

10. The pincer grasp is a fine motor skill that involves the ability to pick up a small object such as a raisin or piece of cereal with the thumb and forefinger and that usually is mastered around:
    a. 4 months
    b. 6 months
    c. 9 months
    d. 16 months

11. You would be concerned about the language development of a child who:
    a. Repeats simple phrases at 32 months
    b. Stutters when excited or tired at the age of 7 years
    c. Has a vocabulary of 10 words at 12 months
    d. Pronounces words that are not understandable at 24 months

12. The most common temperamental profile is:
    a. Easy
    b. Difficult
    c. Slow-to-warm-up
    d. Intermediate

13. The underlying emotion of an insecurely attached (avoidant) relationship is:
    a. Ambivalence
    b. Deprivation
    c. Anger
    d. Conditional love

14. The stage of cognitive development that Piaget described as characteristic of the way preschoolers think is the:
    a. Preoperational stage
    b. Mental combinations stage
    c. Tertiary circular function stage
    d. Sensorimotor stage

15. A preschool boy whose parents have separated and are beginning divorce procedures:
    a. May think that he caused the divorce by misbehaving
    b. Should not be told of the impending divorce until the parents are sure of their decision
    c. Is likely to experience gender identity confusion
    d. Should be able to make a decision about which parent he prefers living with

16. Which behavior would you expect to decrease during the preschool years?
    a. Rough-and-tumble play
    b. Instrumental aggression
    c. Hostile aggression
    d. Cooperative play

17. A preschool child who says that the sky is blue because it is his favorite color is illustrating the concept of:
    a. Symbolic thinking
    b. Egocentrism
    c. Centration
    d. Imaginary audience

18. Which of the following strategies would not be appropriate to include as part of your management of a 9-year-old boy who is obese?
    a. Referral to nutritionist for weight reduction plan
    b. Increase physical exercise
    c. Behavior modification strategies to deal with stress and/or reinforce treatment plan
    d. Involve family in management program

19. Which of the following issues or concepts is relevant to the school-aged child?
    a. Operational thinking
    b. Initiative
    c. Concrete operations
    d. Separation–individuation

20. The first physical sign indicating the onset of female puberty is:
    a. Sparsely distributed, fine, pale pubic hairs
    b. Breast buds
    c. Menarche
    d. Peak height velocity

21. Which of the following findings would be helpful in distinguishing obesity from large body frame in an adolescent who is concerned with her weight?
    a. Tricep skinfold measurement
    b. Weight-for-height ratio
    c. Body mass index
    d. Percent of ideal body weight

22. The most common form of child abuse seen in pediatric primary care is:
    a. Burns
    b. Fractures
    c. Soft tissue injuries
    d. Shaken baby syndrome

23. A differential diagnosis for child abuse would include all of the following except:
    a. Birth marks
    b. Unintentional injury
    c. Inadequate parenting
    d. Prader-Willi syndrome

24. Which of the following symptoms is not typical of a child with ADHD?
    a. Easily distracted
    b. Difficulty playing quietly
    c. Doesn't follow directions
    d. Frequently angry and resentful

25. Which of the following clinical findings would not suggest an eating disorder with a purging component?
    a. Sore throat
    b. Brittle nails
    c. Diarrhea
    d. Finger calluses

26. Which of the following situations does not necessarily warrant immediate mental health assessment and/or referral?
    a. 13-year-old girl who has been "down" for the last month with varied somatic complaints
    b. 9-year-old boy whose parents recently separated and filed for a divorce and who seems to be doing well
    c. 16-year-old girl who has a history of long-standing depression and has started to have "slipping grades" at school
    d. 15-year-old boy who expresses suicidal thoughts

27. Which adolescent would be at greatest risk for developing anorexia nervosa?
    a. 12-year-old female who just had her first period
    b. 14-year-old female gymnast
    c. 16-year-old male runner
    d. 18-year-old female college student

28. Which of the following substances is associated with pupillary constriction?
    a. Amphetamines
    b. LSD
    c. Heroin
    d. Nicotine

29. A risk factor that is common to many psychosocial pediatric problems, including failure to thrive, conduct or oppositional disorders, and childhood depression, is:
    a. Maternal depression or other psychiatric disorder
    b. Substance abuse
    c. Prematurity
    d. History of sexual abuse

30. Which of the following diagnoses is not more common among males?
    a. ADHD
    b. Conduct disorders
    c. Suicide
    d. FTT

31. The diagnostic criteria for autism spectrum disorder include:
    a. A noted lack of back-and-forth conversation
    b. Tolerance of flexibility with routines
    c. Fascination with light or movement
    d. Abnormal eye movements or body language

32. In addition to specific academic skill deficits, learning disabilities are commonly associated with which of the following characteristics?
    a. Perceptual-motor impairments, normal motor function
    b. Perceptual-motor impairments, impulsiveness
    c. Perceptual-motor impairments, Down syndrome
    d. Lack of impulsiveness, perceptual-motor impairment

33. H. O. is a 5-year-old Vietnamese child who has fallen off of his growth curve. The best intervention would be to:
    a. Suggest high-calorie breakfast drinks as supplements
    b. Incorporate traditional foods into a management plan that will provide increased calories and nutrients

c. Educate the family on the need for increased calories and nutrients

d. Refer family to a growth clinic for evaluation

34. While taking the history of 6-month-old E. M., you learn that she is not sleeping through the night and will not fall back to sleep without the parents rocking or feeding her. This is an example of:
    a. Somnambulism
    b. Pavor nocturnus
    c. Learned behavior
    d. Delayed sleep phase

35. Which of the following scenarios is suggestive of a child who may not be ready to enter first grade? An inability to:
    a. Recognize six colors and remember one's phone number
    b. Accurately use pronouns
    c. Empathize with others
    d. Count to five and draw a person with three parts

36. While examining 10-year-old R. M.'s teeth, you note that the upper incisors slightly overlap the lower incisors. The second and lower first molars are absent. Your assessment is:
    a. Malocclusion
    b. Delayed mandibular dentition
    c. Normal dentition
    d. Hyperdontia

37. The mother of 5-year-old D. W. is concerned that her son often cheats when playing board games with his older sister. What is the most appropriate response to D. W.'s behavior?
    a. Encourage the parent to use 5-minute time-outs when cheating occurs.
    b. Explain that D. W. is developmentally unable to comprehend rigid rules.
    c. Make sure that D. W. understands the rules before starting to play the game.
    d. Explain to D. W. that cheating is like lying and is not acceptable behavior.

38. Which of the following physical findings in a 2-month-old child warrants an immediate referral to a neurologist/neurosurgeon?
    a. Head circumference growing faster than height and weight
    b. Unresolved cephalhematoma
    c. Rigid and immobile sagittal suture
    d. Snapping sensation when pressure is applied to parietal bone

39. While listening to 2½-year-old K. L. talk, you note that she frequently omits final consonants and her sentences are two to three words in length. The appropriate plan of care would be:
    a. Routine follow-up at the next well-child visit
    b. Referring for hearing screen
    c. Assessing for developmental delays
    d. Referring to a speech pathologist

40. The mother of 3-year-old G. W. reports that he has begun to stutter. Further probing reveals that the stuttering occurs frequently and lasts 1 to 2 seconds. G. W. does not seem bothered by the stuttering. The appropriate management would be:
    a. Referral to a speech pathologist
    b. Referral for an evaluation for an anxiety disorder
    c. Reassuring the mother that this is a mild problem
    d. Demonstrating to G. W. slow, deep breathing before talking

41. You would expect a school-age child to:
    a. Grow 1.5 inches per year
    b. Grow 0.5 inch per year
    c. Gain about 6 pounds per year
    d. Gain about 3 pounds per year

42. During 8-month-old L. B.'s physical examination, the father boasts that L. B. is going to be a left-handed batter since he prefers doing everything with his left hand. The appropriate response would be to:
    a. Ask if others in the family are left handed
    b. Suggest play activities that require using both hands
    c. Present toys more often to the right hand
    d. Perform a careful neurologic examination

43. Which of the following best describes behavior associated with Piaget's concrete operational phase?
    a. Learning primarily by trial and error
    b. Interpreting events in relationship to themselves
    c. Categorizing information into lower or higher classes
    d. Drawing logical conclusions from observations

44. Jeffrey, at 8 years of age, has been diagnosed with ADHD and is receiving stimulant medication. Which of the following interventions would be least helpful?
    a. Monthly height and weight checks
    b. Small frequent meals and snacks
    c. High-calorie supplemental drinks
    d. Elimination of refined sugar from diet

45. The principle that growth and development become increasingly integrated is best demonstrated by:
    a. Gaining head control before raising the chest
    b. Bringing cup to mouth, tipping, and swallowing
    c. Rolling over before sitting
    d. Grasping with fist before using fingers

46. In males, Tanner stage III can be distinguished from Tanner stage II by:
    a. Fine, downy pubic hair at the base of penis
    b. Adult-like pubic hair not extending to thighs
    c. Penile growth in width
    d. Penile growth in length

47. T. J., 13 years old, reluctantly shares with you that his "chest hurts." On physical examination, you note unilateral breast enlargement, which is tender to palpation. You suspect physiologic gynecomastia. Which Tanner stage would support that diagnosis?
    a. Tanner stage I
    b. Tanner stage III

c. Tanner stage IV
d. Tanner stage V

48. During a physical examination of 10½-year-old Melissa, you note the appearance of breast buds. You tell her that she can expect which of the following in approximately 2 years?
    a. Growth of pubic hair
    b. Peak height velocity
    c. Onset of menses
    d. Axillary hair

49. Adolescents who engage in risky behavior, such as driving without a seat belt, are displaying:
    a. A type of egocentrism
    b. A need for independence
    c. Role experimentation
    d. Low self-esteem

50. An increase in which of the following behaviors is seen more frequently in late rather than in early adolescence?
    a. Value conflict with parents
    b. Focus on physical appearance
    c. Peer group involvement
    d. Understanding inner motivations of others

☐ ANSWERS AND RATIONALES

1. B: These theories address deviations from developmental progress norms.
2. A: Time-out is a practice of behavioral modification as promulgated by B. F. Skinner's model of operant conditioning with a negative consequence for an unacceptable behavior.
3. B: A mesosystem is the link or relationship between the various settings (microsystems) within which a child exists (i.e., home, school, day care, etc.).
4. C: The weight and length are at significantly different percentiles; if the IUGR were symmetrical, these would be at the same percentile.
5. D: Rooting (i.e., moving the head to locate the nipple) is a key survival reflex.
6. A: An infant's weight should approximately triple by the age of 1 year.
7. A: The development of an infant–caregiver bond is key to the prevention of long-term psychological effects associated with deprivation and/or failure to develop secure, stable bonds.
8. C: Transactional theory explains risks and protective factors associated with resilience and vulnerability. It may explain some of the environmental factors associated with FTT.
9. B: These are gross developmental norms associated with the 6-month-old child.
10. C: This is a developmental norm for a child of 9 months.
11. B: Stuttering associated with fatigue or excitement is not unusual in a preschooler but may indicate a more pervasive problem in a 7-year-old.

12. A: Approximately 40% of children are described as having an easy (rhythmic, approachable, adaptive) temperament.
13. C: Attachment is the bond that develops throughout the first year of life; underlying anger characterizes avoidance or an insecure bond.
14. A: Piaget characterizes preschoolers as preoperational thinkers.
15. A: Preschoolers are characterized by egocentrism; they think the world revolves around them and that everything that happens is because they did or did not do something.
16. B: Preschoolers strongly defend what is "theirs," be it a toy or a space or a special privilege; this aggression wanes as they begin to understand sharing and appropriate impulse control.
17. B: Egocentrism is the hallmark of preschoolers; there is little they think they do not control, from the weather to the color of the sky.
18. A: Treatment of obesity in a 9-year-old requires a multifactorial approach, including "eating healthy" and exercise, and needs not necessarily focus on weight reduction. The goal is to prevent weight gain and maintain weight until linear growth catches up.
19. C: Concrete operational thinking is key to successful adaptation to school. It involves the concepts of reversibility, conservation, classification, and seriation.
20. B: The first sign of female puberty is the development of breast buds, closely followed by the development of pubic hair. Peak height velocity and menarche generally occur at age 12½ years.
21. C: Body mass index is generally considered the best index for evaluation of weight; it correlates weight with height.
22. C: Soft tissue injuries, such as bruises, abrasions, and lacerations, are the most common form of abuse, occurring in all age groups.
23. D: Prader-Willi is associated with uncontrolled appetite and obesity; it has no outward sign that could be confused with signs of child abuse.
24. D: Anger is not usually a manifestation of ADHD, whereas high distractibility and inability to sit quietly or follow directions are red flags that a child may have ADHD.
25. C: Eating disorders with a purging component are characterized by constipation, rather than diarrhea, resulting from chronic laxative use.
26. B: This child may be at risk for a mental health issue, but he appears to be coping well and immediate referral is not indicated.
27. B: There is a very high incidence of anorexia nervosa in ballet dancers and gymnasts.
28. C: Opiates cause constricted pupils. Amphetamines and LSD cause dilated pupils, and nicotine generally does not have any effect on the pupils.

29. A: All of these problems have multifactorial etiolo-gies; maternal psychiatric disorders that could affect parenting or development of a secure and stable bond are important factors to consider.
30. D: The incidence of failure to thrive has no predomi-nance in males or females.
31. B: Children with ASD do not tolerate alterations to prescribed routines and may benefit from predictable schedules.
32. B: Children with LD may demonstrate impulsive behaviors as attention-getting behaviors.
33. B: It is important for healthcare professionals to understand the cultural norms and perspectives of others. This often helps in compliance with sug-gestions for improved health. Asian families, out of respect, often do not ask questions or challenge advice. By understanding their food patterns and incorporating that into a diet plan, the healthcare pro-fessional may increase compliance.
34. C: Sleepwalking (somnambulism) and pavor noctur-nus (night terrors) are sleep disturbances that occur in school-age and preschool-age children, respec-tively. Learned behavior is a result of parents interfer-ing with the child's attempts to return to sleep without stimulation from the parents.
35. D: Children entering first grade should have the requi-site skills to master the tasks they will encounter. This includes language, fine and gross motor skills, and personal and social skills. At this age the child should be able to draw a person with at least six parts and count to 10 or more.
36. B: The mandibular (lower) molars usually erupt between ages 6 and 7. Even allowing for individual variation, this is a considerable delay. *Hyperdontia* refers to supernumerary teeth.
37. B: Developmentally, the concept of cheating is not well understood until 7 years of age. The idea of play-ing fairly to ensure everyone an equal chance occurs with maturity and the ability to differentiate among moral choices.
38. C: Ridged and immobile sutures indicate premature fusing resulting in craniosynostosis. For proper brain growth, sutures need to approximate each other yet remain mobile.
39. A: Children aged 2 to 3 years have several articula-tion dysfluencies, among them is the dropping of final consonants. Two- to three-word sentences are normal for the 24- to 30-month-old child.
40. C: This represents a mild stuttering problem but does not warrant immediate referral unless the child or parent is increasingly concerned or if it continues indefinitely.
41. C: The recognized standard of physical growth of school-age children is to gain 5 to 7 pounds per year and grow about 2.5 inches per year.
42. D: Handedness before a year is cause for concern and may indicate cerebral palsy. A neurologic examination

is indicated. The examiner should carefully assess for increase in deep tendon reflexes and tone.
43. C: Concrete operations occur during the school-age years as children begin to understand the character-istics of things and objects. Classification is a thought process that develops during this time.
44. D: Stimulant medication may decrease the appetite, so careful monitoring of growth and a nutritional plan that encourages adequate calories are important. There is no sound evidence that sugar or artificial additives play a role in ADHD.
45. B: Infants must first develop hand–mouth coordina-tion before incorporating tipping and swallowing, which is a more integrated function. Head control before raising the chest demonstrates the principle of cephalocaudal progression. Options C and D suggest proximal-distal progression.
46. D: Most penile growth in Tanner stage III is in length rather than width because of underdevelopment of the corpora cavernosa. Fine, downy pubic hair appears in stage II, and adult-like appearance occurs in stage IV.
47. B: Physiologic gynecomastia is a common clinical finding in young adolescent males. It is usually pres-ent during Tanner stage III.
48. C: Understanding the sequencing of pubertal devel-opment is important, but it must be remembered that individual timing may differ. In the female patient, pubic hair, axillary hair, and the peak height velocity generally occur before menarche.
49. A: The belief that one is immune to poor or bad out-comes (e.g., death, disease) is a form of egocentrism known as personal fable in which adolescents believe that the laws of nature do not apply to them.
50. D: Late adolescence is characterized by increased autonomy and beginning to appreciate the complexi-ties and motivations of other people's behaviors.

☑ BIBLIOGRAPHY

American Academy of Pediatrics. (2007). *Bright futures: Guidelines for health supervision of infants, children, and adolescents.* Washington, DC: Author.

American Dental Association. 2012. Primary Tooth Development. Retrieved from http://success.ada.org/~/media/MouthHealthy/Files/Kids_Section/ADAPrimaryToothDev_Eng.ashx

American Psychiatric Association. (2013). *Diagnostic and statistical manual of mental disorders* (5th ed.). Wash-ington, DC: Author.

Baron-Cohen, S., Wheelwright, S., Cox, A., Baird, G., Char-man, T., Swettenham, J., Drew, A., & Doehring, P. (2000). Early identification of autism by the CHecklist for Au-tism in Toddlers (CHAT). *Journal of the Royal Society of Medicine, 93*(10), 521-525.

Berger, K. S., & Straub, R. (2011). *The developing person through the life span.* (8th ed.). New York, NY: Worth Publishers.

Burns, C. E., Dunn, A. M., Brady, M. A., Starr, N. B., & Blosser, C. (2012). *Pediatric primary care: A handbook for nurse practitioners* (5th ed.). Philadelphia, PA: W. B. Saunders.

Center for Pediatric Therapy. (2015). Child development guide. Retrieved from http://www.spokanecpt.com/68/child-development-guide/

Centers for Disease Control and Prevention. (2015). Autism spectrum disorders: Data and statistics. Retreived from http://www.cdc.gov/ncbddd/autism/data.html

Centers for Disease Control and Prevention. (2015). Injury Prevention & Control: Division of Violence Prevention, Youth Suicide. Retrieved from http://www.cdc.gov/violenceprevention/pub/youth_suicide.html

Child Welfare Information Gateway. (2012). *Child abuse and neglect fatalities: Statistics and interventions*. Retrieved from https://www.childwelfare.gov/pubPDFs/fatality.pdf

Daniels, S. R., Greer, F. R., & the Committee on Nutrition. (2008). Lipid screening and cardiovascular health in children. *Pediatrics, 122*(1), 198–208.

Dixon, S. D., & Stein, M. T. (2005). *Encounters with children: Pediatric behavior and development* (4th ed.). St. Louis, MO: Mosby Year Book.

Feldman, H. M., Coleman, W. L., Carey, W. B., & Crocker, A. C. (2009). *Developmental-behavioral pediatrics* (4th ed.). Philadelphia, PA: W. B. Saunders.

Genel, M., McCaffree, M. A., Hendricks, K., Dennery, P. A., Hay, Jr., W. W., Stanton, B., . . . & Jenkins, R. R. (2008). A national agenda for America's children and adolescents in 2008: Recommendations from the 15th Annual Public Policy Plenary Symposium, annual meeting of the Pediatric Academic Societies, May 3, 2008. *Pediatrics, 122*(4), 843–849.

Johns Hopkins Medicine. (2014). Age-appropriate speech and language milestones. Retrieved from http://www.hopkinsmedicine.org/healthlibrary/conditions/pediatrics/age-appropriate_speech_and_language_milestones_90,P02170/

Johnson, C. P., Myers, S. M., & American Academy of Pediatrics Council on Children with Disabilities. (2007). Identification and evaluation of children with autism spectrum disorders. *Pediatrics, 120*(5), 1183–1215.

Kaakinen, J. R., Gedaly-Duff, V., & Hanson, S. M. H. (2009). *Family health care nursing: Theory, practice and research* (4th ed.). Philadelphia, PA: R. A. Davis.

Kliegman, R. M., Stanton, B. M. D., St. Geme, J., & Schor, N. F. (2011). *Nelson textbook of pediatrics* (19th ed.). Philadelphia, PA: W. B. Saunders.

Mayo Clinic. (2015). Infant and toddler health. Retrieved from: http://www.mayoclinic.org/healthy-lifestyle/infant-and-toddler-health/expert-answers/infant-growth/faq-20058037

McMillan, J. (2006). *Oski's pediatrics: Principles and practice* (4th ed.). Philadelphia, PA: Lippincott Williams & Wilkins.

Monasterio, E. B. (2014). Adolescent substance involvement use and abuse. *Primary Care, 41*(3), 567–585.

Myers, S. M., Johnson, C. P., & American Academy of Pediatrics Council on Children with Disabilities. (2007). Management of children with autism spectrum disorders. *Pediatrics, 120*(5), 1162–1182.

National Coalition for the Homeless. (2009). Homeless families with children. Retrieved from http://www.nationalhomeless.org/factsheets/families.html

Neinstein, L. S., Gordon, C. M., Katzman, D. K., Rosen, D. S., & Woods, E. R. (Eds.). (2007). *Adolescent health care: A practical guide* (5th ed.). Philadelphia, PA: Lippincott.

Ousley, O., & Cormak, T. (2014). Autism spectrum disorder: Defining dimensions and subgroups. *Current Developmental Disorders Report, 1*, 20–28.

Stirling, J., Jr., & American Academy of Pediatrics Committee on Child Abuse and Neglect. (2007). Beyond Munchausen syndrome by proxy: Identification and treatment of child abuse in a medical setting. *Pediatrics, 119*(5), 1026–1030.

Substance Abuse and Mental Health Services Administration. (2012). *Results from the 2012 National Survey on Drug Use and Health: National Findings*. Rockville, MD: Substance Abuse and Mental Health Services Administration Office of Applied Studies.

U.S. Department of Health and Human Services. (2013). *Child maltreatment 2012: Reports from the states to the National Child Abuse and Neglect data system*. Washington, DC: U.S. Government Printing Office.

U.S. Department of Health and Human Services. (2014). *Healthy people 2020*. Washington, DC: U.S. Government Printing Office. Retrieved from https://www.healthypeople.gov/

U.S. Department of Health and Human Services, Administration on Children, Youth and Families. (2007). *Child maltreatment 2007*. Washington, DC: U.S. Government Printing Office. Retrieved from http://www.acf.hhs.gov/programs/cb/resource/child-maltreatment-2007

U.S. Preventive Services Task Force. (2008). Universal screening for hearing loss in infants: U.S. Preventive Task Force recommendation statement. *Pediatrics, 122*(1), 143–148.

U.S. Preventive Services Task Force. (2014). Guide to clinical preventive services, 2014. Retrieved from http://www.ahrq.gov/professionals/clinicians-providers/guidelines-recommendations/guide/

Warikoo, N., & Faraone, S. V. (2013). Background, clinical features and treatment of attention deficit hyperactivity disorder in children. *Expert Opinions in Pharmacotherapy, 14*(14), 1885–1906.

Zero to Three. (2005). *Diagnostic classification: 0–3: Diagnostic classification of mental health and developmental disorders of infancy and early childhood*. Washington, DC: Author.

Health Promotion and Well-Child Care for Infants, Children, and Adolescents

JoAnne Silbert-Flagg

CHAPTER 3

☑ OVERVIEW: HEALTH MAINTENANCE AND HEALTH PROMOTION

Pediatric nurse practitioners (PNPs) have long been on the forefront of promoting and maintaining optimal physical and mental health for children and their families. Their understanding of the multiple factors that influence the overall health and development of children and adolescents enables PNPs to implement evidence-based care and individualize interventions, appropriately involving family members to enhance health outcomes.

One strategy for enhancing health and developmental outcomes in children, adolescents, and their families is the implementation of routine child health supervision. Health supervision comprises those measures that promote health, prevent morbidity and mortality, and facilitate optimal development and maturation within the context of the family and community. It involves routine well-child visits, which include health promotion strategies, anticipatory guidance, as well as specific screening procedures at regular, timed intervals throughout childhood and adolescence.

☑ CHILD HEALTH SUPERVISION

- Components of the Health Visit That Are Age-Appropriate, Health and Developmentally Focused
  1. The parent/child interview
  2. Developmental and educational surveillance (including school performance)
  3. Observation of parent–child interaction
  4. Physical examination specific for each visit
  5. Screening and immunizations

6. Assessment of strengths and vulnerabilities (concerns, problems, and stressors affecting the child and family)
  7. Evidence-based individualized interventions, including health promotion strategies and anticipatory guidance
- General Interviewing Approaches
  1. Determine who will be present for interview
  2. Provide privacy and empathetic environment
  3. Maintain eye contact and relaxed facial expressions
  4. State you will be taking notes during interview to enhance accuracy of recorded data
  5. Obtain history with child clothed
  6. Ask open-ended questions that begin with "why," "how," or "what"
  7. Use direct questions to obtain specific information
  8. Avoid leading questions
  9. Use language parents and child understand
  10. Provide undivided attention; listen carefully, both through verbal and nonverbal actions
  11. Build self-esteem and confidence throughout interview
  12. Conduct interview with cultural sensitivity
- Communication with Parents (in addition to general approach)
  1. Obtain parent's perception of any concerns or problems; if both parents are present, obtain each parent's view of concerns or problems
  2. Restate parental concerns to ensure accuracy and understanding
  3. Be supportive, not judgmental, e.g., avoid "Why didn't you bring your child in earlier?"
- Communication with Young Children (younger than 6 years of age)
  1. Talk to child at his/her eye level
  2. Use play to enhance comfort

3. Use projective techniques to elicit information about how child is feeling, e.g., "Tell me how your bear is feeling today."
4. Use nonthreatening words, e.g., *tube* instead of *needle*, *opening* instead of *cut*, since young children engage in magical thinking
5. Allow adequate time for responses
6. Remember that young children have difficulty giving detailed information
- Communication with Younger School-Age Children
  1. Communicate with parent first if child is initially shy
  2. Ask questions and give explanations using concrete terminology
  3. Use simple diagrams when asking child to describe location of symptoms
  4. Allow time for responses
  5. Give permission to express fears and concerns
- Communication with Older School-Age Children and Adolescents
  1. If parent is present, conduct part of interview (questions dealing with personal or sensitive information) when alone with the older child or adolescent
  2. Interview while child is fully clothed
  3. Start interview with nonthreatening questions
  4. Inform older child/adolescent that all questions you are asking have to do with his/her health; that you ask all older children/adolescents these questions
  5. Acknowledge that although all of your questions are necessary, some may feel uncomfortable to answer
  6. Inform older child/adolescent that information shared is confidential unless he/she tells you about wanting to hurt himself/herself or someone else has hurt him/her
  7. Encourage expression of feelings and concerns
  8. Enhance self-esteem and provide positive feedback during interview
- Confidentiality Issues and Informed Consent
  1. Healthcare providers are required by law to keep the information gathered in the course of a child's care confidential; in 2003, national standards to protect the privacy of personal health information were established as part of the Health Insurance Portability and Accountability Act (HIPAA) of 1996 (U.S. Department of Health and Human Services [DHHS], 2003)
  2. Privileged information may only be shared among healthcare professionals involved in the care of a child when parental consents are signed or in medical emergencies when release of information is in the best interest of the child and absolutely necessary for the provision of care
  3. Many states mandate reporting by healthcare professionals of special circumstances (reasonable cause to suspect child physical or sexual abuse or neglect, suicidal intent, gunshot and stab wounds)
  4. Some states require reporting of births, deaths, certain diseases, and other vital statistics

5. Consents should be signed by child's parent or legal guardian before information concerning child is released; emancipated minor (younger than age 18 years and married, parent of his or her own child, or self-sufficiently living away from home with parental consent) also may sign consents
6. Minor's informed consent laws vary across states by status (emancipated) and conditions
   a. Individual states have statutes allowing access to contraceptives; pregnancy testing/prenatal care; as well as the diagnosis, treatment, and prevention of sexually transmitted diseases per consent of minor
   b. Individual states have statutes allowing HIV testing and treatment per consent of minor

☐ THE PEDIATRIC HISTORY

During the examination of a pediatric patient, the history is critical in the early detection of problems and prevention of long-term negative outcomes. Approximately 80% of the information used to arrive at a diagnosis is derived from the history.
- Complete Patient History
  1. Biographic information—demographic data; name and reliability of person providing the history as well as his/her relationship to child
  2. Chief complaint (CC)—reason for visit
  3. History of present illness (HPI)—if there are symptoms
     PQRST—parameters of symptoms
       P—promoting, preventing, precipitating, palliating factors
       Q—quality or quantity
       R—region or radiation
       S—severity, setting, simultaneous symptoms
       T—temporal factors, onset, duration, intervals, frequency, course over time, has symptom occurred before?
     OLDCARTS
       O—onset
       L—location
       D—duration
       C—characteristics
       A—associated symptoms
       R—relieving/aggravating factors
       T—timing, treatment
       S—severity, sequence, summary
  4. Past medical history (PMH): General state of health—(in child's/parent's words)
     Perinatal history—obtained based on child's age and appropriateness to care
     a. Prenatal history
     b. Planned or unplanned pregnancy
     c. Onset of prenatal care and compliance with recommended care
     d. Medications, drugs, alcohol use during pregnancy
     e. Medical problems during pregnancy

Perinatal history—obtained based on child's age and appropriateness to care

   a. Length of labor and delivery

   b. Type of delivery

   c. Medications or anesthesia

   d. Complications

   e. Birth weight

   f. Gestation at birth, Apgar scores

   g. If multiple births, birth order

Postnatal history—obtained based on child's age and appropriateness to care

   a. Maternal and infant problems

   b. Age and weight at discharge

   c. Early feeding history, including breastfeeding history

5. Common childhood illnesses—list dates and type

6. Serious illnesses—list dates and course of illness

7. Mental health care received—list date and type

8. Hospitalizations—list dates and type

9. Injuries—list dates and course of treatment, recovery

10. Current health status (CHS)—based on child's age

   a. Nutrition—24-hour recall, meal pattern, who eats with whom, how mealtime conducted, fluid type and volume consumed, cultural expectations, special diet, caffeine, artificial sweeteners, carbonated beverages, dietary supplements, and herbal supplements (also known as natural health products). The use of natural health products by pediatric patients is common, yet healthcare providers often do not provide management guidance (Gutierrez, Silbert-Flagg, & Vohra, 2015)

   b. Elimination—toilet training, urinary characteristics, enuresis or encopresis, day and night variations, bowel pattern

   c. Sleep—hours, location, naps, snoring, enuresis, night bottle usage

   d. Development—including school performance, daily activities, recreation and hobbies, social adjustment, behavior, and temperament

   e. Discipline/behavioral concerns—of parent, teacher, childcare provider, relationship with siblings/friends, approaches to discipline

   f. Safety—specific for age (see preventive health care and anticipatory guidance)

   g. Immunizations and screening—specific for age (see preventive health care)

   h. Allergies—specify nature of allergic reaction, medications, food, airborne, transfusion

   i. Current medications—prescription, over the counter, alternative

11. Environmental history assessment of environmental hazards

   a. Arsenic—source is drinking water; used to preserve wood; added to poultry feed

   b. Mercury—source is contaminated fish (swordfish, tuna, and shark), industries that burn fossil fuels

   c. Lead—source is indoor paint, water, soil, or foreign bodies

   d. Polychlorinated biphenyls (PCBs), dioxins, and furans—source is exposure through dietary fat, including in fish, meat, and dairy products

   e. Asbestos—source is through housing construction

   f. Water pollutants—source is drinking water or crop irrigation

   g. Indoor air pollutants—source is carbon monoxide, environmental tobacco smoke (ETS), radon, molds, solvents, and pesticides

   h. Outdoor air pollutants—source is ozone, particulate matter, sulfur dioxide, nitrogen oxides, diesel exhaust, and polycyclic aromatic hydrocarbons

   i. Sun exposure—source is ultraviolet radiation from sun

   j. Solvents—source is gasoline, degreasers, art and craft supplies, nail products, paint, glues, varnishes, newly installed carpeting, dry cleaning products, indoor and outdoor air, and drinking water contaminants

   k. Pesticides—source is household products used in gardens, lawns, fruits and vegetables, some lice removal shampoos, and drinking/bathing water (Physicians for Social Responsibility, n.d.)

12. Assessment of risk prevention—appropriate for age

   a. Smoke detector/radon detector, carbon monoxide detector

   b. Hot water heater setting

   c. Use of car seat/seat belt

   d. Pet safety

   e. Sports safety equipment

   f. Gun safety

   g. Childproofing of household appropriate to age

   h. Use of sunscreen with SPF 15 or higher (Physicians for Social Responsibility, n.d.)

13. Growth and development—based on child's age and appropriateness to care

   a. Physical growth—pattern of height, weight, head circumference, and body mass index

   b. Developmental milestones—language, fine motor, gross motor, social, achievement of milestones, early intervention provided

   c. Mental health/social-emotional development—temperament, relationships, mood state, coping abilities

   d. School—performance, attendance, individualized educational plan (IEP)

14. Family history (FH)

   a. Family profile and medical history (genogram)—include serious, chronic, inherited, and congenital problems in three generational family (blood) relatives; drug and alcohol abuse; mental health problems

   b. Family social history—include household composition/type of dwelling/family support systems

c. Members of household and their relationship to the child, cultural influences, religious affiliation

d. Physical environment of household

e. Employment of parents and work schedule

f. Socioeconomic factors of parents or legal guardian

g. Healthcare coverage

h. Childcare arrangements/after-school care and activities

i. Family stressors—current, recent, or chronic

j. Family travel to high-risk areas

15. Review of systems (ROS)—not addressed in HPI and appropriate for age; ask, "Does this child now, or has this child ever, had problems with any of the following systems?"

a. General—recent weight change, fever, fatigue, weakness

b. Head—injury

c. Eye—last eye examination, visual problems, use of glasses/contacts

d. Ears—last hearing screen, otitis media

e. Nose/sinus—frequent upper respiratory infections, nasal discharge, nosebleeds, sinus pain

f. Throat—frequent tonsillitis/pharyngitis

g. Dentition—last dental examination, problems with teeth, bleeding gums

h. Neck—stiffness, adenopathy, goiter

i. Respiratory—cough, pneumonia, bronchiolitis, wheezing, tuberculosis (TB), chest x-ray, shortness of breath

j. Cardiovascular—murmur, rheumatic fever, palpitations, chest pain, hypertension

k. Gastrointestinal—abdominal pain, vomiting, gastroesophageal reflux, diarrhea, constipation, flatus, hepatitis

l. Genitourinary/reproductive

   (1) Female—menarche, dysmenorrhea, premenstrual syndrome, last menstrual period, sexual activity (age of onset, number of partners, dyspareunia, contraception, condom use), pregnancy, vaginal discharge, history of gynecological examinations, history of screening/treatment for sexually transmitted infections, breast self-examinations, and breast abnormalities

   (2) Male—hernia, testicular pain/self-examination, penile discharge, sexual activity (age of onset, number of partners, condom use)

m. Musculoskeletal—muscle or joint pain, decreased range of motion

n. Neurologic—fainting, seizures, weakness, paralysis, numbness, tremors, dizziness, headache

o. Hematological—anemia, bruising easily

p. Psychiatric—anxiety, depression, mood swing, suicide ideation, anorexia, bulimia, violence, abuse

q. Endocrine—heat or cold intolerance, endocrine disease (thyroid, diabetes, adrenal), polyuria, polydypsia, polyphagia

- Adolescent History Based on Adolescent's Age and Appropriateness to Care
  HEADS—Home, Education/Employment, Activities and Peers, Drugs, Safety

  1. Home—household relationships, family dynamics and relationships, living arrangements

  2. Education/employment—school attendance, grades, attitude about school relationships, best and worst subjects, homework, goals, type of employment and hours worked

  3. Activities and peers—spare time, physical activity, screen time, friends

  4. Disabilities/drugs—tobacco, alcohol, substance use (by self and friends), ability to carry out activities of daily living, sleep, safety, self-image, sexuality, suicide, self-mutilation, history of harm to animals, history of harm to others, Internet use (time, sites, chat rooms, personal profiles, email), communication with strangers, exposure to violence, conflict management, firearm exposure and use, gang membership (self and friends)

- Tools for Screening for Alcohol or Substance Use in Adolescents

  1. RAFFT Tool for Adolescents (alcohol screening)—a single "yes" answer indicates further investigation is needed. Two or more positive responses strongly suggest the probability that an alcohol-dependence problem exists. Four "yes" responses indicates alcohol dependence.
     Do you use alcohol to Relax?
     Do you use alcohol Alone?
     Do you use alcohol with Family?
     Do you use alcohol with Friends?
     Have you experienced any Trouble (problems) as a result of your alcohol use?

  2. CRAFFT Tool for Adolescents (alcohol and/or substance use screening)
     C—Have you ever ridden in a Car driven by someone (including yourself) who was "high" or had been using alcohol or drugs?
     R—Do you ever use alcohol or drugs to Relax, feel better about yourself, or fit in?
     A—Do you ever use alcohol or drugs while you are by yourself, Alone?
     F—Do you ever Forget things you did while using alcohol or drugs?
     F—Do your Family or Friends ever tell you that you should cut down on your drinking or drug use?
     T—Have you ever gotten into Trouble while you were using alcohol or drugs?

- Sexual/Reproductive and Substance Use History Guidelines

  1. Inform child that these questions are asked of all older school-age children and adolescents

  2. Reinforce that although these questions are very personal or sensitive, they are necessary to gain a complete picture of that child's or adolescent's health

3. Reassure child or adolescent that the information he or she shares is confidential unless information about harm to self or others is revealed
4. Progress from least to most sensitive questions
5. It is best to phrase questions as "When was the first time you had intercourse?" instead of "Have you ever had intercourse?"
6. Make sure older child or adolescent understands meaning of terms used
7. Essential elements of sexual/reproductive history
   a. Date of menarche (first menses)
   b. Frequency, length, and quantity of menses with associated symptoms; e.g., cramping, headache, or backache
   c. Date of last menses
   d. Use of tampons or pads
   e. Age of first intercourse, date of last intercourse
   f. Sexual preference, e.g., males, females, or both; same-sex exploration is common in teenagers; number of sexual partners
   g. Types of sexual practices, e.g., male, female; oral sex, intercourse
   h. Reasons for sexual activity, e.g., increases self-esteem; enjoyment; peer pressure
   i. Pregnancies and outcomes
   j. Current contraception
   k. History of any sexually transmitted infections (STIs); naming each disease, e.g., gonorrhea, chlamydia, etc.
   l. Vaginal or penile discharge
   m. Date of last pelvic examination
   n. Contraceptive history, current contraception, use of condoms
   o. Knowledge of STIs, AIDS, pregnancy, and prevention measures
   p. Date of prior test or desire for HIV testing
   q. Performance of self breast or testicular exam
   r. History of sexual abuse
- Interval History
  1. Chief complaint (CC)
  2. Interim health—since last visit
  3. Current health—nutrition, elimination, sleep, development, allergies, immunizations
  4. Update any changes in history since last visit
  5. Review of systems since last history
- Telephone History (telephone triage)
  1. Requires triage decision
     a. Telephone management
     b. Office visit
     c. Refer to emergency department or other health-care provider
  2. Telephone protocol books are helpful in assessment and management of common illnesses and problems encountered by phone
  3. Critical elements
     a. Identify yourself

b. Identify caller, his or her relationship to child, and caller's telephone number
c. Obtain child's name, age, and approximate weight
d. Ascertain thorough history of present illness or problem
e. If not medically necessary to see child, explain rationale and evaluate comfort of caller in home management
f. Tell caller when to call back, which includes advising on signs of worsening status
g. Ask caller to telephone again to give progress report if there are any concerns about the child; if caller does not telephone as requested, IT IS CRITICAL TO MAKE THE FOLLOW-UP CALL
h. Ask caller to write down information that has been given or at least to repeat the information
i. Offer simple, understandable explanations
j. Advise caller to contact you again with any questions
k. Convey warmth, empathy, and support
l. Document all telephone conversations, including history, diagnosis, and management plan

☐ THE PEDIATRIC PHYSICAL EXAMINATION

- General Information
  1. Examination should be comprehensive and systematic
  2. Observation is first critical component of the examination beginning as soon as the child is seen
  3. Use examination to teach child about his or her body
- Age-Related Issues (Infants)
  1. Developmental considerations
     a. Stage of trust versus mistrust
     b. Stranger anxiety develops at 6 to 7 months
     c. Separation anxiety develops at 8 to 9 months
     d. Major fears—separation from parents and pain
  2. Approaches to physical examination
     a. Approach slowly
     b. Conduct as much of examination with infant on parent's lap
     c. Provide infant with security objects, e.g., special blanket or toy
     d. Use distraction and engaging facial expressions during the examination
     e. Conduct examination using noninvasive to invasive sequence, e.g., auscultate heart and lung sounds first, examine ears and throat last
     f. Allow for brief break if infant is hungry or stressed
- Age-Related Issues (Toddlers)
  1. Developmental considerations
     a. Stage of autonomy vs. shame/doubt
     b. Striving for independence
     c. Negativism and temper tantrums (common)
     d. Beginning of magical thinking
     e. Major fears—separation from parents, intrusion of body orifices, loss of control, pain

2. Approaches to physical examination
   a. Use of distraction is helpful
   b. Allow child to touch and hold equipment before examination
   c. Demonstrate examination on doll, toy, or parent before conducting examination on child
   d. Give child choices when possible
   e. When necessary, tell child what you are going to do instead of gaining permission, e.g., "I am going to check your tummy" vs. "Is it OK with you if I check your tummy?"
   f. Conduct as much of examination as possible on parent's lap
   g. Conduct examination using noninvasive to invasive sequence
- Age-Related Issues (Preschool Children)
  1. Developmental considerations
     a. Stage of initiative vs. guilt
     b. Magical thinking
     c. Egocentrism
     d. Major fears—separation from parents, loss of control, body mutilation, pain
  2. Approaches to physical examination
     a. Inform child what you are going to do and what he/she can do to help
     b. Role-play with equipment, e.g., let child examine ears of doll first
     c. Head-to-toe examination sequence can usually be implemented
     d. Choose words carefully because of magical thinking
     e. Allow choices whenever possible
     f. Teach child about his/her body during course of examination
     g. Praise child for helping and attempting to cooperate
- Age-Related Issues (School-Age Children)
  1. Developmental considerations
     a. Industry vs. inferiority
     b. Concrete thinking
     c. Desires to act brave
     d. Enjoys gathering scientific information
     e. Modesty emerges with older school-age child
     f. Major fears—separation from peers, loss of control, pain, death; beginning at age 9 years
  2. Approaches to physical examination
     a. Head-to-toe sequence
     b. Scientific terminology with concrete explanations
     c. Answer questions factually with age-appropriate vocabulary
     d. Explain use of equipment, e.g., otoscope
- Age-Related Issues (Adolescents)
  1. Developmental considerations
     a. Stage of identity vs. role diffusion
     b. Striving for independence and control
     c. Formal operational thinking
     d. Bodily concerns
     e. Concerns about being different
     f. Major fears—change in body image, separation from peers, loss of control, death

2. Approaches to physical examination
   a. Assure privacy
   b. Examine without parent unless adolescent prefers parent remain in room
   c. Inform adolescent of each step of examination
   d. Give choices whenever possible
   e. Cover parts of body not currently being examined
   f. Teach adolescent about his/her body during course of examination
   g. Provide reassurance of "normalcy" during course of examination
   h. Recognize and discuss apprehension about breast, pelvic, and testicular examinations
- Measurement of Vital Signs
  1. Temperature
     a. Rectal temperature is an accurate method, but proper technique must be used to avoid injury. Temporal artery thermometers, which are more expensive, are increasingly becoming available
     b. Tympanic membrane and axillary temperature are quick and noninvasive measurements; reliability may be a problem
     c. Temperature of 38°C and above is considered a fever
     d. A normal newborn's temperature ranges from 36.5°C to 37.5°C rectally
  2. Pulse norms
     a.

Age	Beats per Minute	Mean
Birth to 7 days	95–160	(125)
1 to 3 weeks	105–180	(145)
1 to 6 months	110–180	(145)
6 to 12 months	110–170	(135)
1 to 3 years	90–150	(120)
4 to 5 years	65–135	(110)
6 to 8 years	60–130	(100)
9 to 16 years	60–110	(85)
Older than 16 years	60–100	(80)

     b. Conditions that commonly elevate pulse
        (1) Temperature—for every 1°F elevation, pulse increases by 10 beats per minute
        (2) Anxiety/stress, excitement
        (3) Exercise
        (4) Severe anemia
        (5) Hyperthyroidism
        (6) Hypoxia
        (7) Heart disease
  3. Respiration norms
     a.

Age	Breaths per Minute
Neonate	40–60
Up to 1 year	24–38
1–3 years	22–30
4–6 years	20–24
7–9 years	18–24
10–14 years	16–22
14–18 years	14–20

b. Conditions that commonly elevate respirations
   (1) Temperature—for every 1°F elevation, respirations increase by 4 breaths per minute
   (2) Anxiety/stress, excitement
   (3) Pain
   (4) Respiratory conditions, e.g., pneumonia
   (5) Heart disease
4. Blood pressure
   a. Appropriate cuff size required for accurate reading
      (1) Bladder width should be approximately 40% of the circumference of the arm measured at a point midway between the olecranon and acromion
      (2) Bladder length should cover 80% to 100% of the circumference of the arm
      (3) Blood pressure should be measured with cubital fossa at the heart level; the arm should be supported
      (4) The stethoscope bell is placed over the brachial artery pulse, proximal and medial to the cubital fossa and below the bottom edge of the cuff
   b. Use Korotkoff sound IV (muffling sound) as diastolic blood pressure in children younger than 13 years of age; use Korotkoff sound V (disappearance of sound) as the diastolic blood pressure in children 13 years of age and older
   c. Plot blood pressure on standard blood pressure graphs for boys or girls
   d. Begin to measure blood pressure at well-child visits, starting at 3 years of age
   e. A single elevated blood pressure measurement in an apparently healthy child does not necessarily reflect disease
   f. Hypertension—average systolic and/or diastolic blood pressure 95th percentile for age and sex on at least 3 separate occasions using the same arm, same cuff, and same position

   ■ **Blood Pressure Readings from 50th Percentile Ages Birth to 12 Months**

Age	Systolic (mm Hg)	Diastolic (mm Hg)
Birth to 6 months	76–106	68–66
6 to 12 months	68–65	65–67

   Note: Four limb blood pressure measurements can be used to assess for coarctation of the aorta. Mean difference between upper and lower extremities should be 10 mm Hg or less.
   Data from Engorn, B., & Flerlage, J. (2014). *The Harriet Lane handbook* (20th ed.). St. Louis, MO: Mosby.

   ■ **Blood Pressure Readings from 5th to 95th Percentiles Ages 1 to 17 Years**

Age	Systolic (mm Hg)	Diastolic (mm Hg)
1 to 3 years	98–109	54–67
4 to 6 years	106–117	66–76
7 to 10 years	110–119	74–78
11 to 14 years	117–128	78–84
15 to 17 years	126–136	81–89

   Data from National Institutes of Health & National Heart, Lung, and Blood Institute. (2005). *Fourth report on the diagnosis, evaluation, and treatment of high blood pressure in children and adolescents* (2005). Retrieved from https://www.nhlbi.nih.gov/files/docs/resources/heart/hbp_ped.pdf

   g. Taller, heavier children have higher blood pressure than smaller children of same age
   h. Pulse pressure—difference between systolic and diastolic blood pressures (normal is 20 to 50 mm Hg)
      (1) Wide pulse pressure from high systolic pressure is usually due to fever, exercise, or excitement
      (2) Wide pulse pressure from low diastolic pressure is usually due to patent ductus arteriosus, aortic regurgitation, or other serious heart disease

❐ SPECIFIC NORMAL FINDINGS AND COMMON VARIATIONS

• Head and Neck
  1. History indicating possible abnormalities
     a. Difficult birth; use of forceps, vacuum
     b. Unusual head shape or preferred position at rest
     c. Poor head control for age
  2. Selected physical examination findings
     a. Head circumference is approximately 2 cm larger than chest during first year of life; head and chest circumferences should be equal at 1 year of age; during childhood, chest is usually 5 to 7 cm larger than head
     b. Fontanels—best to assess while infant is sitting up and not crying
        (1) Posterior fontanel rarely palpable at birth; closes by 2 months of age
        (2) Size of anterior fontanel should be no larger than 4 to 5 cm in diameter
        (3) Anterior fontanel closes by 18 months of age
           (a) Early closure usually leads to synostosis
           (b) Late closure is commonly seen with increased intracranial pressure, hypothyroidism, rickets, syphilis, Down syndrome, osteogenesis imperfecta
        (4) Large anterior fontanel may indicate:
           (a) Chronically increased intracranial pressure
           (b) Subdural hematoma
           (c) Rickets
           (d) Hypothyroidism
           (e) Osteogenesis imperfecta
        (5) Bulging anterior fontanel is usually seen with conditions that cause increased intracranial pressure, e.g., meningitis/encephalitis, fluid overload
        (6) Sunken anterior fontanel is usually seen with severe dehydration (more than 10%)

c. Unusual head size or shape
   (1) Hydrocephalus—excessively large head at birth or head that grows abnormally rapid; usually associated with distended scalp veins, widely separated cranial sutures, large and tense anterior fontanel, and "sunset eyes"
   (2) Microcephaly—head circumference >2 standard deviations below the mean for age, sex, and gestation; reflects an abnormally small brain; common causes are intrauterine infections (e.g., herpes, rubella, syphilis); genetic defects; drug usage during pregnancy (especially alcohol)
   (3) Macrocephaly—head circumference >2 standard deviations above the mean for age, sex, and gestation; common causes are hydrocephalus, masses, increased intracranial pressure; skeletal dysplasias (osteogenesis imperfecta)
   (4) Head tilt—common causes include strabismus, central nervous system (CNS) lesions, or short sternocleidomastoid muscle
   (5) Caput succedaneum—diffuse edema of the soft tissue of the scalp that usually crosses suture lines; may be seen with bruising due to traumatic vaginal birth; seen at birth; no specific treatment necessary; usually resolves in 2 to 3 days
   (6) Cephalohematoma—subperiosteal collection of blood that does not cross suture lines; often does not appear until several hours after birth and may increase over 24 hours; no specific treatment indicated; resolves over a few weeks to months; observe for hyperbilirubinemia
   (7) Premature or irregular closure of suture lines can cause unusual head shape (craniosynostosis)
   (8) Bossing (bulging) of frontal area is associated with rickets and prematurity
d. Head control
   (1) By 4 months of age, head should be held erect and in midline
   (2) By 6 months of age, there should be no head lag when infant is pulled from supine to sitting position; if present, may indicate neuromuscular disorder; may be the first sign of cerebral palsy
e. Neck
   (1) Pain and resistance to flexion may indicate meningeal irritation
   (2) Torticollis (restriction of motion)—can result from birth trauma (e.g., injury to the sternocleidomastoid muscle with bleeding into the muscle), muscle spasm, viral infection, or drug ingestion
   (3) Webbed neck—common in Turner's syndrome, a chromosomal abnormality occurring 99% of the time in females that results in webbed neck, widespread nipples, abnormal ears, micrognathia, and lymphedema of hands and feet
   (4) Unusual position of trachea could indicate serious lung problem
   (5) Mass in the neck
      (a) Thyroglossal duct cyst—usually seen near midline of neck; cyst moves up and down with protrusion of tongue; may become infected and present as an abscess; surgical excision recommended
      (b) Brachial cleft cyst—can appear as swelling anterior to sternocleidomastoid (SCM) muscle or as opening along anterior border of SCM; may drain and become infected
      (c) Hematoma (of sternocleidomastoid muscle)—more common in breech deliveries
      (d) Enlarged thyroid—due to hyperthyroidism or hypothyroidism; visible thyroid gland is almost always enlarged
      (e) Enlarged lymph node—most frequent cause of lateral neck mass
- Face
  1. History indicating possible abnormalities
     a. Difficult delivery; use of forceps, vacuum
     b. Asymmetry of face when crying or speaking
     c. Facial features that are unusual or do not match family characteristics
     d. Drug or alcohol use during pregnancy
  2. Selected physical examination findings
     a. Asymmetry of nasolabial folds or drooping mouth indicates facial nerve impairment or Bell's palsy
     b. Child who demonstrates open mouth breathing and facial contortions may have allergic rhinitis
     c. Dysmorphic facial features are hallmark of numerous syndromes (e.g., fetal alcohol syndrome) and diagnosis should be pursued
- Eyes
  1. History indicating possible abnormalities
     a. Premature infant who required resuscitation, needed ventilator or oxygen support, had retinopathy of prematurity
     b. Infant who does not track faces or objects; absent blink in response to bright lights or sudden movements
     c. Children younger than 6 years of age who:
        (1) Rub eyes excessively, squint, have photophobia
        (2) Have difficulty reaching for or picking up small objects
        (3) Engage in head tilting
        (4) Hold objects close to face
     d. School-age children (same as young children) who:
        (1) Sit close to blackboard or TV in order to see
        (2) Are making poor progress in school not explained by intellectual deficit or learning disability
     e. Any age child who:
        (1) Demonstrates white area in pupil visible in photographs (retinoblastoma)

(2) Complains of headaches not present upon awakening but that progress during the day (accommodative errors)

(3) Has problems with excessive tearing—allergies (accommodative errors)

(4) Has an eye that turns in or out (strabismus)

2. Selected physical examination findings

a. Position and placement—inner canthal distance averages 2.5 cm; epicanthal folds present in Asian children; palpebral fissures lie horizontally

(1) Hypertelorism (wide set eyes)—present in Down syndrome

(2) Epicanthal folds can be frequently seen in Down syndrome, renal agenesis, or glycogen storage disease

(3) Ptosis could be normal or may indicate paralysis of oculomotor nerve

(4) Exophthalmos (protruding eyeballs)—can be seen with hyperthyroidism

b. Eyelids normally same color as surrounding skin

(1) "Stork bite" mark—telangiectatic nevi disappear by 12 months

(2) Blocked tear duct (dacryostenosis)—may lead to infection of lacrimal sac evidenced by swelling, redness, and purulent discharge (dacryocystitis)

(3) Periorbital edema—soft swelling that may be associated with renal or cardiac problems or sinusitis; acute onset of unilateral eyelid edema with erythema, induration, and tenderness indicates periorbital cellulitis

c. "Allergic shiners"—bluish discoloration and soft edema below eyes usually indicates allergies

d. Sclera and conjunctiva

(1) Sclera is shiny, clear, and white

(2) Bulbar conjunctiva (covers sclera) is moist and transparent and palpebral conjunctiva (lines the eyelids) is pink and moist

(3) Spots of brown melanin may be seen in dark-skinned races

(4) Yellow sclera indicates jaundice

(5) Redness may indicate bacterial or viral infection, allergy, or irritation, e.g., chemicals

(6) Excessive pallor of the palpebral conjunctiva indicates anemia

(7) Cobblestone appearance of palpebral conjunctiva (lining the eyelids) can indicate severe allergy or contact lens irritation

e. Pupils and iris

(1) Unequal pupils (anisocoria)—usually congenital and normal, but can indicate increased intracranial pressure from head trauma or other intracranial disease processes, e.g., meningitis

(2) Dilated, fixed pupils—usually indicate severe brain damage

(3) Dilated pupils—may result from use of anticholinergic drugs (e.g., atropine) and substance abuse (e.g., amphetamines)

(4) Abnormally small pupils—may result from brain damage, use of morphine, or substance abuse (e.g., cocaine)

f. By 3 to 4 months, infants should have binocular vision (ability to fixate on one visual field with both eyes simultaneously)

(1) Assessment techniques to elicit phoria (movement of eye when covered) or tropia (obvious turning in or out of eye without coverage) (e.g., strabismus)

(a) Cover–uncover test—when eye is covered, it may deviate in (esophoria) or out (exophoria) and return to midline when uncovered

(b) Corneal light reflex (Hirschberg's test)—with light held 12 to 14 inches from eyes, reflection of light should be the same on both corneas; if unequal, it is suggestive of phoria or tropia

(2) Intermittent alternating convergent strabismus—normal from 0 to 6 months of age

3. Ophthalmoscopic examination—red reflex should be elicited before discharge from the nursery and at all subsequent routine health supervision visits

a. The result of the red reflex examination is to be rated as normal when the reflections of the two eyes viewed, both individually and simultaneously, are equivalent in color, intensity, and clarity and there are no opacities or white spots (leukokoria) within the area of either or both red reflexes

b. A child with an abnormal red reflex should be immediately referred to an ophthalmologist for a more complete examination

c. All infants and children with a positive family history of retinoblastoma; congenital, infantile, or juvenile cataracts; glaucoma; or retinal abnormalities should be referred to an ophthalmologist for a more complete eye examination, regardless of the status of the red reflex

• Ears

1. History indicating possible abnormalities

a. Prenatal exposure to maternal infection, irradiation, or drug abuse

b. Birth weight less than 1500 g

c. Anoxia in neonatal period

d. Ototoxic antibiotic usage (e.g., gentamycin)

e. Cleft palate

f. Infections

g. Meningitis

h. Encephalitis

i. Recurrent or chronic otitis media

2. Behaviors suggestive of hearing loss

a. No reaction to loud or strange noises

b. No babbling in infant after 6 months

c. No communicative speech; reliance on gestures after 15 months of age

d. Language delays

3. Selected physical examination findings
    a. Position and placement—low or obliquely set ears may indicate genitourinary or chromosomal abnormality or a multisystem syndrome
    b. Pain
        (1) Pain produced by manipulation of auricle or pressure on tragus may indicate otitis externa
        (2) Pain and tenderness over mastoid process may indicate mastoiditis
    c. Examination of tympanic membrane (TM)
        (1) For best visualization of TM—pull auricle down and back in children younger than 3 years of age; pull auricle up and back for children older than 3 years of age
        (2) Crying produces erythema of TM bilaterally; landmarks are still visible with succinct light reflexes and TM mobility
        (3) Pneumatic otoscopy is critical for assessment of fluid in middle ear
            (a) Decreased TM mobility—indicates fluid in middle ear
            (b) In child with pressure equalization (PE) tubes, decreased mobility of TM indicates obstruction or dysfunction of tubes
- Nose and Sinuses
    1. History indicating possible abnormalities
        a. Inability to move air through both nares
        b. Discharge
        c. Nasal flaring or narrowing on inspection
        d. Hypernasal voice—snoring, hypertrophied adenoids
    2. Selected physical examination findings
        a. Flattened nasal bridge (in other than Asian or African American children) may indicate congenital anomalies
        b. Boggy nasal mucous membranes (bluish, pale, edematous) with serous drainage indicates allergic rhinitis
        c. Persistent copious or purulent discharge is indicative of sinusitis
        d. Unilateral purulent discharge suggests foreign body
- Throat/Mouth
    1. History indicating possible abnormalities
        a. Lack of or excessive fluoride supplementation or fluoridated water
        b. Infant or toddler who goes to sleep with bottle of milk or juice
        c. Thumb sucking or pacifier use beyond 2 years of age
        d. Unusual sequence of tooth eruption
    2. Selected physical examination findings
        a. Lips
            (1) Cherry red color indicates acidosis
            (2) Drooping of one side of lips indicates facial nerve impairment
            (3) Fissures at corners of mouth may indicate riboflavin or niacin deficiency
    b. Teeth
        (1) Mottling may indicate excessive fluoride intake
        (2) Green or black staining can result from oral iron intake
    c. Palate—decay of maxillary incisors may result from baby bottle caries syndrome
        (1) Palpation of palate is important in newborns to detect submucosal cleft
        (2) Uvula rises and remains in midline when saying "ah"; deviation or absence of movement indicates involvement of glossopharyngeal or vagus nerves
        (3) Bifed uvula is suggestive of a submucosal cleft palate
    d. Tonsils
        (1) During childhood, tonsillar hypertrophy is a normal immunological response; largest in size between 8 and 9 years of age and decreases in size after puberty
        (1) Asymmetrically enlarged tonsil without infection may suggest tonsillar lymphoma
    e. Voice
        (1) Nasal quality indicates enlarged adenoids
        (2) Hoarse cry may indicate croup, cretinism, or tetany
        (3) Chronic hoarseness may indicate vocal cord polyps
        (4) Shrill, high-pitched cry may indicate increased intracranial pressure
    f. Temporomandibular joint (TMJ)
        (1) Findings indicative of TMJ dysfunction—pain upon palpation of TMJ, decrease in mandibular movement, TMJ sounds (popping and clicking), malocclusion, and abnormal morphology of mandible (micrognathia)
        (2) Inability to open jaw (trismus) associated with fever and sore throat is suggestive of peritonsillar abscess
- Heart
    1. History indicating possible abnormalities
        a. Infant
            (1) Increased respirations, especially during sleep
            (2) Prolonged feeding time, tires during feedings
            (3) Cyanosis of mucous membranes of mouth
            (4) Eyelid edema
        b. Child
            (1) Increased respirations, especially during sleep
            (2) Squatting or sleeping in knee–chest position
            (3) Eyelid edema
            (4) Cyanosis of mucous membranes of mouth
            (5) Exercise intolerance
    2. Selected physical examination findings
        a. Heart sounds and area of clearest auscultation
            (1) S_1 (closure of mitral and tricuspid valves)—heard best at apex
            (2) S_2 (closure of aortic and pulmonic valves)—heard best at aortic and pulmonic areas

(3) Physiologic splitting of S_2 during inspiration is normal; if fixed (heard upon inspiration and expiration), may indicate atrial septal defect or pulmonic stenosis

(4) S_3—heard best at apex (sounds like "Kentucky"); due to blood rushing through mitral valve and hitting an empty ventricle; normal in almost all children; if loud in character, may indicate high diastolic pressure in involved ventricle as found in acute ventricular failure

(5) S_4—heard best at apex (sounds like "Tennessee"); almost never normal; indicates high pressure in either ventricle as found in pulmonic and aortic stenosis and systemic hypertension

b. Normal variations in heart rhythm—in sinus arrhythmia, heart rate increases with inspiration and decreases with expiration; disappears with exercise or holding breath

c. Innocent (functional) murmurs—present in approximately 50% of children

(1) Characteristics

(a) Usually systolic in timing

(b) Usually soft; never more than Grade III

(c) Rarely transmitted

(d) Low pitched, vibratory, musical, or twangy

(e) Short duration

(f) Usually loudest at left lower sternal border or at the second or third intercostal space

(g) Varies in loudness and presence from time to time

(h) Heard loudest in the recumbent position, during expiration, and after exercise

(i) Diminishes with change in positioning from recumbent to sitting

(j) No cyanosis

(k) Normal pulses, respiratory rate, and blood pressure (BP)

(l) Normal growth and development

(m)Absence of a thrill (vibratory sensation felt over murmur with palm of hand)

(2) Types of innocent heart murmurs in children

(a) Pulmonary ejection murmur (heard at the pulmonic area)—early to mid systole; distinct gap between first heart sound and murmur and end of murmur and second heart sound

(b) Vibratory or Still's murmur—musical or vibratory murmur; heard best at the lower left sternal border

(c) Venous hum—heard best above or below clavicles, second or third interspace; more coarse quality; very dependent upon position; disappears when child lies down or turns neck, which decreases blood velocity through internal jugular veins

(3) Conditions that increase intensity of innocent heart murmurs—exercise, fever, and anemia due to increased cardiac output

(4) Innocent murmurs in the newborn

(a) Transition from fetal to adult circulation may take up to 48 hours

(b) Usually Grade I or II

(c) Systolic

(d) Not associated with other signs and symptoms

(5) Point of maximal impulse (PMI)

(a) Children younger than 8 years—fourth intercostal space, midclavicular line

(b) Children older than 8 years—fifth intercostal space, slightly right of midclavicular line

(c) Displacement of PMI with cardiac enlargement

(d) Increased pulsation of PMI indicates conditions that increase cardiac output, e.g., anemia, anxiety, fever, fluid overload

(6) Peripheral pulses—normally palpable, equal in intensity and rhythm; weak or absent femoral pulses may indicate coarctation of the aorta

- Lungs

1. History indicating possible abnormalities

a. Family history of tuberculosis, cystic fibrosis, allergy, asthma, atopic dermatitis

b. Infants and young children

(1) Premature infant with any respiratory complications

(2) Sudden onset of coughing or difficulty breathing

(3) Difficulty feeding

(4) Apnea episodes

c. Older children and adolescents

(1) Smoking

(2) Cocaine use

(3) Recurrent or chronic cough

(4) Exercise intolerance

2. Selected physical examination findings

a. Normal breath sounds—breath sounds are best heard by having child breathe through mouth

(1) Vesicular—low pitch, soft intensity; inspiration is more than expiration with a ratio of 5:2; heard over peripheral lung fields

(2) Bronchovesicular—medium pitch, moderate intensity; inspiration equals expiration with a ratio of 1:1; heard over main bronchus

(3) Bronchial/tracheal—high pitch, loud intensity; inspiration less than expiration with a ratio of 1:2

b. Abnormal breath sounds

(1) Rhonchi—coarse sounds heard on expiration that are indicative of secretions in the large airways; usually present in bronchitis; clear with coughing; associated with bronchial fremitus (coarse vibrations felt with hand on chest as air passes through exudate in bronchi)

(2) Transmitted rhonchi—coarse sounds that result from the transmission of sound from

congested nasal passages to the chest; can be avoided by having child breathe through mouth

(3) Wheezing—high-pitched musical or whistling sounds produced as air passes through narrowed airways; heard in bronchiolitis, asthma; cystic fibrosis; foreign body aspiration (unilateral wheezing)

(4) Crackles—fine crackling sounds heard upon inspiration indicative of air passing through moisture in alveoli; usually suggests pneumonia or congestive heart failure

(5) Pleural friction rub—creaking or grating sound caused by inflamed parietal and visceral pleural linings rubbing together; usually inspiratory and expiratory; subsides when child holds breath

c. Chest movement

(1) Children younger than 7 years of age are diaphragmatic (abdominal) breathers

(2) Girls older than 7 years of age become thoracic breathers; boys continue as abdominal breathers

(3) Chest structural abnormalities may compromise lung function

(a) Pectus carinatum—protuberant sternum

(b) Pectus excavatum—depressed sternum

• Breasts

1. History indicating possible abnormalities

a. Prepubertal breast enlargement in girls

b. Gynecomastia in boys at any age

c. Breast mass

d. Galactorrhea not associated with childbearing

2. Selected physical examination findings

a. Neonate may have gynecomastia and milky discharge that disappears within 2 weeks (or at least 3 months)

b. Gynecomastia can be normal variant in males due to temporary estrogen/testosterone imbalance (usually begins at Tanner stage II to III and can last for 1 to 2 years); most commonly felt as small, tender, oval subareolar mass measuring up to 2 to 3 cm in diameter

c. Gynecomastia also may be indicative of

(1) Obesity or increased muscle (pseudogynecomastia)

(2) Testicular tumor (testes must be palpated in any male with gynecomastia)

(3) Medication usage—estrogen, steroids, tricyclic antidepressants (e.g., imipramine), respiridol, mellaril, amphetamines, digoxin, cimetidine

(4) Klinefelter's syndrome (47XXY)—associated with small penis and testes, scoliosis, aspermia, decreased testosterone levels, and height greater than 6 feet

d. Asymmetric breast development is normal in the adolescent female

e. Galactorrhea may be indicative of:

(1) Pregnancy

(2) Recent abortion

(3) Pituitary tumor—associated with increased prolactin level, increased headaches, amenorrhea, peripheral vision loss

(4) Drug use—marijuana; opiates (codeine, heroin, morphine); amphetamines; hormones (oral contraceptives); digoxin; valium; cimetidine; phenothiazines (thorazine, mellaril); haloperidol; tricyclic antidepressants; respiridol

(5) Hypothyroidism

f. Breast masses in adolescents

(1) Benign breast masses (obtain ultrasound versus mammogram due to dense breast tissue in adolescents)

(a) Fibroadenoma—most common breast mass in adolescents; increased incidence in African Americans

(i) Characteristics—single, unilateral mass; round or discoid in shape; firm and smooth in consistency; no retraction; mobile; nontender

(ii) No variation with menstrual cycle

(b) Fibrocystic breasts—usually result of hormonal imbalance

(i) Characteristics—breast pain with or without lumps; symptoms worsen a few days before menses and resolve with completion of menses

(ii) Mobile cysts or areas are more dense and fibrous; usually resolve in 1 to 3 months

(2) Neoplastic breast masses (very rare)—firm, nonmobile, painless, overlying skin changes, nipple discharge

• Abdomen

1. History indicating possible abnormalities

a. Birth weight under 1500 g places infant at high risk for necrotizing enterocolitis

b. Failure to pass first meconium stool within 24 hours

c. Jaundice

d. Failure to grow or unexplained weight loss

e. Projectile vomiting or blood in emesis

f. Chronic diarrhea or constipation

g. Enlargement of the abdomen with or without pain

h. Abdominal or pelvic pain

2. Selected physical examination findings—flexion of knees and hips facilitates examination

a. Prominent abdomen (potbelly)—normal in early childhood in sitting and supine positions due to poorly developed musculature; children up to 13 years of age may have prominent abdomen in standing position

b. Liver edge—may be palpable 1 to 2 cm below right costal margin, especially with deep inspiration

b. Poor growth, failure to thrive

c. Maternal HIV infection

d. IV drug use

e. Multiple and indiscriminate sexual contacts

2. Selected physical examination findings

a. Normal size is up to 1 cm in inguinal area; 2 cm in cervical area; in other areas, up to 3 cm is normal

b. Nodes enlarged due to infection are firm or fluctuant, warm, tender, mobile, and may be accompanied by redness of overlying skin

c. "Shotty" nodes (e.g., under 0.5 cm in diameter, firm, mobile, and nontender) can be present at any time in childhood and usually indicate past infection

d. Suspect malignancy or tuberculosis if supraclavicular nodes are palpated

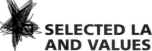

SELECTED LABORATORY TESTS AND VALUES

- General Considerations

1. Cost, pain, and invasiveness vs. need for data to make accurate diagnosis

2. Anesthetic cream used topically can ease venipuncture, especially in highly anxious children

3. Laboratory values should be referenced against specified norms of laboratory conducting the testing since normal values may vary from laboratory to laboratory

- Hematology—CBC with differential

1. Normal range of values for complete blood count (CBC) with differential (see **Table 3-2**)

2. Common causes of variation in CBC with differential

a. Hemoglobin variations

(1) Increased—may indicate polycythemia (an overproduction of RBCs as a result of hypoxia); dehydration, or intravascular hemolysis

(2) Decreased—may indicate anemia, hemodilution, sickle cell anemia, thalassemia, hemorrhage, or hyperthyroidism

b. Hematocrit variations

(1) Increased—may indicate polycythemia, dehydration, or erythrocytosis

(2) Decreased—may indicate anemia, hemorrhage, hyperthyroidism, leukemia, or cirrhosis

c. Red blood cell variations

(1) Increased—may indicate dehydration, hemorrhage, severe diarrhea, acute poisoning

(2) Decreased—may indicate blood loss, low iron intake, lead poisoning, leukemia, rheumatic fever, systemic lupus erythematosis, or subacute bacterial endocarditis

d. White blood cell variations
   (1) Increased—may signal bacterial infection (e.g., tonsillitis, sepsis, meningitis, appendicitis) or indicate acute hemorrhage, serum sickness, steroid use, hemolysis, or leukemia
   (2) Decreased—indicates bone marrow depression that may result from viral infection; rickettsial infection; hypersplenia; leukemia; certain drugs (e.g., antiseizure medications, antibiotics, antihistamines, diuretics, analgesics, tricyclic antidepressants)
e. Neutrophils variations
   (1) Increased—may indicate bacterial infection, ischemic necrosis from burn injuries, metabolic disorders (e.g., diabetic ketoacidosis), stress response, emotional distress, inflammatory diseases (e.g., rheumatic arthritis), or hemolysis
   (2) Decreased (neutropenia)—viral infections (e.g., hepatitis, mononucleosis), chemotherapy or radiation, immune deficiencies, malignancies
f. Band cell or stab (immature neutrophil) variations—increased (known as a shift to the left); usually indicates severe bacterial infection (e.g., sepsis, pneumonia)
g. Lymphocytes variations

j. Basophil variations
   (1) Increased—may indicate certain leukemias, Hodgkin's disease, inflammatory conditions (e.g., ulcerative colitis), polycythemia, chronic hemolytic anemia; infections such as TB, varicella, influenza
   (2) Decreased—may indicate hyperthyroidism, pregnancy, stress, prolonged use of steroids, allergic reaction
k. Platelet variations
   (1) Increased—may indicate acute infection, malignancy, postsplenectomy, trauma, rheumatoid arthritis, Kawasaki disease
   (2) Decreased (thrombocytopenia)—may indicate leukemia, idiopathic thrombocytopenic purpura (ITP), autoimmune disorders, drugs (e.g., penicillin, ampicillin, cephalothin), hemolytic uremic syndrome, disseminated intravascular coagulation (DIC), viral infection, HIV infection
l. Reticulocyte count variations
   (1) Increased—may indicate hemorrhage/blood loss, increased destruction of red blood cells (RBCs), response to initiation of iron therapy
   (2) Decreased—may indicate iron-deficiency anemia, chronic infection, radiation, aplastic anemia

3. Blood urea nitrogen (BUN)
   a. Normal range—5 to 20 mg/dL
   b. Increased—may indicate a high-protein diet, renal or urinary obstruction or disease, gastrointestinal (GI) hemorrhage, malignancies, dehydration, shock
   c. Decreased—hemodilution, pregnancy, nephrotic syndrome, liver failure
4. Creatinine (more sensitive indicator of renal function than BUN)
   a. Normal value—0.3 to 1 mg/dL
   b. Increased—may indicate renal dysfunction, urinary tract obstruction, dehydration, muscle disease
5. Bilirubin (mg/dL)
   a. Birth—1.5
   b. Three to four days postnatal
      (1) Breastfed—7.3
      (2) Formula fed—5.7
   c. Older infant and child
      (1) Total—less than 1.5
      (2) Direct (conjugated)—0.2 to 0.4 (higher levels require investigation for pathology)
      (3) Indirect (unconjugated) bilirubin—0.4 to 0.8 (levels greater than 20 mg/dL may be neurotoxic to brain)
6. Cholesterol (mg/100 mL)
   a. Full-term newborn—45 to 167
   b. Infant—70 to 190
   c. Child and adolescent—less than 170
7. Lead—normal value (less than 10 μg/dL)
- Urine
1. pH
   a. Newborn—5.0 to 7.0
   b. Older infant and child—4.8 to 7.8
   c. Increased (alkaline)—may indicate urinary tract infection, salicylate intoxication
   d. Decreased (acidic)—may indicate acidosis, renal failure, diarrhea, or dehydration
2. Specific gravity
   a. Newborn—1.001 to 1.020
   b. Older infant and child—1.001 to 1.030
   c. Increased—may indicate dehydration, nephrosis, glomerulonephritis
   d. Decreased—may indicate diabetes insipidus, severe renal damage
3. Glucose (should be negative)—presence of sugar may indicate diabetes mellitus or other metabolic disorders; liver disease or renal tubular disorders
4. Protein (should be negative)—presence of protein may indicate renal disease (e.g., nephritis, nephrosis), exercise, SLE, orthostatic proteinuria, asymptomatic proteinuria
5. Ketones (should be negative)—presence of ketones may indicate fever, dehydration, anorexia, diarrhea, fasting, prolonged vomiting, or anorexia
6. Nitrites (should be negative)—presence of nitrites strongly suggests urinary tract infection

7. White blood cells (WBCs)
   a. Normal range—0 to 4 WBCs/HPF
   b. Increased—may indicate urinary tract infection, fever, pyelonephritis, TB, nephrosis
8. RBCs
   a. Normal range 1 to 2 RBCs/HPF
   b. Increased—may indicate urinary tract infection, pyelonephritis, SLE, renal stones, trauma, TB, hemophilia, polyarteritis nodosa, malignant hypertension
9. Bacteria (should be negative)—100,000 colonies/mL or more of a single pathogen on urine culture by clean-catch method confirms a urinary tract infection; repeat urine culture should be obtained for a result of 10,000 to 100,000 colonies/mL For febrile children 2 to 24 months a diagnosis is made on the basis of the presence of both pyuria and at least 50,000 colonies per milliliter of a single uropathogenic organism in an appropriately collected specimen of urine (Subcommittee on Urinary Tract Infection, Steering Committee on Quality Improvement and Management, 2011)
- Cerebrospinal Fluid (CSF)
1. Pressure—70 to 180 mm H$_2$O; higher indicates increased intracranial pressure, which may be the result of a tumor, cerebral hemorrhage, meningitis, obstructed shunt
2. Appearance—clear
   a. Bloody—may indicate traumatic tap, cerebral hemorrhage
   b. Yellow—may indicate hyperbilirubinemia or metastatic melanoma
   c. Cloudy—suggests increased WBCs as found in bacterial meningitis
3. Glucose—60 to 80 mg/dL
   a. Increased—diabetes
   b. Decreased—may indicate bacterial meningitis, TB meningitis, hypoglycemia, leukemia with metastasis
4. Protein—15 to 45 mg/dL; increased in encephalitis, bacterial meningitis, TB meningitis, acoustic neuroma
5. Cell count
   a. Infant—0 to 20 WBCs/mm³
   b. Child and adolescent—0 to 10 WBCs/mm³
   c. Increased—bacterial meningitis, early viral meningitis, cerebral abscess

☐ SELECTED SCREENING TESTS

- Refer to the most recent periodicity schedule: http://pediatrics.aappublications.org/content/133/3/568.full
- Newborns should be screened for critical congenital heart disease using pulse oximetry before leaving the hospital
- Blood pressure screening on all children beginning at age 3 years. If child has renal or cardiovascular abnormality, perform at all visits regardless of age

- Growth Parameters
  1. Height, weight, and head circumference from birth to age 3 plotted on appropriate growth chart at each well-child visit. If head circumference has been appropriate for the first 2 years, routine measurements need not continue being obtained after age 2. Body mass index beginning at age 24 months
     a. Infants should be undressed completely, and young children should be wearing underpants only
     b. Recumbent length is plotted on the chart from birth to 3 years
     c. When the child is old enough to be measured upright, height should be plotted on the chart for ages 2 through 18
  2. Height, weight, and body mass index from age 3 through adolescence plotted on appropriate growth chart at each well-child visit. A BMI higher than the 95th percentile identifies a child who is overweight, and a BMI lower than the 5th percentile identifies a child who is underweight (See http://www.cdc.gov/growthcharts/)
- Newborn Screening
  1. Screening should be conducted according to state law
  2. All states require testing for:
     a. Hypothyroidism
     b. Phenylketonuria (PKU)
     c. Galactosemia
     d. Hemoglobinopathies (e.g., sickle cell disease)
  3. Other tests may include screening for:
     a. Maple syrup urine disease
     b. Homocystinuria
     c. Biotinidase deficiency
     d. Tyrosinemia
     e. Congenital adrenal hyperplasia
     f. Cystic fibrosis
     g. Toxoplasmosis
  4. Initial specimens should be obtained at least 24 hours after birth, but not more than 7 days of age
  5. Most states recommend a second metabolic screening in the first week of life for those infants discharged prior to 24 hours
  6. Infants with a positive screen result should receive close follow-up with additional confirmatory studies performed
- Vision Screening
  1. Identify risk factors
     a. Prenatal infections
     b. Congenital cyanotic heart disease
     c. Structural malformation
     d. Family history of eye or vision problems
     e. Excessive oxygenation in neonatal period
     f. Hearing problems
     g. Parent concern about the child's visual functioning
     h. Deterioration in school performance
  2. Conduct vision screen at ages 3, 4, 5, 6, 8, 10, 12, 15, and 18 years. Rescreen in 6 months if uncooperative at the time of visit

  a. Young infant
     (1) Assess pupillary response to light
     (2) Illicit blink reflex
     (3) Determine ability to fix on and follow an object
     (4) Assess red reflex
  b. Older infant and toddler
     (1) Determine ability to fix on and follow an object
     (2) Perform corneal light reflex test (Hirschberg)
     (3) Perform cover–uncover test
     (4) Assess red reflex
  c. Preschool child (same as toddler, plus)
     (1) Conduct visual acuity tests (Allen figures, HOTV, Sjogren hand, illiterate E)
     (2) Use Ishihara for color perception
     (3) Assess red reflex
  d. School-age child and adolescent (preschool child, plus)
     (1) Far vision—Snellen chart
     (2) Near vision—Rosenbaum or Jaeger card
     (3) Assess red reflex
  e. Refer children for further evaluation with:
     (1) Abnormal or asymmetric red reflex
     (2) Asymmetric corneal light reflex
     (3) Abnormal cover/uncover test
     (4) Structural abnormality
     (5) Failure to follow object equally when covering each eye
     (6) Visual acuity minimal acceptable is 20/40 for age 3 to 5 and 20/30 for age 6 and older
     (7) Two-line difference or more in scores between eyes
- Hearing Screening
  1. Identify infants and children at risk for hearing problems
     a. Neonatal risk criteria
        (1) Affected family member
        (2) Bilirubin >20 mg/dL
        (3) Congenital cytomegalovirus (CMV), herpes, rubella
        (4) Defects in ears, nose, throat (ENT) structure
        (5) Birth weight <1500 g
        (6) Bacterial meningitis
        (7) Use of ototoxic medications for more than 5 days
        (8) Mechanical ventilation for cardiopulmonary disease for more than 48 hours
        (9) Intracranial hemorrhage
     b. Risk criteria for children younger than 2 years of age (neonatal risk factors, plus)
        (1) Parental concerns regarding hearing or language development
        (2) Head trauma with temporal bone fracture
        (3) Infections known to cause sensorineural hearing loss (e.g., measles, mumps)
        (4) Recurrent otitis media or middle ear effusion
  2. Conduct hearing screen at the following intervals and when indicated

a. Newborn performed prior to discharge using auditory brainstem response (ABR) or evoked oto-acoustic emissions (EOAE)

b. Ages 4, 5, 6, 8, and 10 years

   (1) Examine ears using an otoscope with pneumatic otoscopy before conducting audiometry

   (2) Conduct pure tone audiometry—test each ear at 500, 1000, 2000, and 4000 Hz (hand-held audiometers have not proven effective in screening children)

   (3) Use tympanometry to further assess middle ear air pressure and tympanic membrane compliance if pneumatic otoscopy was abnormal

3. Refer children to an audiologist for further evaluation if hearing threshold levels are greater than 20 dB at any of the above frequencies; if the reliability of a test with an individual child is uncertain, repeat screening before referral

- Tuberculosis Screening

1. Mantoux test should be used for testing; use 0.1 cc of purified protein derivative (PPD), which contains 5 tuberculin units; administer via intradermal injection on the volar aspect of the forearm to produce a 6- to 10-mm wheal; multiple-puncture tests do not have adequate specificity and sensitivity

2. Test should be read 48 to 72 hours following injection by a measurement of the area of induration, not redness

3. BCG vaccination is NOT a contraindication to TB skin testing

4. Positive skin tests include children who have reaction of:

a. At least 15 mm *INDURATION* with no risk factors

b. At least 10 mm *INDURATION* who are younger than 4 years of age or those with medical risk factors (e.g., born, or whose parents were born, in areas of prevalent TB [Asia, Middle East, Africa, or Latin America] or exposed to adults who are HIV positive, homeless, illicit drug users, nursing home residents, incarcerated or institutionalized persons, or migrant farm workers)

c. At least 5 mm *INDURATION* who are household contacts of active or previously active TB cases as well as children with immunosuppressive conditions, including HIV infection

5. Current recommendations for TB testing are based on degree of risk rather than routine, universal screening

6. Immediate TB testing should be conducted on children who are contacts of individuals with confirmed or suspected infectious TBI, who have been in contact with persons who have been incarcerated in the last 5 years, who are immigrating from or with a history of travel to endemic countries, and who have clinical or radiologic findings of TB

7. Annual TB testing should be conducted for children at high risk, beginning as early as 3 months of age

a. HIV positive or living with an HIV-infected person

b. Institutionalized and/or incarcerated children and adolescents

8. Testing every 2 to 3 years. Children exposed to the homeless, HIV-infected individuals, nursing home residents, institutionalized or incarcerated adolescents, illicit drug users, and migrant farm workers

9. Periodic TB testing between 4 and 6 years and again between 11 and 16 years for children living in high-prevalence areas or with uncertain history of risk factors

10. See most recent American Academy of Pediatrics (AAP) *Red Book* for specific updated guidelines (http://aapredbook.aappublications.org)

- Lead Screening

1. The Centers for Disease Control and Prevention (CDC) no longer recommends universal screening; targeted screening beginning at age 1–2 years of age should be based on surveillance of risk. All children receiving Medicaid are required by federal regulation to be tested for blood lead levels at 1 and 2 years of age

2. Risk factors include children who live in a house, or are cared for in a house, built before 1950 or built before 1978 that has recently or is undergoing renovation; who have a sibling or playmate being followed for lead poisoning; who live with a person whose job involves exposure to lead; who live near an industrial site; who use pottery that is suspected of having lead content; and/or who have exposure to burning lead-painted wood

3. Most children with lead poisoning are between the ages of 6 months and 6 years

4. Venous blood samples of lead levels are more reliable than capillary samples

5. The CDC recommends that a reference value based on the 97.5th percentile of the National Health and Nutrition Examination Survey (NHANES)-generated blood lead level (BLL) distribution in children 1–5 years old (currently 5 µg/dL) be used to identify children with elevated BLL

6. Children with levels of 5 µg/dL should also be assessed for iron deficiency and general nutrition (e.g., calcium and vitamin C levels), consistent with AAP guidelines. Iron-deficient children should be provided with iron supplements. Children with elevated BLLs will need to be followed over time until the environmental investigations and subsequent responses are complete

7. Chelation of lead is indicated for levels of 45 µg/dL or more and is urgently required for levels over 70 µg/dL

- Cholesterol Screening

1. Universal screening for all children is not recommended. Cholesterol screening is recommended between ages 9 and 11 years

2. Children 2 years of age and older who have a parent with a total cholesterol level of 240 mg/dL or greater should receive a total cholesterol screen

3. Children 2 years of age and older with a family history of premature cardiovascular disease (e.g., a parent

or grandparent with a myocardial infarction, sudden cardiac death, angina pectoris, coronary arteriography for diagnostic purposes, or cardiac bypass surgery at the age of 55 years or younger) should be screened with a serum lipid profile

4. Overweight children are in a special risk category and should be screened regardless of family history or other risk factors
5. There are differences in cholesterol concentrations related to gender; it is higher in females than in males after pubertal development. There may be variations by ethnicity, with African American children having a higher high-density lipoprotein (HDL) cholesterol and lower triglycerides than non-Hispanic white and Hispanic children
6. Children receiving total cholesterol screening may eat a normal diet before the test
7. Children receiving a serum lipid profile should fast for 12 hours (except for water) before their blood is drawn
8. An acceptable total cholesterol level in children and adolescents is less than 170 mg/dL; an acceptable low-density lipoprotein (LDL) level is less than 110 mg/dL
9. An elevated total cholesterol level in children and adolescents is greater than or equal to 200 mg/dL; a high LDL level is greater than or equal to 130 mg/dL

- Urine Screening
  1. Routine screening recommended only if indicated by history and/or physical examination findings
  2. Positive results of bacteriuria from a bagged urine specimen are not acceptable, and children 2 to 24 months should have urine obtained by catheterization or suprapubic aspiration
  3. "Clean-catch" midstream urine specimens in children and adolescents are best for reliable results

- Anemia Screening: Hemoglobin/hematocrit obtained between 9 and 12 months of age and for at-risk children ages 1 through 5 years. A risk assessment for hematocrit or hemoglobin is recommended at ages 15 and 30 months

- Depression Screening: recommended from 11 through 21 years along with suggested screening tools

- Adolescent Screening for Alcohol and Drug Use: recommended with the use of screening tools

- Sexually Transmitted Infections/HIV
  1. All sexually active adolescents (especially females who are often asymptomatic) should be screened for gonorrhea, chlamydia, syphilis, and trichomoniasis
  2. Female adolescents who are sexually active and all females age 21 years and older should have a Pap smear performed at least every 3 years and more frequently if indicated by risk factors
  3. Screening for HIV is recommened between ages 16 and 18 years. High-risk adolescents (e.g., those with multiple sexual partners, who reside in areas with a high prevalence of STI/HIV infection, who have been sexually abused by or have had sexual contact with

individuals with documented STI/HIV infection or parenteral drug use) should be offered HIV testing

☐ SPECIAL EXAMINATIONS

- The Newborn Examination
  1. Immediately after birth, obtain Apgar scores at 1 and 5 minutes; composite scores range from 0 to 10 based on 5 criteria

■ Apgar Scoring System

Criteria	0	1	2
Heart rate	Absent	Slow (<100)	>100
Respiratory rate	Absent	Slow, irregular	Good strong cry
Muscle tone	Limp	Some flexion of extremities	Active motion
Reflex irritability	No response	Grimace	Cough or sneeze
Color	Blue, pale	Body pink, extremities blue	Completely pink

2. Obtain length, weight, head circumference percentiles, and vital signs
3. Assess vision and hearing
4. Assess gestational age (Ballard/Dubowitz exam)
5. HEENT
   a. Palpate anterior and posterior fontanels—note presence of molding, craniosynostosis, cephalohematomas, and asymmetry
   b. Assess presence of red reflex
   c. Note size, shape, and position of ears and characteristics of tympanic membrane (TM)
   d. Assess for patency of nares, intact palate, and any unusual findings in the mouth
6. Assess neck for webbing, palpate for masses
7. Auscultate lungs and assess thorax for shape, symmetry, and character of respirations
8. Perform cardiac evaluation, including auscultation for murmurs and assessment of brachial and femoral pulses
9. Conduct abdominal examination, including the number of blood vessels in cord (two umbilical arteries and one umbilical vein), cord appearance, and condition of stump
10. Assess genitourinary system, including prominence of labia, number of testicles and position, position of urethra
11. Conduct musculoskeletal examination, including hips, feet, range of motion, presence of crepitus, Ortolani and Barlow maneuvers
12. Perform neurologic examination, including assessment of head lag and muscle tone; illicit the following reflexes:
    a. Root/suck
    b. Gag reflex

c. Moro

d. Plantar/palmar

e. Stepping

f. Tonic neck

13. Assess skin for cyanosis, jaundice, meconium staining, rashes, lesions, and birthmarks

a. Major risk factors for jaundice*

(1) Jaundice in first 24 hours

(2) Blood group (ABO) incompatibility

(3) Gestational age less than 37 weeks, LBW

(4) Previous sibling received phototherapy

(5) Cephalohematoma or bruising

(6) Exclusive breastfeeding not going well

(7) East Asian race

b. Minor risk factors for jaundice*

(1) Gestational age 37–38 weeks

(2) Previous sibling with jaundice

(3) Macrosomic IDM

(4) Maternal age. 25

(5) Male

(6) Delayed cord clamping

- The Sports Evaluation

1. Purpose

a. Identify risk factors associated with morbidity and mortality

b. Identify conditions that place the child at risk for injury

c. Identify conditions that could worsen with sports participation

d. Determine appropriate sports activities for child's abilities

2. Preparticipation History

a. Cardiovascular—murmur, chest pain, syncope, shortness of breath, family history of cardiac diseases

b. Hypertension—130/75 mm Hg in a child younger than age 10 or 140/85 mm Hg in a child 10 years of age or older

c. History of chronic diseases

d. Musculoskeletal limitations and prior injuries

e. Menstrual history for females

f. Nutritional factors—recent weight loss or gain, eating patterns

g. Medication history—including performance-enhancing compounds, stimulants, and narcotics

3. The physical examination should be comprehensive with emphasis on:

a. Cardiac examination, including blood pressure

(1) Presence of a systolic murmur that increases on sitting or with Valsalva maneuver requires an echocardiogram

(2) An arrhythmia that does not subside with exercise requires referral to a cardiologist

b. Musculoskeletal examination—including range of motion of neck, shoulders, upper and lower extremities, back, and gait

(1) Perform scoliosis screen

(2) Have child perform the "duck walk" (squat on heels, walk 4 steps, and stand up)

(3) Assess shoulder flexion and rotation

c. Genitalia exam

(1) Tanner stage

(2) Presence of hernias

(3) Presence of both testicles in males

d. Skin for contagious lesions

e. Visual problems

f. Neurologic problems

4. Estimate the relative risk of an acute injury to the athlete by categorizing sports as contact, limited contact, or noncontact sport. Contact sport includes the subset of collision sport. Collision implies greater injury risk. Clinical judgment involving the risk of acquiring a disease as a result of participation. Variables to consider:

a. The advice of knowledgeable experts

b. The current health status of the athlete

c. The sport in which the athlete participates

d. The position played

e. The level of competition

f. The maturity of the competitor

g. The relative size of the athlete

h. The availability of effective protective equipment

i. The availability of efficacy of treatment

j. Whether rehabilitation has been completed

k. Whether the sport can be modified to allow safer participation

l. The ability of the athlete's parent(s) or guardian and coach to understand and to accept the risks involved in participation

5. Exclusion from sports participation include:

a. Carditis

b. Fever

6. Exclusion (until cleared) requiring consultation with a specialist and/or evaluation include:

a. Atlantoaxial instability (as found in Down syndrome or juvenile rheumatoid arthritis with cervical involvement)

b. Bleeding disorder

c. Blood pressure reading at least 5 mm Hg above the 99th percentile

d. Congenital heart disease

e. Dysrhythmia

f. Heart murmur

g. Structural or acquired heart disease

h. Vasculitis/vascular disease

i. Cerebral palsy

j. Diarrhea

k. Eating disorder

l. Eye disorder

m. Conjunctivitis, infectious

n. Gastrointestinal disorder

o. Heat illness, history of

p. Absence of a kidney

---

* AAP Guidelines for high-risk factors for jaundice

q. Hepatosplenomegaly

r. Malignant neoplasm

s. Neurologic disorders

t. Myopathies

u. Recurrent plexopathy and cervical cord neuroo-praxia with persistent defects

v. Seizure disorder, poorly controlled

w. Organ transplant recipient

x. Pregnancy/postpartum

y. Respiratory conditions, including pulmonary compromise such as cystic fibrosis, not asthma

z. Acute upper respiratory infections

aa. Rheumatologic diseases

bb. Sickle cell disease

cc. Skin infections

7. If the athlete participates in sports despite known medical risks and against medical advice, the parents or guardian should be asked to sign a written consent statement indicating they have been advised of the potential dangers of participation and that they understand these dangers. The athlete should also sign the consent statement. It is recommended that the adult write the statement in their own words and handwriting

- Breast and Pelvic Examinations

1. Breast

   a. Although breast disease is rare in adolescent females, assessment of the breasts should be performed routinely as part of the well-child physical examination from the start of puberty (as soon as breast budding occurs)

   b. In addition to detection of disease, the breast examination is an opportunity to teach adolescents about breast development and self-breast examination as well as provide reassurance about the "normalcy" of their breasts

2. Pelvic

   a. Recognize the pelvic examination produces much fear and anxiety for adolescents, especially those who are experiencing it for the first time, have had a prior difficult experience, or have been sexually abused

   b. Prepare the adolescent for the examination by showing her illustrations of the reproductive system and explaining the procedure

   c. Provide concrete objective information about sensations the adolescent will feel during course of the examination, which will help her cope better with the experience

   d. Suggest ways to maintain control and decrease anxiety during examination (e.g., relaxation techniques)

   e. Use largest speculum that will fit comfortably within vagina (usually small plastic or Pederson speculum work best for this age group)

   f. Warm speculum before insertion

   g. Inform adolescent of what you are doing throughout the examination

   h. Encourage the adolescent to become involved with the examination if she desires (e.g., a mirror can be positioned to see the area being examined)

   i. Verbal or visual modes of distraction are helpful (e.g., interesting posters on the ceiling or wall)

   j. Use examination to teach adolescent about her body and to reassure her of "normalcy"

   k. Provide as much privacy as possible, e.g., while dressing

   l. Give positive feedback to the adolescent for her cooperation or assistance

   m. Recognize that cervical ectopy is a normal finding during the examination, especially in adolescents taking hormonal contraceptives

☐ PROBLEM-ORIENTED HEALTH RECORD

- Organized system for recording health visits to allow for thorough, concise data; easy retrieval of data; enhanced communication between health professionals; documentation of problem assessment/management; and decreased risk of liability

- Components of the Problem-Oriented Health Record

1. Database—medical history, physical examination, growth charts, developmental flow sheets, screening and laboratory tests, and problem-specific progress notes

2. Problem list—conditions that require diagnostic work-up or ongoing management

3. Management plan—includes information related to the diagnosis, management, education, and follow-up for specific health problem

4. Progress notes—includes documentation of each patient visit and is usually recorded in SOAP format

   a. S—subjective information provided by child and parent or caregiver

   b. O—objective information that consists of observations, physical examination, and laboratory findings

   c. A—assessment (diagnosis)

   d. P—plan

      (1) Medications

      (2) Treatments

      (3) Further laboratory studies

      (4) Consultations or referrals

      (5) Diet or activity modifications

      (6) Teaching

      (7) Follow-up schedule (visit or telephone contact)

☐ CHILD HEALTH SUPERVISION SCHEDULE OF VISITS WITH KEY ISSUES (NUTRITION, DEVELOPMENT, SCREENING, IMMUNIZATIONS, ANTICIPATORY GUIDANCE, AND HEALTH EDUCATION)

- Prenatal Visit

1. General Considerations: A prenatal visit is recommended for parents who are at high risk, for first-time parents, and for those who request a conference. The

prenatal visit should include anticipatory guidance, pertinent medical history, and a discussion of benefits of breastfeeding and planned method of feeding

    a. Major purposes—ensure the health of the fetus, child, family; establish relationship with family; answer questions; provide anticipatory guidance and plan of care

    b. Timing—between 30 and 35 weeks' gestation

    c. Include both parents and/or grandparents if single parent

2. Family history—parents and siblings' ages; health of parents, siblings, and blood relatives, including chronic illnesses such as asthma, cystic fibrosis, and heart disease, as well as mental disorders

3. Obstetrical history—current gestational age; beginning of prenatal care; ultrasound or amniocentesis results; name of obstetrician; medications, drugs, cigarettes, or alcohol usage during this pregnancy; prior pregnancies and outcomes

4. Preparation for childbirth and infant

    a. Readiness for parenthood

    b. Planned or unplanned pregnancy

    c. Prenatal classes, childbirth preparation

    d. Sibling preparation, if applicable

    e. Choice of infant feeding

    f. Circumcision, if applicable

    g. Genetic testing, if applicable

    h. Arrangements for child care

    i. Special concerns of prospective parents

    j. Current life stressors

5. Social history

    a. Family type—single parent, nuclear

    b. Number and types of pets

    c. Perceived social support

    d. Healthcare practices/religion

    e. Financial information, including insurance

    f. Cultural issues

6. Plan of care and anticipatory guidance

    a. Timing of health supervision visits

    b. Immunizations

    c. Organization of practice, e.g., team approach with nurse practitioners and physicians

    d. How and where to access care when needed; available hours

    e. Fees/medical coverage

    f. Need for transportation

    g. General infant care and supplies needed

    h. Safety information, e.g., car seats, pets

    i. Psychological adjustment of parents and siblings

- Prenatal Breastfeeding Guidance

1. Review the benefits of breastfeeding as appropriate during visit

    a. Species specific

    b. Benefits child's health

    c. Maximizes potential of infant

    d. Assists with birth spacing

    e. Conserves resources

    f. Benefits mother's health

    g. Environmentally friendly

    h. Empowers women

    i. Promotes bonding

2. Promote attainment of Healthy People 2020 breastfeeding goals

    a. 82% ever breastfed

    b. 61% breastfed at 6 months

    c. 34% breastfed at 1 year

3. Identify and clarify contraindications to breastfeeding prior to birth

    a. Mother has active TB

    b. Maternal HIV

    c. Debilitating maternal disease (cancer)

    d. Drug abuse—cocaine, heroin

    e. Mother has HTLV1 (human T-cell leukemia virus type 1)

4. Clarify misconceptions related to what is NOT a contraindication to breastfeeding prior to birth

    a. Hepatitis B or C infection

    b. Exposure to low-level environmental contaminants

    c. Alcohol use (limit to occasional drink)

    d. Tobacco use (encourage to stop smoking or avoid infant exposure)

    e. Cytomegalovirus (CMV) infection unless infant preterm

5. Identify physical conditions of the breast that may inhibit breastfeeding and recommend lactation consult prior to delivery

    a. Hypoplastic/tubular breasts

    b. No increase in breast size during pregnancy a risk factor

    c. Breast surgery (augmentation/reduction)

    d. Previous treatment for breast cancer

    e. Trauma or burns to the breast

6. Identify risk factors for lactation problems related to history/social factors and recommend lactation consult prior to delivery

    a. Early intention to breastfeed and formula feed

    b. History of previous breastfeeding problems

    c. History of hormone-related infertility, intended oral contraceptive pill (OCP) use

    d. Significant medical problems (hypothyroidism, diabetes, polycystic ovary syndrome [PCOS])

    e. Maternal age (adolescent or advanced maternal age [AMA])

    f. Psychosocial problems, especially depression

    g. Anticipated multiple birth or possible preterm delivery

    h. Insufficient prenatal education about breastfeeding

    i. Maternal employment and lack of knowledge about continuation of breastfeeding while employed

    j. Lack of family and societal (workplace) support. Inform mother regarding federal guidelines that support time to express breastmilk using a pump at work until the child is 1 year of age

7. Incorporate best practices for the PNP to promote breastfeeding

    a. Encourage prenatal breastfeeding education

b. Recommend human milk for all infants unless contraindicated

c. Encourage mother to initiate breastfeeding within the first hour of life

d. Encourage exclusive rooming-in of newborn with mother

- Hospital Newborn Visit Breastfeeding Guidance
1. Identify and clarify contraindications to breastfeeding present after birth of infant
   a. Infant has galactosemia/inborn errors of metabolism
   b. Mother has active herpetic lesions on her breast(s)
   c. Mother has varicella that has been determined to be infectious to the infant
   d. Medications including radioactive isotopes, anti-metabolites, cancer chemotherapy
2. Clarify misconceptions related to what is NOT a contraindication to breastfeeding present after birth of infant
   a. Maternal fever in absence of other contraindications
   b. Hepatitis B or C infection
   c. Alcohol use (limit to occasional drink)
   d. Tobacco use (encourage to stop smoking or avoid infant exposure)
   e. CMV infection unless infant preterm
3. Promote breastfeeding in the first 24 hours
   a. Promote skin-to-skin contact
   b. Promote rooming-in, avoid interruptions in breastfeeding
   c. Teach feeding cues or feeding readiness: increased activity, mouthing, rooting
   d. Remember the 4 As
      (1) Alignment—body and head of infant: Positions
         (a) Cross-cradle
         (b) Clutch or football
         (c) Side-lying
         (d) Cradle or Madonna
      (2) Areolar grasp
      (3) Areolar compression
      (4) Audible swallowing
   e. Use positive supportive tone and body language
4. Minimum output AAP guidelines:
   a. First 24 hour: one stool one void
   b. Second 24 hours: 2 stools and 2 voids
   c. Third and fourth days: 3 stools and 5 voids
   d. Meconium stool: days 1–2
   e. Transitional stool: days 3–4
   f. Breastfed stool: days 4–5 on
5. Normal breastfeeding patterns
   a. 1st day: baby will feed 6–8 times in 24 hours
   b. 2nd and 3rd days: baby will cluster feed
   c. 4th and 5th days: baby will feed 10–12 times a day
6. Identify risk factors for lactation problems identified after birth and recommend lactation consult prior to discharge
   a. Nipple trauma
   b. Pain throughout feed

c. Infant weight loss: 8% to 10% of birth weight (less than 2–3% per day). May refer to website such as https://www.newbornweight.org/chart/ to determine percentage of weight loss from birth and guidelines based on type of delivery and feeding method

d. Inadequate output

e. None or little swallowing after 24 hours of age

f. Abnormal infant oral anatomy

g. Mother of NICU infant/separation from infant

h. Late preterm (34–36 6/7), small for gestational age (SGA), large for gestational age (LGA)

i. Jaundice infant

j. Multiple births

k. Birth interventions

l. Unrelieved fullness or engorgement

7. Pumping guidelines requiring a hospital pump
   a. Infants in NICU
   b. Infants with weight loss > 8%
   c. Infants close to 24 hours old and have not breastfed
   d. Inverted, flat, or sore nipples
   e. Using breast shield
   f. History of breast surgery
   g. Medical conditions, i.e., hemorrhage or shock

8. Provide information to mother regarding milk volume at week 2 if exclusively providing pumped breastmilk
   a. Ideal: 750 to 1000 mL/day
   b. Adequate: 500 mL/day
   c. Borderline: <350 mL/day

9. Breastmilk storage guidelines

a. Room temperature	4–8 hours
b. Refrigerator	3–5 days
c. Freezer	3–6 months
d. Deep freeze	1 year
e. Thawed, refrigerated	24 hours

   f. Store in opaque, clear, or brown glass or breast-milk storage bags to maintain maximum number of functional cells

10. Signs of good feeding after discharge
   a. Feeling good, strong deep sucking, without sharp pain
   b. Audible swallowing (at 18 hours of life)
   c. Breast softer
   d. Adequate output
   e. Seeing milk in baby's mouth
   f. Leaking from other breast

11. Signs of poor feeding after discharge
   a. Sleepy baby
   b. Baby has difficulty latching on
   c. Pain throughout feeding
   d. Clicking or popping sounds in baby's mouth
   e. Inadequate output
   f. Less than 8 feedings per day or more than 12 feedings per day

12. Incorporate best practices for the PNP to promote breastfeeding
   a. Avoid supplementation unless medically indicated
   b. Avoid pacifier use until breastfeeding well established
   c. Provide timely hospital follow-up

- Newborn Visit
  1. Purposes—obtain complete history, physical examination, anticipatory guidance, and plan of care
  2. Initial history—from chart review and parent(s)
     a. General health of mother
        (1) Mother's age and gestation at first prenatal visit, regularity of visits
        (2) History of maternal infection and prenatal complications
        (3) Substance abuse, tobacco use
        (4) History of chronic disease
        (5) Medications during pregnancy
        (6) Weight gain, nutritional status
        (7) Number of weeks of gestation
        (8) Number of living children
     b. Labor and delivery
        (1) Length of labor
        (2) Medications used—anesthesia
        (3) Type of facility—birthing center, hospital, other
        (4) Type of delivery—spontaneous, C-section (explanation needed if yes)
        (5) Blood type, including Rh factor
     c. Infant's status at delivery
        (1) Identification verified
        (2) Term, preterm (number of weeks)
        (3) Determination of gestational age (Ballard/Dubowitz exam)
        (4) Apgar scores
        (5) Complications
        (6) Oxygen or any other treatment(s) required
        (7) Blood type, Rh factor; other values
        (8) Length, weight, head and chest circumference (including percentiles)
        (9) Physical examination results—note any abnormal findings
        (10) Correct date of birth
     d. Nursery course—presence of jaundice; type of treatments; medications, immunizations; length of stay; circumcision/cord condition
     e. Family history—maternal/paternal
        (1) Review of systems (ROS)—includes physical and mental health problems
        (2) Home environment—members of household, pets, smokers, infant supplies, and sleeping arrangements
     f. Common parental concerns
        (1) Initial weight loss, appearance of infant (cephalohematoma, molding), normalcy of infant
        (2) Rashes, skin markings—telangiectasis, café-au-lait, hemangiomas
        (3) Infant's habits—feeding, stooling, sleeping, development, normal crying
        (4) Female infant—breast engorgement, vaginal discharge
     g. Objective data
        (1) Verify identification of mother, infant
        (2) Parent–infant interaction—eye contact; holding; response to crying, vocalization
        (3) Behavioral—consolability, self-quieting
        (4) Physical examination (refer to "Newborn Examination" in the "Special Examinations" section earlier in this chapter)
     h. Plan of care
        (1) Reinforce infant care, cord care, circumcision care, instructions on when to seek medical advice
        (2) Emphasize individual variability of infant temperament, noting positive aspects and challenges
        (3) Breastfeeding mothers
           (a) Quiet alert state optimal time for nursing
           (b) Initial feedings 3 to 5 minutes/each breast every 1½ to 2 hours; increase time as tolerated
           (c) Supplemental formula unnecessary
           (d) Colostrum present first 2 to 4 days
           (e) Increase maternal fluid intake especially at 6 weeks and 3 months during infant growth spurts
           (f) Adequate infant intake indicated by 6 or more voids/day
           (g) Vitamin D supplementation of 400 IU daily in breastfeeding infant or infant receiving combination of any amount of breastfeeding and formula feeding (Taylor, Geyer, & Feldman, 2010)
        (4) Formula-feeding mothers
           (a) Amount and frequency varies
              (1) 0 to 1 month—2 to 4 oz every 3 to 4 hours
              (2) 2 to 4 months—5 to 7 oz every 4 to 5 hours
           (b) Inform them that iron-fortified formulas are best
           (c) Suggest partial hydrolysate formula if infant at risk for atopic disease, e.g., strong family history of atopic disease
        (5) Crying—infant's first way of communicating needs
           (a) Less than 2 hours/day during first month; peaks at 6 weeks
           (b) Decreases as infant learns other ways to communicate
        (6) Colic—excessive crying in otherwise healthy infants beginning at 2 to 3 weeks; may last 3 to 4 months
           (a) Rule out physical problems
           (b) Assess for over/underfeeding
           (c) Acknowledge stressful situation; encourage breaks from infant if possible; reassure that it usually subsides by 3 to 4 months
           (d) Avoid sudden overstimulation of infant

(e) If nursing, eliminate possible offending sources from maternal diet, e.g., coffee, spices, chocolate, milk, gas-forming foods

(f) Soothing techniques—rocking, walking, background "white noise," car rides

(g) Antiflatulent if indicated by history and examination

(7) Sleep patterns

(a) Usually sleeps 8 hours by 3 months

(b) Early introduction of solids—doesn't cause infants to sleep through the night

(c) Position on side or supine as sudden infant death syndrome (SIDS) preventive measure unless medically contraindicated

(8) Bowel movements

(a) Usually after feeding (especially if breast-fed); normal variation may be up to one/week

(b) Avoid laxatives; use stool softener if constipated

(9) Reminder to schedule office visit for 2 weeks of age

- Newborn Breastfeeding Guidance

1. Promote exclusive breastfeeding for approximately the first 6 months

2. Provide a formal evaluation of breastfeeding, including observation, position, latch, milk transfer

3. Identify maternal risk factors for breastfeeding problems

   a. Inverted, short, or flat nipple

   b. Sore nipples/nipple pain and causes

      (1) Overly full breasts—engorgement

      (2) Poor positioning and/or latch or improper pumping

      (3) Not breaking suction correctly

      (4) Anatomic oral variations of newborn or poor fit of mother to infant or inappropriate infant sucking

      (5) Inappropriate cleaning of nipples (alcohol/drying agents)

      (6) Infection due to bacterial or candidal infection

   c. Engorgement

      (1) Normal breast fullness typically peaks days 4–5, resolving without treatment

      (2) Signs of engorgement are evidenced by continual breast fullness/edema, breast pain, and/or flattened nipples often causing difficulty latching

      (3) Predisposing factors for engorgement

         (a) Mother—delayed or missed breastfeeding, early supplements, flat or inverted nipples, breast surgery, abrupt weaning

         (b) Infant—ineffective or poor latch, sleepy infant or poor feeder, prematurity/SGA, jaundice, physical abnormalities of mouth (tight frenulum/tongue-tie [ankyloglossia])

      (4) Overproduction or pathologic engorgement

         (a) Continual breast fullness at 3 weeks post-partum and beyond, usually with forceful milk ejection

         (b) Possible infant signs include:

            (1) Chokes, coughs, sputters, arches with feeding

            (2) Gassy, irritable, restless, frequent crying

            (3) Green, thin, frothy stools

            (4) Rapid weight gain (note that many symptoms similar to reflux in infant)

         (c) Milk duct obstruction

         (d) Mastitis—cause

            (1) Infrequent or missed feedings

            (2) Poor latch leading to insufficient milk removal

            (3) Nipple damage

            (4) Illness in mother or baby

            (5) Oversupply of milk

            (6) Rapid weaning

            (7) Pressure on the breast—tight bra, car seat belt

            (8) Blocked milk duct or blocked nipple pore

            (9) Maternal stress and fatigue

            (10) Maternal malnutrition or anemia

   d. Insufficient milk supply—causes

      (1) Most common cause is infrequent feedings or early introduction of formula (without pumping)

      (2) Insufficient milk transfer as evidenced by poor output or inadequate weight gain in infant

      (3) Conditions of mother—fatigue, stress, medications that inhibit milk production (estrogen-containing contraception, Sudafed [pseudoephedrine]), psychological inhibition, pregnancy, or smoking

      (4) Fussy infant for other reasons or growth spurt of infant

      (5) At 4 weeks postpartum breasts naturally less full prior to feeding

   e. Bleb, vasospasm

   f. Maternal medical problems—separation

4. Identify infant risk factors for breastfeeding problems

   a. Jaundice (physiologic and pathologic) or other medical problems (hypoglycemia, respiratory distress, infection)

   b. Ankyloglossia (tongue-tie) or other oral abnormality

      (1) Incidence in the population is predicted to be 4.8%

      (2) Genetic prevalence

      (3) More prevalent in males, 2.6 to 1.0

   c. Late preterm/low birth weight

   d. Multiples

   e. Neurologic problems/genetic syndromes

- First Newborn Office History Questions Related to Breastfeeding
  1. Number of feedings/wet diapers/stools in last 24 hours
  2. Does newborn wake for feedings?
  3. Does newborn easily latch and breastfeed eagerly?
  4. Is breastfeeding painful or uncomfortable?
  5. Is newborn receiving any supplements?
  6. Has mother previously breastfed, and if yes, successful?
  7. Is mother taking any medications or dietary supplements?
  8. How is mother's nutrition/weight reduction/special diet?
  9. Family support at home
- Examining Newborn and Mother Related to Breastfeeding
  1. Calculate newborn's weight gain or loss since birth
  2. Perform routine exam and oral motor assessment
  3. Assess state of hydration
  4. Observe for jaundice
  5. Observe breastfeeding
  6. Examine mother's breasts or refer for examination if necessary
  7. Consider test weight to estimate milk volume consumed
- Anticipatory Guidance Related to Breastfeeding
  1. Encourage breastfeeding on demand
  2. Review normal breastfeeding patterns
  3. Discourage use of pacifiers and discuss potential risks
     a. AAP recommends avoiding use until breastfeeding is established (about 3 weeks) as use is associated with:
        (a) Decreased weight gain
        (b) Nipple confusion
        (c) Early weaning
  4. Avoid long nighttime intervals without feeding
  5. Review normal elimination patterns
  6. Reinforce the importance of care of the mother
  7. Avoid maternal use of alcohol, tobacco, and caffeine
  8. Discuss maternal use of medications
     a. Drugs may transfer into human milk if they:
        (1) Attain high concentrations in maternal plasma
        (2) Are low in molecular weight (<500)
        (3) Are low in protein binding (drugs that circulate are either bound to albumin or freely soluble in plasma). Look for levels >90%
        (4) Are very lipid soluble
     b. General guidelines for medications and breastfeeding
        (1) Premature infants may not be able to tolerate medications like full-term infants can
        (2) During early lactation (days 1–3) and late-stage lactation (the amount of milk produced, 30–100 mL a day) is so low that infant receives limited amounts in milk

        (3) Avoid nursing at times of peak drug concentration
        (4) Administer the drug before the infant's longest sleep period
     c. Lactation risk categories
        (1) L1 safest
        (2) L2 safer
        (3) L3 moderately safe
        (4) L4 possibly hazardous
        (5) L5 contraindicated
- Breastfeeding Interventions
  1. Attempt to determine and treat the cause of inadequate milk supply before supplementing
  2. Consider referral to lactation consultant if problems ongoing
  3. Identify an appropriate peer support group
- How Father of Baby or Support Can Help with Breastfeeding
  1. Assist with positioning
  2. Help with sleepy baby
  3. Assist mother into comfortable position
  4. Get the baby ready for feed by changing diaper
  5. Monitor mom's fatigue level
  6. Monitor visitors
- Closing the Visit Related to Breastfeeding
  1. Congratulate parents on decision to breastfeed their infant
  2. Review some of the benefits of breastfeeding
  3. Remind mother to take the time to establish regular food and fluid intake to meet her needs
  4. Arrange for appropriate follow-up until weight gain is adequate and breastfeeding is going well
- Interim Visits: 2 Weeks to 1 Year (2 Weeks; 2, 4, 6, 9, and 12 Months)
  1. Subjective information
     a. Feeding—type, amounts, time at breast, name of formula
     b. Elimination—frequency, color, consistency of stools, number of saturated diapers per day
     c. Sleep
     d. Development, including behavior and temperament
     e. Concerns of parent, caregiver
     f. Interval history—health since last visit, emergency care, illnesses, medications used
  2. Objective data
     a. Caregiver–infant interaction
     b. Length, weight, head circumference; including percentiles
     c. Vital signs
     d. Vision and hearing screening (refer to screening guidelines this chapter)
     e. Physical examination
     f. Developmental screening—Denver II or equivalent and results; autism screening at 9 months

g. Laboratory
   (1) Newborn screening (metabolic screen)
   (2) Hematocrit at 12 months or sooner if indicated
   (3) Lead screening by 12 months as appropriate based on well-child surveillance of risk (CDC)

3. Plan of care, including health promotion strategies and anticipatory guidance
   a. Administer immunizations as indicated after obtaining consent and assessing response to previous immunizations—contact CDC and the AAP for updated recommended childhood and adolescent schedules
      (1) Inform parents of common side effects of immunizations; there is a website designed and maintained by the CDC that has the most up-to-date information about immunization and possible side effects: http://www.cdc.gov/vaccines/schedules/index.html
      (2) The National Childhood Vaccine Injury Act of 1986 requires all health providers who administer vaccines to report occurrences of certain adverse events stipulated in the act—the Vaccine Adverse Event Reporting System (VAERS) website has the most up-to-date listing of reportable events and the associated time intervals from vaccine administration. Additionally, providers may report adverse effects online using this website: http://vaers.hhs.gov
   b. Inform parents of any medications prescribed, including name, rationale, dosage, frequency, course, and potential side effects
   c. Implement health promotion strategies and anticipatory guidance appropriate for age and developmental level (ideally should be done before or at the very beginning of a developmental stage or problem); best to focus on one or two per visit with input from the parent or caregiver

4. Anticipatory guidance—nutrition and feeding
   a. Nutritional requirements are 110 to 120 calories/kg/day
   b. Consumption of more than 32 oz of formula per day usually indicative of need for solids once an infant is at least 4 months of age
   c. Formula recommended up to 1 year of age; whole milk until 2 years of age
   d. Judicious use of juices, some fortified with vitamin C; best to place in cup versus bottle
   e. Best to avoid giving infants a bottle in bed, especially containing formula or juice (leads to dental caries)
   f. Introduction of solids
      (1) Usually best to delay introduction of solids until 6 months of age; earlier introduction may lead to overfeeding and allergies
      (2) Cereal usually first food added to diet followed by vegetables, fruits, and meats
      (3) Add only 1 new food every 3 to 5 days
      (4) Do not give common allergenic foods until 1 year of age, e.g., cow's milk, egg whites, wheat, citrus fruits, peanut butter
      (5) Avoid the following until 3 years of age to prevent choking—nuts; potato chips; popcorn; raw celery and carrots; hot dogs; fish with bones; tough meat; small, hard candies
   g. Introduction of cup—when infant loses interest in bottle (7 to 10 months), spout cup may be used initially
   h. Weaning (breast or bottle)—gradually decrease number of feedings over several weeks; night feeding usually last to be eliminated

5. Anticipatory guidance—sleep
   a. 2- to 4-month-old infant—8 to 12 hours at night; 2 to 3 naps
   b. 6- to 12-month-old infant—11 to 12 hours at night; 2 to 3 naps
   c. Side-lying or supine sleep position through 6 months
   d. Strategies for parents
      (1) Put infant in crib when drowsy rather than asleep
      (2) Quiet, nonstimulating night feedings
      (3) Night waking once night feedings stop—briefly stroke infant lightly; don't pick infant up
      (4) Avoid pattern of placing infant in parent's bed

6. Anticipatory guidance—infant stimulation
   a. Provide variety of age-appropriate stimulation
   b. Formal infant stimulation programs for infants at risk for developmental delays

7. Anticipatory guidance—teeth
   a. Eruption typically begins at approximately 6 months of age
   b. Signs and symptoms—local sensitivity and inflammation, increased drooling, biting, irritability
   c. No evidence that teething causes fever, diarrhea, or other systemic illnesses
   d. Comfort measures—hard rubber teething toy, chilled teething ring, wet wash cloth, avoid liquid-filled teething rings

8. Stranger/anxiety—emerging awareness and preference for mother/primary caregiver; early indicator of healthy attachment process emerging around 6 months

9. Separation anxiety—emerging awareness that infant is an individual distinct from primary attachment figure/caregiver
   a. Develops around 9 months; peaks at around 18 months
   b. Suggestions for parents
      (1) Recognize that bedtime, going to child care, having a child care provider at home are all separations
      (2) Gradually introduce child to new situations and caretakers
      (3) The child learns to accept separation through multiple, brief separations and reunions

(4) Games such as "peek-a-boo" and "hide-and-seek" may be helpful

10. Safety—prevention of ingestion/aspiration of foreign objects
    a. Keep pins, buttons, and other small objects off the floor and out of reach
    b. Do not feed infants hard foods (e.g., nuts, hard candies)
    c. Discard broken or cracked rattles with beads
    d. Do not give infant balloons
    e. Do not prop infant's bottle
    f. Select pacifier with shield too large to enter infant's mouth
    g. Learn emergency procedure for dealing effectively with choking

11. Injury prevention
    a. Keep electrical wires out of reach; outlets covered; cabinet safety locks; medicines, poisons out of reach
    b. Install smoke detectors in household
    c. Keep Poison Control telephone number available, other emergency phone numbers
    d. Use car seat appropriate for infant's weight and age; rear facing until 12 months and 20 pounds
    e. Avoid walkers and stairs; use gate to barricade doorways and unsafe areas, e.g., kitchen and bathroom
    f. Do not place necklaces or pacifier cords around infant's neck
    g. Discourage infant jewelry
    h. Position crib or playpen away from window blind or curtain cords
    i. Use a crib with side rails spaced no more than 2 inches apart
    j. Secure infant with belt on changing table
    k. Lower crib mattress when infant begins to stand

12. Water safety—prevention of drowning and burns
    a. Set hot water heater temperature at 120°F or lower
    b. Do not leave infant unattended in bathtub
    c. Do not allow child to play in water unattended, e.g., toilet bowls, sinks, buckets of water
    d. Use of safety devices around swimming pools, lakes, and in boats, e.g., life jackets
    e. Lock fences around swimming pools
    f. Continuous supervision around water
    g. Do not leave other children in charge of infants around any body of water

13. Sun safety and sunburn protection—use lotion with sun protective factor (SPF) of at least 15; avoid use around eyes; use caps with sun visors or bonnets to protect eyes; keep infants in shaded areas, even with sunscreen; sun avoidance for infants, 6 months

14. Alternative child care arrangements—discuss child care provider options; appropriate supervision and stimulation/activities (language, visual, and motor)

15. Emphasize positive qualities of the infant and the parent–child relationship and mutually agree upon a plan with the parent to strengthen needed areas

16. Initiate referrals to other nurse practitioners, physicians, clinics, and community resources as needed

17. Schedule for next visit

- Infant Breastfeeding Guidance: 2 Weeks to 1 Year
  1. Early infancy
     a. Discuss stool pattern/feeding pattern/night waking
     b. Discuss mother's plans to return to work and breastmilk expression and storage
     c. Provide 400 IU of oral vitamin D at 2 months of age
     d. Discuss maternal use of medications
     e. Assess milk supply
     f. Encourage exclusive breastfeeding until 6 months of age
  2. Six months
     a. Discuss stool pattern/feeding pattern/night waking/distractibility/teething
     b. Discuss mother's plans/adjustment to return to work and breastmilk expression and storage
     c. Provide supplementary fluoride at 6 months of age
     d. Discuss maternal use of medications
     e. Assess milk supply
     f. Introduction solids/high-iron foods
  3. Nine months
     a. Discuss stool pattern/breastfeeding pattern/decreasing frequency/fluids in cup
     b. Assess milk supply
     c. Assess pressures to wean
     d. Discuss maternal use of medications
  4. Twelve months
     a. Discuss stool pattern/breastfeeding pattern/decreasing frequency/fluids in cup
     b. Discuss weaning techniques if desired, benefits of breastfeeding a toddler

- Interim Visits: Toddler (1 to 3 Years—12, 15, 18, and 24 Months)
  1. Subjective data—nutrition/appetite, elimination, sleep, development, parental concerns, health since last visit
  2. Objective data
     a. Assess parent–child interaction and parenting style
     b. Height, weight, head circumference (up to 2 years), including percentiles; body mass index (BMI) starting at 24 months, including percentiles
     c. Vital signs
     d. Vision and hearing screening (refer to screening guidelines earlier in this chapter)
     e. Physical examination
     f. Developmental screening—Denver II, Ages and Stages or equivalent and results; autism screening at 18 and 30 months
     g. Laboratory
        (1) Hematocrit at 1 year of age
        (2) Lead screening as appropriate based on well-child surveillance of risk (CDC)
  3. Management
     a. Update immunizations—contact CDC and AAP for updated recommended childhood and adolescent

schedules; inform parents of common side effects of immunizations: http://www.cdc.gov/vaccines/schedules/index.html

b. Advise parents of any medications prescribed, including vitamins and fluoride, e.g., name, rationale, dosage, frequency, course, and potential side effects

c. Nutrition appropriate for age
  (1) Nutritional requirements are 102 cal/kg
  (2) Provide foods from the five major food groups in realistic amounts; ¼ to ⅓ of adult portion or one measuring tablespoon for each year of the child's age
  (3) Physiologic anorexia is common between 15 and 18 months of age
  (4) Parental concerns regarding nutrition—decreased appetite, food jags, rituals, variable intake, definite likes and dislikes
  (5) Potential nutritional problems—iron-deficiency anemia (especially if toddler is drinking more than 32 oz of milk per day); low intake of calcium, vitamin A, zinc, ascorbic acid; obesity
  (6) Provide regular meals and snacks
  (7) Avoid food battles

d. Toilet training
  (1) Most children are psychologically and physiologically ready between 18 and 30 months
  (2) Majority of children achieve daytime bowel and bladder training simultaneously; average age is 28 months
  (3) Nighttime control generally occurs about 1 year after daytime control is achieved
  (4) Toilet training should not be started when family is unduly stressed (e.g., new baby, moving, holidays, divorce)
  (5) Suggestions for parents—praise all efforts; expect accidents to happen; don't punish; if child is resistant, try again in a few weeks; follow usual pattern of elimination; limit time on potty to 5 to 10 minutes

e. Sleep
  (1) One- to 3-year-olds usually sleep 10 to 12 hours at night and take 1 to 2 naps
  (2) Toddlers need rituals and consistency at bedtime as well as security objects, e.g., blanket, special toy
  (3) Nightmares start at approximately 3 years; child generally wakens and remembers dream
  (4) Night terrors generally occur between 2 and 4 years; child does not waken
  (5) Tips for parents—quietly reassure child; let child fall asleep in own bed

f. Negativism
  (1) Normal behaviors in toddlers as they strive to develop sense of autonomy
  (2) Expressed as "no," temper tantrums, breath holding

  (3) Tips for parents
    (a) Give child as much control as possible (e.g., offer choice of two acceptable objects or actions); allow independence when possible
    (b) Ignore temper tantrums; however, expect a "response burst" initially when ignored

g. Sibling rivalry
  (1) Can occur throughout childhood; is often most troublesome just after birth of new baby if older sibling is younger than 2 years
  (2) Tips for parents
    (a) Involve children in preparation for new baby
    (b) Praise "big-kid" behaviors; ignore regression
    (c) Provide special time for each child every day
    (d) Stay out of minor sibling conflicts, but discipline if aggression occurs
    (e) Foster individual interests of each child and avoid comparing children

h. Thumb sucking—peaks between 18 and 21 months; ignore before age 4 years unless child is not thriving

i. Safety—apply recommendations given earlier that are appropriate for toddlers, plus:
  (1) Emphasize street safety—begin teaching the basic rules of pedestrian and traffic safety
  (2) Avoid strangers—teach child methods to avoid encounters with strangers, which can be harmful
  (3) Continued use of car seats according to weight—all toddlers should ride forward facing and upright (studies show safest place for the child is middle of back seat)
  (4) Keep medicine and poisons out of reach in locked cabinets—highest incidence of poisoning occurs in 2-year-olds
  (5) Use of helmets with any type of bicycle use, either as a passenger or alone
  (6) Enroll child in swimming lessons and always supervise when in or around water

j. Dental care—every child should begin to receive oral health risk assessments by 6 months, and the AAP recommends establishment of the dental home by 1 year of age. Children at risk for dental caries Include:
  (1) Children with special healthcare needs
  (2) Children of mothers with a high caries rate
  (3) Children with demonstrable caries, plaque, demineralization, and/or staining
  (4) Children who sleep with a bottle or breastfeed throughout the night
  (5) Later-order offspring
  (6) Children in families of low socioeconomic status

k. Parenting and discipline
   (1) Use limit setting and time-out for inappropriate behavior—1 minute of time-out for each year of age
   (2) Praise good behavior
   (3) Emphasize consistency, especially between parents
   (4) Spend time with child; read to child on a daily basis
   (5) Parents set example as role models
   (6) Assign chores appropriate for age, e.g., put toys away
   (7) Begin socialization with other children
l. Television
   (1) Limit television viewing to appropriate children's programs
   (2) Limit time spent watching TV
   (3) Strong correlation between viewing aggression-type programs and child's level of aggressive play
   (4) TV fosters negative outcomes—rapid paced, superficial problem solving; obesity
   (5) Watch TV with child and provide reality base; opportunity to discuss values and stereotypes
   (6) Set good example through parental TV habits
m. Child care arrangements—discuss child care provider options; head start programs, nursery school, preschool programs
n. Emphasize positive qualities of the child and the parent–child relationship and mutually agree upon a plan with the parent to strengthen needed areas
o. Initiate referrals to other nurse practitioners, physicians, clinics, and community resources as needed
p. Schedule for next visit
• Interim Visits: Preschool Children (Ages 3, 4, and 5 Years)
1. Subjective information—nutrition/appetite; elimination; sleep; development, including behavior and temperament; caregiver concerns; interim health since last visit, including stressful life changes, e.g., move, divorce
2. Objective data
   a. Assess parent–child interaction and parenting style
   b. Height, weight, body mass index, including percentiles
   c. Vital signs, including blood pressure
   d. Vision and hearing screening (refer to screening guidelines earlier in this chapter)
   e. Physical examination
   f. Developmental screening—Denver II or equivalent and results
   g. Laboratory
      (1) Mantoux test for TB screening between 4 and 6 years of age if at risk
      (2) Hematocrit if indicated
      (3) Cholesterol screening if indicated

3. Management
   a. Immunizations—contact CDC and AAP for updated recommended childhood and adolescent schedules; review status and update as indicated; inform parents of common side effects of immunizations: http://www.cdc.gov/vaccines/schedules/index.html
   b. Advise parents of any medications prescribed, including vitamins and fluoride, e.g., name, rationale, dosage frequency, and potential side effects
   c. Nutrition appropriate for age
      (1) Nutritional requirements are 90 cal/kg
      (2) Provide foods from the five major food groups in realistic amounts
      (3) Provide nutritious snacks (e.g., fruits, vegetables) instead of high-fat foods (e.g., potato chips, cookies)
      (4) Potential nutritional problems (same as in the toddler years)
   d. Elimination—expect occasional nighttime accidents until 4 years of age; do not punish or embarrass child
   e. Sleep
      (1) The 3- to 5-year-old child usually sleeps 8 to 12 hours per night and gradually eliminates naps
      (2) Prepare parents for an increase in nightmares
   f. Development
      (1) Discuss the change from the pleasing 3-year-old to the sometimes aggressive, frustrating behavior of the 4-year-old; provide reassurance that "calmness" usually begins at age 5 years
      (2) Emphasize the "magical thinking" of the preschool child and how it places the child at risk for unintentional injury and an increase in fears
      (3) Discuss the child's rigid superego and how children this age feel guilty for negative events
      (4) Inform parents that they can expect "tall tales," the use of "toilet talk," and the construction of imaginary playmates
      (5) Discuss need for peer companionship and school readiness
   g. Sex education—begins in infancy and toddlerhood when parents label the genitals and accept genital exploration and masturbation as normal activities
      (1) Preschool children are curious about gender differences and "how babies are made"; their questions should be answered briefly and accurately
      (2) Explore parents' feelings about masturbation and prepare for a possible increase in this behavior
      (3) Talk with child about inappropriate touch; encourage parents to reinforce prevention
   h. Dental care
      (1) Brush teeth after each meal if possible and at bedtime

      (2) Recommend first dental visit if not previously done

      (3) If thumb sucking is persistent at age 4, have dental evaluation to rule out malocclusion; speech evaluation if tongue thrust is suspected

  i. Safety—apply recommendations given earlier that are appropriate for preschool children, plus:

      (1) Reinforce pedestrian safety—children ages 3 to 7 years are more frequently involved in pedestrian-related motor vehicle accidents

      (2) Teach guidelines for bicycle safety; avoid busy streets

      (3) Devise fire escape plan and teach the child; conduct routine fire drills

      (4) Teach child to stop, drop, and roll if clothing catches on fire

      (5) Teach safety—the danger of matches, open flames

      (6) Always supervise child when swimming or near any water

      (7) Frequently check playground equipment for stability, loose nuts and bolts, and suitable landing surface

      (8) Keep child away from power equipment, including lawn mowers

      (9) Never clean or handle a gun in the presence of the child

     (10) Discard old refrigerators and other large appliances or remove all doors during storage to avoid entrapment during play or exploration

     (11) Do not allow chewing gum or eating while running or jumping; parent should be aware of intervention for choking

  j. Exercise—encourage frequent periods of outdoor activities and limit television viewing

  k. Emphasize positive qualities of the child and the parent–child relationship and mutually agree upon a plan with the parent to strengthen needed areas

  l. Initiate referrals to other nurse practitioners, physicians, clinics, and community resources as needed

  m. Schedule for next visit

- Interim Visits: School-Age Children—Annual Visit (6 to 12 Years)

1. Subjective data
  a. Nutrition/appetite
  b. Elimination—especially constipation and enuresis
  c. Sleep
  d. Development—include school, activities, exercise, friends, behavior, and family relationships
  e. Allergies and reactions
  f. Medications
  g. Drug, alcohol, cigarette, and caffeine usage (for older school-age child)
  h. Concerns of child and caregiver; current/recent stressors, e.g., move, divorce
  i. Interim health since last visit (include review of systems); for older school-age children, obtain sexual/reproductive history as indicated

2. Objective
  a. Assess parent–child interaction and child behavior
  b. Height, weight, body mass index, including percentiles
  c. Vital signs, including blood pressure
  d. Vision and hearing screening (refer to screening guidelines earlier in this chapter)
  e. Physical examination, including assessment for scoliosis and Tanner staging
  f. Laboratory
      (1) Mantoux test for TB screening of high-risk child
      (2) Hematocrit if indicated
      (3) Cholesterol if indicated

3. Management
  a. Immunizations—review status and update as indicated—contact CDC and AAP for updated recommended childhood and adolescent schedules; inform parents of common side effects: http://www.cdc.gov/vaccines/schedules/index.html
  b. Advise parents of any medications prescribed, including vitamins and fluoride, e.g., on name, rationale, dosage, frequency, and potential side effects
  c. Nutrition
      (1) Nutritional requirements are approximately 70 cal/kg
      (2) Most behavioral problems with food resolved
      (3) Potential nutritional problems—obesity, iron deficiency
      (4) Encourage good nutritional practices (e.g., balanced meals, nutritious snacks, no meal skipping)
  d. Development characteristics and behaviors
      (1) Ages 6 to 7—nervous mannerisms, restless activity, egocentric thinking, rigid superego
      (2) Ages 8 to 10—takes on idols and heroes, friends serve as allies against adults, less rigid superego
      (3) Ages 10 to 12—increased self-awareness and self-consciousness; body image concerns; mood swings, stormy behavior; need for independence
      (4) Inform parents that use of inappropriate language may occur
      (5) Prepare for pubertal changes and menstruation in girls
      (6) Discuss with parents the importance of and strategies for bolstering the child's self-esteem
  e. Good health habits—assist child and parents to establish early patterns of behavior, e.g., regular exercise; sufficient sleep; regular dental care; avoidance of drugs, alcohol, tobacco
  f. Communication—encourage parents to assist child in developing good communication skills, problem-solving strategies, and stress management
  g. Drugs, smoking, and alcohol—encourage parent–child discussions

h. Sex education—anatomy and physiology, sexual activity, values clarification, decision making, contraception, prevention of STIs and HIV

i. Parenting strategies

   (1) Although the child is maturing, quality time, attention, and affection from parents is important (evidence exists supporting "connectedness" to parents and/or another adult decreases risk-taking behaviors)

   (2) Encourage independence and decision making

   (3) Promote responsibility and accountability by assigning appropriate chores

   (4) Maintain adequate supervision

   (5) Discuss methods of discipline; use positive reinforcement and appropriate consequences for inappropriate behavior

   (6) Establish fair rules

   (7) Respect the child's need for privacy

   (8) Set example by being a good role model

   (9) Provide child with an allowance

   (10) Encourage movies and TV programming and video games that are appropriate for child's developmental level

   (11) Praise child for achievements

   (12) Encourage consistent school attendance

   (13) Refer parents to resources that can assist them in building assets and preventing psychosocial morbidities (Lewin & Graham, 2012). KySS is a national effort by the National Association of Pediatric Nurse Practitioners (NAPNAP) to decrease emotional and behavioral problems in children and adolescents

j. Safety

   (1) Bicycle, skateboarding, rollerblading; use of helmets and protective padding

   (2) Seat belt use

   (3) Prevention of sexual abuse, e.g., inappropriate touching; what to do if it occurs

   (4) Water safety; swimming

   (5) Fire prevention safety; home fire drill, proper use of appliances

   (6) Sunburn prevention

   (7) Prevention of violence in home; lock up guns, ammunition; teach child firearm safety (avoidance of firearms)

   (8) Pedestrian safety

k. Lying and cheating (common in school-age children)

   (1) School-age children lie to avoid trouble or gain an advantage

   (2) Appropriate response—confront child in a positive way, try to understand reason for lie, follow through with age-appropriate discipline when needed

   (3) Adults should model honesty

l. Sports

   (1) For 6- to 8-year-olds, sports participation should be noncompetitive and focused on learning rules, teamwork, and having fun

   (2) Older school-aged children and teenagers should have a preparticipation physical examination

m. Emphasize positive qualities of the child and the parent–child relationship and mutually agree upon a plan with the parent to strengthen needed areas

n. Initiate referrals as needed

o. Schedule for next visit

- Interim Visits: Adolescents—Annual Visit (13 to 18 Years)

1. Subjective information—gather "sensitive" information when alone with the adolescent

  a. Nutrition—especially appetite; meal-skipping

  b. Elimination—especially use of aids such as laxatives, diuretics

  c. Sleep practices

  d. Development—special emphasis on assessment of mental and emotional health (including school performance and attendance; self-esteem, friends and relationships; family functioning and "connectedness"; hobbies; activities; work; stress and anger management; coping skills; risk-taking behaviors, such as driving while drinking and use of weapons; violent or aggressive behavior; ideations about hurting self or others)

  e. Allergies

  f. Medications

  g. Drug, alcohol, cigarette, and caffeine consumption

  h. Sexual activities, reproductive issues

  i. Concerns/worries; current and recent stressors

  j. Interim health since last visit—include review of systems, with special emphasis on gathering psychological and sexual/reproductive data

  k. Specific questions when alone with parent

    (1) Family communication patterns and relationship with the adolescent

    (2) Parent's description of the adolescent's strengths and areas needing improvement; attitudes and behaviors

    (3) Discipline practices and response

    (4) Specific concerns and worries about the adolescent

2. Objective data

  a. Observation of parent–adolescent interaction (e.g., parental support of adolescent; does the parent allow the adolescent to answer questions)

  b. Height and weight, including percentiles

  c. Vital signs, including blood pressure

  d. Vision and hearing screening (refer to screening guidelines earlier in this chapter)

  e. Physical examination—including scoliosis screen, Tanner stage, and breast examination; pelvic examination if adolescent female is sexually active, is having irregular menses, or is older than 16 years of age

  f. Laboratory

    (1) Urinalysis if sexually active

    (2) Hematocrit if indicated

    (3) VDRL, GC, chlamydia, and HIV if sexually active or history of sexual abuse

(4) Pap smear if pelvic examination performed

(5) Liver function tests (if history of drug usage); cholesterol, if indicated

(6) Mantoux test for TB screening if at risk

3. Management

a. Update immunizations—contact CDC and AAP for updated recommended childhood and adolescent schedules; http://www.cdc.gov/vaccines/schedules/index.html

b. Advise regarding any medications prescribed, e.g., include name, rationale, dosage, frequency, course, and potential side effects

c. Nutrition appropriate for age

(1) The adolescent diet should be similar to an active adult, with extra calories during rapid growth periods; prudent consumption of high-fat foods, e.g., red meats, butter, and eggs

(2) Nutritional issues—irregular meals, chaotic lifestyle; increase in meals eaten away from home; increase in snacks; skipping of meals; fad diets; vegetarianism

(3) Potential nutritional problems—increased need for calcium, iron, zinc; eating disorders; obesity

(4) Encourage well-balanced meals and nutritious snacks

(5) Discuss adolescent's perception of his/her weight

(6) Encourage healthy weight loss strategies if indicated, e.g., healthy food choices, regular exercise

d. Safety—same as school-age child, plus:

(1) Emphasize the possible consequences of drinking and use of drugs while driving

(2) Discourage being a passenger when the driver has been drinking or using drugs

(3) Discuss typical high-risk situations and how to avoid them; role-play healthy behaviors to use in high-risk situations

(4) Encourage safe swimming and diving practices

(5) Discuss proper use of safe sports equipment and maintenance

(6) Instruct adolescent in proper training and warm-up exercises for sports and physical activities

(7) Educate regarding safe and proper use of firearms and other potentially dangerous objects such as firecrackers

(8) Discuss use and misuse of over-the-counter medications

e. Developmental Issues

(1) Discuss dating and peer pressure

(2) Encourage open communication with parents, peers, and school personnel

(3) Teach stress reduction techniques and coping skills

(4) Educate regarding healthy outlets for anger

(5) Discuss plans for the future—further education, work, recreation, hobbies, marriage, parenthood

(6) Educate regarding acne—e.g., cause, myths, and proper skin care

f. Discuss issues related to sexuality—decision making; mature relationships; assertiveness; safe sex/prevention of STIs, including HIV; pregnancy and contraception; implications of potential parenthood; "normalcy" of occasional masturbation

g. Encourage good health habits—e.g., regular exercise, sufficient sleep, regular dental care

h. Continue education regarding use of drugs, alcohol, cigarettes, and caffeine

i. Inform parents of major developmental characteristics of adolescents

(1) Increased self-awareness, self-consciousness, and self-appraisal

(2) Body image concerns

(3) Mood swings and stormy behavior

(4) Need for independence

(5) Using peer values as criteria with which to judge own values, but still needing family to provide acceptance and feeling of self-worth

(6) Interest in opposite sex

j. Parenting strategies with adolescents

(1) Fairness in rules and reasonable limit setting

(2) Allow decision making

(3) Respect adolescent's privacy

(4) Expect periods of estrangement (be available; adolescent needs supportive family)

(5) Praise achievements at home, school, extracurricular activities

(6) Bolster self-esteem

(7) Supervision as needed

(8) Encourage independence, new experiences, after-school activities, including part-time job

(9) Promote family communication

(10) Serve as role model—practice good health habits, e.g., parents should not smoke if they do not want child to imitate their behavior

(11) Recognize signs of probable substance abuse—drop in school performance, personality change, mood swings, sleepiness or fatigue, depression

k. Emphasize positive qualities of the adolescent and the parent–adolescent relationship and mutually agree upon a plan to strengthen needed areas

l. Make referrals as needed

m. Refer parents to resources that can assist them in building their teen's assets as well as with their parenting skills

n. Schedule for next visit

☐ QUESTIONS

Select the best answer.

1. Sixteen-year-old Sarah makes the following statements to you during a health visit. Which of the following pieces of information should not be kept confidential?
   a. "I have been sexually active with three of my boyfriends."
   b. "I sometimes smoke marijuana."
   c. "I want to get pregnant."
   d. "Sometimes I feel like ending my life."

2. In performing a physical examination of a 9-month-old infant, which of the following developmental fears would not be appropriate for you to consider?
   a. Stranger anxiety
   b. Pain
   c. Separation from parents
   d. Bodily harm

3. When performing a physical examination of a toddler, which of the following body parts would you examine last?
   a. Heart and lungs
   b. Abdomen and genitals
   c. Ears and throat
   d. Hips and extremities

4. Role-play with equipment during the course of a physical examination would be most beneficial with which of the following age groups?
   a. Toddlers
   b. Preschoolers
   c. Young school-age children
   d. Older school-age children

5. Providing reassurance of "normalcy" during the course of an examination would be most important for:
   a. Preschool children
   b. Young school-age children
   c. Older school-age children
   d. Adolescents

6. Which of the following would not elevate the pulse of a child?
   a. Fever
   b. Anemia
   c. Hypothyroidism
   d. Exercise

7. The PNP recognizes which of the following signs as indicators that a baby is not receiving sufficient breastmilk?
   a. Sleepiness, jaundice, and decreased urine and stool
   b. Diarrhea, nausea, and vomiting
   c. Bulging fontanel and irritability
   d. Sleeplessness and excitability

8. Blood pressure should be measured at well-child visits beginning at age:
   a. 2 years
   b. 3 years
   c. 4 years
   d. 5 years

9. A wide pulse pressure that results from a high systolic blood pressure is usually not due to which of the following?
   a. Fever
   b. Exercise
   c. Excitement
   d. A patent ductus arteriosus

10. Head and chest circumferences should be equal at:
    a. 6 months of age
    b. 1 year of age
    c. 2 years of age
    d. 3 years of age

11. The anterior fontanel usually closes by:
    a. 2 months of age
    b. 6 months of age
    c. 18 months of age
    d. 24 months of age

12. Diffuse edema of the soft tissue of the scalp that usually crosses suture lines in the newborn is:
    a. Bossing
    b. Caput succedaneum
    c. Cephalohematoma
    d. Macrocephaly

13. An infant should no longer have a head lag when pulled from the supine to sitting position at what age?
    a. 2 months
    b. 4 months
    c. 6 months
    d. 9 months

14. "Boggy" nasal mucous membranes with serous drainage upon examination usually suggest:
    a. Sinusitis
    b. Polyps
    c. URI
    d. Allergic rhinitis

15. A white instead of red reflex upon eye examination of a 1-year-old child would suggest:
    a. An accommodative error
    b. Retinoblastoma
    c. Papilledema
    d. Retinal detachment

16. A cobblestone appearance of the palpebral conjunctiva usually indicates:
    a. Bacterial infection
    b. Chemical irritation
    c. Viral infection
    d. Severe allergy

17. An eye that deviates in when covered but that returns to midline when uncovered is an:
    a. Esophoria
    b. Exophoria
    c. Esotropia
    d. Exotropia

18. Pain produced by manipulation of the auricle or pressure on the tragus suggests:
    a. Acute otitis media
    b. Otitis externa
    c. Otitis media with effusion
    d. Mastoiditis
19. A hypernasal voice and snoring in a child is suggestive of:
    a. Polyps of the larynx
    b. Nasopharyngeal tumor
    c. Hypertrophied adenoids
    d. Cleft palate
20. Physiologic splitting of the second heart sound during inspiration in a child:
    a. Is normal
    b. Should be evaluated with an EKG
    c. Suggests an ASD
    d. Should be referred to a cardiologist
21. Which of the following is not characteristic of innocent heart murmurs in children?
    a. Systolic in timing
    b. Varies in loudness with positioning
    c. Usually transmitted to the neck
    d. Usually loudest at lower left sternal border or at second or third intercostal space
22. A Grade II musical or vibratory murmur heard best at the lower left sternal border that changes with positioning is suggestive of a:
    a. Pulmonary ejection murmur
    b. Ventricular septal defect
    c. Venous hum
    d. Vibratory or Still's murmur
23. Wheezing in a child may not be found in which of the following conditions?
    a. Asthma
    b. Bronchiolitis
    c. Pleural friction rub
    d. Cystic fibrosis
24. Gynecomastia in a male may not be a finding in which of the following?
    a. Normal pubertal development
    b. Steroid usage
    c. Hypothyroidism
    d. Testicular tumor
25. Which of the following would usually not be considered a sign of a pituitary tumor in an adolescent female?
    a. Dysfunctional uterine bleeding
    b. Galactorrhea
    c. Loss of peripheral vision
    d. Increase in headaches
26. Which of the following is not a specific examination test for a dislocated hip?
    a. Barlow's test
    b. Ortolani's test
    c. Trendelenburg test
    d. Gower's test

27. In addition to the knee, which of the following should be examined in a child complaining of knee pain?
    a. Foot
    b. Ankle
    c. Hip
    d. Spine
28. Which of the following infant reflexes should not disappear by 6 months of age?
    a. Moro
    b. Rooting
    c. Tonic neck
    d. Plantar grasp
29. Spasticity in an infant may be an early sign of:
    a. Neurofibromatosis
    b. Hydrocephalus
    c. Cerebral palsy
    d. Muscular dystrophy
30. A shift to the left is present when which of the following are elevated?
    a. Neutrophils
    b. Bands or stabs
    c. Lymphocytes
    d. Eosinophils
31. Which of the following is usually elevated with viral infections?
    a. Neutrophils
    b. Eosinophils
    c. Lymphocytes
    d. Basophils
32. Decreased platelets may not be found in which of the following?
    a. Leukemia
    b. Anemia
    c. ITP
    d. Medication usage (e.g., ampicillin, cephalothin)
33. Which of the following does not suggest a urinary tract infection?
    a. Increased protein
    b. Increased WBCs
    c. Increased RBCs
    d. Increased nitrites
34. A Mantoux test in a child with no risk factors is considered positive with a reaction of:
    a. At least 5 mm induration
    b. At least 8 mm induration
    c. At least 10 mm induration
    d. At least 15 mm induration
35. The PNP teaches new parents that when breastfeeding is well established they can expect baby to have:
    a. As many as 4 wet diapers each day
    b. A stool every 2–3 days
    c. One wet diaper an hour
    d. Five to 6 wet diapers and 2–3 stools each day
36. Cholesterol screening should be done:
    a. On children 2 years of age and older who have a parent with a total cholesterol level of 240 mg/dL or greater
    b. Once for all children at 6 years of age

c. On overweight children with a family history of premature cardiovascular disease

d. Once for all children at 12 years of age

37. For which of the following screening tests should children fast for 12 hours before the test is administered?
a. Total cholesterol
b. Serum chemistry profile
c. Serum lipid profile
d. Hematocrit

38. Which of the following is the most important history-taking question for a sports evaluation?
a. Has the child ever had a head injury?
b. Has the child ever fainted or lost consciousness during exercise?
c. Does the child ever get short of breath with exercise?
d. Has the child ever undergone surgery?

39. Which of the following conditions would not exclude a child from participating in contact collision sports?
a. Fever
b. Absence of a paired organ
c. Atlantoaxial instability
d. Prior head injury

40. Which of the following topics would not be appropriate to include when providing anticipatory guidance to the parent of a 6-month-old infant?
a. Introduction of solid foods
b. Teething
c. Negativism
d. Introduction of a cup

41. Which is the correct order for introduction of solid foods to an infant?
a. Fruits, cereal, vegetables, and meats
b. Cereal, meats, vegetables, and fruits
c. Fruits, cereal, meats, and vegetables
d. Cereal, vegetables, fruits, and meats

42. Which of the following topics is not appropriate to include when providing anticipatory guidance to the parent of an 18-month-old?
a. Temper tantrums
b. Toilet training
c. Dental care
d. Stranger anxiety

43. Appropriate anticipatory guidance for the parents of an 8-year-old girl should not include:
a. Preparation for an increase in nervous mannerisms and restless activity
b. Preparation for pubertal changes
c. Information that friends begin to serve as allies against adults
d. Information that their daughter will take on idols and heroes

44. A new mom calls the PNP on postpartum day 5. She reports her newborn wants to nurse for 30 minutes every 2 hours. Which of the following is your best response?
a. "This is a very healthy breastfeeding pattern. Be sure to rest when you can. You are doing a great job."

b. "Your baby is too demanding. If you continue to feed that often, you will spoil your child."
c. "You are not making enough milk, and your baby will need to go to the ER to be evaluated."
d. "Your baby has an oral fixation, and you should offer a pacifier to relieve stress."

45. A pelvic examination should not be performed on which of the following adolescents?
a. A 14-year-old who is sexually active
b. A 15-year-old who has just started menarche
c. A 17-year-old who is having irregular menses
d. A 21-year-old healthy female

46. A 2-month-old infant at your clinic received a combined DTaP/HepB/IPV vaccine, and the parents are in need of teaching about possible side effects. Which of the following is not an adverse effect following administration of the DTaP vaccination?
a. Local reaction
b. Fever
c. Increased fussiness
d. Transient morbilliform rash

47. When reviewing immunization protocols at your clinic, you are aware that the varicella vaccine can be administered to susceptible children beginning at what age?
a. 4 months
b. 6 months
c. 12 months
d. 15 months

48. The mother of a 15-month-old child informs you that she feeds the baby skim milk. You advise the mother to change to whole milk primarily because skim milk:
a. Is not as easily digested as whole milk
b. Contains an insufficient amount of calcium
c. Contains too little protein
d. Provides an inadequate amount of essential fatty acids

49. A 12-year-old boy is brought into the clinic for an urgent visit after having ingested 10 diazepam tablets. Following the initial emergent care and stabilization of the child, the most important aspect of your management is:
a. Referring the case to social services
b. Assessing the family supports available to the child
c. Obtaining a psychiatric consultation
d. Reviewing the history for signs of depression

50. You are seeing a 15-month-old boy with leukemia for a check-up. If indicated, this child may receive all of the following vaccines except:
a. Inactivated polio vaccine (IPV)
b. *H. influenzae* type B (Hib)
c. Diphtheria, tetanus, acellular pertussis (DTaP)
d. Varicella (VAR)

51. While conducting the Denver II developmental screening test, the mother of an 18-month-old child reports to you that the toddler does not imitate

activities. You decide to assess the child's development further by giving him tasks from which sector?
a. Personal-social
b. Fine motor-adaptive
c. Language
d. Gross motor

52. You have ordered routine blood screening for a 2-year-old girl who, because of dietary habits, is at risk for iron-deficiency anemia. Which of the following findings is not associated with iron-deficiency anemia?
a. Hypochromic RBC
b. Microcytic RBC
c. Low reticulocyte count
d. Low free erythrocyte protoporphyrin (FEP) level

53. During a prenatal visit, you review the mother's record for routine prenatal screening results. While educating the mother, you explain that the screening of maternal serum for alpha-fetoprotein (MSAFP) between the 15th and 21st weeks of pregnancy is done primarily to screen for:
a. Phenylketonuria
b. Galactosemia
c. Cystic fibrosis
d. Neural tube defects

54. A tenderness is detected over the tibial tuberosity of a 10-year-old boy during a routine examination at a school-based clinic. The PNP knows this may be a sign of:
a. Osgood-Schlatter disease
b. Blount's disease
c. Plantar fasciitis
d. Effusion in the joint space

55. The parents of a 1-week-old infant are concerned about the unusual shape of their child's head. In the physical examination of the infant, which of the following signs would not support a diagnosis of craniosynostosis?
a. Palpation of a ridge along a given suture line
b. Unusual skull configuration
c. A palpable lesion at the occipital region
d. Abnormal head circumference

56. In the emergency room, you encounter a toddler whose injuries are not consistent with the history that is given. Which of the following would be the best step you could take to foster communication with abusive parents?
a. Realize that abusive parents have essentially different goals for their children than other caregivers do
b. Understand that parental hostility and resistance are potent symptoms of fear and inadequacy
c. Consider referring the parents to a substance abuse program
d. Be cautious when sharing the results of medical findings

57. You are preparing a drug prevention program for middle school students. Your educational approach is based on the knowledge that the most common substance of abuse in adolescence is:
a. Marijuana
b. Cocaine
c. Heroin
d. Alcohol

58. During a check-up of a 15-month-old girl, you note that the child has dropped significantly in percentile for weight over the past few months. In evaluating a child with failure to thrive, the most important part of your assessment involves:
a. The history
b. The physical examination
c. Laboratory studies
d. Observation of family interactions

59. A 7-year-old child in your caseload has recently been placed on methylphenidate for behavioral concerns associated with ADHD. Which of the following side effects is not associated with this drug?
a. Decreased appetite
b. Weight gain
c. Irritability
d. Decreased heart rate

60. The parents of an 8-year-old child are concerned that their son does not want to attend school. Which of the following historical findings are not usually associated with the diagnosis of school phobia?
a. Sporadic school absence
b. Chronic medical illness
c. Vague physical symptoms
d. Depression and anxiety

61. A 17-year-old girl is referred to your clinic by the school nurse to be assessed for an eating disorder. Which of the following dynamics is not characteristic of anorexia nervosa?
a. Excessive eating followed by purging
b. A pervasive sense of helplessness and ineffectiveness
c. Weight loss that gives the patient a sense of mastery and control
d. Low body temperature, pulse rate, and blood pressure

☐ ANSWERS AND RATIONALES

1. D: Any statements a patient makes that entail harm of self or others are not covered by patient confidentiality guidelines.

2. D: A 9-month-old infant is not capable of such higher-order thinking.

3. C: Ears and throat examination is most threatening to the toddler and likely to produce resistance during the examination.

4. B: Preschoolers engage in imaginative play and are more easily engaged in this activity.

5. D: Adolescents have heightened concerns regarding body image. They fear that they are abnormal and would be reassured by this behavior.

6. C: Hypothyroidism decreases body metabolism, and the others cause an increase in body metabolism and subsequent pulse rate.

7. A: Decreased intake would cause decreased alertness and decreased excretion of bilirubin due to decreased urine and stool output.

8. B: At age 3 years, per AAP recommendations for preventive pediatric health care.

9. D: Pulse pressure is the difference between systolic and diastolic blood pressures (normal is 20 to 50 mm Hg). A wide pulse pressure from high systolic pressure is usually due to fever, exercise, or excitement. A wide pulse pressure from low diastolic pressure is usually due to patent ductus arteriosus, aortic regurgitation, or other serious heart disease.

10. B: Head circumference is approximately 2 cm larger than chest during the first year of life; head and chest circumferences should be equal at 1 year of age; during childhood, chest is usually 5 to 7 cm larger than head.

11. C: The posterior fontanel closes at 2 months, and the anterior fontanel closes at 18 months.

12. B: Caput succedaneum crosses the suture lines, whereas a cephalohematoma does not. Macrocephaly is enlarged head circumference, and bossing is fullness of the frontal area.

13. C: By 6 months of age, there should be no head lag when infant is pulled from supine to sitting position; if present, it may indicate neuromuscular disorder; may be the first sign of cerebral palsy.

14. D: Boggy nasal mucous membranes (bluish, pale, edematous) with serous drainage indicates allergic rhinitis.

15. B: White spots (leukokoria) within the area of either or both red reflexes is an abnormal red reflex and should be immediately referred to an ophthalmologist for a more complete examination to rule out a retinoblastoma.

16. D: A cobblestone appearance of the conjunctiva is consistent with allergic conjunctivitis.

17. A: Esophoria is inward (*eso*) as opposed to outward (*exo*) movement of the eye when covered (*phoria*, as opposed to *tropia*, which is a movement of the eye without coverage).

18. B: Otitis externa is inflammation of the external auditory canal and is painful with movement of the ear structure.

19. C: A hypernasal voice and/or snoring is characteristic of hypertrophied adenoids.

20. A: Physiologic splitting of the second heart sound during inspiration in a child is normal (refer to cardiac section in this chapter).

21. C: Innocent murmurs rarely transmit to other areas of the body.

22. D: The description is that of an innocent murmur, which is termed vibratory or Still's murmur based on its grade, location, and sound.

23. C: A pleural friction rub causes grating or squeaking sounds as the pleural lining rubs together. It does not cause wheezing.

24. C: Hypothyroidism produces less thyroxine and would not be a risk factor for increasing male estrogen levels, which are responsible for gynecomastia.

25. A: Less frequent or no menstrual periods are a sign of a pituitary tumor, so dysfunctional uterine bleeding would not occur in that disorder. The other symptoms can occur with a pituitary tumor.

26. D: Gower's test is a sign described when a child has to use his hand to "walk" up his own body from a squatting position due to a weakness of the proximal muscles of the lower legs.

27. C: Disorders of the hip often present as knee pain, so hip deformities should be ruled out with a complaint of knee pain.

28. D: Moro reflex is present from birth to 4–6 months, rooting reflex is present from birth to 3–4 months, tonic neck reflex is present from birth (or at 6 weeks) to 4–6 months, and plantar grasp reflex is present from birth to 10–12 months.

29. C: Spasticity is the most common symptom of cerebral palsy. It results from damage to the motor cortex of the brain before, during, or after birth. This part of the brain is responsible for the control of body movements.

30. B: Bands, which are immature WBCs, are elevated with bacterial infections.

31. C: Lymphocytes are WBCs that are elevated with viral infections.

32. B: Anemia is indicated by a decreased hemoglobin/hematocrit and is not a platelet disorder.

33. A: Increased protein may be an indication of a kidney disorder and is not an indication of a urinary tract infection.

34. D: At least 15 mm induration is a positive screen, per the AAP.

35. D: Five to 6 wet diapers and 2–3 stools each day are expected by age 5 or 6 months and beyond.

36. A: Children 2 years of age and older who have a parent with a total cholesterol level of 240 mg/dL or greater are at risk for elevated cholesterol level. It is a recommended screening test for children between 9 and 11 years of age.

37. C: A lipid profile requires fasting to ensure fats ingested prior to the test have been metabolized.

38. B: Fainting or lost consciousness during exercise may indicate an underlying cardiac condition.

39. A: Fever in most cases is a sign of a short-lived illness and does not restrict sports participation unless the underlying cause is a contraindication.

40. C: Negativism is a toddler behavioral characteristic.

41. D: Cereal, because it is easily digested and iron fortified, is good to introduce initially to infants, followed vegetables and fruits, which are good sources of vitamins, followed by meats, which have a high protein

load and are best introduced after the kidneys are more mature.

42. D: Stanger anxiety occurs before 12 months of age.
43. A: Nervous mannerisms and restless activity are not normal behaviors of this age group.
44. A: Breastfeeding patterns can vary the first month, and the infant may feed from 8 to 12 times a day. Mother can monitor void and stool pattern, and pediatric provider can monitor weight gain.
45. B: Initiation of menses is not an indication for a pelvic examination if there are no other concerns.
46. D: A transient morbilliform rash is an adverse effect associated with the MMR vaccine.
47. C: According to the recommended Childhood Immunization Schedule approved by the ACIP and AAP, the varicella vaccine can be administered at 12 months of age.
48. D: All milk (human and cow) is deficient in iron. Skim milk should be avoided until 2 years of age because it provides too few calories, an excess of protein, and an inadequate amount of essential fatty acids.
49. C: Every actively suicidal patient, regardless of apparent seriousness, requires psychiatric consultation and, in some cases, hospitalization.
50. D: Children with cancer and children receiving high-dose corticosteroids or other immunosuppressive agents should not be immunized with live virus or live bacteria vaccines.
51. A: Imitating activities is considered to be a personal-social task.
52. D: Iron-deficiency anemia is a microcytic, hypochromic anemia associated with a low reticulocyte count and elevated FEP level.
53. D: The MSAFP is used primarily to screen for neural tube defects. The other diseases are usually screened for at birth.
54. A: Tenderness over the tibial tubercle may be a sign of Osgood-Schlatter disease. Blount's disease is characterized by severe bowing of the legs, and plantar fasciitis is associated with painful heels.
55. C: Diagnosis of craniosynostosis is suspected as a result of skull configuration, a ridge along a suture line, and abnormal head circumference. Other palpable lesions, which often occur in the occipital region, are not indicative of craniosynostosis.
56. B: Parental fear and inadequacy may be manifested as hostility. Abusive parents generally have similar goals for their children as others and are not any more likely to be substance abusers than nonabusive parents are. Medical findings should be shared with the parents (without necessarily promoting an etiologic conclusion).
57. D: Alcohol is the most common substance of abuse consumed by teenagers.
58. A: The two major causes of poor growth, inadequate intake and social problems, are detected through the history.
59. D: A common side effect of stimulants is a small increase in heart rate or blood pressure.
60. B: Children with chronic medical illness typically strive actively to remain in school. The findings listed in the other answer choices are more likely to be associated with school phobia.
61. A: Excessive eating followed by purging is a sign of bulimia.

☐ BIBLIOGRAPHY

Academy of Breastfeeding Medicine. (n.d.). Home page. Retrieved from http://www.bfmed.org/

Academy of Breastfeeding Medicine. (n.d.). Statements and clinical protocols. Retrieved from http://www.bfmed.org/Resources/Protocols.aspx

Alaria, A. J., & Birnkrant, J. D. (Eds.). (2008). *Practical guide to the care of the pediatric patient* (2nd ed.). Philadelphia, PA: Mosby Elsevier.

American Academy of Pediatrics. (2003). Oral health risk assessment timing and establishment of the dental home. *Pediatrics, 111*(5), 1113–1116. Retrieved from http://pediatrics.aappublications.org/content/111/5/1113.full

American Academy of Pediatrics. (2008). Red reflex examination in neonates, infants and children. *Pediatrics, 122*(6), 1401–1404.

American Academy of Pediatrics. (2014a). Recommendations for pediatric preventive health care. *Pediatrics, 133*(3), 568–570. Retrieved from http://pediatrics.aappublications.org/content/133/3/568.full

American Academy of Pediatrics. (2014b). Screening for nonviral sexually transmitted infections in adolescents and young adults. *Pediatrics, 134*(1), e302–e311. Retrieved from http://pediatrics.aappublications.org/content/134/1/e302

BiliTool. (n.d.). Nomogram for bilirubinemia in newborns. Retrieved from http://bilitool.org/

Centers for Disease Control and Prevention. (2012). Recommendation of the Advisory Committee on Childhood Lead Level Prevention Poisoning. Retrieved http://www.cdc.gov/nceh/lead/acclpp/acclpp_main.htm

Centers for Disease Control and Prevention. (2015). Immunization schedules. Retrieved from http://www.cdc.gov/vaccines/schedules/index.html

Daniels, S. R., Greer, F. R., & the Committee on Nutrition. (2008). Lipid screening and cardiovascular health in children. *American Academy of Pediatrics, 122*(1), 198–208.

Engorn, B., & Flerlage, J. (2014). *The Harriet Lane handbook* (20th ed.). St. Louis, MO: Mosby.

Gutierrez, E., Silbert-Flagg, J., & Vohra, S. (2015). Management of natural health products in pediatrics: A provider-focused quality improvement project. *Journal of Pediatric Health Care, 29*(3), 137–144. DOI: http://dx.doi.org/

Hagan, J. F., & Duncan, P. (Eds.). (2008). *Bright futures: Guidelines for health supervision of infants, children, and adolescents* (3rd ed.). Elk Grove Village, IL: American Academy of Pediatrics.

Hale, T. W., & Rowe, H. (2014). *Medications and mothers' milk* (16th ed.). Amarillo, TX: Hale Publishing.

Hay, W., Levin, M., Deterin, R., & Azbug, M. (2014). *Current diagnosis and treatment pediatrics* (22nd ed.). New York, NY: McGraw-Hill/Appleton & Lange.

Lewin, L., & Graham, G. (2012). Interpersonal violence: Secondary analysis of the Keep Your Children/Yourself Safe and Secure (KySS) data. *Journal of Pediatric Health Care, 26*(2), 102–108.

National Institutes of Health & National Heart, Lung, and Blood Institute. (2005). *Fourth report on the diagnosis, evaluation, and treatment of high blood pressure in children and adolescents.* Retrieved from https://www.nhlbi.nih.gov/files/docs/resources/heart/hbp_ped.pdf

Newborn Weight Tool. (n.d.). Nomogram newborn weight. Retrieved from https://www.newbornweight.org/chart/

Nice, F. J. (2011). *Nonprescription drugs for the breastfeeding mother* (2nd ed.). Amarillo, TX: Hale Publishing.

Physicians for Social Responsibility. (n.d.). Pediatric environmental health toolkit. Retrieved from http://www.psr.org/resources/pediatric-toolkit.html

Pickering, L. K., Baker, C. J., Kimberlin, D. W., & Long, S. S. (Eds.). (2012). *Red book online.* Retrieved from http://redbook.solutions.aap.org/book.aspx?bookid=886

Rice, S. G., & Council on Sports Medicine and Fitness. (2008). Medical conditions affecting sports participation. *Pediatrics, 121*(4), 841–847.

Schanler, R. J. (*Ed.*). (2013). *Breastfeeding handbook for physicians* (2nd ed.). Elk Grove Village, IL: American Academy of Pediatrics & American College of Obstetricians and Gynecologists.

Seidel, H. M., Rosenstein, B. J., Pathak, A., & McKay, W. H. (Eds.). (2006). *Primary care of the newborn* (4th ed.). Philadelphia, PA: Saunders Elsevier.

Subcommittee on Urinary Tract Infection, Steering Committee on Quality Improvement and Management. (2011). Urinary tract infection: Clinical practice guideline for the diagnosis and management of the initial UTI in febrile infants and children 2 to 24 months. *Pediatrics, 128*(3), 595–610. Retrieved from http://pediatrics.aappublications.org/content/early/2011/08/24/peds.2011-1330.full.pdf

Taylor, J., Geyer, L., & Feldman, K. (2010). Use of supplemental vitamin D among infants breastfed for prolonged periods. *Pediatrics, 125*(1), 105–111.

U.S. Department of Health and Human Services. (2003, May). *Summary of the HIPAA Privacy Rule.* Washington, DC: Author. Retrieved from http://www.hhs.gov/ocr/privacy/hipaa/understanding/summary/privacysummary.pdf

Vaccine Adverse Event Reporting System. (2015). Home page. Retrieved from http://vaers.hhs.gov/index

☐ ADDITIONAL BIBLIOGRAPHY

Health Insurance Portability and Accountability Act (HIPAA) of 1996 (U.S. Department of Health and Human Services [DHHS], 2003) http://www.hhs.gov/ocr/privacy/hipaa/understanding/summary/privacysummary.pdf

b. Nonobstructive or communicating hydrocephalus
   (1) Impairment of CSF absorption within sub-arachnoid space
   (2) Usually caused by scarring due to subarachnoid hemorrhage (result of intraventricular hemorrhage in the premature infant) or meningitis
- Signs and Symptoms: Presentation is variable depending on age and etiology
  1. Birth to 12 months—apparent large head, sluggish feeding, vomiting, piercing cry, and irritability
  2. 12 months through adolescence—signs of increased intracranial pressure (ICP), headache following sleep, lethargy or irritability, confusion, personality changes, possible decline in academic performance, signs and symptoms related to specific focal lesion or tumor, possible sixth nerve palsies, chronic papilledema
- Differential Diagnosis
  1. Macrocephaly
  2. Megalencephaly
  3. Benign large head
  4. Macrocrania
  5. Meningitis
  6. Sepsis
  7. Tumor
- Physical Findings
  1. Infancy—bulging anterior fontanel, scalp vein distention, bossing, "setting sun sign," separated skull sutures, slow PERRL (pupils equal, round, reactive to light), hypertonia, hyperreflexia, spasticity
  2. Childhood—strabismus, extrapyramidal tract signs (ataxia), papilledema, optic atrophy, growth failure from endocrine dysfunction
- Diagnostic Tests/Findings
  1. Cranial radiograph—separated sutures
  2. CT scan/ultrasound—impaired CSF circulation causing ventricular enlargement
  3. Ventriculography—obstruction detection
- Management/Treatment
  1. Most cases require extracranial shunts, particularly ventriculoperitoneal types
  2. Treatment of underlying cause, e.g., mass or lesion, inflammation, infection, vasogenic edema
  3. Anticipatory guidance for families and caregivers throughout child's life
     a. Referral to support groups
     b. Teaching signs and symptoms of ICP
     c. Daily head circumference measurements
     d. Management of psychomotor challenges

Caput Succedaneum

- Definition: Diffuse swelling of soft tissue of the newborn's scalp, which usually crosses suture lines with possible bruising
- Etiology/Incidence: Result of compression or trauma to scalp during descent of the baby through birth canal, causing edema of scalp

- Signs and Symptoms
  1. Nonpitting swelling of the scalp, typically present at birth, tending to overlie the occipital bones and some of the parietal bones
  2. Some cases with bruising; often with molding
  3. Typically disappears within the first few days of life
- Differential Diagnosis
  1. Cephalohematoma
  2. Subgaleal hematoma
- Diagnostic Tests/Findings: None
- Management/Treatment
  1. Usually unnecessary with spontaneous resolution within a few days
  2. If extensive ecchymosis, may require phototherapy for hyperbilirubinemia

Cephalohematoma

- Definition: Subperiosteal collection of blood bound by suture lines, usually those surrounding the parietal bones
- Etiology/Incidence
  1. Approximately 0.4% to 2.5% of all deliveries
  2. Most commonly due to a low subperiosteal bleed, secondary to trauma from a difficult delivery (e.g., large infant, prolonged labor, forceps use, abnormal presentation)
  3. Uncommonly may be due to a coagulopathy or intracranial hemorrhage
  4. 25% overlie a linear skull fracture—not depressed; rarely of any clinical significance
- Signs and Symptoms
  1. Not evident at birth but typically presents hours to days after delivery
  2. Limited to periosteum at suture margins; usually unilateral, but occasionally bilateral
  3. May prolong neonatal jaundice from the resorption of a large hematoma
- Differential Diagnosis
  1. Caput succedaneum
  2. Cranial meningocele
- Physical Findings: Nonecchymotic swelling of parietal area that does not cross suture lines; soft, fluctuant
- Diagnostic Tests: None
- Management/Treatment
  1. Usually unnecessary with slow resolution over a few weeks/months
  2. Calcification of hematoma possible; may be felt as bony prominence
  3. Observance for hyperbilirubinemia

Craniosynostosis

- Definition: Premature closure of one or more of the cranial sutures, resulting in a skull deformity. Normally, suture line should remain open until 2–3 years of age.

The craniosynostosis is named according to the suture that has closed prematurely

- Etiology
  1. Primary—due to pathology at the suture line; cause unknown in majority of cases but in approximately 10% to 20% of cases due to a genetic syndrome or familial pattern
  2. Secondary—due to underlying brain pathology such as failure of brain growth (microcephaly); uncommon cause
- Signs/Symptoms
  1. Abnormal head shape
  2. Head size often small but depends on which suture is closed
  3. Typically no symptoms unless part of a genetic syndrome or multiple suture closures; rarely may develop signs/symptoms of increased intracranial pressure
  4. FH of abnormal head shape and/or genetic syndrome
- Differential Diagnosis
  1. Molding in newborn
  2. Pseudosynostosis positional plagiocephaly
- Physical Exam
  1. Abnormal head shape
  2. Palpable bony ridge along affected suture line
  3. Anterior fontanel may be large or small depending on suture closing
- Diagnostic Tests/Findings
  1. Plain skull x-rays can identify
  2. Chromosomal analysis if indicated
- Management
  1. Surgery to open fused suture
  2. Performed primarily for cosmetic reasons, unless neurologic complications

☐ EYE

Conjunctivitis of the Newborn (Ophthalmia Neonatorum)

- Definition: Infection and/or inflammation of conjunctiva in first month of life
- Etiology/Incidence
  1. Chemical—irritation from use of ophthalmic preparations at birth. Decreased incidence since the discontinuation of silver nitrate. Erythromycin ophthalmic ointment 0.5% is now the recommended and only agent used for this purpose. (Recommended alternatives can be found on the Centers for Disease Control and Prevention [CDC] website if shortages of erythromycin occur as happened in 2009)
  2. Gonococcal—perinatal transmission of *Neisseria gonorrhoeae*; prophylactic treatment with erythromycin ophthalmic ointment. Previously used agents such as silver nitrate 1% tetracycline and povidone-iodine 2.5% are no longer used or available
  3. Chlamydia (Inclusion)—perinatal transmission of *Chlamydia trachomatis* during vaginal birth; most

common cause of neonatal conjunctivitis in the United States with an incidence of 8.2/1000 births.
  4. Herpes simplex virus (HSV)—uncommon cause but may result in loss of vision and requires immediate attention. Mothers may be asymptomatic.
  5. Other pathogens include the same bacteria that causes childhood conjunctivitis such as *Haemophilus influenzae* and streptococcus pneumonia
- Signs and Symptoms
  1. Chemical—mild injection of conjunctiva, presents several hours following ophthalmic ointment instillation lasting no longer than 3 to 4 days
  2. Gonococcal—acute purulent discharge 2 to 4 days after birth
  3. Chlamydia—usually presents with mild mucopurulent discharge (may be profuse) a few days to several weeks after birth (typically 5th to 14th days)
  4. Herpes—symptoms variable; eye redness, watery discharge usually begins within 2 weeks. May have systemic symptoms
  5. Other bacteria—purulent discharge normally seen on 2nd to 5th days
- Differential Diagnosis
  1. Dacryostenosis
  2. Foreign body
  3. Corneal abrasion
  4. Congenital glaucoma
- Physical Findings
  1. Chemical—conjunctival hyperemia, minimal lid edema, scanty discharge
  2. Gonococcal—chemosis, significant lid edema, profuse purulent discharge
  3. Chlamydia—minimal lid edema, conjunctival hyperemia, chemosis, possible concomitant pneumonia (afebrile, repetitive staccato cough, tachypnea, and rales)
  4. Herpes—usually unilateral, may have small eyelid vesicles, mild conjunctivitis; possible neurologic or systemic symptoms (lethargy, poor feeding)
  5. Other bacteria—mucopurulent discharge, mild symptoms
- Diagnostic Tests/Findings
  1. Gonorrhea tests:
     a. Gram stain of conjunctival scrapings and purulent discharge may reveal Gram-negative intracellular diplococci
     b. Verify by culture (chocolate agar or Thayer Martin medium)
  2. Chlamydia tests
     a. Giemsa stain of conjunctival scrapings may reveal intracytoplasmic inclusion bodies
     b. Direct immunofluorescent antibody staining of conjunctival scrapings for chlamydial inclusions; highly sensitive and specific
     c. Culture using special tissue culture
  3. Herpes simplex virus (HSV)
     a. Fluorescein staining of eye may detect ocular dendritic ulcers

b. Culture—swab submitted in tissue culture media for virus isolation

- Management/Treatment
  1. Chemical—no treatment necessary; resolves spontaneously without sequelae
  2. Gonococcal
     a. Ocular emergency (can cause blindness); hospitalization is necessary
     b. Eye irrigation with normal saline until eye discharge is cleared
     c. Systemic antibiotics, IV or IM cefotaxime or ceftriaxone. Avoid ceftriaxone in newborns with hyperbilirubinemia
     d. Topical eye medication ineffective and unnecessary when systemic therapy is given
  3. Chlamydia
     a. Oral erythromycin—treats the conjunctivitis and may prevent subsequent pneumonia
     b. Oral sulfonamides (trimethoprim, sulfamethoxazole) may be used after the neonatal period if infant is intolerant to erythromycin
     c. Topical treatment ineffective and unnecessary
  4. Herpes simplex virus
     a. Hospitalization is required
     b. Acyclovir is first line (parenteral)
     c. Topical ophthalmic preparations adjunct therapy; 0.1% iododeoxyuridine, 1–2% trifluridine, or 3% vidarabine
  5. Other bacteria—topical antibiotics such as erythromycin, polymixin-bacitracin, and tobramycin are adequate; warm compresses to remove exudate
  6. Stress thorough hand washing, no sharing of washcloths or towels
  7. Mothers and sexual partner(s) should also be treated appropriately

Conjunctivitis of Childhood

- Definition: Inflammation and/or infection of palpebral (lining of eyelids) and bulbar (layer of tissue over the sclera) conjunctiva in children 1 month or older
- Etiology/Incidence
  1. Most frequent ocular disorder in children
  2. Very contagious, especially in day care and school settings
  3. Infectious causes
     a. Bacterial conjunctivitis—most common pathogens include *Staphylococcus aureus, H. influenzae, Streptococcus pneumoniae,* and *Moraxella catarrhalis;* Conjunctivitis-otitis syndrome occurs in about 25% of young children (<3 years) and most often associated with *H. influenzae;* typically in ipsilateral eye/ear
     b. Viral conjunctivitis primarily due to adenoviruses 3, 4, and 7; uncommonly caused by herpes simplex and varicella zoster; adenoviral conjunctivitis can occur in isolation or as part of a viral illness (e.g., pharyngoconjunctival fever)

4. Allergic and vernal (chronic allergic) conjunctivitis—commonly associated with seasonal allergens (pollens, grasses), but other allergens such as mold and animal dander may cause symptoms. The cause may be unknown

- Signs and Symptoms
  1. Redness of eyes
  2. Pruritus, foreign body sensation
  3. Mild eye discomfort (burning); severe pain suggests another diagnosis
  4. Discharge
     a. Viral, allergic—watery or thick/stringy mucoid
     b. Bacterial—purulent, glued eyes (lids stuck together after sleeping)
- Differential Diagnosis
  1. Nasolacrimal duct obstruction in infants
  2. Blepharitis in older children
  3. Keratitis—can be seen with herpes simplex conjunctivitis or severe adenovirus (e.g., epidemic keratoconjunctivitis); painful
  4. Systemic infection presenting with conjunctivitis (e.g., rubella, rubeola, Kawasaki); illness symptoms present
  5. Periorbital cellulitis
  6. Eye injury—foreign body, corneal abrasion, chemical or sunlight damage
- Physical Findings
  1. Conjunctival redness, varying degree, one or both eyes. Perilimbal erythema suggests a deeper infection such as uveitis
  2. Discharge may or may not be present
  3. Mild eyelid edema and mild redness; caution—can also be early signs of periorbital cellulitis
  4. Preauricular adenopathy—most commonly seen with viral
  5. Cobblestone-like papillary hypertrophy along inner aspect of upper lid (vernal conjunctivitis)
  6. Follicular changes in the palpebral fornix, especially with viral infections
  7. Systemic symptoms: Allergic (nasal congestion, eczema) infection (fever, pharyngitis)
- Diagnostic Tests/Findings
  1. Cultures and sensitivities usually unnecessary unless *Pseudomonas, Neisseria,* or other virulent organism suspected
  2. Rule out corneal involvement with fluorescein stain
- Management/Treatment
  1. Bacterial—most respond readily to topical ophthalmic antibiotics, e.g., tobramycin, erythromycin, sulfacetamide, polymyxin B sulfate-trimethoprim, or fluoroquinolone drops or ointment; if concomitant otitis media, also treat with oral antimicrobials
  2. Viral—artificial tears for lubrication, topical steroids (only by ophthalmologist) if keratitis present
  3. Herpes—ophthalmology referral in all suspected cases. Any child with a history of a herpes ocular infection who presents with red eye, lid vesicles, or dendritic findings on fluorescein corneal staining

should be referred immediately; treatment includes topical and systemic antivirals. Initial infection self-limited, virus remains latent; can recur with worsening eye damage

4. Allergic—avoidance of known allergens, cold compresses, systemic or topical antihistamines, ophthalmic nonsteroidal anti-inflammatories (e.g., ketorolac/Acular) or topical mast cell stabilizers (e.g., cromolyn sodium); refer to ophthalmologist for chronic conjunctivitis
5. Good hand washing and hygiene; stress control of cross contamination; avoid shared linens and towels; cleanse eyelashes with warm sterile water, wiping from inner canthus outward
6. Temporarily stop wearing any contact lenses until conjunctivitis resolved
7. Discard old eye makeup
8. More serious eye infections can occur with contact lens users; use caution
9. Ophthalmologist referral needed:
   a. If conjunctivitis is unresponsive to treatment within 2 to 3 days; especially if patient wears contact lenses
   b. If associated with loss of vision, pain, photophobia
   c. If severe conjunctivitis or with corneal involvement

Dacryostenosis

- Definition: Unilateral or bilateral obstruction of the nasolacrimal duct, usually at nasal punctal opening ("blocked tear ducts")
- Etiology/Incidence
  1. Due to failure of duct canalization during gestation
  2. May also occur secondary to trauma or infection
  3. 90% spontaneous resolution by 12 months; after this age, spontaneous resolution less likely
  4. Most common lacrimal disorder in infants; occurs in approximately 30% of newborns
- Signs and Symptoms
  1. Onset typically 1 to 2 weeks of age (range newborn to 1 month)
  2. Continuous or intermittent tearing (wet looking eye) with crusting of lashes
  3. Conjunctiva clear (no redness)
- Differential Diagnosis
  1. Ophthalmia neonatorum, conjunctivitis
  2. Dacryocystitis—infection of obstructed nasolacrimal duct (fever, erythema, and swelling over lacrimal sac or duct)
  3. Glaucoma
  4. Intraocular inflammation
  5. External irritation
- Physical Findings
  1. Tearing or moist-appearing eye
  2. Expression of thin mucopurulent exudate from lacrimal sac
  3. Conjunctiva clear and no eyelid swelling

- Management/Treatment
  1. Gently massage lacrimal sac and nasolacrimal duct by frequently stroking skin from brow area along lateral aspect of nose (no clear supporting data for effectiveness but often recommended)
  2. For purulent discharge, intermittent use of erythromycin ointment (when drainage becomes clear again, stop ointment)
  3. Referral to ophthalmologist by 6 to 12 months of age or earlier for evaluation and treatment if no improvement with antibiotics and massage
  4. Persistent obstruction and recurrent purulent drainage beyond 6 to 12 months may require surgical probing of duct and/or silicone tube intubation
  5. Severe dacryocystitis requires referral to ophthalmologist and systemic antibiotics

Chalazion

- Definition: Chronic granulomatous inflammation of the meibomian glands, occurring on the conjunctival aspect (inner lining) on the midportion of the eyelid; results in a well-defined, nontender cyst
- Etiology/Incidence: Unknown cause but may be related to chronic inflammation, especially related to hordeolum
- Signs and Symptoms
  1. Slow-growing round, painless, nonpigmented mass in the eyelid (most often the mid upper eyelid)
  2. Possible slight discomfort at onset for few days
  3. Possible minimal redness at onset for few days
- Differential Diagnosis
  1. Blepharitis
  2. Hordeolum
  3. Sebaceous cell carcinoma (rare)
- Physical Findings
  1. Firm, nontender, localized nodule; often at the midportion of the lid or at the lid margin
  2. Occasionally a chalazion will become secondarily infected
  3. Large chalazions may cause chronic pressure on cornea, leading to astigmatism
- Diagnostic Tests/Findings: None indicated
- Management/Treatment
  1. Small chalazions may resolve without treatment
  2. Warm compresses 2 to 3 times a day for 20 minutes for 2 to 3 days
  3. Treat large, recurrent, or infected lesions with local antibacterial drops or ointments (sulfacetamide sodium 10%), four times daily for 1 week; recurrent chalazions may benefit from systemic antibiotics
  4. If unresponsive to treatment, refer to ophthalmologist for surgical excision, curettage, or corticosteroid injections

Blepharitis

- Definition
  1. Common acute or chronic bilateral inflammation of the eyelid margins

2. Types
   a. Seborrheic
   b. Staphylococcal—bacterial infection of eyelash follicles
   c. Mixed—combination of both types
- Etiology/Incidence
  1. Seborrheic blepharitis may be associated with seborrheic dermatitis, psoriasis, eczema, or allergies; chemicals, smoke, air pollution, and cosmetics can aggravate condition
  2. *S. aureus* is primary causative pathogen
- Signs and Symptoms
  1. Irritation, burning sensation to eyes
  2. Sensation of foreign body
  3. Erythema of eyelid margins
  4. Itching of eyelid margin
  5. Loss of eye lashes (especially with staph)
- Differential Diagnosis
  1. Chalazion, conjunctivitis, superficial keratitis
  2. Hordeolum
  3. Pediculosis of eyelashes
- Physical Findings
  1. Scaliness to eyelid margin and scales on eyelashes
     a. Seborrheic—greasy scales
     b. Staphylococcal—dry scales
  2. Redness to lid margin—more marked with staph, less red in seborrheic type
  3. Loss of eyelash—seen with staphylococcal type
  4. Ulcers—tiny ulcerated areas on lid margin with staph type; may lead to eyelid margin distortion and possible ectropion
  5. May be associated with conjunctivitis and superficial keratitis
- Diagnostic Tests/Findings: None indicated
- Management/Treatment: Similar for both forms
  1. Warm, moist compresses to lid margins several times per day
  2. Daily mechanical scrubbing and cleansing of lid margins with cotton-tipped applicator or soft cloth dipped in dilute baby shampoo
  3. Application of topical antibiotic ointment massaged into lid margins (sulfacetamide sodium 10% or polymyxin B-bacitracin)
  4. When seborrheic dermatitis of the scalp is present, frequent shampooing with selenium sulfide recommended
  5. Continue treatment for several weeks if necessary; recurrences are common

Hordeolum (Stye)

- Definition: An acute localized inflammation of one or more sebaceous glands (meibomian or zeisian) of eyelids
- Etiology/Incidence: Most common infectious pathogen is *S. aureus*; highest incidence in children/adolescents
- Signs and Symptoms
  1. Sudden onset of a tender, red papule; typically on the lid margin
  2. Foreign body sensation, occasional
- Differential Diagnosis
  1. Chalazion
  2. Blepharitis
  3. Inclusion cyst
- Physical Findings
  1. Painful erythematous swelling on either side of the eyelid (external stye) or conjunctival (internal stye) surface
  2. May suppurate and drain spontaneously
- Diagnostic Tests/Findings: Culture not necessary
- Management/Treatment
  1. Warm, moist compresses for 15 minutes three to four times daily
  2. Antibiotic ophthalmic ointment or drops. Sulfacetamide sodium 10%, polymyxin B-bacitracin, or erythromycin ophthalmic ointment
  3. Cleanse eyelids with diluted baby shampoo once a day
  4. Refer for incision and drainage if unresponsive to treatment (rarely needed)
  5. Dispose of old eye makeup; discourage use of eye makeup until hordeolum is resolved; stress good hand and eye hygiene

Orbital/Periorbital Cellulitis

- Definition
  1. Orbital—infection of the soft tissues of the orbit posterior to the orbital septum. May involve the extraocular muscles and optic nerve
  2. Periorbital (preseptal)—inflammation/infection of the skin and subcutaneous tissue surrounding eye (without involvement of the eye or orbital contents)
- Etiology/Incidence
  1. Orbital cellulitis
     a. More common in older children. Average age is 12 years
     b. Primary etiology is an extension of a bacterial sinusitis (into the orbital tissues)
     c. Life-threatening and vision-threatening complications may occur and include brain abscess, cavernous venous thrombosis, orbital abscess, retinal detachment, and optic neuropathy
     d. All suspected cases require hospitalization
  2. Periorbital cellulitis
     a. More common than orbital cellulitis
     b. Most commonly seen in younger children (<6 years of age) with the average age of 2 years
     c. Commonly associated with skin diseases of the eyelid or face such as insect bites, impetigo, styes, but can also occur as a result of an extension of a sinusitis
  3. Most common organisms are *S. aureus*, *S. pneumoniae*, *H. influenzae*, group A strep, and anaerobic organisms

4. *S. pneumoniae* (Prevnar) and *H. influenzae* (Hib) vaccines have decreased the annual case rate of periorbital and orbital cellulitis
- Signs and Symptoms
  1. Orbital cellulitis
     a. Insidious onset of unilateral eyelid swelling
     b. Orbital pain, headache
     c. Decreased vision
     d. Fever
     e. Potentially devastating consequences
  2. Periorbital cellulitis
     a. Acute onset of unilateral eyelid swelling (usually the upper eyelid)
     b. Warmth, swelling, and tenderness of overlying skin
     c. Eye itself and vision are usually normal
     d. Systemic symptoms may or may not be present. Most common are fever 102°F and rhinorrhea
     e. Skin lesions on the face or eyelid may be present
- Differential Diagnosis
  1. Differentiate between orbital (within true orbit), periorbital, or preseptal (surrounding orbital septum) cellulitis
  2. Edema secondary to trauma
  3. Allergic periorbital edema
  4. Insect bite on eyelid with local allergic reaction (swelling of eyelid)
  5. Orbital malignancies such as neuroblastoma, retinoblastoma need to be distinguished from orbital cellulitis
- Physical Findings
  1. Orbital cellulitis
     a. Lid edema and redness—not extending onto the eyebrow (as in periorbital cellulitis)
     b. Unilateral
     c. Chemosis
     d. Proptosis
     e. Decreased ocular mobility
     f. Decreased visual acuity
     g. Ophthalmoplegia (paralysis of eye muscles) and proptosis (protrusion of eyeball)—classic findings and distinguish orbital from periorbital cellulitis
  2. Periorbital cellulitis
     a. Unilateral eyelid edema
     b. Erythema
     c. Tenderness of overlying skin
     d. Visual acuity and ocular mobility usually normal
- Diagnostic Tests/Findings
  1. Visual acuity exam—decreased vision with orbital cellulitis only
  2. CT scan of sinuses—determine sinus involvement
  3. Oral contrast enhanced CT scan of orbit—to differentiate orbital from periorbital and determine if any orbital complications
  4. Complete blood count (CBC) with differential—leukocytosis may be present with both; more common with orbital cellulitis
  5. Blood and/or eye cultures—R/O concurrent sepsis and identify pathogen

  6. Lumbar punctures with infants for possible meningitis
- Management/Treatment
  1. Prompt assessment and management
  2. Hospitalization for IV antibiotics:
     a. All patients with suspected orbital cellulitis
     b. Patients younger than 1 year of age
     c. Anyone with signs or symptoms of sepsis
     d. Immunocompromised
     e. Uncertain follow-up
     f. No improvement after 48 hours of outpatient management
  3. Outpatient management with IM ceftriaxone, followed by oral antibiotics and close follow-up. First-line antibiotics would include amoxicillin with clavulanic acid and cefixime. Candidates for this approach would include:
     a. Older than 1 year of age
     b. Early periorbital cellulitis
     c. Not sick appearing
     d. Adequate follow-up

Cataracts

- Definition: Partial or complete opacity of the lens
- Etiology/Incidence: May be congenital or acquired, unilateral or bilateral; can result in amblyopia, partial or complete blindness; some are not clinically significant
  1. Congenital—may result from congenital infections (e.g., rubella, toxoplasmosis, cytomegalovirus), genetic anomalies, prematurity and/or drug exposure, or metabolic abnormalities such as hypocalcemia; may be present at birth or develop in first few months of life
  2. Acquired cataracts due to:
     a. Trauma to the eye; cataracts may be a manifestation of child abuse
     b. Systemic disease—diabetes mellitus, trisomy 21, hypoparathyroidism, galactosemia, atopic dermatitis, hypocalcemia, Marfan's syndrome, neurofibromatosis
     c. Various toxins, drugs, radiation; long-term systemic corticosteroid or ocular steroid drops; require routine ophthalmology exams
     d. Complications from other ocular abnormalities, e.g., glaucoma, uveitis, strabismus, pendibular nystagmus with severe amblyopia
     e. Approximately 30% are hereditary, 30% syndrome/disease related, and the remaining are the other etiologies noted or undetermined
- Signs and Symptoms: Severity of visual acuity deficits depends on location and degree of opacity; cataracts alone may produce no symptoms except possible decreased visual acuity; no associated pain but may experience light sensitivity, evaluate for underlying systemic disease or other eye disorders
- Differential Diagnosis
  1. Retinoblastoma
  2. Glaucoma

- Physical Findings
  1. Decreased visual acuity
  2. Strabismus—may be initial sign of cataract in child
  3. Absent red reflex (leukocoria), black dot(s) surrounded by red reflex, or white plaque-like opacities
  4. Signs of other systemic diseases and ocular abnormalities as noted in etiology
- Management/Treatment
  1. Prompt referral to ophthalmologist for diagnosis/treatment
  2. Surgical measures indicated if vision unable to develop due to extent of cataract; visual correction (e.g., eyeglasses/contact lenses)
  3. Determine etiology; any positive family history of congenital cataracts; treat any underlying disorder

Glaucoma

- Definition: Increased intraocular pressure from disruption of aqueous fluid circulation involving one or both eyes resulting in optic nerve damage with loss of visual acuity and eventual blindness if untreated
  1. Congenital—glaucoma that occurs in the first 3 years of life; 40% present at birth and 85% by 1 year; incidence 1 in 12,500 births
  2. Juvenile—glaucoma that begins between the ages of 3 and 30 years
  3. Two-thirds are males
- Etiology/Incidence
  1. Primary—the cause is an isolated anomaly of drainage apparatus; 50% of infantile glaucoma is primary; incidence 0.03%
  2. Secondary—other ocular or systemic abnormalities are associated such as trauma, intraocular hemorrhage, intraocular tumor, cataracts, corticosteroid use; syndromes such as Marfan's, neurofibromatosis, congenital rubella syndrome, Pierre Robins syndrome
- Signs and Symptoms
  1. Classic triad—photophobia, abnormal overflow of tears (epiphora), blepharospasm (eyelid spasm); triad occurs in about 30%
  2. Decreased vision (peripheral first) leading to tunnel vision
  3. Persistent, extreme pain (occasionally)
- Differential Diagnosis: Cataracts
- Physical Findings
  1. Corneal and ocular enlargement; corneal diameter >12 mm (smaller if infant, >10 mm); eventually entire eye enlarges
  2. Other findings may include corneal haziness and edema; conjunctival injection; irregular corneal light reflex
  3. Deep cupping of optic disc; enlargement of the optic cup and increase of cup: disc ratio greater than 0.5
  4. Hallmark of glaucoma—increase in intraocular pressure (IOP)—can be measured or suspected with firmness to palpation of the eye

- Diagnostic Tests/Findings: Glaucoma pressure test will show increased pressure
- Management/Treatment
  1. Immediate referral to ophthalmologist to confirm diagnosis and initiate therapy
  2. Surgery is often first line, followed by medical therapy; postop steroids and cycloplegic drops are essential to prevent adhesions
  3. Same treatments as with adults: topical beta blockers, adrenergic agents, and carbonic anhydrase inhibitors; miotics not used
  4. Even with treatment, still has high risk for visual impairment; refer early for services for visually impaired

Strabismus

- Definition:
  1. Ocular misalignment ("lazy eye or cross eyed"); eyes may deviate outward (exotropia), inward (esotropia), downward (hypotropia), or upward (hypertropia); causes the eyes to not simultaneously view the same object (causes a diplopia); response to diplopia is visual axis suppression (to eliminate diplopia)
  2. Constant strabismus is termed "tropia"; intermittent is termed "phoria"; esotropia is most common
- Etiology/Incidence
  1. Affects approximately 4% of children younger than 6 years of age; 30–50% develop amyblyopia with some visual loss; requires early detection for normal visual outcome
  2. Intermittent exotropia is a normal variant in first 4 to 6 months of life
  3. Historical risk factors include prematurity, family history, cerebral palsy, many chromosomal and other major genetic anomalies, prenatal drug exposure, fetal alcohol syndrome, major head trauma, major congenital or acquired structural ocular defects
  4. Acquired strabismus occurring after 6 months of age usually from cataracts, retinoblastoma, anisometropia, or high refractive errors
  5. Paralytic strabismus—often due to a tumor
  6. Pseudostrabismus (gives an illusion of strabismus)—eyes appear to be crossed due to prominent epicanthal folds on either side of bridge of nose; no ocular deviation
- Signs and Symptoms
  1. Vary with age
  2. Squinting
  3. Decreased vision
  4. School problems
  5. Head tilting
  6. Face turning
  7. Overpointing
  8. Awkwardness
- Differential Diagnosis
  1. Cataracts
  2. Retinoblastoma

3. Anisometropia
4. High refractive errors
5. Amblyopia
6. Head trauma
7. Other congenital eye muscle syndromes
- Physical Findings
  1. Misalignment of eye(s)—asymmetrical Hirschberg
  2. Intermittent, alternating, or continuous esotropia, exotropia, hypertropia, or hypotropia
- Diagnostic Tests/Findings
  1. Abnormal Hirschberg (unequal corneal light reflex)
  2. Cover-uncover test (abnormal movement of eye)
  3. Vision screen—decreased visual acuity, may reveal refractive errors, amblyopia, or anisometropia
  4. Photoscreener can be used
- Management/Treatment
  1. Referral to ophthalmologist
     a. Ocular misalignment after 4 months of age
     b. Immediate referral for constant or fixed strabismus or hyper- or hypotropia at any age
  2. Urgent referral to neurosurgery if an underlying CNS abnormality suspected (i.e., tumor) such as occurs with a paralytic strabismus
  3. Treatment determined by ophthalmology
     a. Surgery—mainstay of treatment for congenital esotropia (done between 6 months and 2 years of age)
     b. Patching (occlusion therapy)—covering the unaffected eye ("the good eye")
     c. Pharmacologic—0.5–1% atropine sulfate (dilating the unaffected eye forces use of the deviating eye)
     d. Corrective lenses (eyeglasses)—may or may not be indicated
     e. Orthoptic exercises—indicated only on certain forms of intermittent strabismus

Nystagmus

- Definition: Involuntary, horizontal, vertical, rotary, or mixed rhythmic movement of eyes
- Etiology/Incidence
  1. Caused by abnormality in one of three basic mechanisms—fixation, conjugate gaze, or vestibular mechanisms
  2. May be familial
  3. Associated with albinism, aniridia, refractive errors, congenital cataracts, central nervous system (CNS) abnormalities, and various diseases of inner ear and retina
  4. Classified according to direction of movement
  5. Congenital nystagmus accounts for 80% of all nystagmus. The child may have a birth history or prematurity, intraventricular hemorrhage, intrauterine drug exposure
  6. Mild nystagmus of the newborn's eyes is common and exists for few days after birth (normal variant then)
  7. Acquired nystagmus is concerning and requires prompt evaluation

- Signs and Symptoms
  1. Irregular eye movements
  2. Abnormal head movements; may be rhythmic
- Differential Diagnosis: Underlying cause
- Physical Findings
  1. Involuntary rhythmic eye movements
  2. Vision screen may be abnormal
- Diagnostic Tests/Findings: Abnormal visual acuity test
- Management/Treatment
  1. Refer to ophthalmologist and neurologist (as necessary)
  2. Treat underlying cause
  3. Monitor closely

Retinoblastoma

- Definition: Congenital malignancy of retina. Most common malignant intraocular tumor of childhood

Refractive Errors

- Definition: Impaired vision that can be corrected by glasses
- Etiology/Incidence:
  1. Most common cause of decreased visual acuity in children
  2. Four types: myopia, hyperopia, astigmatism, anisometropia with myopia most common in children
  3. For clear vision, light must focus directly on the retina (myopia, light focuses in front of the retina; hyperopia, light focuses behind the retina)

Hyperopia (Farsightedness)

- Definition: Alteration in refractive power when visual image is focused behind the retina; ability to see objects clearly at a distance, but not at close range
- Etiology/Incidence
  1. Axial length of eye too short and/or insufficient convexity of the refracting surfaces of the eye especially the cornea
  2. Familial pattern common
- Signs and Symptoms
  1. Often asymptomatic due to children's ability to easily accommodate for hyperopia
  2. Headache, eye strain, squinting, and eye rubbing during prolonged periods of close work in older children
  3. Strabismus often seen with severe hyperopia
- Differential Diagnosis
  1. Astigmatism
  2. Myopia
  3. Anisometropia
  4. Amblyopia
- Physical Findings: Abnormal vision screen
- Diagnostic Tests/Findings
  1. Vision screen shows hyperopia
  2. Passing vision screen is 20/40 (age 3 to 4 years), 20/30 (older children)

3. A difference of two lines between the two eyes is significant
- Management/Treatment
    1. Refer to ophthalmologist or optometrist
    2. If strabismus present, see previous section for management
    3. May not need correction unless strabismus is present or causes reduced vision
    4. Annual eye examinations

Myopia (Nearsightedness)

- Definition: Alteration in refractive power when visual image is focused in front of retina; ability to see objects clearly at close range, but not at a distance
- Etiology/Incidence
    1. Axial length of eye too long and/or increased curvature of the refracting surfaces of the eye, especially the cornea
    2. Familial pattern common and children of myoptic parents need early vision exams
    3. Rarely present in infancy except with a history of retinopathy of prematurity
    4. Myopia usually appears around 8 to 10 years of age with the degree of myopia increasing during the growing years; corrective lenses may need changing yearly or sometimes every few months; often stabilizing in the mid-older teen years
- Signs and Symptoms
    1. Distant objects blurred
    2. Squinting forms physiologic pinhole to improve acuity
    3. Difficulty reading blackboard
- Differential Diagnosis
    1. Hyperopia
    2. Astigmatism
    3. Anisometropia
    4. Amblyopia
- Physical Findings: Abnormal vision screen
- Diagnostic Tests/Findings: Abnormal vision screen (see hyperopia)
- Management/Treatment
    1. Refer to ophthalmologist or optometrist
    2. Importance of annual eye examinations

Astigmatism

- Definition: Refractive error due to an irregular curvature of the cornea or changes in the lens causing light rays to bend in different directions
- Etiology/Incidence
    1. Familial developmental variations in the curvature of the cornea
    2. Depending on severity of curvature variation, retina cannot focus regardless of distance
    3. Increased risk secondary to injury, periorbital or eyelid hemangiomas, or ptosis (Behrman, Kliegman, & Jenson, 2007)

- Signs and Symptoms
    1. Commonly found in conjunction with other refractive errors
    2. Pain in and around eyes, headache, fatigue, reading problems, frowning
- Differential Diagnosis
    1. Myopia
    2. Hyperopia
    3. Amblyopia
    4. Anisometropia
- Physical Findings: Possible abnormal vision screen; asymmetrical Hirschberg
- Diagnostic Tests/Findings: Vision screen with possible abnormality
- Management/Treatment
    1. Refer to ophthalmologist or optometrist
    2. Corrective lenses or contacts may be prescribed; patching may be recommended

Anisometropia

- Definition: Difference in the refractive error of the two eyes. The visual differences between the two eyes may result in suppression strabismus or amblyopia
- Etiology: May be congenital or acquired (asymmetric age changes, disease, or eye injury)
- Signs and Symptoms: May be none depending on the degree; if significant, double vision, tilting head, or closing one eye to see out of the better eye
- Differential Diagnosis
    1. Myopia
    2. Hyperopia
    3. Amblyopia
    4. Anisometropia
- Physical Findings: Normal except abnormal vision screen
- Diagnostic Tests/Findings: Difference of two lines or more (on the eye chart) between the eyes
    1. Management/Treatment: Refer for corrective lenses to correct vision to see the same image (brain will not process two images)

Blindness (Amaurosis)

- Definition
    1. Varies from inability to distinguish light from darkness to partial vision
    2. Low vision is defined as visual acuity between 20/70 and 20/200 corrected
    3. Legal blindness is distant visual acuity of less than 20/200 corrected
    4. Primary blindness—present at birth
- Etiology/Incidence
    1. Incidence—approximately 2.5 per 100,000 children
    2. Variety of causes—cataracts, glaucoma, retinopathy of prematurity (ROP); retinoblastoma, trauma, detached retina, cranial nerve II problems, infection,

hydrocephalus, genetic problems. Prenatal and genetic causes are the most common etiologies

- Signs and Symptoms: Varies with age and mode of onset, abilities of child, and severity of deficit
  1. Developmental delays, e.g., gross motor, walking often delayed to 18 to 24 months
  2. Social skills—increased passivity, increased anxiety around strangers
  3. Decreased social communication and school performance
  4. Increased self-stimulating behavior, e.g., hand flapping, rocking, rubbing eyes
  5. Language delay; cognitive delays, understanding of object permanence, cause/effect
  6. Delay in development of conversational skills
  7. Photophobia, chronic tearing, wandering eyes
  8. Lack of smiling response to visual stimuli
- Differential Diagnosis: If primary or from birth
  1. Developmental malformations
  2. Damage consequent to gestational/perinatal infection
  3. Anoxia, hypoxia, perinatal trauma
  4. Genetically determined diseases
- Physical Findings: In primary blindness
  1. Nystagmus (may be first clue)
  2. Enlarged or cloudy cornea; abnormal or absent red reflex
  3. Lack of pupillary reflex; optic disc pallor; pigmentary deposits
  4. Fixed or intermittent strabismus beyond 6 months of age
  5. History of retinopathy of prematurity (ROP)
  6. Possible neurologic disorder
- Diagnostic Tests/Findings
  1. Ophthalmologic examination—abnormal as described above
  2. Developmental testing—delays as outlined
  3. CT or MRI—rule out physiologic abnormalities
- Management/Treatment
  1. Obtain complete family genetic visual impairment history
  2. Address family issues, social and emotional needs of child
  3. General medical and developmental history
  4. Metabolic and genetic studies
  5. Prompt referral to ophthalmologist, neurologist, and developmental specialist

Amblyopia (Lazy Eye)

- Definition
  1. Decreased visual acuity in one or both eyes that cannot be attributed to any structural abnormality and cannot be immediately corrected with any glasses
  2. Occurs in visually immature children, during the "sensitive" period for visual development; amblyopia is caused by a lack of a clear image onto the retina of

the immature visual system, which results in suppression of vision in that eye; vision can likely be restored if identified and corrected early; important to identify anything that would cause obstruction of a clear image onto the retina (e.g., strabismus, tumor, and cataract)

- Etiology/Incidence
  1. Organic—trauma, organic lesion, cataract, diseases of the eye or visual pathways, ptosis
  2. Nonorganic—sensory stimulation deprivation or disuse; abnormal binocular interaction during infancy and early childhood (greatest risk between 2 to 3 years of age but can continue until 9 years of age); large difference in refractive errors between both eyes (anisometropia)
  3. Rarely bilateral; associated with strabismus
  4. Occurs in 2% to 2.5% of general population (nearly 6 million Americans)
  5. Five types—deprivation (ptosis, opacities), strabismic, anisometropic, occlusion (patching good eye too much), ametropic (both eyes large refractive errors, typically hyperopic and/or astigmatism)
- Signs and Symptoms: Often asymptomatic; identified only on visual acuity tests
- Differential Diagnosis
  1. Cataracts
  2. Blindness
  3. Ptosis
- Physical Examination
  1. Specific ophthalmic findings with underlying causes; abnormal red reflex with tumor, cataracts; presence of ptosis and strabismus are also causes
  2. May have other physical exam findings if underlying disorder
- Diagnostics Tests/Findings: Abnormal vision test—decreased visual acuity
- Management/Treatment
  1. Early detection, prompt intervention, referral to ophthalmologist
  2. Effective vision screening before 3 years of age
  3. Corrective lenses
  4. Therapy forcing stimulation of amblyopic eye; patching or use of atropine in good eye
  5. Occasionally surgery
  6. Close monitoring and follow-up

Eye Injuries

General information regarding corneal abrasion, foreign body, hyphema, ecchymosis, and chemical injuries
- Definition/Incidence/Etiology
  1. About one-third of all blindness in children younger than 10 years of age is due to trauma
  2. Sports and activities in which ocular trauma is common include BB guns (most common), archery, darts, motorcycling, bicycling, racquet sports, boxing, basketball, and baseball

3. Injury prevention (e.g., protective eyewear) will reduce ocular trauma by 90%
- Physical Examination
  1. Steps in proper evaluation include:
     a. Recognizing life-threatening nonocular conditions, e.g., airway compromise, chemical injuries
     b. Taking adequate history to assess potential risk of injury
     c. Examining in detail (visual acuity, external ocular motility unless ruptured globe suspected), pupil, anterior segment, and fundus
     d. Referral for signs and symptoms or history of severe ocular injury
  2. Use caution—severe intraocular injury may be concealed behind minimal external trauma
  3. Examine lids, lacrimal system, adnexa, sclera, and conjunctiva for lacerations, foreign body, or perforation
  4. Palpate orbital rim for crepitus and obtain a CT scan when orbital fracture suspected; can be associated with significant intracranial and ocular injuries
  5. A dislocated lens presents with a quivering iris
  6. Topical anesthetic recommended for examination only; slows healing of cornea
- Management/Treatment
  1. Ocular injuries requiring immediate referral include:
     a. Chemical injuries
     b. Globe lacerations, severe lacerations of lid
     c. Hyphemas
     d. Penetrating intraocular injury
  2. Avoid pressure to globe by placing a protective shield over injured eye
  3. Nonaccidental trauma or child abuse should be considered with presence of lid ecchymosis, conjunctival hemorrhages, hyphema, or retinal hemorrhages; ideally injuries should be photographed when possible
  4. Acetaminophen for pain, no acetylsalicylic acid (ASA)
  5. Tetanus vaccine if longer than 5 years since last vaccine in a tetanus-prone wound
  6. Rabies prophylaxis if trauma from animal bite
  7. Refer to ophthalmologist for further assessment

Corneal Abrasion

- Definition: Loss of epithelial lining from corneal surface of one or both eyes
- Etiology/Incidence: Abrasions can occur from, paper, brushes, toys or fingernails, tree branches, contact lenses, airbag deployment, sports injury or foreign body in the conjunctival sac; most common ocular injury in children
- Signs and Symptoms
  1. Pain
  2. Tearing
  3. Photophobia
  4. Decreased vision
  5. Injection of sclera
  6. Blepharospasm

- Physical Findings: Epithelial injury visible with use of fluorescein stain and cobalt blue light (e.g., Wood's lamp). The dye stains the area of the missing epithelium (the abraded area)
- Management/Treatment
  1. Topical anesthetic for evaluation only
  2. Remove any foreign body via irrigation with normal saline or moistened cotton swab
  3. Broad spectrum ophthalmic antibiotic ointment such as erythromycin and bacitracin
  4. Topical cycloplegic agent such as cyclopentolate to help alleviate ciliary spasm 2 to 3 times/day for large abrasions
  5. Nonsteroidal anti-inflammatory drugs (NSAIDs) oral or topical (ketorolac 0.5%) can be used for pain control
  6. The trend is away from patching, but if applied, make certain the eye is closed and patch is applied properly; do NOT patch if possible infection or foreign body exists
  7. Most abrasions heal within 24 to 48 hours; follow up in 24 hours and restain to evaluate abrasion
  8. Refer to ophthalmologist if large abrasion, unable to remove a foreign body, no healing within 48–72 hrs.

Foreign Body Eye Injury

- Definition: Foreign body in the eye
- Etiology/Incidence
  1. Surface—nonadherent/loosely adherent to cornea or conjunctival epithelium (most likely sources dirt, sand, grass); organic material has a higher rate of infection and metal can cause a reaction in the vitreous
  2. Penetrating—into but not through cornea or sclera
  3. Perforating—through cornea or sclera and into globe
- Signs and Symptoms
  1. Foreign body sensation
  2. Pain
  3. Sensitivity to light
  4. Tearing
  5. Eye rubbing
- Differential Diagnosis
  1. Corneal abrasion
  2. Chemical injury
- Physical Findings
  1. Foreign body may be visualized
  2. Positive fluorescein examination if corneal abrasion present
  3. Epiphora
  4. Possible visual acuity abnormality
- Diagnostic Tests/Findings
  1. Visual acuity—to determine any deviation from normal
  2. Fluorescein test—to determine presence of corneal abrasion
  3. Possible radiographs to visualize foreign body
- Management/Treatment
  1. Refer to ophthalmologist all intraocular foreign bodies (both penetrating and perforating), persistent corneal abrasion after 24 hours with treatment

2. Topical ophthalmic anesthetic drops only for examination and removal except perforating wounds. Never prescribed or given for home management
3. Remove foreign body via irrigation with normal saline or moistened cotton-tipped applicator
4. After removal, examine for corneal abrasion, treat appropriately

Hyphema

- Definition: Accumulation of blood in anterior chamber
- Etiology/Incidence
  1. Due to blunt or perforating trauma to the globe with hemorrhage from the vessels of the anterior chamber
  2. Most frequently caused by balls, fists, elbows, rocks, and sticks. Less commonly by airbags and child abuse
  3. Nontraumatic causes include hematologic abnormalities such as sickle cell disease, leukemia, and hemophilia
  4. Seventy-five percent of injuries occur in males
  5. Approximately 30% of patients will have rebleeding, which typically occurs 3–5 days after the initial injury and is usually more severe, causing greater loss of vision
- Signs and Symptoms
  1. Ocular injury
  2. Eye pain
  3. Light sensitivity
  4. Blurring of vision
  5. Drowsiness (but also consider head injury)
- Physical Findings
  1. Blood in anterior chamber can be seen on gross inspection with patient sitting up (dark red fluid level visible)
  2. Visual acuity changes
- Management/Treatment
  1. Refer to ophthalmologist
  2. Reduce activity for several days, bed rest in supine position with head of bed elevated 30 to 40 degrees to promote reabsorption of blood; hospitalization often necessary; no reading or activities
  3. Eye patch with a metal shield for 5 days on injured eye (to protect from reinjury); patch must have holes or clear plastic so patients can assess their vision because worsening of vision first sign of rebleed
  4. Surgery may be necessary to remove blood
  5. Close follow-up for complications: rebleed is most common complication, usually 3 to 5 days after the injury (>50% chance in patients with sickle cell trait or anemia); glaucoma, cataracts, and sympathetic ophthalmia (inflammation that occurs in the uninjured eye weeks to years later) are other complications

Ecchymosis ("Black Eye")

- Definition: Bruising of periorbital region
- Etiology/Incidence: Blunt contusion injury; due to isolated periorbital injury or other orbital/ocular injury

- Signs and Symptoms
  1. Pain
  2. Visual impairment if occlusion from edematous eyelid
- Differential Diagnosis: Other orbital/ocular injury (e.g., lens dislocation, globe rupture, retinal detachment)
- Physical Findings
  1. Edema
  2. Ecchymosis
- Diagnostic Tests/Findings
  1. Ophthalmic examination—determine other orbital/ocular injuries
  2. Visual acuity
- Management/Treatment
  1. Uncomplicated—cold compresses for 24 to 48 hours, then warm compresses until swelling resolves; elevate head; inform parents/patient that ecchymosis and edema may spread
  2. Refer to ophthalmologist if black eye is accompanied by other injuries such as a closed head injury or skull or facial fractures. Also refer to neurology or neurosurgery

Chemical Injuries

- Definition: Burns of the eyelids, conjunctiva, and/or cornea
- Etiology/Incidence
  1. Steam, intense heat, and common household agents; deployment of airbags can release chemicals potentially causing alkaline chemical damage
  2. Severe alkali injuries characterized by corneal opacification
  3. Amount of damage directly related to duration of exposure
- Management/Treatment
  1. Acute ocular emergency
  2. Copious irrigation with normal saline for 20 to 30 minutes—patch and refer to ophthalmologist immediately to rule out corneal or other ocular trauma
  3. Severe chemical injury to eye(s) requires hospitalization
  4. Topical anesthetic may reduce pain from injury and irrigation
  5. Pseudomonal contamination common with any burn, possibly leading to corneal ulceration; prevention—antibiotic preparation containing polymyxin B, gentamicin, tobramycin, or colistin should be instilled into the injured eye(s) 3 to 4 times a day

☐ EAR

External Otitis Media (EOM)

- Definition: Acute infection and/or inflammation of external auditory canal; "swimmer's ear"
- Etiology/Incidence
  1. More common in summer months due to excessive wetness (swimming, bathing, or increased environmental

humidity), which changes the acidic environment and promotes bacterial/fungal growth

2. More common in tropical environments (with constant high humidity)
3. Common organisms are *Pseudomonas aeruginosa* (most common), *S. aureus, Streptococcus pyogenes, Enterobacter aerogenes, Proteus mirabilis, Klebsiella pneumoniae, Staphylococcus epidermis*, and fungi, e.g., *Candida, Aspergillus, Trichophyton*
4. Loss of protective cerumen or chronic irritation
5. Trauma disrupting lining of auditory canal, e.g., foreign body, digital irritation, cotton-tipped swabs, hearing aids
6. Excessive dryness (eczema, psoriasis); contact dermatitis, e.g., poison ivy, medications, hair spray, perfumes
7. Results from irritation and/or maceration from excessive moisture in the canal

- Signs and Symptoms
1. Ear pain, accentuated by manipulation of pinna/tragus, lying on the affected ear or performance of otoscopic examination. Varying degrees of pain, which can be severe
2. Pressure/fullness in ear, possible hearing loss related to swelling and debris in the canal
- Differential Diagnosis
1. Acute otitis media with perforation
2. Dental infection
3. Mastoiditis
4. Foreign body in the ear canal
5. Temporomandibular joint (TMJ) inflammation
6. Parotitis
7. Cervical adenitis
- Physical Findings
1. Edematous/erythematous external canal; with or without exudate
2. If present, exudate appears as clumpy or fluffy whitish
3. Tympanic membrane (TM) is normal; may be difficult to visualize due to swelling and exudate in the canal
4. Possible pre- or postauricular lymphadenopathy
5. Observe for signs of mastoiditis or facial cellulitis (extension of the infection)
6. Necrotizing (malignant) otitis externa—a rare, life-threatening complication usually seen only in immunocompromised patients and diabetics
- Diagnostic Tests/Findings: Culture of discharge unnecessary unless unresponsive to treatment
- Management/Treatment
1. Withdraw any foreign bodies or debris from external canal by gentle irrigation with warm water or normal saline; do not irrigate if perforated TM is suspected. (Medicated ear drops must be able to be in contact with the canal wall in order to be effective)
2. Topical antibiotic otic drops are sufficient: those containing combinations of neomycin, polymyxin, and fluoroquinolone are effective (ofloxacin is safe with PE tubes or TM perforation); the addition of

hydrocortisone (e.g., Cipro HC) is helpful when canal is edematous

3. If significant swelling, insert cotton wick saturated with antibiotic solution for first 24 to 48 hours
4. Systemic analgesic often required for severe pain (e.g., NSAIDs, acetaminophen)
5. Avoid swimming and getting ear wet during the acute phase
6. Reexamine 1 to 2 weeks for evaluation of TM and removal of any debris
7. Prevention
   a. Instillation of white vinegar and rubbing alcohol (50/50) in both ear canals after swimming
   b. Avoid water in canals, vigorous cleaning, scratching, or prolonged use of cerumenolytic agents
   c. Properly fitted ear plugs may be helpful
8. Systemic antibiotics when OE accompanied by fever, lymphadenitis, facial cellulitis (uncommon)
9. Refer to ENT if no improvement after 2–3 days; sooner if worsening

Acute Otitis Media (AOM)

- Definition: Inflammation of the middle ear with inflammatory fluid in the middle ear space (suppurative otitis media). Recent American Academy of Pediatrics (AAP) guidelines use more stringent otoscopic findings for diagnosis: (1) moderate to severe bulging of the tympanic membrane, (2) new onset of otorrhea not caused by otitis externa, or (3) mild bulging of the tympanic membrane associated with recent onset of ear pain (48 hours) or erythema
- Etiology/Incidence
1. Fluid/pathogen accumulation in middle ear due to Eustachian tube (ET) dysfunction
   a. ET allows for proper ventilation and drainage of middle ear space; without this, an effusion develops in the middle ear space with subsequent bacterial contamination
   b. ET dysfunction can be due to age-related characteristics of the ET (e.g., floppy ET) or obstruction of the ET (e.g., inflammation from allergies, viral infections, or enlarged adenoids), and/or other mechanical factors
   c. Most ET dysfunction corrects with age; temporary ventilation tubes (PE tubes) provide ventilation of the middle ear until child is older
2. Common pathogenic agents—varies according to geographic location; has recently shifted with the use of Hib and pneumococcal conjugate vaccines
   a. *S. pneumoniae* (approximately 40%)
   b. *H. influenzae* (25% to 30%)
   c. *M. catarrhalis* (10% to 20%)
   d. Less common pathogens—*S. aureus*, group A beta-hemolytic streptococcus, and *P. aeruginosa* (more common in chronic otitis media)
   e. Viruses—influenza, respiratory syncytial virus (RSV; most common), adenovirus, parainfluenza, and coronavirus

f. Prevalence of b-lactamase producing strains highest in past 15 years

g. Increase in drug-resistant bacteria, especially in children younger than 24 months, those who recently were treated with b-lactamase antibiotics, and children exposed to large numbers of children

h. No growth found in approximately 16% of AOM

3. One of the most common pediatric diagnoses—approximately 80% of children will have at least one episode of acute otitis media

4. Otitis media is the most common reason for antibiotics and surgery in children

5. Natural history of untreated otitis media—70% to 90% spontaneous resolution

6. The highest incidence is between 6 and 36 months of age

7. Highest incidence in winter/spring; males, Caucasians, American Indians, Eskimos, and lower socioeconomic groups

8. Risk factors include age, craniofacial abnormalities (e.g., cleft palate, Down syndrome), upper respiratory infections, allergic rhinitis, environmental smoke exposure, day care and bottle-feeding in the supine position

9. Mild to moderate hearing loss with concomitant language delays may occur with OME, contributing to subsequent behavioral difficulties, including poor attention and school performance

- Signs and Symptoms
  1. Pain, or discomfort; infants may pull on ears or be fussy
  2. Fever in 30% to 50% of cases
  3. Poor appetite/feeding, irritable with sleep disturbances (especially in infants)
  4. Rhinorrhea and/or nasal congestion—frequent
  5. Less frequently gastrointestinal (GI) symptoms—nausea, vomiting, diarrhea
  6. Purulent otorrhea with TM rupture

- Differential Diagnosis
  1. Crying infant/toddler (TM will become erythematous with intense crying)
  2. Serous otitis media
  3. Tympanosclerosis
  4. Cholesteatoma
  5. Otitis externa
  6. Rare complications—mastoiditis, sepsis in young infant, hearing loss, developmental/speech delay

- Physical Findings: Diagnosis is determined by changes in color, contour, and mobility of TM
  1. Color is erythematous
  2. Contour may be bulging; light reflexes and bony landmarks usually distorted
  3. Mobility decreased or absent via tympanometry or pneumatic otoscopy
  4. Conductive hearing loss (to varying degrees; may not be evident to parent)

- Diagnostic Tests/Findings: Usually not necessary with acute otitis media. Use depends on age of child and stage of middle ear disease
  1. Pneumatic otoscopy—to visualize degree of mobility impairment
  2. Tympanometry using electroacoustic impedance bridge to measure compliance of the TM—identifies middle ear effusion, perforation, patent ventilation tubes, or excessive hard-packed cerumen
  3. On follow-up, can consider:
     a. Hearing test—to determine if any hearing loss
     b. Language screen—assess for language delay
     c. Allergy evaluation and immunologic evaluation for children with recurrent OM and other supporting symptoms (e.g., allergy symptoms)

- Management/Treatment
  1. Antibiotic therapy—mainstay of treatment; however, judicious use recommended because of an increase in antibiotic resistance and spontaneous resolution of OM in 70% of children
     a. Option to observe may be indicated if older than 6 months of age and nonsevere illness. Close follow-up is essential if no treatment
     b. Initiate antibiotics if younger than 6 months of age and any age with severe illness (high fever; bilateral OM)
     c. Antibiotics: First line high-dose amoxicillin (80–90 mg/kg/day) or amoxicillin-clavulanate. If allergic cefdinir, cefuroxime, cefpodoxime, and ceftriaxone are acceptable.
        Second line for treatment failures are amoxicillin-clavulanate and ceftriaxone with clindamycin as an alternative treatment
  2. Maintain realistic expectations—90% to 95% symptom relief within 48 to 72 hours; if no better, initiate antibiotics or change antibiotic to second-line therapy
  3. Length of treatment is controversial; typically 10 days; however, in older children (>2 years) and with milder cases, may consider shorter courses (5–7 days)
  4. Use tympanocentesis sparingly, only used for retreatment failures with severe symptoms (performed by ENT)
  5. Monitor residual OME—may last for several months; persistent OME for 6 to 8 weeks, consider treatment with second-line antibiotics
  6. Pain and fever control
     a. Analgesics—acetaminophen, ibuprofen. Ibuprofen is preferred because of earlier onset and longer duration of action
     b. Local anesthetic otic drops such as benzocain (contraindicated in acute/chronic perforations and ventilation tubes)
  7. Decongestant use not recommended
  8. Recheck AOM after 10 to 21 days
  9. Prevention
     a. Proper feeding techniques for infants
     b. Encourage breastfeeding—possible protective effect

c. Eliminate exposure to environmental smoke

d. Antibiotic prophylaxis—not typically recommended; only considered for control of chronic AOM, e.g., 3 or more episodes in 6 months or 4 episodes in 12 months

e. Immunizations including influenza vaccines

10. Referral to otolaryngologist

a. Persistent AOM resistant to treatment over 1 to 2 months

b. Frequent recurrent OM—3 in 6 months, 4 to 5 episodes in 1 year

c. Persistent/chronic OME persisting longer than 3 months

d. Evidence of hearing deficit and/or language delay

e. Determine need for tympanostomy tube placement

Otitis Media with Effusion (OME)

- Definition: Inflammation/fluid accumulation in middle ear (serous, not purulent fluid) with decreased TM mobility on pneumatic otoscopy but without signs and symptoms of ear infection; also referred to as serous, secretory, mucoid, and allergic otitis media or "glue ear"

- Etiology/Incidence

1. Caused by Eustachian tube dysfunction (negative pressure in the middle ear produces an effusion in the middle ear space); also occurs as a frequent sequelae of acute otitis media

2. OME accounts for 25% to 35% of all cases of OM

3. 30% to 40% have OME associated with allergic rhinitis

4. Majority (50% to 80%) clear spontaneously within 2 to 3 months

- Signs and Symptoms

1. Sometimes none or mild discomfort, crackling or full sensation in ear

2. Behavioral changes, e.g., hearing loss, decreased attention span

- Differential Diagnosis: Same as AOM

- Physical Findings

1. Color—yellow, dull, opaque, or translucent TM; possible presence of fluid level or air bubbles

2. Contour—appears retracted due to negative pressure in middle ear

3. Vascularity—none visible

4. Mobility—decreased; tympanometry reveals high negative pressure or flat line

5. Assess for complications more commonly seen with OME; cholesteatoma and persistent TM perforation

- Diagnostic Tests/Findings: Same as AOM

- Management/Treatment

1. Most cases resolve without antibiotics

2. Limit use of antibiotic prophylaxis due to marginal benefit

3. Limit passive smoking exposure, treat other infections, control allergies

4. Referral to otolaryngologist: if persists longer than 3 months or associated hearing loss

5. Consider surgery (PE tubes, adenoidectomy if indicated) for chronic OME accompanied by pain, recurrent AOM, speech or hearing problems

6. Decongestants and antihistamines not recommended except if allergy symptoms present

7. Follow up every 3 to 4 weeks

8. Prevention and education, same as AOM

Tympanostomy Tubes (PE Tubes)

- Definition: Surgical incision of eardrum (myringotomy with placement of ventilation tube) to relieve pressure and drain pus/fluid from middle ear

- Etiology/Incidence

1. One million tubes inserted annually

2. With increasing number of resistant bacteria, possibility of more frequent use of tubes

- Signs and Symptoms

1. History of PE tube surgery

2. No symptoms normally. Hearing often improved

3. Otorrhea with otitis media

4. Rarely may bleed with expulsion of tube from TM

Differential Diagnosis: Small colorful foreign body in ear

3. Labrynthitis
4. Lateral sinus thrombophlebitis
5. Otitis externa
6. Air bubbles from SOM
- Physical Findings
  1. Thickened, inflamed middle ear mucosa; with or without discharge
  2. May contain granulation tissue or polyps
  3. Conductive hearing loss dependent on size of perforation
  4. Site of perforation important to note
- Diagnostic Tests/Findings
  1. Culture discharge—*P. aeruginosa* and *S. aureus* most often seen
  2. CT scan of mastoid—rule out mastoiditis
- Management/Treatment
  1. Oral antibiotics (see **Table 4-1**) for 14 days plus antibiotic eardrops (3 to 4 drops four times a day for 7 days); if not responsive, suspect mastoiditis or cholesteatoma

2. Refer to otolaryngologist
3. Hospitalization may be necessary if serious complications or underlying disorder exists
4. Follow up every week to 3 months; most heal within 2 weeks
- Prevention of Recurrent Infection
  1. Cotton plugs with petroleum jelly (on outer surface) when bathing and hair washing
  2. Discourage swimming (use fitted earplugs if unavoidable)
  3. Diving, jumping into water, and underwater swimming forbidden

Mastoiditis

- Definition: Infection of the mastoid bone, more specifically the periosteum of the mastoid; can lead to destruction of the mastoid air system and abscess formation; considered an extension of a middle ear infection; a suppurative complication of otitis media
- Etiology/Incidence
  1. Uncommon, due to successful antibiotics for AOM; incidence 0.2% to 0.4%
  2. Develops secondary to OM, leading to periostitis and osteitis with abscess formation
  3. About 60% are between 6 and 24 months of age
  4. Common pathogens
     a. Most common—*S. pneumoniae*, *S. pyogenes*, *S. aureus*
     b. Less common—*H. influenzae*
     c. Other agents—*Pseudomonas* (chronic mastoiditis), *Mycobacterium tuberculosis* (rare), *M. catarrhalis*, enteropathic Gram-negative rods
- Signs and Symptoms
  1. Pain, tenderness behind ear
  2. Fever or irritability
  3. Otorrhea
- Differential Diagnosis
  1. Meningitis
  2. Extradural abscess
  3. Subdural empyema
  4. Focal otic encephalitis
  5. Otitis externa
  6. Parotitis
- Physical Findings
  1. Tenderness over mastoid bone
  2. Mastoid area often edematous with erythema
  3. Presence of AOM, but may be normal if on antibiotics
  4. Pinna displaced downward and outward (late finding)
  5. Narrowing of ear canal in posterior superior wall due to pressure from mastoid abscess
  6. Purulent drainage and debris may be present in ear canal
- Diagnostic Tests/Findings
  1. CT scan of the mastoid/temporal bone—diffuse clouding of mastoid cells; later in disease, bony destruction and resorption of the mastoid air cells; CT also done if brain abscess is suspected

2. CBC—elevated white blood cells (WBCs)
3. Blood culture—rule out sepsis
4. PPD—rule out exposure to tuberculosis
5. Tympanocentesis—identify pathogen
- Management/Treatment
  1. Prompt referral to ENT and hospitalization
  2. Systemic intravenous antibiotics; surgical drainage of any abscess
  3. Oral systemic antibiotics for 4 to 6 weeks after discharge
  4. Complications—meningitis, brain abscess, cavernous sinus thrombosis, acute suppurative labyrinthitis, facial palsy

Cholesteatoma

- Definition: Cystlike growth within the middle ear with lining of stratified squamous epithelium filled with desquamated debris
- Etiology/Incidence
  1. Congenital or acquired
  2. Various theories explaining formation, e.g., inflammatory process, perforation, or failure of desquamated tissue to clear from middle ear
  3. Most common cause of acquired cholesteatoma is long-standing chronic serous otitis media
  4. If surgery is delayed, it can invade and destroy other structures of the temporal bone and possibly spread to intracranial cavity, with life-threatening consequences
  5. If untreated, may lead to facial nerve paralysis, intracranial infection
- Signs and Symptoms
  1. Dizziness
  2. Hearing loss
- Differential Diagnosis: Aural polyps, tympanosclerosis
- Physical Findings
  1. Pearly white, opacity, on or behind tympanic membrane
  2. History of chronic OM with foul-smelling purulent otorrhea
- Diagnostic Tests/Findings
  1. CT scan of the temporal bone—detects presence and extent of the disease
  2. Audiogram to rule out hearing deficit
- Management/Treatment
  1. Referral to ENT for surgical excision
  2. Complications
     a. Irreversible structural damage
     b. Permanent bone damage
     c. Facial nerve palsy
     d. Hearing loss
     e. Intracranial infection

Hearing Loss

- Definition: A deficit in hearing process classified as conductive, sensorineural, or mixed; can range from mild to severe, may be congenital or acquired; quantified by measured hearing threshold
  1. Conductive loss—normal bone conduction and reduced air conduction due to obstruction of transmission of sound waves through external auditory canal and middle ear to the inner ear; usual range of 15 to 40 dB loss
  2. Sensorineural loss—cochlea hair cells and/or auditory nerve damage; may range from mild to profound
  3. Mixed—components of conductive and sensorineural hearing loss present
  4. Hearing loss criteria in children differs from adults since children are in the process of speech and language development
     a. Mild—15 to 30 dB
     b. Moderate—30 to 50 dB
     c. Severe—50 to 70 dB
     d. Profound—70 dB and above
- Etiology/Incidence
  1. Hearing loss can be classified in five ways
     a. Age of onset
     b. Type—conductive, sensorineural, mixed, or central
     c. Degree—ranging from mild to profound
     d. Configuration—decibel (dB) loss
     e. Hearing status of parent(s)
  2. Congenital
     a. Sensorineural—moderate to profound loss; 1–2/1000 live births (Behrman et al., 2007)
        (1) Genetic—autosomal dominant (80%), autosomal recessive (20%)
        (2) In utero infections—TORCH, CMV, and rubella most common causes in newborn
        (3) Erythroblastosis fetalis
        (4) Anoxia
        (5) Birth trauma
        (6) Birth weight less than 1500 g
        (7) Exposure to ototoxic drugs
        (8) Prolonged mechanical ventilation
     b. Conductive—congenital atresia, deformities, or stenosis of ossicles
  3. Acquired
     a. Sensorineural
        (1) Meningitis
        (2) Mumps, measles
        (3) Labyrinthitis, ototoxic drug exposure
        (4) Severe head trauma
        (5) Noise-induced hearing loss (NIHL) from loud music, firecrackers, firearms, toy cap pistols, squeaking toys, recreational vehicles, farm equipment, lawn mowers, inappropriate hearing aids
     b. Conductive
        (1) Otitis media with middle effusion—75% of children have one episode of AOM with conductive hearing loss
        (2) Cerumen impaction; foreign bodies in external canal

(3) Perforated/damaged tympanic membrane; severe head trauma

(4) Cholesteatoma, otosclerosis

- Signs and Symptoms
  1. Infants
     a. Failure to elicit startle or blink reflex to loud sound
     b. Failure to be awakened by loud sounds
     c. General indifference to sound
     d. Lack of babbling by 7 months
  2. Children
     a. Substitution of gestures for words, especially after 15 months
     b. Failure to develop intelligible speech by 24 months
     c. Asking to have statements repeated
     d. Inappropriate response to questions
     e. Markedly inattentive
- Differential Diagnosis
  1. Mental retardation
  2. Profound deprivation
  3. Communication disorder—articulation disorders, expressive language delay, global language disorder, autism
- Physical Findings
  1. Physical exam may be normal
  2. Careful evaluation of TM, e.g., decreased mobility, bulging, opacity
  3. Assess for congenital abnormalities—external canal abnormalities, craniofacial malformations, structural abnormalities of external ear
- Diagnostic Test/Findings
  1. Audiogram—if appropriate for age to rule out hearing loss
  2. CT scan—rule out physiologic abnormalities
  3. Weber and Rinne tests—abnormal response
- Management/Treatment
  1. Check newborn hearing test results
  2. History screening at 2-week-old visit—family history of hearing loss, perinatal infections (TORCH), anatomic malformations involving head or neck, birth weight less than 1500 g, hyperbilirubinemia, bacterial meningitis, asphyxia
  3. Detect hearing loss as young as possible, take parental suspicions seriously; many tests available for all age groups (otoacoustic emissions—OAE, auditory brainstem response—ABR)
  4. Referral for full audiological testing and language evaluation as soon as deficit is suspected; since the institution of universal newborn hearing screening, early detection of hearing loss has resulted in higher scores for language at school age
  5. Psychosocial considerations—rehabilitation, hearing aids, educational programs
  6. Prevention
     a. Early identification and intervention; periodic hearing and language screening (birth to 4 months—responds appropriately to loud noises; 4 to 24 months—responds to noise out of field of vision; older children—pure tone audiometry)

b. Appropriate management and treatment of auditory canal obstruction and middle ear disease
c. Avoid repeated exposure to loud noises to prevent NIHL
d. Control erythroblastosis with use of RhoGAM; hyperbilirubinemia with phototherapy and exchange transfusions
e. Prevent mumps and measles with immunization
f. Avoid ototoxic medications

☐ NOSE

Allergic Rhinitis

- Definition: IgE-mediated response to inhaled allergens or irritants producing nasal mucosa inflammation
- Etiology/Incidence
  1. Types—seasonal or perennial depending on exposure/sensitization to allergen
     a. Seasonal—inhaled pollens, e.g., trees, grasses; more common after age 6
     b. Perennial—house dust mites, mold spores, animal dander; may occur in children younger than age 6, uncommonly seen younger than 24 months
  2. Most common pediatric allergic disease; commonly associated with conjunctivitis, sinusitis, OME, and/or atopic dermatitis
  3. Strong genetic predisposition
- Signs and Symptoms
  1. Chronic, intermittent, or daily nasal congestion; clear rhinorrhea
  2. Episodes of sneezing with itching of eyes, ears, nose, palate, pharynx
  3. Frequent sniffing and/or throat clearing
  4. Open mouth facies, snoring with sleep
  5. Excessive tearing
  6. Halitosis
  7. Sinus headaches
  8. Symptoms year-round with perennial rhinitis
  9. Purulent secretions indicate secondary infection (e.g., sinusitis, foreign body)
- Differential Diagnosis
  1. Bacterial or viral upper respiratory infection, e.g., strep pharyngitis, influenza, OM, sinusitis
  2. Vasomotor rhinitis
  3. Congenital or anatomical abnormalities leading to obstruction, e.g., nasal polyps, foreign body
- Physical Findings
  1. Allergic "shiners" of eyes and allergic "salute" with nasal crease
  2. Hypertrophied turbinates
  3. Nasal mucosa pale, boggy, and edematous with watery or mucoid secretions
- Diagnostic Tests/Findings
  1. Nasal smear for eosinophils—10% considered confirmatory

2. RAST and skin testing—elevations or reactions to specific allergens
3. CBC differential—elevated eosinophils and total IgE
- Management/Treatment: Referral to allergist may be necessary
  1. Allergen avoidance—first line of therapy
  2. Environmental controls—removal of carpets, drapes, and stuffed animals; plastic covers for mattresses and pillows; decrease humidity with air conditioner; use of air purifiers; avoidance of environmental and tobacco smoke
  3. Drug therapy—several classes of medications are effective:
     a. Antihistamine-loratidine, cetirizine, fexofenadine, diphenhydramine
     b. Nasal sprays
        (1) Nasal steroids-beclomethasone, fluticasone
        (2) Nasal antihistamines—azelastine
        (3) Nasal ipratropium spray—for older than age 6 years
        (4) Nasal cromolyn sodium—limited by need for frequent (4 times per day) dosing
        (5) Normal saline—helps to clean away allergens
     c. Leukotriene antagonist—montelukast useful, especially with concurrent asthma
     d. Oral decongestants/sympathomimetic (pseudoephedrine—for short-term relief of nasal congestion)
  4. Referrals if symptoms not responsive to avoidance and/or medication
     a. Allergist for skin testing for possible long-term immunotherapy
     b. Immunotherapy effective in relieving symptoms due to dust mites, animal dander, pollens, molds, insect stings, and drug sensitivities
     c. ENT specialist for consultation and possible surgical interventions, e.g., myringotomy tubes

Chronic Rhinitis

- Definition: Chronic nasal discharge with or without acute exacerbations
- Etiology/Incidence
  1. May reflect underlying disorder, e.g., allergic rhinitis, nasal polyps, chronic sinusitis, chronically infected tonsils, cystic fibrosis, foreign body, deviated septum, congenital malformation
  2. May result from prolonged topical nasal decongestant use
- Signs and Symptoms: Variable
  1. Nasal discharge—variable; may be foul smelling or clear or mixed
  2. Possible bloody discharge, e.g., with foreign body
  3. Disturbances in taste and smell
  4. Fever with superimposed infection
- Differential Diagnosis: Allergic rhinitis

- Physical Findings
  1. Excoriation of anterior nares and upper lip
  2. Nasal discharge—usually clear
- Management/Treatment: Treat underlying cause
  1. Antibiotic for bacterial infection
  2. Environmental controls to minimize exposure to allergens
  3. Medications—can try medications used for allergic rhinitis

Foreign Body in Nose

- Definition: Foreign body in either nostril
- Etiology/Incidence: Common items include food, crayons, small toys, erasers, paper wads, beads, beans and stones, alkaline button batteries (batteries may release small amounts of chemicals, leading to chemical burns/perforations, and need immediate removal)
- Signs and Symptoms
  1. Initial—sneezing, mild discomfort, rarely pain; can increase with time
  2. Infection usually follows—unilateral purulent, malodorous, or bloody discharge is always suggestive of a foreign body
- Differential Diagnosis
  1. Nasal polyps, nasal tumors
  2. Purulent rhinitis, sinusitis
- Physical Findings
  1. Unilateral foul-smelling nasal discharge
  2. Visualization of foreign body
- Diagnostic Tests/Findings: None usually; head mirror or light will provide visualization of object
- Management/Treatment
  1. Remove promptly with forceps or nasal suction
  2. Generally infection resolves after removal
  3. Referral to otolaryngologist if unable to remove

Epistaxis

- Definition: Bleeding from the nose
- Etiology/Incidence
  1. Most cases are benign and frequent in childhood due to increased vascularity of nasal mucosa
  2. Trauma and inflammation of mucosal lining (sudden onset) most common cause—nose picking, foreign body insertion, direct blunt trauma, violent sneezing
  3. Nasal mucosal drying (intermittent bleeding) from poorly humidified air, e.g., heating systems
  4. Chronic infection/inflammation of nasal tissue—viral/bacterial or allergies
  5. Substance abuse, e.g., cocaine, cannabis
  6. Systemic diseases—consider with bleeding that is severe, prolonged, or recurrent or concurrently bilateral
     a. Hypertension—exacerbates problem
     b. Clotting abnormalities, e.g., hemophilia, aplastic anemia, leukemia, idiopathic thrombocytopenia, platelet dysfunction

c. ASA and NSAID overuse, neoplasms (gradual onset), cancer treatments, hormonal influences, e.g., menses, birth control pills (BCP), pregnancy
- Signs and Symptoms
  1. Bleeding from nares—usually unilateral
  2. Tarry stools—occasionally with frequent bleeds
- Differential Diagnosis
  1. Foreign bodies
  2. Infection
  3. Substance abuse
  4. Allergies
  5. Chronic rhinitis
  6. Chronic nasal spray use
- Physical Findings
  1. Determine location of bleeding
     a. Anterior bleed—most common site (90%) Kiesselbach's plexus
     b. Posterior bleed—can see only if nose is normal, no inflammation, and with special instruments; may see posterior oropharynx blood flow
     c. High nasal bleed—may represent nasoethmoid or orbit fracture
     d. Recurrent—consider bleeding disorder or chronic irritation
  2. Assess nares for growths, septal hematoma (requires immediate attention)
  3. Assess for other signs of bleeding, excess bruising, petechiae/purpura
- Diagnostic Tests/Findings
  1. CBC with differential, platelets, PT, PTT; coagulation profile (if bleeding disorder is suspected)
  2. Stool for occult blood—determine if child is swallowing blood
  3. Roentgenograms to determine if nasal fracture, foreign body
- Management/Treatment
  1. Complete history including—recurrent or acute, unilateral or bilateral, duration, recent upper respiratory infection (URI), allergic rhinitis, ASA or NSAID use, signs of underlying disease
  2. Monitor vital signs, especially blood pressure
  3. Apply pressure to anterior nasal septum with patient sitting in upright position with head tilted forward (most stop within 10 to 15 minutes); application of ice; avoid nose blowing immediately after nose bleed.
  4. Antibiotics (topical and oral) may be indicated if infection is suggested
  5. Topical nasal vasoconstrictor drops (phenylephrine) and packing may be needed
  6. Prevention: Increase humidity of home, especially in bedroom; avoiding nose picking
  7. Recurrent or severe cases—refer to otolaryngologist

Sinusitis

- Definition: Acute, subacute, or chronic inflammation of mucosal lining in one or more of paranasal sinuses
  1. Acute—persistent symptoms for 10–30 days
  2. Chronic—persistent symptoms for >30 days

- Etiology/Incidence
  1. Common pathogens (also commonly found in AOM)
     a. Predominately in acute sinusitis—*S. pneumoniae*, *H. influenzae*, and *M. catarrhalis*
     b. Prevalent in chronic sinusitis are group A beta-hemolytic streptococcus and *S. aureus* and anaerobes
     c. Viruses—less common
  2. 5% to 10% of URIs in children develop into sinusitis
  3. May be secondary to allergies, adenoidal hypertrophy, anatomical abnormalities, dental abscess, diving and swimming
  4. Patients with cystic fibrosis and immune deficiencies are at a higher risk for sinus infections
  5. Maxillary and ethmoid sinuses most frequently involved
  6. Complications are uncommon overall but are serious; orbital cellulitis is the most common, intracranial abscesses and osteomyelitis of the frontal bone (Potts puffy tumor) can also occur
  7. Adolescent males are at higher risk for intracranial abscesses
- Signs and Symptoms: Children have less specific complaints; adolescents usually present with classical symptoms
  1. Persistent URI (beyond 7 to 10 days) with purulent or watery drainage
  2. Cough, low-grade fever
  3. Facial pain, toothache, headache, or tenderness over involved sinus
  4. Postnasal drip, bad breath, sore throat
  5. Increased pain with cough, bending over, or abrupt head movement
  6. Fatigue, malaise, anorexia
  7. Periorbital swelling in morning
- Differential Diagnosis
  1. Dental infections, foreign bodies, tumors and polyps, nasal trauma, malformations
  2. Allergic and purulent rhinitis, common cold
  3. Cystic fibrosis, immunodeficiency states, allergy, or asthma
- Physical Findings
  1. Clear or mucopurulent rhinorrhea and/or postnasal drainage
  2. Erythema of nasal mucosa and/or throat
  3. Pain on percussion with possible erythema/edema in area of affected sinus
  4. Purulent postnasal drip on posterior pharyngeal wall
  5. OME common finding—especially in younger child
  6. Assess for complications—eyelid swelling with orbital cellulitis, persistent, recurrent, or worsening fever/headache, vomiting, neurologic deficits (intracranial abscess)
- Diagnostic Tests/Findings
  1. Screening CT scan of sinuses—primary diagnostic tool to diagnose sinus disease and complications; obtained if recurrent, uncertain of diagnosis, unresponsive to treatment, assess for complications
  2. Culture of nasal discharge, nasal scrapings for eosinophilia, routine sinus x-rays—not routinely obtained

- Management/Treatment
  1. Antibiotic therapy—same as used in AOM
     a. Chronic sinusitis many require antibiotics for 3 weeks
     b. Clindamycin and trimethoprim/sulfamethoxazole can be used but has limitations; clindamycin is not effective against Gram-negative organisms such as *Haemophilus influenza*, and trimethoprim/sulfamethoxazole is not effective against group A streptococci
  2. Decongestants/antihistamines not proven effective except with concomitant allergic manifestations or nasal congestion
  3. Nasal sprays—topical inhaled steroids (budesonide) and normal saline nasal spray; nasal decongestants can be used with caution, but not for more than 3 days
  4. Comfort measures—analgesics, increase humidity, increase oral fluids
  5. Diving/swimming in moderation; consider elimination of activity during an acute episode or with chronic cases
  6. Refer to otolaryngologist and/or allergist for chronic sinusitis and allergy control

Nasal Polyps

- Definition: Benign pedunculated tumors
- Etiology/Incidence
  1. Originate from edematous, chronically inflamed nasal mucosa
  2. Common in children with cystic fibrosis; 25% develop nasal polyps
- Signs and Symptoms
  1. Nasal obstruction
  2. Mouth breathing
- Differential Diagnosis
  1. Chronic sinusitis
  2. Cystic fibrosis
  3. Chronic allergic rhinitis
- Physical Findings
  1. Nasal obstruction
  2. Mucoid/mucopurulent rhinorrhea
  3. Shiny gray, grape-like mass(es) between nasal turbinates and septum
- Diagnostic Tests/Findings: Sweat test to rule out cystic fibrosis on every child with polyps
- Management/Treatment
  1. Care in distinguishing swollen turbinates from polyps
  2. Antihistamines if allergy related
  3. Local/systemic decongestants/corticosteroids not helpful
  4. Refer for surgical removal in those with complete obstruction or uncontrolled deformity

❑ MOUTH

Oral Candidiasis (Thrush)

- Definition: Common yeast infection of oral mucosa
- Etiology/Incidence
  1. *Candida albicans* (monilial)
  2. More common in neonate and infant than in other age groups (transmission during vaginal delivery), affecting 2% to 5% of newborns
  3. Predisposing factors
     a. Steroid therapy
     b. Antibiotic therapy
     c. Compromised immune system
     d. Diabetes
- Signs and Symptoms
  1. White patches in mouth
  2. May be painful or produce no discomfort
- Physical Findings
  1. Characteristic white, curdlike adherent plaques that are not easily removed; found on the buccal mucosa, tongue, pharynx, and/or tonsils
  2. Bleeding occurs with attempts to remove plaques
- Diagnostic Tests/Findings: Systemic/immune status evaluation if persistent or recurrent
- Management/Treatment
  1. Anti-yeast therapy—nystatin oral suspension applied to oral mucosa 4 times/day for 10 days; if not responding, consider oral fluconazole; gentian violet can be used but is less effective than the newer antifungals and is messy (stains clothes permanently)
  2. If breastfeeding, consider examining and treating mother for candidiasis of breast (cross-infection)
  3. Check diaper area for concurrent monilial diaper rash and treat with nystatin ointment
  4. Sterilize nipples, pacifiers if bottle-fed; apply nystatin to nipples if breastfeeding; if recurrent, look for other causes, e.g., HIV

Cleft Lip and Cleft Palate

- Definition
  1. Cleft lip—failure to join of embryonic structures surrounding oral cavity
  2. Cleft palate—failure of palatal shelves to fuse
  3. Occurs in various degrees
  4. Submucous cleft—bony defect of the palate covered by normal oral mucosa (appears normal but palpation of palate reveals the cleft)
- Etiology/Incidence
  1. Genetic influence with cleft lip more than palate
  2. Both can occur sporadically
  3. More common to have combination of both than one without the other
  4. Cleft lip with or without palate—1:800 births
  5. Cleft palate alone—1:1750 births
  6. More common in males, Asians, and with maternal drug exposure
  7. Lower incidence in African Americans
  8. Increase in middle ear/nasopharyngeal/sinus infections with associated hearing loss
  9. Recurrent otitis media is common
- Signs and Symptoms: Separation of lip and/or palate
- Differential Diagnosis: None

- Physical Findings
  1. Degree of cleft varies from small notch to complete separation
  2. Unilateral or bilateral
  3. Involves soft and/or hard palate
  4. Bifid uvula indicates submucosal cleft palate; can palpate defect on hard palate
- Diagnostic Test/Findings: Audiogram to rule out hearing deficit (because of frequent otitis media associated with cleft palate)
- Management/Treatment
  1. Surgical repair; timing individualized—lip usually by 2 months, palate by 9 to 12 months
  2. Teach feeding techniques (breast or bottle) before and after repair
  3. Referral for dental restoration if needed
  4. Referrals to otolaryngologist, plastic surgeon, pediatric dentist, prosthodontist, orthodontist, speech therapist, psychiatrist, social worker, and genetic counselors
  5. Support family adjustment and management

Dental Caries

- Definition: Demineralization of tooth surface secondary to production of organic acids by bacterial fermentation of dietary carbohydrates
- Etiology/Incidence
  1. In the United States, more than 40% of children have dental cavities by 5 years of age
  2. Mutans streptococci are primary etiological organism responsible for human dental caries
  3. Rate of formation depends on frequency of acid environment in mouth, availability of fluoride for remineralization, and oral hygiene
  4. Early childhood caries
     a. Tooth decay resulting from repeated/prolonged contact with milk, formula, or juice
     b. Babies who are put to bed with bottle or sleep at the breast or use either the breast/bottle as pacifier are at increased risk
  5. Most pediatric dental caries occur on the occlusal surfaces of posterior and lingual aspect of the maxillary incisors, molars, and cuspids; nursing bottle caries affect the upper central and lateral incisors
  6. New teeth are at greater risk for caries than established teeth
  7. Fluoride is critical in the process of remineralization
  8. Incidence has decreased in past 30 years but remains high in low-income children
- Signs and Symptoms
  1. Sensitive or painful tooth
  2. Severe decay—pain, edema, and infection
  3. Weight loss—if severe
  4. Feeding problems
- Physical Findings
  1. Initial decalcification of enamel appears as opaque white spots that turn light brown, progressing to dark brown with destruction of tooth

  2. Left untreated, caries can progress to dental abscess (pain, facial swelling) and, rarely, to sepsis/death
- Management/Treatment
  1. Prevention of dental caries/periodontal disease
     a. Well-balanced diet with appropriate feeding practices; low sugar and complex carbohydrate consumption
     b. Wean from bottle, pacifier, and breast at 1 year of age
     c. Brush/clean/wipe teeth as soon as they appear
     d. Daily brushing and flossing of teeth; for children younger than 8 years, parental involvement needed
     e. Oral fluoride supplement if no fluoride in local water; topical fluoride varnish every 3–6 months can be done in dental or primary care office; dental sealants to occlusal surfaces of the posterior teeth
     f. Early dental visits—American Academy of Pediatric dentists recommend starting dental visits at 12 to 18 months of age for initial discussion of oral hygiene, weaning, and fluoride supplementation; routine dental checkups starting at 3 years
  2. Dental referral for identified caries

Aphthous Ulcers (Canker Sores)

- Definition: Shallow, painful mouth ulceration, prone to recurrence, two types: minor and major
- Etiology/Incidence
  1. Minor aphthous ulcers, more common, occur on the unattached gingiva; major ulcerations are larger and appear on attached gingiva or palate
  2. Appearance: Well-defined lesion, appears as an ulcer with yellow/white necrotic base with surrounding erythema
  3. Cause is unknown but multiple theories—trauma, stress, sun, food allergies, endocrine or hematologic disorders, infectious agents (viral), autoimmune basis
  4. Onset often in adolescence (20%) and recurrent
  5. "Minor"—1 to 5 lesions, 1 cm, lasting 7 to 14 days
  6. "Major"—10% of cases; defined as lesions that are greater than 1 cm, lasting greater than 6 weeks
- Signs and Symptoms
  1. Burning or tingling before appearance of lesion
  2. Pain at lesion site
  3. Afebrile
- Differential Diagnosis
  1. Herpetic lesions (simplex zoster)
  2. Herpangina (coxsackievirus A)
  3. Trauma
  4. Chemical burns
  5. Hand, foot, and mouth disease (coxsackievirus A5, A10, A16)
- Physical Findings
  1. Single or multiple, small, oval, indurated papules with erythematous halo; develops pale center that erodes into ulcers
  2. No systemic symptoms

- Diagnostic Test/Findings: None
- Management/Treatment
  1. Oral analgesics, e.g., 6 to 12 years use chloraseptic spray; greater than 12 years use viscous xylocaine solution, steroid in Orabase (i.e., triamcinolone in Orabase)
  2. Antibacterial (tetracycline) rinses may shorten disease course in children greater than 9 years of age
  3. Referral to pediatric dentist if condition lasts more than 14 days

Herpes Labialis (Cold Sore, Fever Blister) and Herpes Simplex Stomatitis

- Definition
  1. Ulceration and inflammation of oral mucosa from the herpes virus
  2. Acute primary herpetic gingivostomatitis (APHGS) occurs in previously unexposed children
- Etiology/Incidence
  1. Virus acquired from individual who has mouth sore or herpetic whitlow on a finger or toe; caused by herpes simplex virus 1 (HSV-1)
  2. Illness starts 5 to 10 days after exposure
  3. Spontaneous recovery in 7 to 10 days
  4. 50% develop subsequent cold sore episodes after primary acute episode; reactivated from the sensory neurons, by sunlight, stress, fevers
- Signs and Symptoms
  1. Initial infection (APHGS) includes fever, chills, irritability, tender submandibular adenopathy, ulcerative exanthem of the gingiva and mucous membranes of the mouth, sore throat. Anorexia and mouth pain could lead to dehydration
  2. Recurrent herpes simplex limited to a few lesions on the lips—may erupt without symptoms but sometimes have prior tingling in lips before blisters appear
- Differential Diagnosis
  1. Aphthous ulcers
  2. Hand, foot, and mouth syndrome
  3. Herpangina
- Physical Findings
  1. Cold sores—grouped vesicles on erythematous base; commonly found on mucocutaneous border of lips
  2. Primary gingivostomatitis—vesicles on oral mucosa, gingiva, tongue, and lips; ulcers that bleed easily form following vesicle stage; diffuse erythematous, edematous gingiva, especially the interdental papillae
  3. Cervical and/or submandibular adenopathy with gingivostomatitis
  4. May spread to perioral skin
- Diagnostic Tests/Findings: None; rarely if needed, can obtain a viral culture
- Management/Treatment
  1. Treatment is primarily for pain relief (comfort). Once the blisters/vesicles are out, no treatment will hasten resolution
  2. Over-the-counter (OTC) cold sore treatment

3. Pain management—acetaminophen or ibuprofen; topical relief with occlusive gels, e.g., infant oral anesthetic agents; 1:1 mixture of diphenhydramine combined with antacid preparations consisting of magnesium and aluminum hydroxide *or* antidiarrheal preparations to provide a protective coating for the oral mucosa (severe cases add 2% viscous lidocaine sparingly)
  4. Acyclovir may be considered in select patients for primary episodes but is not routinely used; must be started in first 72 hours
  5. Spontaneous recovery within 2 weeks, rarely complications; dehydration is a concern in primary herpes

Hand, Foot, and Mouth Disease

- Definition: Acute viral illness presenting with vesicular exanthem on tongue, gums, palate, oral mucosa; papulovesicular exanthem on hands, feet, and commonly the buttocks in diapered children; less commonly may occur on the trunk and extremities
- Etiology/Incidence
  1. Coxsackievirus A16 (most common), A5, and A10
  2. Enterovirus 71—frequently more severe illness (aseptic meningitis, encephalitis, and paralytic disease)
  3. Seasonal, predominant in summer and fall
  4. Incubation 4 to 6 days
  5. Spontaneous resolution in one week
- Signs and Symptoms
  1. Fever; if present, typically low-grade
  2. Anorexia
  3. Dysphagia
- Differential Diagnosis
  1. Acute primary herpetic gingivostomatitis
  2. Aphthous stomatitis, herpangina
  3. Trauma, burns
- Physical Findings
  1. Small vesicles erode to ulcers on buccal mucosa, hard palate, tonsils, and tongue
  2. Vesicular lesions appear as blanching red lesions on anterior pillars, palms, and soles, less commonly on trunk and extremities
  3. Lesions on buttocks are not usually vesicular
- Diagnostic Tests/Findings: Unnecessary
- Management/Treatment: See Herpangina

Herpangina

- Definition: Acute viral illness presenting with ulceration and inflammation of oral mucosa
- Etiology/Incidence
  1. Coxsackievirus group A (most common)
  2. Coxsackie B viruses and echoviruses (less common)
  3. Seasonal in United States—predominant in summer months
  4. Resolves spontaneously in 3 to 5 days
- Signs and Symptoms
  1. Fever in moderate range
  2. Headache, myalgia, malaise

3. Dysphagia, vomiting (25%), anorexia, significant oral discomfort, drooling
- Differential Diagnosis
  1. Acute primary herpetic gingivostomatitis
  2. Aphthous stomatitis
  3. Trauma or burns
  4. Hand, foot, and mouth disease
  5. Pharyngitis/tonsillitis
- Physical Findings: Small vesicles or punched-out ulcers, especially on soft palate and tonsillar pillars; anterior structures (i.e., gingiva, buccal mucosa, and hard palate) are typically not affected
- Diagnostic Tests/Findings: Unnecessary
- Management/Treatment
  1. Fever and/or pain control—acetaminophen, ibuprofen
  2. Topical relief with 1:1 mixture of diphenhydramine combined with antacid preparations consisting of magnesium and aluminum hydroxide *or* antidiarrheal preparations to provide a protective coating for the oral mucosa (severe cases add 2% viscous lidocaine; use sparingly)
  3. Encourage fluids to ensure adequate hydration

☐ THROAT

Pharyngitis and Tonsillitis

- Definition: Acute inflammation and infection of the throat; when tonsils are main focus of inflammation, *tonsillitis* is more appropriate term to use
- Etiology/Incidence
  1. Causes vary by geographic location, season, age; most common in 5- to 15-year-olds
  2. Viruses
     a. Approximately 80% to 90% of sore throats are viral; numerous viruses, most are not distinguishable from each other
     b. Virus is probable cause when other viral symptoms are present such as nasal congestion, rhinorrhea, cough, hoarseness, conjunctivitis, diarrhea
     c. Adenovirus is common; other viruses include influenza, RSV, parainfluenza, and cytomegalovirus
     d. Epstein-Barr virus—associated with infectious mononucleosis
     e. Enteroviruses (e.g., coxsackievirus A and echovirus) seen in summer and fall
  3. Bacteria
     a. Group A beta-hemolytic streptococcus (GABHS) accounts for 15% to 30% of all pharyngitis cases; typically occurring in late winter and early spring
     b. *Neisseria gonorrhoeae*—in sexually active adolescents or sexually abused children
     c. *Corynebacterium haemolyticum* and *Corynebacterium diphtheriae*—characteristic presence of gray pseudomembranous exudate on pharynx and tonsils that bleeds with attempts at removal; quite rare in United States; seen in developing countries

4. Noninfectious causes (no fever or illness symptoms)
   a. Trauma from tobacco smoke, heat, alcohol
   b. Allergic rhinitis or postnasal drainage
5. Transmission—through exposure to infected respiratory secretions, shared silverware
6. Complications—most are complications of GABHS
   a. Peritonsillar or retropharyngeal abscess or cellulitis
   b. Cervical adenitis, AOM, sinusitis, pneumonia
   c. Acute rheumatic fever in untreated group A beta-hemolytic streptococcal pharyngitis—prevented if treatment started within 9 days of initial complaints of sore throat
   d. Glomerulonephritis—host/immune response to infection with GABHS; not all strains are nephrogenic; manifests in 1–3 weeks after pharyngeal or skin infection of GABHS; unrelated to treatment
- Signs and Symptoms: Common symptomatology with some variability by causative organism
  1. Sudden or gradual onset of symptoms
  2. Sore throat
  3. Fever, variable
  4. Headache, anorexia, occasional nausea, vomiting, abdominal pain, and malaise
  5. Viral pharyngitis—hoarseness, conjunctivitis, runny nose, cough, cold symptoms
  6. GABHS pharyngitis—usually seen 2 years of age and older, sudden onset of fever with complaints of headache, abdominal pain, and vomiting; scarlatina rash, "strawberry tongue" may be present
- Differential Diagnosis
  1. Stomatitis
  2. Peritonsillar or retropharyngeal abscess, epiglottitis
  3. Allergic rhinitis, postnasal drainage
- Physical Findings
  1. Erythema of pharynx, of varying degrees; one presentation of GABHS is a beefy red appearance; petechial lesions on the soft palate can be seen with GABHS
  2. Enlarged tonsils with exudate can be seen with both viral and strep infections
  3. Erythema of nasal mucosa with coryza—more consistent with viral sore throats
  4. Cervical nodes usually enlarged with possible tenderness—tonsillar nodes can be enlarged with GABHS; posterior cervical nodes often enlarged with infectious mononucleosis
- Diagnostic Tests/Findings
  1. Rapid strep test to determine presence of GABHS
     a. Rapid strep tests 90% to 99% sensitive
     b. Treat if positive; throat culture obtained to confirm negative rapid strep test
  2. CBC—WBC may be elevated with bacterial infection and normal or decreased with viral infections, but not entirely reliable. Not routinely obtained unless mono suspected—lymphocytes often increased with infectious mono
  3. Obtain CBC, mono spot, and EBV titers when infectious mono is suspected

4. Consider other studies—dependent on history, age, and clinical presentation, such as culture for gonorrhea, diphtheria culture, CMV titers

- Management/Treatment
  1. Viral pharyngitis/tonsillitis—symptomatic/supportive care
     a. Saline gargles, throat lozenges
     b. Analgesics for fever/pain (acetaminophen, ibuprofen)
     c. Encourage fluids for maintaining hydration
  2. Bacterial pharyngitis/tonsillitis
     a. GABHS—oral penicillin drug of choice. IM penicillin G benzathine (600,000 U for less than 60 pounds, 1.2 million U for greater than 60 pounds); amoxicillin often substituted for penicillin because of better taste
     b. Erythromycin or first-generation cephalosporin for those with penicillin allergy (cephalosporins can be substituted if nonanaphylactic reaction)
     c. Second-line therapy includes macrolides, cephalosporins, or clindamycin. Zithromax is dosed differently for strep than for other conditions such as pneumonia—10 mg/kg/day × 5 days (double dose daily for 5 days)
     d. Considered noncontagious after 24 hours on antibiotic, and if afebrile, patients may return to school. Stress importance of completing antibiotic
     e. Recurrent strep—evaluate for compliance, possible carrier state, or nontreated family member. Not transmitted by family pets or other animals
     f. Gonococcal pharyngitis—one IM injection of ceftriaxone
     g. Diphtheria—hospitalization and treatment with erythromycin or penicillin G

Acute Nasopharyngitis (Common Cold)

- Definition: Acute viral infection of upper respiratory tract with potential involvement of nasal passages, sinuses, Eustachian tubes, middle ears, conjunctiva, and nasopharynx
- Etiology/Incidence
  1. Causative pathogens
     a. More than 100 infectious pathogens—respiratory syncytial virus (RSV) most common
     b. Other common pathogens include parainfluenza viruses, corona viruses, adenoviruses, enterovirus, influenza viruses, *Mycoplasma pneumoniae*
  2. Pathogen shed in large amounts through nasal secretions and easily spread through self-inoculation from fingers and hands to objects (clothing, environmental surfaces)
  3. Universal susceptibility; children average 5 to 8 infections/year with a peak incidence during first 2 years
  4. Increased susceptibility associated with active/passive smoke exposure
  5. More frequent in day care settings and crowded environments
  6. Occurrence in cooler months in temperate climates—peaks in early fall, late January, and early April
- Signs and Symptoms: Generally lasts 1 week; dry cough with rhinorrhea, may persist up to 3 weeks
  1. Infants
     a. Irritability, restlessness, fever (100°F to 102°F)
     b. Rhinorrhea
     c. Occasional diarrhea
     d. Changes in feeding and sleep patterns
  2. Older children
     a. Afebrile or low-grade fever, stuffy nose, watery nasal discharge
     b. Sore throat, sneezing, cough, chills
     c. Occasional headache, malaise
- Differential Diagnosis
  1. Underlying secondary bacterial infection—sinusitis, OM, pharyngitis, lower respiratory tract disease
  2. Allergic rhinitis
  3. Foreign body
  4. Substance abuse in older children and adolescents
  5. Overuse of medicated nasal spray
- Physical Findings
  1. Coryza
  2. Inflamed, moist nasal mucosa and oropharynx
  3. Chest clear
- Diagnostic Tests/Findings
  1. Viral cultures expensive, generally unnecessary
  2. If suspicious of differential diagnosis, consider additional tests such as throat culture, chest or sinus x-rays, allergy testing
- Management/Treatment: Symptomatic/supportive care
  1. Analgesics for sore throat, muscle aches, and general discomfort
  2. Relief of nasal congestion
     a. Saline nose drops or saline spray with nasal bulb syringe
     b. Cool mist humidification
     c. Antihistamines and decongestants not routinely recommended
     d. Antibiotics are not indicated in viral infections
  3. If symptoms persistent beyond 7 to 10 days, consider secondary infection
  4. Maintain hydration
  5. Prevention
     a. Good hygiene and cleaning of clothes, toys, and play areas
     b. Limited exposure to crowded situations

Retropharyngeal Abscess

- Definition: Infection of the retropharyngeal lymph nodes; inflammation of posterior aspect of pharynx with suppurative retropharyngeal lymph nodes
- Etiology
  1. Usually preceded by URIs, pharyngitis, sinusitis, and cervical lymphadenitis
  2. In older children—usually superinfection from penetrating injury to posterior wall of oropharynx

3. Most common organisms—GABHS and staph aureus
4. Relatively rare infection, most common in children younger than 6 years of age; peak incidence at age 3
- Signs and Symptoms
  1. Acute onset of high fever with persistent severe throat pain
  2. Drooling due to difficulty in swallowing
  3. Tachypnea, dyspnea, stridor
  4. Neck and head hyperextension
- Differential Diagnosis
  1. Epiglottitis
  2. Peritonsillar abscess
  3. Laryngotracheobronchitis (croup)
  4. Acute infectious mononucleosis
  5. Acute pharyngitis
  6. Bacterial tracheitis
  7. Meningitis
- Physical Findings
  1. Toxic-appearing child; neck and head in hyperextension
  2. Noisy, gurgling respiration
  3. Drooling, meningismus
  4. Stridor, airway obstruction
  5. Possible neck swelling, torticollis
  6. Prominent swelling of posterior pharyngeal wall—confirms diagnosis
- Diagnostic Tests/Findings
  1. Lateral neck radiography—retropharyngeal space wider than C4 vertebral body or greater than 6 mm at C2
  2. CBC—elevated WBCs common
  3. CT scan to visualize abscess
- Management/Treatment
  1. Emergency hospitalization necessary
     a. Transported by ambulance to hospital
     b. ENT consult immediate at hospital
     c. Admission to pediatric ICU for continuous monitoring for airway obstruction and possible respiratory arrest
     d. Surgical incision and drainage necessary
     e. IV antibiotics—penicillin, clindamycin

Peritonsillar Abscess

- Definition: Infection of tonsils spreading to tonsillar fossa and surrounding tissues (peritonsillar cellulitis); if left untreated, tonsillar abscess forms
- Etiology/Incidence
  1. GABHS (most common)
  2. *S. aureus*, anaerobic microorganisms
  3. Can occur at any age; more common in preadolescent or adolescent age groups
  4. Complication of untreated peritonsillar abscess—lateral pharyngeal abscess leading to possible airway obstruction; aggressive early treatment needed
- Signs and Symptoms
  1. Severe sore throat with high fever
  2. Toxic appearance, muffled voice, spasms of jaw muscles

3. Difficulty swallowing and drooling in severe cases
4. Bad breath
- Differential Diagnosis
  1. Retropharyngeal abscess
  2. Epiglottitis
- Physical Findings
  1. Unilateral enlargement of tonsil(s), bulging medially with anterior pillar prominence (most common)
  2. Soft palate and uvula edematous, erythematous, with uvula displaced toward unaffected side
  3. Extreme tonsillar tenderness on palpation
  4. Trismus can occur, making visualization of the pharynx difficult
  5. May have limited range of motion of neck
- Diagnostic Tests
  1. CBC—increased WBCs
  2. Rapid strep test to rule out GABHS
- Management/Treatment
  1. Immediate referral to ENT
  2. Surgical incision and drainage often necessary
  3. Hospitalization common for 24 hours; if not hospitalized, daily follow-up visits until stable
  4. Antibiotics (penicillin or clindamycin), IV initially, and discharged on oral antibiotics

Cervical Lymphadenitis (Cervical Adenitis)

- Definition: Inflammation/infection affecting one or more cervical lymph nodes
- Etiology/Incidence
  1. Pathogens
     a. *S. pyogenes* and *S. aureus* account for approximately 80% of cases
     b. *M. tuberculosis*
     c. Other organisms (e.g., viral, fungal, or parasitic)
  2. Secondary to local infections of the ear, nose, and throat (most common)
  3. Prevalent among preschool children
- Signs and Symptoms
  1. Complaints of swollen neck or face
  2. Fever commonly present
  3. Rare—stridor, hoarseness, drooling if adenopathy impinges on airway
- Differential Diagnosis
  1. Bilateral cervical adenitis—mononucleosis, tularemia, diphtheria
  2. Subacute or chronic adenitis—cat scratch fever, nonspecific viral infections
  3. Atypical mycobacterium—tuberculosis
  4. Cervical node tumors, e.g., leukemia
  5. Parotitis, cyst, hematoma
- Physical Findings
  1. Large unilateral cervical mass, 2 to 6 cm
  2. Overlying erythema may be present
  3. Likely tenderness on palpation

- Diagnostic Tests/Findings
  1. CBC—may be normal or elevated; depending on the etiology
  2. PPD—rule out tuberculosis
  3. Mono spot and EBV titers to rule out mononucleosis
  4. Throat culture—rule out GABHS
  5. Serology tests if not resolving (e.g., toxoplasmosis, CMV, *Bartonella henselae* for cat scratch)
  6. Aspiration of node if fluctuant—aerobic/anaerobic culture
- Management/Treatment
  1. With no evidence of sepsis, treat empirically with oral antibiotics—dicloxacillin, amoxicillin clavulanate, or cephalexin for a minimum of 10 days
  2. Measure and follow size of node; may take several weeks to regress even with adequate treatment
  3. Analgesics for fever and pain; application of cold compresses
  4. Reevaluation after 36 to 48 hours; if no improvement, possible hospitalization for IV antibiotics, especially with infants and young children
  5. Referral to otolaryngologist if not improving
  6. Surgical aspiration may be necessary
  7. Persistent unexplained, symptomatic node, increasing in size despite treatment, refer for biopsy

Epiglottitis (Supraglottitis)

- Definition: Severe, rapidly developing inflammation and swelling of the supraglottic structures leading to life-threatening upper airway obstruction
- Etiology/Incidence
  1. Can occur at any age, highest incidence 2 to 7 years of age
  2. Pathogens—group A beta-hemolytic streptococci, pneumococci, *H. influenzae*
  3. Decreasing incidence from *H. influenzae* with use of Hib vaccine by 99% in children younger than 5 years but can still occur even with a complete set of vaccines
- Signs and Symptoms
  1. Acute, sudden onset of high fever, severe sore throat, muffled voice, drooling, poor color, labored breathing in a previously well child
  2. Choking sensation, refuses to speak
  3. Restless, irritable, anxious, apprehensive, frightened
  4. Hyperextension of neck, leaning forward and chin thrust out, prostration; "sniffing dog" or tripod position—provides best possible airway
- Differential Diagnosis
  1. Acute laryngeal edema, croup syndrome, foreign body aspiration
  2. Pertussis, diphtheria, Kawasaki syndrome
  3. Bacterial tracheitis, retropharyngeal abscess
- Physical Findings
  1. Rapidly progressive respiratory distress—suprasternal and subcostal retractions, soft inspiratory stridor, nasal flaring leading to possible respiratory arrest

  2. Toxic, distressed appearance
  3. Beefy erythematous epiglottis
  4. If epiglottitis suspected, do not attempt to visualize
- Diagnostic Tests/Findings: Often deferred until airway secured to minimize acute respiratory distress
  1. CBC—WBCs (greater than 18,800); laboratory examination is low priority in child with severe respiratory distress
  2. Cultures of blood, tracheal, or epiglottis secretions—identifies pathogen
  3. Radiograph—lateral neck shows a thickened/swollen epiglottis ("thumb sign"); may elect not to perform radiograph due to possibility of airway obstruction and respiratory arrest; airway can be safely visualized in surgery
- Management/Treatment
  1. Requires prompt recognition and treatment; represents a true medical emergency; death can occur within hours
  2. While waiting for emergency transport: provide oxygen, keep child calm, be prepared for emergency cardiopulmonary resuscitation
  3. Following diagnosis, airway must be established by nasotracheal or endotracheal intubation or elective tracheotomy immediately; usually extubated within 24 to 48 hours after reducing epiglottis and afebrile
  4. IV antibiotic therapy for 2 to 3 days
     a. Third-generation cephalosporins until initial pathogen identified; antibiotics most commonly used include ceftriaxone and ampicillin-sulbactam
     b. In areas with penicillin- and cephalosporin-resistant pneumococci, vancomycin is drug of choice
  5. Oral antibiotics will follow IV antibiotics to complete 10-day course
  6. Corticosteroid therapy to reduce swelling
  7. Prevention—*H. influenzae* type b vaccine at 2, 4, 6 or 12, and 15 months of age; no vaccines against other pathogens

❏ QUESTIONS

Select the best answer.

1. Which one of the following may cause microcephaly?
   a. Hypocalcemia
   b. Craniosynostosis
   c. Skull fracture
   d. Seizure disorder
2. What finding may accompany macrocephaly?
   a. Pulsating anterior fontanel
   b. Sunken fontanel
   c. Premature closure of suture lines
   d. Widened suture lines
3. Obtaining a CT of the head would be indicated in which of the following conditions?
   a. Macrocephaly
   b. Cephalohematoma
   c. Craniosynostosis
   d. Caput succedaneum

4. Which one of the following conditions increases the risk of developing hydrocephalus?
   a. Bilateral cephalohematomas
   b. Craniosynostosis
   c. Prematurity
   d. Familial macrocephaly

5. A conjunctivitis appearing in a 2-day-old newborn is likely due to:
   a. Chemical irritation from eye drops
   b. Group B streptococcus
   c. Chlamydia
   d. Gonorrhea

6. Confirming the diagnosis of chlamydia conjunctivitis in a newborn would best be done by obtaining which one of the following?
   a. Cervical swab of the mother
   b. Urine PCR from the mother
   c. Culture of the eye discharge
   d. Culture of the conjunctival scrapings

7. Which one of the following eye findings would be considered an ophthalmic emergency?
   a. Unilateral vesicular lesions on the upper eyelid in a 3-week-old
   b. Presence of chemosis in a 5-year-old with bilateral upper eyelid edema
   c. Cobblestone-like appearance along the inner aspect of the upper eyelid in a 15-year-old
   d. Bilateral redness along eyelid margins with tiny ulcerated areas in a 16-year-old

8. The most appropriate management of a 5-year-old with a firm, nontender nodule in the mid-upper eyelid for 3 weeks would be:
   a. Cool compresses
   b. Topical ophthalmic ointment
   c. Oral antibiotics
   d. Oral steroids

9. Daily eyelid cleansing with diluted baby shampoo and a cotton-tipped applicator would be appropriate in the treatment of which one of the following conditions?
   a. Dacryostenosis
   b. Chalzion
   c. Hordeolum
   d. Blepharitis

10. A 3-year-old has an edematous, mildly erythematous right upper eyelid for 1 day with a fever of 103°F. An important eye assessment would be:
    a. Ocular mobility
    b. Conjunctival inflammation
    c. Pupillary reaction
    d. Optic disc papilledema

11. Concurrent otitis media and conjunctivitis is likely due to which organism?
    a. *Streptococcus pneumoniae*
    b. *Haemophilus influenzae*
    c. *Moraxella catarrhalis*
    d. *Staphylococcus aureus*

12. All but which one of the following is consistent with glaucoma?
    a. Photophobia
    b. Epiphora (increased tears)
    c. Blepharospasm
    d. Leukokoria (white red reflex)

13. All but which one of the following assessments is used to determine the presence of a strabismus?
    a. Hirschberg test
    b. Cover–uncover test
    c. Extraocular movements
    d. Pupillary response

14. A 3-month-old has a mild asymmetrical corneal light reflex on physical exam. What is the next appropriate step?
    a. Observe and reevaluate at the next well check
    b. Refer immediately to ophthalmology
    c. Begin atropine drops or eye patching
    d. Protect eyes from sunlight

15. Prematurity increases the risk of developing which one of the following?
    a. Nystagmus
    b. Astigmatism
    c. Myopia
    d. Glaucoma

16. Fluorescein staining of the eye is used to detect a:
    a. Keratitis
    b. Foreign body
    c. Corneal abrasion
    d. Hyphema

17. Trauma to the eye increases the risk of developing all but which one of the following?
    a. Strabismus
    b. Glaucoma
    c. Cataracts
    d. Hyphema

18. Corneal abrasions can be managed with topical application of which one of the following?
    a. Anesthetic to control pain
    b. Steroids to prevent adhesions
    c. Antibiotics to prevent infection
    d. Atropine to prevent ciliary spasm

19. The greatest risk in a patient with a hyphema is which one of the following?
    a. Glaucoma
    b. Infection
    c. Rebleed
    d. Cataracts

20. A 16-year-old was hit in the eye 1 day ago and now has ecchymoses on the upper and lower lids with 5 out of 10 eye pain. All but which of the following would be appropriate to obtain at this time?
    a. Visual acuity
    b. Intraocular pressure
    c. CT scan
    d. Fluorescein stain

21. A 10-year-old has marked ear pain, not wanting anyone to touch his ear. The canal is edematous and exudate is present. TM is normal. How should this be managed?
    a. Topical fluoroquinolone
    b. Oral steroids and topical neomycin
    c. Oral amoxicillin and topical anesthetic
    d. Oral amoxicillin and topical steroid

22. Patients with otitis externa should be instructed to do which one of the following?
    a. Keep ear dry until symptoms improve
    b. Limit swimming for remainder of summer
    c. Wear earplugs at all times with swimming
    d. Use alcohol drops before swimming each day

23. All but which one of the following patients are at an increased risk of developing otitis media?
    a. 2-year-old with cleft palate repair at 1 year of age
    b. 15-month-old with Down syndrome
    c. 9-month-old with lactose intolerance
    d. 3-year-old with IgA immune deficiency

24. A 15-month-old failed treatment with amoxicillin for otitis media. At his 2-week recheck, his TM remained red with distorted landmarks, and he persisted with nasal congestion and poor nighttime sleeping, and he has had a 101°F fever for the past 2 days. The next best step would be to treat with:
    a. A 10-day course of Augmentin
    b. A 3-week course of a cephalosporin
    c. A higher dose amoxicillin and topical antibiotics
    d. Ceftriaxone and an antihistamine

25. A 2-year-old male with a history of chronic serous otitis media is noted to have a pearly white opacity in the upper outer quadrant of his TM. He currently has no symptoms and appears to hear adequately. The most likely diagnosis and appropriate management would be:
    a. Tympanosclerosis; no treatment is necessary
    b. Persistent perforation; prescribe topical antibiotic drops
    c. Foreign body; perform an ear wash for removal
    d. Cholesteatoma; refer to otolaryngology

26. A 7-year-old has experienced recurrent nosebleeds in the past 2 months. What finding on the physical exam would suggest an underlying medical cause for the epistaxis?
    a. Wheezing
    b. Grade II murmur
    c. Petechiae
    d. Tonsil hypertrophy

27. An 8-year-old has chronic intermittent nasal congestion. All but which one of the following would support allergic rhinitis?
    a. Pale boggy turbinates
    b. Darkened areas on lower eyelids
    c. Increased basophils on CBC
    d. Itchy, watery eyes

28. Acceptable management options for allergic rhinitis include all of the following except:
    a. Oral cetirizine
    b. Oral montelukast
    c. Nasal beclomethasone
    d. Nasal neosynephrine

29. Which foreign body in the nose requires immediate removal?
    a. Bean
    b. Bead
    c. Stone
    d. Battery

30. What complication of sinusitis are adolescent males more prone to?
    a. Intracranial abscess
    b. Potts puffy tumor
    c. Orbital cellulitis
    d. Dental infection

31. Patients with sinusitis should be instructed not to participate in which activity?
    a. Swimming/diving
    b. Boxing/wrestling
    c. Weight lifting
    d. Cross-country running

32. All of the following may predispose a patient to thrush except:
    a. Age
    b. Steroid therapy
    c. Antibiotics
    d. Poor oral hygiene

33. A 9-month-old is noted to have a bifed uvula. This would increase his risk of developing which disorder?
    a. Otitis media
    b. Retropharyngeal abscess
    c. Sinusitis
    d. Dental malocclusion

34. A 10-year-old has a single painful ulcerated lesion on an erythematous base on the inner buccal mucosa. The most likely diagnosis and treatment would be:
    a. Herpes simplex stomatitis—oral acyclovir
    b. Herpangina—viscous xylocaine
    c. Aphthous ulcer—triamcinolone in Orabase
    d. Hand, foot, mouth syndrome—antibiotic mouthwash

35. Initial exposure to the herpes virus may produce all of the following except:
    a. Fever and dehydration
    b. Submandibular lymph nodes
    c. Vesicular lesions on tonsils
    d. Friable and edematous gingiva

36. The organism that causes hand, foot, mouth syndrome is what virus?
    a. Cytomegalovirus
    b. Parainfluenza
    c. Varicella-zoster
    d. Coxsackie

37. Which one of the following complications of strep pharyngitis cannot be prevented with antibiotics?
    a. Peritonsillar abscess
    b. Cervical adenitis
    c. Glomerulonephritis
    d. Acute rheumatic fever

38. In addition to penicillin, all of the following antibiotics can be used to treat strep pharyngitis except:
    a. Clindamycin
    b. Erythromycin
    c. Bactrim
    d. Ceftriaxone

39. Retropharyngeal abscess is typically seen in what age group and includes which mainstay treatment?
    a. Neonates; hospitalization for IV antibiotics
    b. 2- to 6-year-olds; ICU admission and IV antibiotics
    c. 6- to 12-year-olds; outpatient oral antibiotics
    d. Adolescents; ENT drainage of abscess

40. Findings consistent with peritonsillar abscess include all of the following except:
    a. Muffled voice
    b. Unilateral enlargement of tonsil
    c. Trismus
    d. Exudate on tonsils

41. Appropriate lab tests to obtain in assessment of cervical adenitis include all of the following except:
    a. Throat culture
    b. Mono test
    c. PPD test
    d. Blood culture

42. The incidence of epiglottitis has decreased because of which vaccine?
    a. Hib
    b. Prevnar
    c. Varicella
    d. Meningococcal

43. Patients with epiglottitis prefer to sit in which position?
    a. Sitting up and leaning forward
    b. Left lateral position
    c. Supine with neck hyperextended
    d. 45-degree upright, resting back

44. All but which one of the following conditions requires urgent inpatient admission?
    a. Cervical adenitis
    b. Retropharyngeal abscess
    c. Epiglottitis
    d. Orbital cellulitis

45. Conductive hearing loss can be caused by:
    a. Brain tumor
    b. Ototoxic drug exposure
    c. Loud noises
    d. Serous otitis

☐ ANSWERS AND RATIONALES

1. B: None of the other conditions is associated with microcephaly in any way.

2. D: A large head can widen the suture lines. Pulsating anterior fontanel can be a normal variant or due to increased ICP. Sunken fontanel can accompany dehydration, and premature closure of suture lines often results in a small head.

3. A: Macrocephaly has numerous underlying causes such as hydrocephalus that need to be identified so appropriate treatment can be initiated. A CT scan would be necessary for that identification. A routine skull x-ray could be used to identify craniosynostosis or an underlying skull fracture if suspected with cephalohematoma or caput succedaneum but is rarely indicated.

4. C: Prematurity is a known risk factor for hydrocephalus, but the other conditions are not. Bilateral cephalohematomas may result in an underlying skull fracture, but not hydrocephalus. Craniosynostosis, if severe, can result in increased intracranial pressure but is not associated with the development of hydrocephalus. Familial macrocephaly is a normal variant and not associated with any underlying pathology.

5. A: A conjunctivitis developing on day 2 of life is most likely due to a chemical irritation from the routine prophylactic eye medication. Although this is being seen less frequently now with the use of erythromycin ophthalmic ointment instead of silver nitrate, it still does occur. The other causes of conjunctivitis listed in the answers tend to occur later than day 2 of life. Chlamydia can be seen at age 2 weeks or later.

6. D: *Chlamydia* is an intracellular organism, and therefore any sample for testing must include epithelial cells. Conjunctival scrapings collect epithelial cells and eye discharge would not. Testing the mother would not definitively determine what is causing the infant's discharge.

7. A: Unilateral vesicular lesions would indicate a possible herpetic infection of the eye and in a 3-week-old this could spread to the CNS, potentially causing severe, permanent CNS damage and/or death. Chemosis is swelling on the conjunctiva, often associated with allergies and is not life or vision threatening. This is the same with cobblestone appearance of the inverted upper eyelid. Answer D is suggestive of blepharitis, which is not an emergency disorder.

8. B: The history describes a chalazion, which often resolves without treatment. However, topical antibiotic ointment is an appropriate and recommended treatment for chalazions. Chalazions can become infected and topical antibiotics may help to prevent this from happening. Warm compresses, not cool, can also be used. Oral antibiotics are not used except if chalazions become recurrent; the oral antibiotics are used to prevent another reoccurrence. Oral steroids have no part in the treatment of chalazions. Rarely, an ophthalmologist may inject a chalazion with a steroid, but this is not done routinely and only then by an ophthalmologist.

9. D: Daily lid scrubs with dilute baby shampoo is one of the primary treatments for blepharitis. None of the other disorders is treated with this modality. Dacryostenosis (a blocked tear duct) is treated with time,

antibiotic eye ointment, and massage. The treatment for chalazions is described in question 8, and styes (hordeolums) are treated with warm compresses and topical ophthalmic ointments.

10. A: The description given is of an early orbital or periorbital cellulitis. These two disease entities have some similarities but are very different with respect to complications and treatment; therefore, they need to be distinguished. Ocular mobility is absent or significantly decreased with orbital cellulitis; however, it is not affected in periorbital cellulitis. This symptom would therefore be helpful to distinguish between these two disorders. None of the other three assessment points would be helpful with diagnosing these two disorders.

11. B: There is a known association with *Haemophilus influenzae* and concurrent OM and conjunctivitis. The other organisms are not associated with this ear–eye connection.

12. D: The classic triad for glaucoma is photophobia, epiphora, and blepharospasm. The cornea may be hazy with glaucoma, but it is not associated with a white red reflex (leukocoria).

13. D: The Hirschberg test and the cover–uncover test assess for a nonparalytic strabismus, and the EOMs assess for a paralytic strabismus. Pupillary response does not assess for strabismus at all.

14. A: A mild asymmetrical corneal light reflex (Hirschberg test) can be a normal variant until 4 months of age. Therefore, it can safely be reevaluated at the next well visit (4 months of age) and does not need a referral. Only ophthalmologists should prescribe atropine drops and these would not be indicated now. Strabismus (which is the disorder indicated in the test question) is not associated with photophobia or sun exposure.

15. C: Myopia of prematurity is a known association. Prematurity is not a risk factor for the other conditions.

16. C: Most corneal abrasions cannot be seen (except if they are very large). A fluorescein stain placed in the eye will reveal an abrasion (the stain will pool in the gap and be visible). A keratitis is an inflammation of the cornea, but there is no abraded area for the stain to pool in. An exception to that is with herpetic keratitis, which may produce ocular dendritic ulcers that can be seen with a fluorescein stain (but keratitis has many causes, most of which do not stain). A foreign body does not need staining to be seen. Even if very small, fluorescein staining will not enhance its appearance. In a hyphema, there is bleeding into the anterior chamber (behind the cornea) that is usually visible as a blood level in the eye. The area of damage is not accessible to the stain.

17. A: Trauma to the eye does not increase the risk of strabismus. Cataracts and glaucoma may develop years after eye trauma. In contrast, hyphemas, if they occur, develop soon after eye trauma and may reoccur.

18. C: Corneal abrasions are susceptible to infection; therefore, topical ophthalmic antibiotics would be indicated in their management. Topical ophthalmic anesthetic is used only once and in a healthcare setting to assist in diagnosing and treating eye disorders. Repeated use can cause severe and irreversible eye damage. Pain control can be obtained with topical or oral NSAIDs. Ophthalmic steroids and atropine are prescribed only by ophthalmologists for specific disorders, and neither is indicated for treatment of corneal abrasions.

19. C: The greatest imminent risk from a hyphema is a rebleed, which often leads to more eye damage (vision loss) than the initial bleed. There is an increased risk for the development of glaucoma and cataracts following various causes of eye trauma not specific to hyphemas. With hyphemas, the bleeding occurs in the anterior chamber and is not as susceptible to outside organisms like a corneal abrasion would be. Therefore, infection is not as imminent a problem as it would be with a corneal abrasion.

20. B: This is used to test for glaucoma, which, if it occurs, would be years later. Almost all eye injuries, except the most serious such as a ruptured globe, should have a visual acuity done. An eye injury can produce more than one injury. Therefore, a person with a "black eye" could also have other injuries such as an orbital fracture and a corneal abrasion. A CT scan would be appropriate to assess for an orbital fracture. A fluorescein stain could be used to assess for a concurrent corneal abrasion.

21. A: This patient has an otitis externa (OE) by the description of the canal (edematous with exudate). One of the most common organisms is *Pseudomonas*, which is susceptible to the fluoroquinolones. The antibiotic needs to be in contact with the canal, which is why topical antibiotics are used. Oral antibiotics, which are very helpful with acute otitis media, are not effective in the treatment of OE. Oral steroids are not indicated for otitis externa. However, topical steroids can be used, especially when used with a topical antibiotic.

22. A: One of the primary causes of otitis externa is overhydration of the external ear canal. Therefore, part of management is keeping the ear canal dry to enhance healing. Swimming does not need to be limited for the entire summer but just during the acute phase. Earplugs, especially if they are not individually fitted, do not keep all water out. When a small amount of water does get around the earplugs, it can become trapped in the canal and delay healing. Alcohol and white vinegar drops (equal parts) are used to prevent swimmer's ear, instilled at the end of each swimming day to help evaporate any remaining water droplets. These types of drops are not effective in treating an actual otitis externa.

23. C: Lactose intolerance is not a risk factor for the development of otitis media. Food allergies can be a risk factor, but a lactose intolerance is not a true food allergy. Cleft palate, Down syndrome, and IgA immune deficiency are known risk factors for otitis media.

24. A: According to AAP guidelines on treatment of OM, Augmentin (amoxicillin) is recommended for second-line management (failed treatment) or first-line if the child is with significant signs/symptoms (high fever). In this case, Augmentin would appropriately be used second line. A higher dose of amoxicillin would be inappropriate. First-line management starts with high-dose amoxicillin (80–90 mg/kg/day), and dosing higher than this would be potentially dangerous. Topical antibiotics have no role in the treatment of AOM unless there is a perforation of the TM or a PE tube in place. Ceftriaxone is an acceptable alternative for failed therapy but is third-line treatment. Antihistamines are not effective or recommended in the treatment of OM. Three weeks of an antibiotic (i.e., cephalosporin) is not a recommended treatment regime for failed OM therapy.

25. D: A cholesteatoma typically appears as a pearly white opacity in the upper outer quadrant of the TM. Chronic serous otitis media is a risk factor for the development of a cholesteatoma (which this patient had). An immediate referral is needed because it can continue to grow and be very destructive and potentially spread into the brain. The child may appear to hear well because the other ear may be compensating and all hearing in the affected ear is not destroyed immediately. Tympanosclerosis (scar tissue) is also whitish appearing but more cloud-like in appearance and typically located in the lower quadrants of the TM. The patient usually has a history of PE tubes or TM perforations. A foreign body will likely be laying in the canal and not embedded in the TM. Not all foreign bodies are best removed with an ear wash; some are best removed with small forceps. Last, a perforation will typically appear like a round hole in the TM. The patient usually has a history of PE tubes, TM perforation, or ear injury. Topical antibiotics can be used with perforations; however, a referral to ENT would be indicated initially.

26. C: Most children with nosebleeds do not have an underlying medical cause. If they do, it is often hematologic such as bleeding disorders or leukemia. Petechiae can be an indicator of various hematologic disorders. None of the other symptoms listed (wheezing, murmur, or tonsil hypertrophy) are associated with hematologic disorders or other underlying causes of nosebleeds.

27. C: Patients with allergic rhinitis or other allergic disease can have an increase in eosinophils, not basophils. Pale, boggy nasal turbinates, darkened areas under the eyes (allergic shiners), and itchy, watery eyes are all consistent findings with allergic rhinitis.

28. D: Nasal neosynephrine (OTC nasal spray such as Afrin) is indicated only for short-term use (3 days maximum) because extended use leads to rebound chronic nasal congestion. Allergic rhinitis is usually chronic and will need safe long-term management.

Nasal steroid sprays such as beclomethasone, oral cetirizine, and montelukast are recommended treatment modalities for allergic rhinitis and can be used long term.

29. D: All nasal foreign bodies should be removed quickly; however, batteries require immediate removal because they can leak corrosive chemicals that can do irreparable damage to the nasal septum and entire nasal cavity.

30. A: All of the answers are potential complications of sinusitis. However, for unclear reasons, adolescent males have a higher incidence of brain abscesses with their sinusitis. This is one reason why close follow-up is essential for persistent headaches after initiating antibiotics for sinusitis.

31. A: Swimming and diving are known contributing factors to the development of sinusitis as well as exacerbating factors during treatment. This may be due to contaminated water entering the nasal cavities and sinuses at an increased pressure as may occur with both diving and swimming. The other activities (boxing, weight lifting, and running) do not have any association with sinusitis.

32. D: Poor oral hygiene is a risk factor in the development of dental carries, but not thrush. Infants, because of their age, are at an increased risk for developing thrush. Antibiotics alter the balance of microbes in the mouth, allowing yeast to increase above their normal count (bacteria and yeast normally maintain a balance; with antibiotics decreasing the number of good bacteria, yeast can then increase). Steroids can alter normal immune functioning as well as glucose levels.

33. A: A bifed uvula is an indicator of a possible submucous cleft. All cleft palates, whether visible or not visible, increase the risk of otitis media. A submucous cleft is not visible but can be felt by palpating the hard palate. Neither a submucous cleft nor a bifed uvula is a risk factor for the development of a retropharyngeal abscess, sinusitis, or dental malocclusion.

34. C: Aphthous ulcers tend to occur as single, ulcerated lesions and are most often located on the unattached gingiva (i.e., lower, inner buccal mucosa), as described in this case. Triamcinolone in Orabase is an acceptable treatment in a 10-year-old. The other three disorders listed are definite differentials but have different characteristics. Herpes simplex stomatitis tends to occur in younger children (toddlers) and often is associated with high fevers. There is diffuse swelling of the gingiva and very superficial (not deeply ulcerated) lesions on the gingiva. Herpangina tends to occur in older patients, such as in this case, but is usually accompanied by high fevers and a severe sore throat (not a single area of mouth soreness). The intraoral lesions are ulcerative lesions located posteriorly (usually on the anterior pillars), not in the front of the mouth like aphthous ulcers. Last, hand, foot,

mouth syndrome is usually seen in younger children (toddler and preschool age). Fever is usually absent or low grade. Diffuse small and painful blisters can occur throughout the mouth, including the tongue as well as the hard and soft palates. Nonpainful papules can appear on the palms and soles as well as in areas not indicated in the name such as the buttocks.

35. C: The first exposure to the herpes virus is very different from the subsequent intermittent outbreaks of fever blisters on the lips. With the first exposure, the child is usually quite ill. The intraoral lesions of herpes occur in the front of the mouth, primarily involving the gingiva. The gingiva are typically painful, friable (bleed easily), and edematous (the swelling can be so severe as to almost completely cover the teeth). The lesions do not extend to the tonsils. If lesions were seen on the anterior pillars and/or tonsils, another diagnosis should be considered. With the first exposure to the herpes virus, fever is common and can be fairly high (104°F). The illness causes anorexia as a result of the painful mouth lesions that interfere with eating and drinking, potentially leading to dehydration. The submandibular nodes drain the mouth and often become enlarged and tender with herpetic infections of the mouth and the lips.

36. D: The Coxsackie virus is the virus that causes hand, foot, mouth syndrome. The other organisms are not associated with this syndrome. CMV can cause a pharyngitis and fever, but no rash. Parainfluenza virus is a common organism with croup. Varicella-zoster virus is the causative organism with chickenpox and shingles (zoster).

37. C: Even with prompt and adequate treatment with antibiotics, acute glomerulonephritis (AGN) cannot be prevented. Not all strains of strep are nephrogenic, however. All the other potential complications of strep (peritonsillar abscess, cervical adenitis, and acute rheumatic fever) can be prevented with antibiotics.

38. C: The antibiotic Bactrim has no effect on strep and can therefore never be used to treat strep infections. The other antibiotics do provide the needed coverage.

39. B: Retropharyngeal abscesses are usually seen in children younger than 6 years of age, with an average of 3 years of age. Because of changes in lymphatics, they do not usually occur after age 6. They are a life-threatening condition because of potential airway compromise, and the patient is always admitted to the ICU and treated with IV antibiotics.

40. D: Although a pharyngeal abscess would consist of exudate, it is under the surface and not visible. Pharyngeal abscesses are typically unilateral and often associated with a muffled voice ("potato voice") and trismus (difficulty opening mouth).

41. D: The causes of cervical adenitis (swollen cervical node or nodes) include strep pharyngitis, infectious mononucleosis, and, to a lesser extent, tuberculosis. Therefore, it would be appropriate to test for these conditions if indicated. Obtaining a throat culture and mono spot would be helpful. A PPD test would be indicated initially if the history is suggestive (i.e., exposure, cough) or later if the enlarged lymph node did not resolve with antibiotics. Cervical adenitis is not associated with sepsis and therefore a blood culture would not be useful.

42. A: *Haemophilus influenzae* was one of the primary organisms causing epiglottitis. With the advent of the Hib vaccine, there has been a significant decline in the incidence of epiglottitis. But it has not been entirely eradicated. Other organisms can cause epiglottitis, but not any of the organisms associated with the Prevnar, varicella, or meningococcal vaccines.

43. A: Patients who are experiencing airway compromise due to a swollen epiglottis find breathing is easier by sitting up and leaning forward. This is a very common finding in patients with epiglottitis. Lying down, whether supine or lateral, or leaning back does not help open the airway to its maximum potential, and therefore patients with epiglottitis typically do not adopt these positions.

44. A: Cervical adenitis is not a life-threatening condition and is typically treated on an outpatient basis with oral antibiotics and close follow-up to make certain the lymph node or nodes have improved. The other three conditions (retropharyngeal abscess, epiglottitis, and orbital cellulitis) can be life threatening. Retropharyngeal abscess and epiglottitis can cause airway compromise. Orbital cellulitis can be life and vision threatening.

45. D: There are two types of hearing loss—conductive and sensorineural. A conductive hearing loss occurs with a problem in the outer ear, such as impacted cerumen, or in the middle ear, such as fluid in the middle ear. Both these conditions (cerumen and fluid) impede the conduction of sound from the environment to the inner ear. In contrast, a sensorineural hearing loss stems from a problem in the inner ear and extending to the hearing center in the brain, such as a tumor on the acoustic nerve (8th cranial nerve). Ototoxic drugs and loud noises damage parts of the inner ear such as the cochlea and can result in sensorineural hearing loss.

❏ BIBLIOGRAPHY

Behrman, R., Kliegman, R., & Jenson, H. (2007). *Nelson textbook of pediatrics*. Philadelphia, PA: Saunders.

Berger, C., Bachman, J., Casalone, G., Farberman, S., & Fish, A. (2014). An oral health program for children. *Nurse Practitioner, 39*(2), 48–53.

Block, S. (2013). Improving the diagnosis of acute otitis media: Seeing is believing. *Pediatric Annals, 42*(12), 485–490.

Block, S. (2014). Streptococcal pharyngitis: Guidelines, treatment issues, and sequelae. *American Family Physician, 43*(1), 11–16.

Bradfield, Y. (2013). Identification and treatment of amblyopia. *American Family Physician, 87*(5), 348–352.

Burns, C., Dunn, A., Brady, M., Starr, N., & Blosser, C. (2013). *Pediatric primary care*. Philadelphia, PA: Elsevier Saunders.

DeMuri, G., & Wald, E. (2013). Acute bacterial sinusitis in children. *Pediatrics in Review, 34*(10), 429–436.

Friedmann, A. (2008). Evaluation and management of lymphadenopathy in children. *Pediatrics in Review, 29*(2), 53–59.

Gausche-Hill, M., Fuchs, S., & Yamamoto, L. (2007). *The pediatric emergency medicine resource*. Sudbury, MA: Jones and Bartlett.

Gelston, C. (2013). Common eye injuries. *American Family Physician, 88*(8), 515–519.

Gereige, R., & DeSautu, C. (2011). Throat infections. *Pediatrics in Review, 32*(11), 459–468.

Harmes, K., Blackwood, A., Burrows, H., Cooke, J., VanHarrison, R., & Passamani, R. (2013). Otitis media: Diagnosis and treatment. *American Family Physician, 88*(7), 435–440.

Hay, W., Levin, M., Deterding, R. & Abzug, M. (2014). *Current diagnosis and treatment: Pediatrics*. (24th ed.). New York, NY: McGraw-Hill.

Kamat, D., Adam, H. M., Cain, K. K., Campbell, D., Holston, A., Kelleher, K. J., . . . Wolraich, M. L. (2010). *American Academy of Pediatrics: Quick reference to pediatric care*. Washington, DC: American Academy of Pediatrics.

Krouse, H., & Krouse, J. (2014). Allergic rhinitis diagnosis through management. *Nurse Practitioner, 39*(4), 20–27.

Langlosis, D., & Andreae, M. (2011). Group A streptococcal infections. *Pediatrics in Review, 32*(10), 423–429.

Lieberthal, A., Carroll, A., & Chonmaitree, T. (2013). The diagnosis and management of acute otitis media. *Pediatrics, 131*(3), e964–e999.

Morris, P., & Leach, A. (2009). Acute and chronic otitis media. *Pediatric Clinics of North America, 56*, 1383–1399.

Nicoteri, J. (2013). Adolescent pharyngitis: A common complaint with potentially lethal complications. *Journal for Nurse Practitioners, 9*(5), 295–300.

Prentiss, K., & Dorfman, D. (2008). Pediatric ophthalmology in the emergency department. *Emergency Medical Clinics of North America, 26*(1), 181–198.

Saccomano, S., & Ferrara, L. (2013). Infectious mononucleosis. *Clinician Reviews, 23*(6), 42–49.

Schaefer, P., & Baugh, R. (2012). Acute otitis externa: An update. *American Family Physician, 86*(11), 1055–1061.

Sicherer, S., & Sher, L. (2011). Diagnosing allergic diseases. *Contemporary Pediatrics, 28*(8), 34–46.

Wipperman, J., & Dorsch, J. (2013). Evaluation and management of corneal abrasions. *American Family Physician, 87*(2), 114–120.

Zitelli, B., & Davis, H. (2012). *Atlas of pediatric physical diagnosis*. Philadelphia, PA: Mosby Elsevier.

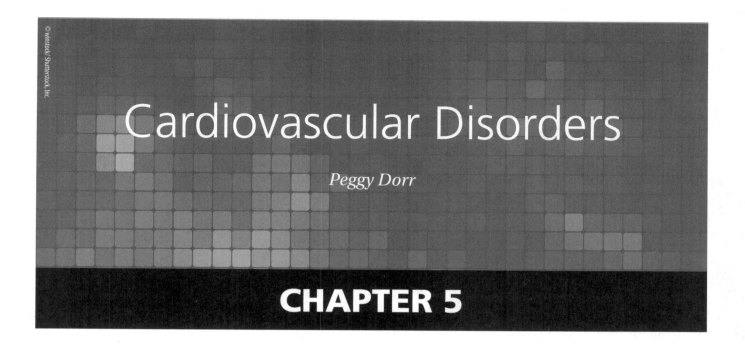

Cardiovascular Disorders

Peggy Dorr

CHAPTER 5

☐ CONGENITAL HEART DEFECTS

- Definition: Cardiovascular malformations that result from abnormal structural development of the heart and/or vessels; most heart defects occur within first 8 weeks of gestation
- Etiology/Incidence
  1. Etiology of most defects unknown
  2. Probable genetic predisposition interacting with environmental trigger
  3. Chromosomal abnormalities account for nearly 10% of cardiac malformations (Down syndrome, Turner's syndrome, DiGeorge syndrome, and others)
  4. Environmental or adverse maternal conditions account for 2% to 4%
     a. Maternal diabetes mellitus, phenylketonuria, systemic lupus erythematosus, rubella, or other viruses
     b. Maternal ingestion of alcohol, lithium, anticonvulsant agents, and other drugs
  5. Approximately 8 per 1000 live births; about 32,000 new cases of congenital heart disease per year in the United States
  6. Ventricular septal defect (VSD) is most common (25% to 30% of all lesions)
- Signs and Symptoms: Presentation of congenital heart defects varies. Some symptoms of distress, failure, or cyanosis may not present until pulmonary vascular resistance drops after birth at approximately 4 weeks of life or the ductus arteriosus closes or there is adequate shunting of blood to cause hemodynamic significance. Common symptoms of a congenital heart defect can include:
  1. Increased respiratory rate and/or effort at rest or with activity, including feeding
  2. Poor feeding; fatigue during feeding
  3. Excessive sweating in infant, unrelated to the environment, especially while feeding
  4. Recurrent respiratory infections
  5. Cyanosis—usually apparent at oxygen saturation of 85% or less. Not all congenital heart defects will manifest with cyanosis
     a. Central (arterial desaturation)—generalized, mucous membranes
     b. Peripheral
  6. Poor perfusion as evidenced by cool extremities, pale/mottled extremities, decreased pulse intensity, decreased capillary refill
  7. Decreased exercise tolerance
- Differential Diagnosis
  1. Pulmonary disease
  2. Arrhythmias
  3. Myocardial diseases
  4. Rheumatic fever
  5. Sepsis
  6. Hypoglycemia, anemia, polycythemia, especially in neonates
  7. Central nervous system disorders
- Physical Findings
  1. Poor growth/weight gain
  2. Abnormal respiratory patterns
     a. Tachypnea
     b. Dyspnea
  3. Tachycardia
  4. Hepatic enlargement with some defects
  5. Cyanosis (central or peripheral); pallor
  6. Precordial prominence or increased precordial activity
  7. Palpable thrill if murmur is classified as IV/VI

8. Abnormal heart sounds
   a. Increased intensity
   b. Abnormal splitting
   c. Murmurs (may be absent or soft in spite of serious heart defect)
   d. Ejection clicks
   e. Fourth heart sound (gallop)
9. Abnormal peripheral pulses
   a. Decreased as a result of poor cardiac output
   b. Bounding (seen with defects that increase blood volume to left heart, i.e., patent ductus arteriosus [PDA])
   c. Unequal (decreased lower extremity pulses suggest coarctation of the aorta)
10. Abnormal blood pressure
    a. Hypotension
    b. Upper extremity blood pressure (systolic) 10 mm Hg or more higher than lower extremity blood pressure, suggestive of coarctation of aorta
11. Peripheral edema, uncommon in infants
12. Clubbing of the fingers or toes (with long-standing arterial desaturation)

- Diagnostic Tests/Findings
  1. Chest radiograph to evaluate heart size and pulmonary vascular markings
  2. Electrocardiogram to evaluate rhythm, chamber enlargement, or hypertrophy
  3. Arterial blood gas and hemoglobin in infant with cyanosis—if decreased pO_2 in room air, repeat arterial blood gas after 10 to 15 minutes in 100% inspired oxygen (oxygen challenge) to help differentiate between cardiac and pulmonary cyanosis; if minimal increase in pO_2, cardiac etiology suggested
  4. Echocardiogram for diagnosis of specific congenital heart defect; evaluate function, estimate right heart and pulmonary pressures
  5. Imaging studies (CT/MRI—evaluate cardiac structure, including pulmonary veins, coronary arteries, aortic arch abnormalities)
  6. Cardiac catheterization
- Management/Treatment
  1. Prompt referral to pediatric cardiologist or institution with pediatric cardiology and/or cardiothoracic surgical services
     a. Symptomatic infant or child
     b. Infant with cyanosis
  2. Initiation of prostaglandin infusion for cyanosis in the newborn, until congenital heart disease (CHD) ruled out
  3. Monitoring and counseling to promote optimal growth and development
  4. Primary care, immunizations per routine
  5. Endocarditis prophylaxis with dental or surgical procedures only recommended in select situations. See Table 5-3 for detailed recommendations
  6. Psychosocial support of child and family
  7. Surgical management/treatment of most common congenital heart defects—see **Table 5-1**

■ **Table 5-1** Complex Congenital Heart Defects Requiring Surgical Intervention

Transposition of the Great Arteries (Cyanotic)
Anatomy: The aorta arises from right ventricle; pulmonary artery from the left ventricle; have PDA at birth; usually create/enlarge atrial septal opening (BAS) to allow for unrestricted mixing until surgery. This is traditionally done as a catheterization procedure.
Surgical Management: Arterial switch (Jatene) operation in neonatal period (within first 14 days of life optimal) or intra-atrial baffle (Mustard or Senning procedure) if anatomy does not allow for switch procedure (rare). Arterial switch entails dissection of great vessels above the valve, and then reattachment of the aorta above the left ventricle and attachment of the pulmonary artery above the right ventricle. The coronary arteries are also removed from root of original aorta to root of "new" aorta coming off of the left ventricle.
Tetralogy of Fallot (Cyanotic)
Anatomy: Combination of four findings: (1) pulmonary stenosis, (2) ventricular septal defect, (3) overriding aorta, and (4) right ventricular hypertrophy
Surgical Management: • *Palliative:* BT shunt (subclavian artery to pulmonary artery) or other aortopulmonary shunt in infancy if necessary to increase pulmonary blood flow and allow child time to grow prior to full repair; infrequently performed today, most children undergo the complete repair only.   • *Repair:* Patch closure of VSD and resection of infundibular pulmonary stenosis ± pulmonary valvulotomy if needed. If performed, this leaves the child with no pulmonic valve and free pulmonary insufficiency. This will be surgically addressed in late childhood/early adolescence.
Atrioventricular Septal Defect (Also AV Canal, Endocardial Cushion Defect) (Cyanotic)
Anatomy: Failure of central portion of heart to form, resulting in a primum (low) ASD, high VSD, and abnormal mitral and tricuspid valves due to failure of endocardial cushion to develop appropriately.

■ **Table 5-1** Complex Congenital Heart Defects Requiring Surgical Intervention (*continued*)

Surgical Management:
Repair: Patch closure of septal defects, repair of mitral valve to ensure competence (limit leakage without causing more damage or obstruction to valve, trying to prevent need for valvar replacement).
Coarctation of the Aorta (Acyanotic)
Anatomy: Congenital narrowing of the aorta, usually distal to the origin of the left subclavian artery, opposite the area of the ductus arteriosus.
Surgical Management:
Repair: Performed via thoracotomy, several types of repair possible; typically "end-to-end anastamosis" where narrowed area is cut out and ends of aorta are sewn back together, or a "subclavian flap repair" where the subclavian artery is isolated and opened longitudinally and extended over narrowed portion of aorta.
Total Anomalous Pulmonary Venous Connection
Anatomy: Pulmonary veins do not enter left atrium but are connected either directly or indirectly to right atrium; if veins return below the diaphragm, emergency surgery is usually required.
Surgical Management:
Repair: Pulmonary venous confluence connected to left atrium in infancy or the anomalous veins are rerouted to drain to the left atrium.
Truncus Arteriosus
Anatomy: Single arterial trunk that did not divide completely in utero; single vessel provides blood flow to both pulmonary and systemic circulation, overrides ventricles and receives blood from them through a ventricular septal defect.
Surgical Management:
Repair: Closure of ventricular septal defect, removing origin of the pulmonary arteries from trunk, and connecting pulmonary arteries to right ventricle with a conduit in infancy; the original truncus portion becomes the aorta.
Single Ventricle Physiology (Secondary to Pulmonary Atresia with Intact Ventricular Septum, Tricuspid Atresia, Hypoplastic Left or Right Heart Syndrome, Etc.)
Anatomy: Abnormal cardiac anatomy and development result in only one functioning ventricle; anatomic bases for this are numerous, but the repair is essentially the same.
Surgical Management:
Repair: Repair is broken out into three stages. The first stage, the Norwood procedure, consists of an augmentation of the aorta as necessary, ligation of the PDA, and placement of a shunt that provides consistent pulmonary blood flow. This is accomplished by placement of either a BT shunt or a Sano shunt (RV-PA conduit). The second stage is a bidirectional Glenn, which involves removing the SVC from the right atrium and attaching it to the branch pulmonary artery and taking down the initial shunt. The final stage is the Fontan, which involves directing IVC blood flow directly to the branch pulmonary artery, typically through an extracardiac conduit. The goal of these surgeries is to allow venous return to flow directly to the lungs and use the single ventricle as the systemic ventricle.

Note: ASD, atrioventricular septal defect; BAS, balloon atrial septostomy; BT, Blalock-Taussig; IVC, inferior vena cava; PDA, patent ductus arteriosus; RV-PA, right ventricle to pulmonary artery; SVC, superior vena cava; VSD, ventricular septal defect

☐ CONGESTIVE HEART FAILURE (CHF)

- Definition: Clinical syndrome that reflects the inability of the heart to meet metabolic requirements of the body; failure may initially be left- or right-sided, but if left untreated, the entire heart will fail
- Etiology/Incidence
  1. Congenital heart defects with volume or pressure overload (most common cause in pediatric age group)—see **Table 5-2**
     a. Ventricular septal defect (alteration in volume)
     b. Atrioventricular septal defect (AV canal)
     c. Patent ductus arteriosus
     d. Coarctation of the aorta (obstruction to flow)
     e. Hypoplastic left heart syndrome
  2. Defects that decrease pulmonary blood flow such as tetralogy of Fallot will not cause congestive heart failure unless the degree of pulmonary stenosis is very mild. Other defects that do increase pulmonary blood flow (transposition of the great arteries, truncus arteriosus) do not usually progress to CHF because they are repaired early in infancy
  3. Acquired heart disease (less common cause)
     a. Myocarditis

■ **Table 5-2** Heart Defects Commonly Causing Congestive Heart Failure in Infancy

Defect	Etiology of Heart Failure
Ventricular septal defect (VSD)	Opening between right and left ventricles that may cause excess blood flow to pulmonary system if defect is large enough.
Atrioventricular septal defect (ASD)	The combined atrial and ventricular septal defects allow excessive pulmonary blood flow to occur. This defect commonly occurs in children with Down syndrome, and these children have a propensity toward elevated pulmonary vascular resistance, which could affect right heart function.
Patent ductus arteriosus (PDA)	If large enough, the excess blood flow through the PDA to the pulmonary system increases volume load on the lungs and alters the pulmonary pressures and resistance over time.
Coarctation of the aorta	Severe or chronic coarctation causes obstruction to left ventricle (increased afterload) and alters function over time.
Single ventricle defects	Cardiac output must be balanced between pulmonary and systemic circulations. Decreases to pulmonary pressures or an increase in systemic blood pressure increases pulmonary blood flow. Once a shunt is in place, there is some restriction to pulmonary blood flow due to the size of the shunt. But children with single ventricle lesions should not be treated with high concentrations of oxygen therapy because they are still at risk for increased pulmonary blood flow until after their Glenn surgery.

   b. Metabolic abnormalities
   c. Cardiomyopathy
   d. Rheumatic heart disease
 4. Other causes
   a. Tachyarrhythmias, sustained at any age
   b. Complete heart block in infancy
   c. Severe anemia, hydrops fetalis
   d. Acute hypertension
   e. Infection/sepsis
   f. Endocrinopathies, renal failure
   g. Arteriovenous malformations
 5. Incidence unknown because congestive heart failure is secondary to other disease processes
• Signs and Symptoms
 1. Increased respiratory rate and/or effort at rest or with activity
 2. Poor feeding
 3. Excessive sweating, especially with feeding in infants
 4. Decreased exercise tolerance
 5. Fatigue, persistently tired
 6. Poor weight gain
 7. Orthopnea in older child, chronic cough
• Differential Diagnosis
Note: Congestive heart failure is not a disease unto itself. It is secondary to other disease processes that affect heart function and/or metabolic demands.
 1. Pulmonary diseases
 2. Cardiac diseases (see Etiology/Incidence)
• Physical Findings
 1. Tachycardia (common)
 2. Tachypnea (common)
 3. Hepatomegaly (right-sided failure)
 4. Periorbital edema common in infants, peripheral edema less common in children

 5. Wheezing, pulmonary rales may be present (with left-sided failure)
 6. Pallor, mottling of extremities
 7. Weakly palpable peripheral pulses; cool extremities related to peripheral vasoconstriction and/or poor cardiac output
 8. Gallop rhythm with myocardial failure
 9. Cyanosis with alveolar edema
• Diagnostic Tests/Findings
 1. Chest radiograph—cardiomegaly almost always present; pulmonary vascular congestion dependent on etiology
 2. Echocardiogram to assess ventricular function, chamber enlargement, anatomy
 3. Electrocardiogram not diagnostic, but may help define etiology
• Management/Treatment
 1. Referral to cardiologist to determine etiology if heart disease suspected; may require referral for cardiac transplantation if refractory, end-stage heart failure
 2. Increase oxygen supply (supplemental oxygen, correct anemia); decrease oxygen demand
 3. Drug therapy
   a. Inotropic agents—usually digoxin or vasopressors in acute care setting to increase cardiac output
   b. Diuretics to address pulmonary overcirculation
   c. Afterload-reducing agents (angiotensin-converting-enzyme [ACE] inhibitors such as captopril or enalapril for systemic afterload reduction to aid with cardiac output)
 4. Caloric supplementation up to 30 kcal/oz of formula; can use breast milk fortifier
 5. Treatment of underlying condition if specific therapy available

6. Other measures
   a. Prostaglandin E_1 if systemic perfusion is dependent on patency of ductus arteriosus
   b. Mothers may need to pump breast milk and feed the infant with a bottle rather than breastfeed to conserve calories
   c. Frequent rest periods

☐ MURMURS

- Definition: A murmur is the result of turbulent blood flow through the heart. The turbulence can be caused by normal or excess flow of blood through a defect within the heart, or through an abnormal or obstructed area, or it can be the result of vibrations from normal heart structures. Murmurs are evaluated based on timing within the normal heart cycle (systolic vs. diastolic), intensity (I–VI scale), location, radiation, pitch, and quality. Murmurs can be innocent or pathologic
  1. Innocent murmurs are murmurs not associated with any anatomic abnormality
  2. Innocent murmurs are also referred to as functional, Still's, or vibratory
- Etiology/Incidence
  1. Heard in more than 50% of children with no underlying heart disease from infancy through adolescence
  2. Still's (innocent) murmur most common; heard most frequently from 3 to 7 years of age
  3. Changes in intensity of sound in innocent murmurs associated with increased cardiac output state (fever, acute illness, anemia, anxiety, exercise); best to reevaluate murmur after illness resolved; frequently murmur is not audible at that time
  4. Four diagnoses account for majority of murmurs noted in children:
     a. Patent ductus arteriosus (PDA)
     b. Ventricular septal defect (VSD)
     c. Innocent murmur
     d. Peripheral pulmonic stenosis (PPS) of the newborn
- Signs and Symptoms: Asymptomatic if innocent; if pathologic, symptoms related to underlying disease process or defect
- Differential Diagnosis
  1. Congenital heart disease
  2. Conditions associated with high cardiac output
- Physical Findings
  1. Innocent murmurs
     a. No cyanosis or other cardiovascular abnormalities
     b. Normal blood pressure, and equal peripheral pulses in upper and lower extremities
     c. Normal heart sounds, including normal splitting (not fixed) of second heart sound
     d. No clicks
     e. Characteristics of a typical Still's murmur:
        (1) Systolic, noted at left lower sternal border out to apex
        (2) Low intensity (grade 1 to 3)
        (3) Short duration, not holosystolic; never associated with precordial thrill
        (4) Well localized, poorly transmitted
        (5) Intensity typically varies with position change (louder when supine) or respiration
  2. Pathologic murmurs: Abnormal heart sounds in systole and/or diastole
     a. May be associated with thrill, gallop, click, lift, or heave
     b. Sound does not change with body position or respiration
     c. Diastolic murmurs are *always* pathologic
     d. For a murmur to be graded IV/VI, there must be a palpable thrill
  3. Common innocent murmurs
     a. Still's murmur—vibratory, groaning, or musical systolic murmur heard best between lower-left sternal border and apex; some theories attribute the murmur to turbulence in left ventricular outflow tract or vibration of the tendonae in the ventricles
     b. Physiologic peripheral pulmonary stenosis—low-intensity systolic ejection murmur heard best at upper left sternal border, axillae, and back in neonates until 3 to 6 months of age; attributed to relative hypoplasia of branch pulmonary arteries at birth and anatomy of left pulmonary artery
     c. Venous hum—humming continuous murmur usually heard best at upper right sternal border in sitting position with marked decrease of murmur with change in head position (turn head sideways) or disappearance of murmur in supine position; result of blood flow returning through the superior vena cava (SVC) to the heart with gravity acceleration
     d. Pulmonary or aortic flow murmur—slightly harsh systolic ejection murmur heard best at second to third left intercostal space; attributed to turbulent flow in right or left ventricular outflow tract
     e. Supraclavicular arterial bruit—early systolic murmur heard above clavicles, attributed to turbulence at site of branching of brachiocephalic arteries
  4. Pathologic murmurs are related to the turbulence caused by altered blood volume, pressure differences across a site and/or the size of a chamber or vessel, or pathologic changes in function or size of heart (cardiomyopathies)
- Diagnostic Tests/Findings
  1. Testing not routine
  2. May be indicated to rule out congenital heart defect
     a. Electrocardiogram can be normal
     b. Echocardiogram if recommended by cardiologist
- Management/Treatment of an Innocent Murmur
  1. Inform parents of murmur finding
  2. Provide reassurance that child's heart is normal
  3. Inform them that murmur may come and go; may sound louder if the child is sick
  4. Child does *not* require subacute bacterial endocarditis (SBE) prophylaxis

5. Referral to cardiologist if:
   a. Symptomatic
   b. Cardiovascular abnormalities on physical examination, including pathologic murmur findings
   c. Uncertainty regarding innocence of murmur; change in murmur intensity
   d. Persistent parental concern

☐ DISTURBANCES OF RATE AND RHYTHM

- Definition: Occur as a result of abnormalities in, or insults to, the cardiac conduction system or heart tissues
- Etiology/Incidence
  1. May be congenital or acquired
  2. Bradyarrhythmias and heart block are uncommon causes of electrocardiogram (ECG) abnormalities in children without congenital heart disease
     a. Bradycardia—a heart rate (HR) below the lower limits of normal for age
        (1) Athletes frequently have heart rates below normal as a result of conditioning of heart muscle
        (2) Symptomatic bradycardia is associated with symptoms of poor perfusion and requires immediate attention
        (3) Most common pre-arrest rhythm
  3. Tachyarrhythmias cause nonspecific signs and symptoms if there are extreme rates or it persists for an extended period; type and extent of symptoms vary with age
     a. Tachycardia—an HR above the upper limits of normal for age
        (1) May be normal response to fever or stress
        (2) Supraventricular tachycardia (SVT) is the most common symptomatic tachycardia in first year of life
        (3) SVT is defined as an HR greater than 220 in infants and greater than 180 in children; narrow QRS complex with hidden P waves; no rate variability
        (4) SVT can be associated with Wolff-Parkinson-White (WPW) syndrome (short PR interval, slurring of initial segment of QRS complex creating the "delta wave," wide QRS complex)
  4. Atrioventricular block—a disturbance of impulse conduction from the atria to the ventricles
     a. Congenital complete heart block (CHB); 1 in 25,000 live births; associated with maternal systemic lupus erythematosus or other connective tissue diseases
     b. Acquired heart block caused by damage to conduction system during cardiac surgery; severe myocarditis, acute rheumatic fever, mumps, tumors in conduction system, endocrine/metabolic disorders
  5. Isolated premature atrial contractions (PACs) and premature ventricular contractions (PVCs) common in healthy children

6. Prolonged QT syndrome—defined as a QT_c interval greater than 0.45 seconds
   a. The QT interval measures the duration of activation and recovery of the ventricles; leading evidence supports derangements in cardiac ion flows that result in prolongation of the action potential as the underlying pathophysiologic derangement that leads to potentially fatal dysrhythmia (torsades de pointes) in susceptible individuals with specific triggers:
      (1) Bradycardia
      (2) Increased sympathetic activity
      (3) Hypokalemia
      (4) Antiarrhythmic medications
   b. Must correct the QT interval for heart rate; the formula to calculate the QT_c is the QT interval (in seconds) / square root of the previous R-R interval (in seconds)
   c. May be hereditary; look for family history of sudden death; genetic testing is available for numerous long QT mutations that may help confirm diagnosis
   d. Syncope may be the presenting symptom; all syncope patients should get an ECG
7. Other causes for rate disturbances
   a. Drugs (beta agonists, cocaine, antipsychotics, many others)
   b. Electrolyte imbalance
   c. Acidosis/hypoxia
   d. Increased intracranial pressure
   e. Endocrine disorders (hyper/hypothyroidism)
   f. Cardiomyopathy, structural heart disease, or surgery
   g. Pheochromocytoma
- Signs and Symptoms
  1. Children are usually asymptomatic
  2. Symptoms of low cardiac output or congestive heart failure if bradycardia or tachycardia is severe and/or prolonged
  3. Irritability, pallor, poor feeding in infants
  4. Palpitations (feeling or awareness of an irregular, rapid, or strong beating of the heart)
  5. Dizziness, syncope
  6. Chest pain
  7. Seizures
  8. Rare sudden cardiac arrest (with ventricular tachycardia or fibrillation)
- Differential Diagnosis
  1. Sinus arrhythmia (phasic acceleration and deceleration of heart rate with respiration; normal in children)
  2. Sinus tachycardia with associated noncardiac causes
     a. Anemia
     b. Fever
     c. Hyperthyroidism
     d. Hypoglycemia
     e. Hypovolemia or dehydration

f. Neurocardiogenic syncope

g. Pheochromocytoma

3. Psychiatric causes
   a. Anxiety
   b. Panic attacks

4. Drugs/medications/substance abuse
   a. Alcohol
   b. Caffeine/energy drinks
   c. Drugs of abuse (cocaine, PCP, marijuana, tobacco)
   d. Prescription medications (stimulants, beta agonists)

5. Sinus bradycardia and associated noncardiac causes
   a. Physical training
   b. Hypothyroidism

6. Cardiac conditions associated with heart rate disturbances (see Etiology/Incidence)

- Physical Findings
  1. Bradycardia, tachycardia, or irregular rhythm
  2. Signs of heart failure (tachypnea, hepatomegaly, poor perfusion, especially in infants) if rate disturbance severe and/or prolonged

- Diagnostic Tests/Findings
  1. 12-lead electrocardiogram
  2. Other tests based on clinical findings and symptoms (i.e., to evaluate for anemia, dehydration, hyperthyroidism, etc.)
  3. Further ECG monitoring (24-hour Holter monitor or 30-day event monitor), echocardiogram if concerns for heart failure or structural abnormalities

- Management/Treatment
  1. Referral to cardiologist for evaluation and treatment if:
     a. Symptomatic with sensation of abnormal heart rhythm
     b. Symptoms occur with activity
     c. Sustained dysrhythmia
     d. Recurrent dysrhythmia
  2. Treatment of underlying condition if noncardiac cause

❒ SYNCOPE

- Definition: Abrupt, transient loss of consciousness associated with loss of postural tone that is usually followed by spontaneous recovery

- Etiology/Incidence
  1. Fairly common with 15% to 25% of children experiencing at least one syncopal event by adulthood; peaks in females aged 15–19 years old (Friedman & Alexander, 2013)
  2. Noncardiac causes include metabolic, neurologic, and psychological disorders
  3. Most common cause is neurocardiogenic, which is "a transient reflex failure of peripheral vascular tone in combination with relative bradycardia" (Friedman & Alexander, 2013). This type of syncope is also called

vasovagal or neurally mediated and is a benign cardiac etiology

4. More pathologic cardiac causes of syncope include arrhythmias, long QT syndrome, Wolff-Parkinson-White (WPW) syndrome, hypertrophic cardiomyopathy, coronary artery anomaly, myocarditis

- Signs/Symptoms
  1. Neurocardiogenic:
     a. Associated with orthostatic intolerance
     b. Dizziness
     c. Nausea
     d. Tunnel vision, vision changes
     e. Pallor, diaphoresis
     f. Fairly quick recovery
  2. Cardiac:
     a. Abrupt onset with no prodromal symptoms
     b. Frequently associated with activity/exertion
     c. May not have spontaneous recovery

- Differential Diagnosis: Must be categorized based on clinical history, physical examination, and ECG. A thorough history (event, patient, and family) guides the differentiation into benign cardiac cause, pathologic cardiac cause, or other cause such as pure neurologic, metabolic, or psychogenic

- Physical Findings: Usually benign physical examination. If murmur noted, must pursue structural cardiac anomaly as cause of syncope

- Diagnostic Tests/Findings
  1. 12-lead ECG
  2. Echocardiogram if indicated by physical examination or family history
  3. Laboratory sampling may include viral panel to rule out prodrome for myocarditis or Lyme carditis, complete blood count (CBC) to evaluate for anemia
  4. 24-hour or 30-day monitor
  5. Genetic testing

- Management/Treatment
  1. Neurocardiogenic:
     a. Increase fluid intake
     b. Increase sodium/salt intake
     c. Avoiding caffeine
     d. Education regarding postural techniques to prevent venous blood pooling (isometric extremity contraction, toe raises, leg crossing)
     e. Assume supine position if possible at onset of symptoms
     f. Fludrocortisone (Florinef): Mineralocorticoid to enhance sodium absorption and fluid retention. Dose recommendation 0.1 mg PO daily; may use 0.2 mg if not responsive or during times of fluid loss (heavy menses)
     g. Midodrine: Alpha-adrenergic activator to enhance vascular tone and decrease venous pooling. Dose recommendations 2.5–10 mg PO TID
  2. Cardiac:
     a. Restrict from activity until evaluated by cardiologist

☐ CHEST PAIN

- Definition: A sensation of pain or discomfort experienced by the child anywhere in the chest/thorax. Can be acute or chronic, vary in description, severity, associated symptoms, precipitating and alleviating factors. May be pathologic but is most commonly benign in children
- Etiology/Incidence
  1. Most recently, accounted for 5.2% of all cardiology consults and 15% of all outpatient visits at a large, tertiary care pediatric cardiology practice
  2. Less than 5% are associated with a cardiac condition
  3. Usually divided into cardiac and noncardiac causes
- Signs/Symptoms
  1. Noncardiac chest pain
     a. Sharp, stabbing pain along two or more contiguous costochondral joints
     b. Pain exacerbated by deep breathing or coughing
     c. May occur at rest or with activity
     d. Short duration (seconds to a few minutes)
     e. May have history of recent upper respiratory infection, asthma, pain after eating, recent injury or trauma to chest
  2. Cardiac chest pain
     a. Can be associated with palpitations
     b. Exertional
     c. Radiating
     d. Associated nausea, dizziness, fatigue
- Differential Diagnosis
  1. Noncardiac chest pain
     a. Costochondritis
     b. Idiopathic
     c. Trauma/muscle strain
     d. Slipping rib syndrome
     e. Scoliosis
     f. Asthma
     g. Pneumonia
     h. Chronic cough
     i. Gastroesophageal reflux disease (GERD)/gastritis/esophagitis
     j. Pneumothorax/pneumomediastinum
     k. Psychogenic
     l. Sickle cell disease
  2. Cardiac chest pain
     a. Arrhythmia (supraventricular tachycardia, ventricular tachycardia)
     b. Pericarditis
     c. Coronary artery vasospasm
     d. Anomalous origin of the coronary artery
     e. Left ventricular outflow tract obstruction (related to varying degrees of aortic stenosis or hypertrophic cardiomyopathy)
     f. Cocaine use
- Physical Findings: Observe for dysmorphic features, chest wall abnormalities, scoliosis, signs of trauma
  1. Noncardiac chest pain

a. Reproducible pain with palpation at costosternal junctions
b. Localized inflammation of a costochondral joint
c. Typically a benign physical examination
  2. Cardiac chest pain
     a. Recent history of febrile illness
     b. History of Kawasaki disease
     c. Murmur will be noted if there is underlying cardiac disease
- Diagnostic Tests/Findings: Will depend on history, presenting symptoms, and examination results
  1. 12-lead electrocardiogram if concern for arrhythmia or chest pain with exertion
  2. Echocardiogram for chest pain associated with activity, syncope, or an abnormal cardiac examination
- Management/Treatment
  1. Noncardiac chest pain
     a. Education
     b. Ibuprofen as indicated for inflammatory conditions
     c. Activity restrictions until inflammatory condition resolves
     d. Use of bronchodilator as needed
     e. Referral to appropriate specialist for concerns of pulmonary or gastrointestinal systems
  2. Cardiac chest pain
     a. Referral to cardiology
     b. Restriction from all activities until seen by cardiology

☐ HYPERTENSION

- Definition: "Average systolic blood pressure (SBP) and/or average diastolic blood pressure (DBP) greater than or equal to the 95th percentile for gender, age, and height, with measurements obtained on at least three occasions" (National High Blood Pressure Education Program Working Group on High Blood Pressure in Children and Adolescents, 2004)
  1. Prehypertension: Defined as average SBP or DBP levels that are greater than/equal to the 90th percentile but less than the 95th percentile
  2. Children with BP levels greater than 95th percentile in an office or clinic setting who are normotensive outside a clinical setting ("white coat syndrome") should be followed using their ambulatory BP readings
  3. At 12 years of age, the BP range that defines prehypertension includes any reading greater than 120/80 mm Hg, even if it is less than the 90th percentile
  4. Children 3 years of age and older should have their BP measured routinely
  5. Preferred method of BP measurement is auscultation; measures obtained by oscillometric devices (automatic blood pressure machines) should be repeated by auscultation if abnormal
  6. *Must have* a correct size BP cuff to obtain an accurate measurement; width of the cuff bladder should be

40% of the arm circumference; if an appropriate cuff size is not available, the next larger size is used

- Etiology/Incidence: 1–5% prevalence in children, with higher rates among minority adolescents
  1. Primary hypertension (essential hypertension)
     a. No known underlying disease present to cause hypertension
     b. May be related to factors such as heredity, salt intake, stress, sleep disorders/apnea, and obesity
     c. Obese children are three times more likely to develop hypertension
     d. May be recognized in childhood; it is characterized by mild hypertension and is often associated with a positive family history of hypertension or cardiovascular disease; these children are frequently overweight
  2. Secondary hypertension—more common in children than in adults
     a. Etiology varies with age
        (1) Newborn infants—renal artery thrombosis, renal artery stenosis, congenital renal malformations, coarctation of the aorta, bronchopulmonary dysplasia
        (2) Infancy to adolescence—renal parenchymal diseases, coarctation of the aorta, renal artery stenosis
        (3) Other causes—endocrine disorders, neurogenic tumors, drugs or toxins, increased intracranial pressure
- Signs and Symptoms
  1. Primary hypertension—usually no symptoms
  2. Secondary hypertension—symptoms related to underlying disease and may include:
     a. Congestive heart failure
     b. Respiratory distress (infants)
     c. Failure to thrive
     d. Irritability
     e. Convulsions
     f. Feeding problems
  3. Severe hypertension—may complain of headaches, dizziness, visual disturbances, epistaxis (rare); infants may show irritability, failure to thrive, vomiting, or feeding problems
- Differential Diagnosis: Causes of secondary hypertension (see Etiology/Incidence)
- Physical Findings
  1. Elevated blood pressure on at least three separate occasions (without acute illness)
  2. Related to underlying disease if secondary hypertension—may include edema, pallor, increased sweating, signs of specific syndrome, including absent or diminished femoral pulses seen with coarctation of the aorta
- Diagnostic Tests/Findings
  1. Based on history, age, other clinical findings
  2. Complete blood count (to evaluate for anemia)
  3. Urinalysis
  4. Blood urea nitrogen (BU), creatinine (to evaluate renal function)
  5. Renal ultrasound (renal scarring, disparate kidney size, congenital anomalies)
  6. Lipid profile (evaluated as a comorbidity risk factor)
  7. Echocardiogram
     a. For baseline measurements of left ventricular dimensions and function
     b. To rule out coarctation of the aorta
     c. To evaluate for left ventricular hypertrophy as an indicator of end-organ damage
     d. Prior to initiation of drug therapy
  8. Additional tests based on suspected cause
- Management/Treatment
  1. Depends on cause and degree of elevation
  2. General counseling regarding cardiovascular risk factors such as family history, obesity, lack of exercise, smoking
  3. Nonpharmacologic therapy
     a. Weight reduction if indicated
     b. Regular aerobic exercise programs (especially in adolescents)
     c. Dietary modification—heart healthy, sodium reduction
  4. Antihypertensive drug therapy indicated for secondary hypertension and insufficient response to lifestyle modifications for primary hypertension or if evidence of end-organ damage is noted
     a. Therapy should be initiated with a single drug; acceptable drug classes for use in children include:
        (1) ACE inhibitors (captopril, enalapril, lisinopril)
        (2) Angiotensin receptor blockers (losarten)
        (3) Beta blockers (atenolol, metoprolol)
        (4) Calcium channel blockers (amlodipine, isradipine, nifedipine)
        (5) Diuretics (hydrochlorothiazide [HCTZ], furosemide, spiranolactone)
     b. Goal of therapy should be reduction of blood pressure to less than 95th percentile
     c. Severe, symptomatic hypertension should be treated with IV antihypertensive agents in an acute care setting until controlled, then transition patient to PO medications
  5. If secondary hypertension, focus is on therapy for underlying disease
  6. Long-term follow-up: Referral to subspecialist (cardiologist, nephrologist) for management of underlying disorder and/or for difficulty maintaining normotensive state

☐ HYPERLIPIDEMIA

- Definition: Elevated serum lipid and lipoprotein concentrations
  1. Total cholesterol of 200 mg/dL or above

2. Total cholesterol of 170 to 199 mg/dL considered "borderline high"

3. Low-density lipoprotein (LDL) cholesterol of 130 mg/dL or above

- Etiology/Incidence

1. High tracking correlations for total and LDL cholesterol levels from childhood to adulthood

2. Potential increased risk for developing atherosclerotic or coronary heart disease as adults, especially in association with other risk factors

   a. Positive family history of premature coronary heart disease (before 55 years of age), peripheral vascular disease, or hypercholesterolemia (above 240 mg/dL)

   b. Diabetes

   c. Hypertension

   d. Obesity

   e. Smoking

   f. Physical inactivity

3. Among children aged 2 to 11 years in United States, about 25% with cholesterol levels in borderline high or high range

4. Familial hypercholesterolemia is an autosomal dominant condition resulting in deficient or defective LDL receptors, impairing clearance of circulating LDL

5. Secondary causes of hypercholesterolemia

   a. Obesity

   b. Endocrine and metabolic conditions

   c. Obstructive liver disease

   d. Nephrotic syndrome

   e. Anorexia nervosa

   f. Collagen disease

   g. Drugs

      (1) Corticosteroids

      (2) Isotretinoin (Accutane)—increases triglycerides

      (3) Thiazide diuretics

      (4) Some beta blockers

      (5) Some oral contraceptives

- Signs and Symptoms: Asymptomatic during childhood
- Differential Diagnosis: Causes of secondary hypercholesterolemia (see Etiology/Incidence)
- Physical Findings

1. Rare xanthomas with familial hypercholesterolemia and very high cholesterol levels

2. Signs of risk factors (hypertension, obesity)—the metabolic syndrome is a clustering of risk factors (abnormal waist circumference, lipid levels, BP, and fasting glucose level) for cardiovascular disease and diabetes mellitus that seem to be more prevalent in overweight children and adolescents. "Pathology studies have clearly shown that the presence of an increasing number of risk factors (as seen in Metabolic Syndrome) is associated with increased risk of fatty streaks and fibrous plaques in the aorta and coronary arteries" (deFerranti & Washington, 2012)

- Diagnostic Tests/Findings

1. Measurement of fasting lipid panel in children between 2 and 8 years of age and 12 and 16 years of age with a positive family history of early heart disease or known dyslipidemia or if child demonstrates other risk factors such as diabetes, hypertension, or body mass index (BMI) ≥95th percentile

   a. Recommend performing two profiles and averaging results

   b. Non-HDL cholesterol levels have been identified as a significant predictor of the presence of atherosclerosis in children and adolescents. This level is more predictive of persistent dyslipidemia than total cholesterol, LDL cholesterol, or high-density lipoprotein (HDL) cholesterol levels alone

2. Universal screening with either a nonfasting lipid profile (use calculated non-HDL cholesterol) or a fasting lipid profile recommended between 9 and 11 years of age and between 17 and 21 years of age

3. Additional studies to evaluate causes of secondary hypercholesterolemia, as indicated

- Management/Treatment

1. Trans fatty acid intake is limited to less than 1% of total calories; these fats tend to increase LDL and do not raise HDL

2. Intake of fruit juice, sugar-sweetened beverages and food, and salt needs to be reduced

3. In general, children need to consume more fruits, vegetables, fish, whole grains, and low-fat dairy products

4. Dietary therapy guidelines for children older than 2 years of age:

   a. If LDL cholesterol >130 mg/dL, follow recommendations in the Cardiovascular Health Integrated Lifestyle Diet (CHILD-1) and limit total calories from fat to no more than 30%, less than 10% of total calories as saturated fat, and less than 300 mg of cholesterol per day; adequate calories to reach or maintain desirable body weight

   b. If LDL cholesterol >130–189 mg/dL after 6 months of CHILD-1 with modifications, CHILD-2 diet is prescribed—saturated fatty acid intake reduced to less than 7% of calories and cholesterol intake to less than 200 mg per day; adequate amounts of nutrients, vitamins, and minerals provided

   c. If LDL cholesterol ≤190 mg/dL after initial diet modifications, statin therapy should be considered for children 10 years of age and older

   d. Fat- and cholesterol-restricted diets have been well studied and are safe, but frequently result in only modest improvements in hyperlipidemia

5. Drug therapy in children age 10 years and older if after an adequate trial of diet therapy or moderately elevated (160–189 mg/dL) LDL cholesterol levels *plus* a positive family history of premature cardiovascular disease *or* two or more other cardiovascular risk factors are present in the child. Refer to National Heart,

Lung, and Blood Institute (NHLBI) guidelines for details regarding lipid profile levels, specific diet, and medication therapy recommendations

a. HMG CoA reductase inhibitors (statins)—work by inhibiting the rate-limiting enzyme hydroxymethylglutaryl coenzyme A (HMG CoA) reductase for the endogenous synthesis of cholesterol; ultimately lead to increased clearance of LDLs from circulation; pediatric studies have been done; has demonstrated excellent ability to lower LDLs with few side effects

b. Bile acid binding resins—previously advocated as first-line treatment but high incidence of gastrointestinal (GI) complaints; poor palatability; low compliance and limited effectiveness have led to these drugs not being prescribed as first-line therapy

c. Cholesterol absorption inhibitors—new class preventing the intestinal absorption of cholesterol; used in conjunction with statins for severe hyperlipidemia. No pediatric studies of monotherapy with this group have been performed as of the last guideline publication. Suggest use of these agents only in consultation with a lipid specialist

6. Increase exercise—regular physical activity is the best approach; data support exercise as a factor that has a favorable impact on multiple lipoprotein aspects

7. Prevention—anticipatory guidance during all well-child maintenance visits to maintain well-balanced diet, encourage daily exercise, and avoid known risk factors

☐ KAWASAKI DISEASE (MUCOCUTANEOUS LYMPH NODE SYNDROME)

- Definition: Acute febrile syndrome associated with generalized vasculitis affecting all blood vessels throughout the body, preferentially involving the coronary arteries
- Etiology/Incidence
  1. Etiology uncertain, but epidemiology and clinical presentation highly suggestive of infectious etiology
  2. Most frequently (80%) affects children younger than 5 years of age; leading cause of acquired heart disease in United States
  3. Male to female ratio 1.5:1
  4. All racial backgrounds affected; highest incidence in children of Asian ancestry
  5. Approximately 20% risk of developing coronary artery abnormalities with decreased risk if intravenous gamma globulin therapy instituted before 10th day of illness; 2–3% of untreated cases will die due to coronary vasculitis
- Signs and Symptoms
  1. Vary in severity and over course of illness
  2. Acute phase—lasts about 10 days; most of diagnostic criteria are noted at some point during this time period

a. Preceding or concurrent respiratory symptoms—runny nose, cough, ear infection
b. Diarrhea, vomiting, or abdominal pain (common)
c. Irritability
d. Persistent high fever for a minimum of 5 days
e. Reddened eyes
f. Red tongue and throat
g. Redness and/or swelling of hands and feet
h. Rash
i. Swollen lymph nodes
j. Fast and/or irregular pulse
k. Arthritis or arthralgia involving multiple joints

3. Subacute phase—lasts from approximately day 11 to day 21
a. Decrease in fever
b. Skin desquamation (dry, peeling skin on lips, fingers, and toes) begins about day 14; not painful
c. Joint pain

4. Convalescent phase—begins about day 21
a. Coronary artery aneurysms are often detected by echocardiography at this time if present
b. Acute phase reactants subside

- Differential Diagnosis
  1. Measles
  2. Scarlet fever
  3. Toxin-mediated disease related to staphylococcal or streptococcal disease
  4. Drug reactions
  5. Juvenile rheumatoid arthritis
  6. Other febrile viral illness (adenovirus, Epstein-Barr, enterovirus)
  7. Stevens-Johnson syndrome
  8. Rocky Mountain spotted fever
  9. Staphylococcal scalded skin syndrome
  10. Toxic shock syndrome

- Physical Findings
  1. Diagnostic criteria includes presence of:
     a. Fever (typically high 39°C/102°F) for at least 5 days *and* four of the five following clinical features:
        (1) Bilateral, painless bulbar conjunctival injection without exudate
        (2) Changes of mucous membrane—dryness and cracking of lips, strawberry tongue, erythema of oropharyngeal mucosa
        (3) Changes to extremities—acute erythema and/or edema of hands/feet
        (4) Polymorphous nonvesicular exanthem within 4 to 5 days of fever onset
        (5) Cervical nonfluctuant lymphadenopathy; at least one lymph node more than 1.5 cm in diameter; usually unilateral (least common symptom)
  2. Coronary artery abnormalities (usually beyond 10 days of illness onset) with fever and fewer than five clinical features is diagnostic; more common in young infants

3. Other physical findings
   a. Arthritis or arthralgia
   b. Tachycardia out of proportion to degree of fever; gallop rhythm (signs of myocarditis); new murmur (less common)
   c. Sterile pyuria
   d. Aneurysm of peripheral arteries (less common)

- Diagnostic Tests/Findings
  1. No specific diagnostic test for Kawasaki disease; "diagnosis of exclusion"
  2. Leukocytosis with left shift during acute phase
  3. Thrombocytosis, may be marked; frequently seen after first week of illness (subacute phase—peaks in 3rd week)
  4. Erythrocyte sedimentation rate (ESR) elevated
  5. C-reactive protein (CRP) positive
  6. Mild anemia in acute phase
  7. Serum transaminase levels may be high (approximately 40%)
  8. Hypoalbuminemia (associated with more severe, more prolonged disease)
  9. Electrocardiogram changes are nonspecific and related to secondary myocarditis; may see ST-T wave changes and prolonged PR interval
  10. Echocardiogram—coronary artery dilation/ectasia or aneurysms; occasional pericardial effusion or decreased contractility; coronary artery dilation may be present as early as the end of the first week of illness

- Management/Treatment
  1. Immediate referral to tertiary care facility and subspecialist (immunologist, pediatric cardiologist) if suspected
  2. Management goals
     a. Reducing inflammation in the coronary arterial wall
     b. Preventing coronary thrombosis
     c. Long-term therapy for individuals who develop coronary aneurysms is aimed at preventing myocardial ischemia or infarction
  3. Therapy during acute phase
     a. Intravenous gamma globulin (2 g/kg IV) within 10 days of onset of illness (shown to reduce frequency of coronary aneurysms)
        PLUS
     b. High-dose aspirin (80 to 100 mg/kg/day) for its anti-inflammatory and antithrombotic effects until patient is afebrile; then reduced to 3 to 5 mg/kg/day for 6 to 8 weeks
     c. If fever persists 36 hours after first IVIG dose, may repeat same dose
     d. The use of steroids in treating Kawasaki disease has been studied, but the results are not consistent. Based on the available data, Eleftheriou et al. (2014) recommend the use of corticosteroids for:
        (1) Patients who were not responsive to the first dose of IVIG

        (2) Patients with features of the most severe disease (less than 1 year old, persistent signs of severe inflammation despite IVIG, liver dysfunction, hypoalbuminemia, or shock states)
        (3) Patients with evolving coronary and/or peripheral aneurysms with ongoing inflammation at presentation
  4. If coronary arterial abnormalities detected
     a. Low-dose aspirin until aneurysms resolve; continued indefinitely for giant aneurysms (>8 mm)
     b. Anticoagulation therapy—considered if coronary artery abnormality >8 mm or stenosis noted (high risk for myocardial infarction)
        (1) Warfarin
     c. Long-term follow-up by pediatric cardiologist; may require cardiac catheterization or surgical intervention
  5. Administration of live virus vaccines (measles and varicella) delayed at least 11 months after intravenous gamma globulin treatment unless risk of exposure is high; may give earlier, but then be reimmunized at 11 months after IVIG administration. IVIG decreases the effectiveness of these immunizations
  6. Administration of annual influenza vaccine in patients on long-term aspirin therapy
  7. Activity restrictions beyond initial 6 to 8 weeks based on severity of coronary artery involvement

☐ ACUTE MYOCARDIAL INFLAMMATORY DISEASE

- Definition: Focal or diffuse inflammation of the layers of the heart (pericardium, myocardium, or endocardium); myocarditis
- Etiology/Incidence
  1. Precise etiology usually unknown (idiopathic)
  2. May be caused by virtually any bacterial, viral, rickettsial, fungal, or parasitic organism—viral infections are the most common etiology, especially parvovirus B19, adenovirus, enterovirus (coxsackie viruses), or human herpesvirus 6
  3. Other causes include autoimmune, hypersensitivity reactions, or drug reactions (rare)
  4. Possible genetic predisposition with viral trigger
  5. Survival to discharge does not imply recovery; myocarditis can progress to dilated cardiomyopathy or there may be persistent myocardial dysfunction requiring ongoing medical management
- Signs and Symptoms
  1. Great variability—from no distress to severe congestive heart failure or shock
  2. Often fever or history of antecedent "flu-like" viral illness
  3. Suspect myocarditis if onset of congestive heart failure with no obvious structural or functional etiology
     a. Persistent tachycardia (out of proportion to fever if present)

b. Tachypnea, dyspnea

c. Abnormal respiratory exam

d. Easy fatigue, poor feeding in infant

e. Gallop rhythm, usually no murmur

f. Poor perfusion

g. Isolated gastrointestinal symptoms such as anorexia, abdominal pain, vomiting

4. Can also present as new onset arrhythmias, syncope, or sudden death event

- Differential Diagnosis
  1. Carnitine deficiency
  2. Idiopathic dilated cardiomyopathy (myocarditis accounts for up to one-third of dilated cardiomyopathy cases)
  3. Endocardial fibroelastosis
  4. Hereditary mitochondrial defects
  5. Anomalies of the coronary arteries
  6. Metabolic or endocrine disorders (hyperthyroidism)
- Physical Findings: See section on congestive heart failure
- Diagnostic Tests/Findings
  1. Erythrocyte sedimentation rate, C-reactive protein, and troponin may be elevated
  2. Viral cultures, antibody titers, and polymerase chain reaction (PCR) may suggest viral etiology
  3. Laboratory studies to rule out metabolic causes of cardiomyopathy
  4. Echocardiography to assess ventricular structure and function and rule out other cardiac anomalies (30–35% present with a dilated cardiomyopathy)
  5. Chest radiograph to assess cardiac enlargement, which is variable
  6. Electrocardiogram may show tachycardia, ST segment and T wave abnormalities, possibly reduced QRS voltage, or dysrhythmias
  7. Cardiac MRI may be most helpful to diagnose myocarditis. Can accurately assess LV ejection, chamber size, and wall thickness as well as localize tissue injury, edema, hyperemia, or fibrosis
  8. Endomyocardial biopsy for possible confirmation of diagnosis; only recommended in patients with new onset failure of 2 weeks to 3 months duration with a dilated LV, ventricular arrhythmia, and high-grade atrioventricular block
- Management/Treatment
  1. Immediate referral to pediatric cardiologist and/or emergency department if the disease is suspected and acute care services are needed
  2. Supportive measures for congestive heart failure
     a. Inotropic agents, including digoxin, at reduced dosage (may be arrythmogenic)
     b. Diuretics
     c. Afterload reduction (ACE inhibitors such as captopril, lisinopril)
  3. Treatment of dysrhythmias
  4. Use of immunosuppressive medication in myocarditis is supported with some research, but no large, randomized controlled study at this time

5. Possible administration of intravenous immunoglobulin—effectiveness not proven; risk of anaphylaxis

6. Psychosocial support of child and/or family—usually sudden onset of illness in previously healthy child

7. Outcome from myocarditis varies from complete resolution and recovery to development of chronic cardiomyopathy or death without cardiac transplantation

☐ RHEUMATIC FEVER/HEART DISEASE

- Definition: A postinfectious inflammatory disease in genetically predisposed individuals to group A beta-hemolytic streptococcal pharyngitis. It is a self-limited disease that is diagnosed using the Jones criteria. Although the Jones criteria were last published in 1992, a recent workgroup reaffirmed the validity of the major and minor Jones criteria and stated that these criteria should continue to be considered the accepted standard for the diagnosis of initial attacks of acute rheumatic fever (Ferrieri, 2002)
- Etiology/Incidence
  1. Follows a group A streptococcal infection of the upper respiratory tract
  2. Probably involves abnormal immune response of certain individuals with genetic predisposition to this complication
  3. Incidence of acute rheumatic fever (ARF) approximately 3% of individuals with untreated or inadequately treated group A streptococcal tonsillopharyngitis (greater risk of recurrence)
  4. Most common in children between 5 and 15 years of age; rarely seen before 3 years in the United States; rare in adults
  5. Seasonal incidence follows that of streptococcal pharyngitis; peak incidence in winter and early spring
  6. Greater frequency of rheumatic heart disease in patients who had severe cardiac involvement during initial attack or recurrence of ARF
     a. Mitral valve damage and regurgitation most common
     b. Tricuspid and pulmonary valve involvement rare
- Signs and Symptoms
  1. Diagnosis of the initial attack of acute rheumatic fever based on evidence of preceding group A streptococcal pharyngitis *plus* two major manifestations *or* one major and two minor manifestations of the following:
  2. Major manifestations
     a. Carditis (approximately 50% of patients)
        (1) Valvulitis usually—evidenced by development of new murmur, especially apical systolic murmur of mitral regurgitation
        (2) Myocarditis rare in absence of valvulitis—evidenced by tachycardia; other signs of congestive heart failure
        (3) Pericarditis rare in absence of valvulitis—evidenced by distant heart sounds, friction rub, chest pain

b. Polyarthritis (approximately 70% of patients)
   (1) Several joints may be intermittently involved, ranging from vague arthralgia to florid swelling, heat, and redness
   (2) Most frequently larger joints—knees, hips, ankles, elbows, wrists
c. Chorea (Sydenham's chorea)
   (1) Purposeless, involuntary, rapid movements of trunk and/or extremities
   (2) Often associated with muscle weakness and emotional lability
d. Erythema marginatum (rare)
   (1) Macular, nonpruritic rash with irregular, geometric morphology; areas have pale centers and rounded margins
   (2) Lesions most commonly located on trunk and proximal limbs, never on face
e. Subcutaneous nodules (rare)
   (1) Firm, painless nodules over the extensor surfaces of certain joints, particularly elbows, knuckles, knees, ankles, occiput, and vertebrae
   (2) Skin overlying nodules is not inflamed and moves freely
3. Minor manifestations
   a. Arthralgia without objective evidence of inflammation
   b. Fever usually at least 39°C (102.2°F)
   c. Elevated acute phase reactants
   d. Prolonged PR interval on electrocardiogram
- Differential Diagnosis
  1. Juvenile rheumatoid arthritis
  2. Myocardial disease
  3. Infective endocarditis
  4. Septic arthritis
  5. Sickle cell disease
- Physical Findings: No single specific finding; see Signs and Symptoms
- Diagnostic Tests/Findings
  1. No specific diagnostic test
  2. Elevated acute phase reactants

a. Erythrocyte sedimentation rate
b. C-reactive protein
c. Leukocyte count
3. Elevated or rising antistreptolysin-O (ASO) titer
4. Electrocardiogram may demonstrate prolonged PR interval (first-degree heart block)
5. Echocardiogram may show mitral valve damage resulting in valvular regurgitation and/or mitral valve stenosis
- Management/Treatment
  1. Referral to cardiologist if suspected
  2. Antibiotic treatment of group A streptococcal infection—benzathine penicillin G IM or oral penicillin V (started even as late as 9 days after acute onset has demonstrated effectiveness)
  3. Anti-inflammatory agents for treatment of arthritis and discomfort
     a. Salicylates or nonsteroidal agents
     b. Possible steroids if congestive heart failure and/or carditis severe; no definitive data, most are anecdotal and not based on well-designed randomized controlled trials
  4. Activity restrictions during acute phase may be appropriate (competitive sports); continued activity restrictions will depend on degree of cardiac disease
  5. Treatment of congestive heart failure if present
  6. Prevention of further streptococcal infection and recurrence of rheumatic fever; persons with previous group A streptococcal (GAS) pharyngitis are at greater risk of recurrent attack of rheumatic fever; recurrent ARF attacks can be associated with worsening of the severity of current rheumatic heart disease
     a. Prompt and adequate treatment of streptococcal pharyngitis
     b. Administration of monthly injections of long-acting benzathine penicillin (most reliable) or daily oral antibiotic regimen (penicillin)
     c. Antibiotics for endocarditis prophylaxis prior to dental work or surgical procedures are *not* recommended anymore (see **Table 5-3**)

■ **Table 5-3** Prevention of Bacterial Endocarditis: American Heart Association Guidelines 2007

Antibiotic prophylaxis with dental procedures is recommended only for patients with cardiac conditions associated with the highest risk of adverse outcomes from endocarditis. These include:
1. Prosthetic cardiac valve
2. Previous endocarditis
3. Congenital heart disease only in the following categories:
   a. Unrepaired cyanotic congenital heart disease, including those with palliative shunts and conduits
   b. Completely repaired congenital heart disease with prosthetic material or device, whether placed by surgery or catheter intervention, during the first 6 months after the procedure
   c. Repaired congenital heart disease with residual defects at the site or adjacent to the site of a prosthetic patch or prosthetic device that would inhibit endothelialization
4. Cardiac transplantation recipients with cardiac valvular disease

Antibiotic prophylaxis solely to prevent bacterial endocarditis is no longer recommended for patients who undergo a GI or GU tract procedure, including patients with the highest risk of adverse outcomes.

Reprinted with permission. *Circulaton.2007*;116:1736–1754. ©2007, American Heart Association, Inc.

d. Rheumatic fever without carditis: Prophylaxis should continue for 5 years or until 21 years of age, whichever is longer

e. Rheumatic fever with carditis but *no* valvular disease: Prophylaxis should continue for 10 years or until patient is 21 years of age, whichever is longer

f. Rheumatic fever with carditis *and* persistent valvular disease: Prophylaxis should continue for 10 years or until 40 years of age, whichever is longer

☐ QUESTIONS

Select the best answer.

1. The most common congenital heart defect in children is:
   a. Tricuspid atresia
   b. Ventricular septal defect
   c. Aortic stenosis
   d. Pulmonary atresia

2. The mother of a 4-month-old infant reports that he turned "blue" and seemed to have fast, labored breathing after vigorous crying soon after awakening. He settled down and his color and breathing seemed to improve. On physical examination, the mucous membranes of the lips and mouth appear mildly cyanotic. A systolic murmur is heard best at the upper and lower left sternal border. Vital signs are normal with normal peripheral pulses. There is no hepatomegaly. A likely diagnosis is:
   a. Congestive heart failure
   b. Apnea
   c. Coarctation of the aorta
   d. Cyanotic spell related to tetralogy of Fallot

3. Management of the infant with suspected heart disease and a reported cyanotic spell should include:
   a. Prompt referral to a cardiologist
   b. An apnea monitor
   c. Instructing the parent to keep a diary of these episodes
   d. Continuous administration of oxygen

4. Chest pain in young children is usually:
   a. A symptom of congenital heart disease
   b. Noncardiac in origin
   c. A sign of hypercholesterolemia
   d. A symptom of congestive heart failure

5. A common cause of congestive heart failure in the first year of life is:
   a. Pulmonary stenosis
   b. Ventricular septal defect
   c. Rheumatic fever
   d. Complete heart block

6. The least likely physical finding in a 2-month-old with congestive heart failure is:
   a. Tachypnea
   b. Tachycardia
   c. Hepatomegaly
   d. Pedal edema

7. A vibratory systolic ejection murmur is heard at the lower left sternal border in a healthy 4-year-old at her preschool physical. The cardiovascular exam is otherwise normal. A likely diagnosis is:
   a. Venous hum
   b. Still's murmur
   c. Transposition of the great arteries
   d. Rheumatic heart disease

8. Characteristics of a venous hum include:
   a. A systolic murmur
   b. Radiation over the precordium
   c. A marked decrease or disappearance of the murmur when the child is supine
   d. Heard best at the lower left sternal border

9. Which of the following is true regarding innocent murmurs?
   a. The murmur is often holosystolic.
   b. Prompt referral to a cardiologist is indicated.
   c. A precordial thrill is present.
   d. The murmur is low intensity, grade 1–3.

10. SBE prophylaxis is recommended for:
    a. All children with congenital heart disease on a daily basis
    b. All children with congenital heart disease before dental, GI, and genitourinary (GU) procedures
    c. Children with repaired congenital heart disease with a residual defect at the repair site
    d. Five (5) years after repair of all congenital heart disease

11. A 12-year-old girl seen at a routine visit has a blood pressure of 138/90 mm Hg. This blood pressure (systolic and diastolic) is in the 99th percentile for a height at the 95th percentile. She denies any symptoms such as headache or blurred vision; there is no family history of hypertension. The initial management would include:
    a. Intravenous pyelogram
    b. Return for two repeat blood pressure measurements
    c. No follow-up needed—blood pressure probably related to anxiety
    d. Diuretic therapy

12. A 9-year-old boy presents with a fever of 102°F and complaints of leg pains. His mother reports that he had an upper respiratory infection with a sore throat approximately 2 weeks ago, which subsided without therapy. On physical examination, he has tender, swollen knees bilaterally. His heart rate is 120 beats per minute and a blowing systolic murmur is heard at the apex. No murmur was noted at a previous well-child visit. The most likely diagnosis is:
    a. Kawasaki disease
    b. Rheumatic fever
    c. Sickle cell anemia
    d. Viral illness

13. The most useful test for evaluation of suspected acute rheumatic fever is:
    a. Antistreptolysin-O (ASO) titer
    b. Electrocardiogram

c. C-reactive protein (CRP)

d. Urinalysis

14. The initial attack of acute rheumatic fever is preceded by:
    a. A viral illness
    b. A group A streptococcal infection
    c. Exposure to mites
    d. Exposure to chickenpox

15. A 3-week-old infant has a 1-day history of irritability, pallor, and poor feeding. He is afebrile. On physical examination, his heart rate is 240 beats per minute while asleep. The most likely diagnosis is:
    a. Supraventricular tachycardia
    b. Premature ventricular contractions
    c. Sinus tachycardia
    d. Cyanotic heart defect

16. Congenital complete heart block may be associated with:
    a. Maternal lupus erythematosus
    b. Wolff-Parkinson-White syndrome
    c. Alcohol consumption during pregnancy
    d. Kawasaki disease

17. The most common cause of myocarditis in North America is:
    a. Bacterial
    b. Viral
    c. Drug reaction
    d. Radiation therapy

18. Which of the following is not an expected finding in a child with myocarditis?
    a. Persistent tachycardia
    b. History of antecedent illness with nonspecific cold symptoms
    c. A gallop rhythm
    d. A significant heart murmur

19. Hypercholesterolemia in children older than 2 years is defined as a total cholesterol at or above:
    a. 100 mg/dL
    b. 130 mg/dL
    c. 160 mg/dL
    d. 200 mg/dL

20. A potential childhood risk factor for development of atherosclerotic or coronary heart disease as an adult is:
    a. Obesity
    b. Tachycardia
    c. Easy fatigability
    d. Aerobic exercise

21. Which of the following is not likely to cause secondary hypercholesterolemia?
    a. Nephrotic syndrome
    b. Hypertension
    c. Corticosteroids
    d. Obstructive liver disease

22. Which of the following is a common cause of acquired coronary artery disease during childhood?
    a. Rheumatic fever
    b. Hypertension

c. Systemic lupus erythematosus

d. Kawasaki disease

23. Kawasaki disease is most common in:
    a. Neonates
    b. Children younger than 5 years of age
    c. Children older than 6 years of age
    d. Females

24. Principal clinical features of Kawasaki disease are:
    a. Low-grade fever for 24 hours and a pruritic rash
    b. Conjunctivitis with exudate and facial rash
    c. Arthritis and chorea
    d. Fever persisting at least 5 days and acute erythema and/or edema of hands and feet

25. An essential test in the evaluation of a 2-year-old being managed for Kawasaki disease is:
    a. An echocardiogram
    b. Electrolytes
    c. Cholesterol
    d. Antistreptolysin-O titer

26. A 14-year-old female, otherwise healthy, presents to your office with a complaint of syncope at school. She had just stood up from her chair at the end of the day, felt dizzy and nauseous, and then woke up on the floor. She did not hit her head and woke up within 30 seconds. Based on this description of the event, your initial impression is:
    a. Concern for an arrhythmia that precipitated the event
    b. She was experiencing an anxiety attack
    c. This was an attention-getting event and she should receive behavioral therapy
    d. This appears to be a case of neurocardiogenic syncope

27. Initial therapy for neurocardiogenic syncope is:
    a. Ensuring adequate hydration
    b. Pharmacologic therapy with a beta blocker
    c. A 24-hour Holter monitor to ensure there are no arrhythmias
    d. Antiepileptic therapy

28. A new patient presents at the age of 4 years. He has a BMI of 19, which is greater than the 95th percentile for his age. His family relates a history of early heart attacks in both sets of grandparents (before the age of 55 years), and the parents state they have recently been diagnosed with elevated cholesterol levels. On the basis of this information, you will:
    a. Counsel the family on limiting the child's saturated fat intake to <7% and cholesterol intake to 200 mg/day.
    b. Do nothing; he is too young for testing to be helpful, and a child this age should not have any dietary modifications implemented.
    c. Perform two fasting lipid profiles and average the results because the child presents with several high-risk factors.
    d. Perform one fasting lipid profile and initiate statin therapy immediately given the high BMI.

☐ ANSWERS AND RATIONALES

1. B: Ventricular septal defect (VSD) is the most common defect, either in isolation or in association with other defects. The incidence of VSD ranges from 1.56 to 53.2 per 1000 live births. VSD occurs in 50% of all children with congenital heart disease and 20% as an isolated defect (Minette & Sahn, 2006). Tricuspid atresia and pulmonary atresia are fairly rare (approximately 4–6/100,000 live births) as is aortic stenosis (approximately 8 per 1000 live births, accounting for 3–5% of all congenital heart defects).

2. D: This child is presenting with a fairly typical hypercyanotic spell and the presence of a systolic murmur at the left sternal border is consistent with the pulmonary stenosis murmur (upper sternal border) and the ventricular septal defect (VSD) murmur (lower sternal border) of tetralogy of Fallot. Congestive heart failure would not necessarily produce cyanosis, would be consistently present, and typically would present with hepatomegaly. The child was breathing throughout the event, so it was not triggered by apnea, and coarctation of the aorta is an acyanotic lesion with a murmur that is typically noted while auscultating along the left scapular area.

3. A: Although instructing the parents to keep a diary of the time and duration of the episodes is a good idea, it should not preclude a cardiology referral. Because the event is associated with a congenital heart defect, the administration of oxygen will not treat the cyanosis; the apnea monitor would be helpful only to document apneic episodes, not cyanotic events.

4. B: The most common etiology of chest pain in children is noncardiac, typically idiopathic or musculoskeletal. Only rare congenital heart disease such as anomalous origin of the left coronary artery has been noted to cause chest pain. Although children may demonstrate evidence of hypercholesterolemia, they do not present with the associated coronary artery disease that causes chest pain. Chest pain is not seen in congestive heart failure.

5. B: As ventricular septal defects are the most common defect in children and lead to increased pulmonary blood flow, over time they can cause congestive heart failure if not medically or surgically managed. Pulmonary stenosis causes decreased pulmonary blood flow and could cause right heart failure, but not typical signs of congestive heart failure. Infants who do contract a streptococcal infection do not get rheumatic fever (Keane, Lock, & Fyler, 2006); the average age for acute rheumatic fever is 5 to 15 years. Complete heart block is also rare and typically diagnosed and treated soon after birth as a result of the low heart rates noted.

6. D: Tachycardia and tachypnea are early signs of congestion and increased work of the heart. Hepatomegaly is also an early finding. Children may develop peripheral edema, but there must be a 10% increase in weight and the edema is initially noted in eyelids; it can be a very subtle finding.

7. B: This is a classic definition of an innocent, Still's murmur. A venous hum is a continuous murmur noted at the right upper sternal border. Even with septal shunts, a child born with transposition of the great arteries would not appear healthy and go undiagnosed for 4 years, and rheumatic heart disease typically has a mitral valve murmur that is noted at the apex, radiates to the axillae, and is holosystolic.

8. C: A venous hum is associated with drainage of the blood from the upper body through the superior vena cava to the right atrium. By turning the head or having the child lie down, the course of the blood is altered, and so the quality of the murmur changes. It is a continuous murmur, not a systolic murmur, and it does not radiate but is heard only in the right upper sternal border area.

9. D: Innocent murmurs are always very low in intensity and grading and do not require urgent referral to a cardiologist. Holosystolic murmurs are always pathologic and are associated with ventricular septal defects or mitral valve regurgitation; a thrill is always associated with a pathologic disease state and mandates a minimum scoring of IV/VI for the murmur.

10. C: The 2007 American Heart Association (AHA) recommendations include antibiotics for bacterial endocarditis prophylaxis for children only within 6 months of a surgical repair or catheterization procedure that left a closure device (septal or ductal occluder, vascular plug) and for any child with a residual defect at a repair site (surgical or catheterization based), regardless of the time since the procedure.

11. B: A diagnosis of hypertension must be pursued given the data at this visit, so two more blood pressure measurements must be documented at different times. If the child does seem anxious, the measurements could be obtained in school by the nurse. It is not appropriate to start any diuretic therapy or perform invasive imaging studies until a diagnosis is confirmed and further preliminary testing is performed.

12. B: This is a classic presentation of rheumatic fever: previous viral illness typically with pharyngitis, subsequent fever, polyarthritis, tachycardia, and carditis manifested by the appearance of a murmur. Kawasaki disease would include a fever higher than 102°F for at least 5 days and to be diagnosed must include clinical manifestations other than joint pain. Typically, a pathologic murmur is not associated with Kawasaki disease. Although sickle cell anemia may produce a new murmur and tachycardia, joint pain and fever would not be seen. A recurrent viral illness may produce a new murmur, but it is typically an innocent murmur that is systolic, low frequency, vibratory in quality, and heard at the left lower sternal border.

13. A: Antistreptolysin-O titer (ASO) evaluates for a recent or current infection with beta-hemolytic, group A

streptococci. A rise in titer begins about 1 week after infection, peaks 2 to 4 weeks later, and will usually fall to preinfection levels within 6 to 12 months (Jacobs, DeMott, & Oxley, 2004). Although an electrocardiogram (ECG) may identify complications secondary to the rheumatic fever, it does not identify an underlying organism. C-reactive protein can be used to identify infectious diseases and inflammatory states, such as active rheumatic fever, but it is a marker of nonspecific acute phase reactants found in a variety of inflammatory disease processes and would not confirm a streptococcal infection and allow appropriate therapy. A urinalysis would not provide data specific to a streptococcal infection.

14. B: Rheumatic fever is considered to be a delayed autoimmune reaction in genetically predisposed individuals to group A, beta-hemolytic streptococcal pharyngitis. No other organism has been associated with rheumatic fever.

15. A: Supraventricular tachycardia (SVT) in an infant is defined as a heart rate greater than 220 beats per minute with no variability and no other underlying pathologic states. Premature ventricular contractions (PVCs) are intermittent and would not produce a heart rate this high. Sinus tachycardia does not typically reach rates greater than 220 beats per minute and is associated with an etiology that causes the heart rate to increase such as fever, pain, or anxiety. Congenital heart defects, cyanotic or acyanotic, do not cause altered rate response such as this.

16. A: Congenital complete heart block is associated with fetal exposure to maternal antibodies related to connective tissue disorders, primarily systemic lupus erythematosus. Wolff-Parkinson-White syndrome is associated with supraventricular tachycardia. Maternal alcohol consumption has not been shown to affect the cardiac conduction system but rather affects growth patterns and neurologic development. Kawasaki disease has not been associated with congenital complete heart block.

17. B: Viral infections are the most common cause of myocarditis in North America, with typical agents including enteroviruses, adenovirus, and parvovirus B19. Diphtheria often causes myocarditis in countries without widespread immunizations. Hypersensitivity and toxic reactions to medications can cause myocarditis, but these are less common.

18. D: The sympathetic response attempting to compensate for poor contractility will cause an elevated heart rate and frequently a gallop rhythm due to the rapid filling of a noncompliant, poorly contractile left ventricle. Murmurs are less common unless there is valvular insufficiency. The most common etiology of myocarditis is a preceding viral illness.

19. D: The most recent guidelines from the National Cholesterol Education Program (NCEP) Expert Panel on Cholesterol Levels in Children list a cholesterol value

greater than or equal to 200 mg/dL as high. An acceptable total cholesterol level is less than 170 mg/dL.

20. A: It is well documented that obesity has a strong association with cardiovascular disease and specifically accelerated atherosclerosis (Balakrishnan, 2014). Prevalence of overweight and obesity has increased in all age groups, with the most dramatic increase in the 6- to 11-year-old cohort. According to the 2013 Heart Disease and Stroke Statistics Update, 31.8% of children aged 2 to 19 years are overweight or obese, and 16.9% are obese (Go et al., 2013). Tachycardia and easy fatigability can be symptoms of an overweight state and may be reversible with routine exercise and a healthy diet.

21. B: Nephrotic syndrome, obstructive liver disease, and the use of corticosteroids are known to increase the risk of dyslipidemias and contribute to accelerated atherosclerosis in children and young adults. These are all risk factors for children and should demand close monitoring of the child's lipid levels. Hypertension can be seen with elevated cholesterol levels, but it does not cause elevated cholesterol levels.

22. D: The defining factor of Kawasaki disease is coronary ectasia (dilation) and/or aneurysms. Rheumatic fever and systemic lupus erythematosus (SLE) do not affect the coronary arteries or cause long-term changes in the coronary arteries. Hypertension can cause changes to the left ventricle but has not been noted to have a direct impact on the coronary arteries.

23. B: Classic age for presentation of Kawasaki disease is in children younger than 5 years of age. If a child older or younger than this is diagnosed with Kawasaki disease, it would be characterized as atypical. Males are more frequently affected with Kawasaki disease than are females.

24. D: Diagnosis of Kawasaki disease includes a high fever for at least 5 days and erythema of hands and feet. Although the eyes may be injected, there is not necessarily exudate; joints may be sore, but chorea is not associated with this process. Any rash associated with Kawasaki disease is not typically pruritic.

25. A: An echocardiogram must be performed if a diagnosis of Kawasaki disease is given to a child. Coronary artery involvement may confirm the diagnosis, but it is also necessary to have a baseline evaluation of the coronary arteries for future reference. Coronary involvement may be noted at presentation, but aneurysms rarely form before day 10 of the illness. Kawasaki disease itself does not directly affect electrolytes, is not caused by an elevated cholesterol level, and has no known pathogen, so an antistreptolysin-O (ASO) titer to test for streptococcal antibodies would not assist with the diagnosis of Kawasaki disease.

26. D: This brief description meets the common complaints seen with neurocardiogenic syncope. Cardiac syncope does not routinely have a prodrome event. There was no description of a nervous state or

hyperventilation to support anxiety or psychogenic syncope, but further history taking can work toward these differential diagnoses if necessary.

27. A: Adequate oral fluid therapy (and salt intake) will help improve symptoms in up to 90% of patients. By achieving adequate fluid balance, the blood pressure changes associated with changes in position are minimized. A beta blocker can be used if tachycardia is persistently described as a prodromal symptom. There is no need for a 24-hour monitor unless the patient complains of palpitations prior to a syncopal event, and then a 30-day monitor will be more effective in diagnosing a possible arrhythmia. Antiepileptic therapy is not indicated for neurocardiogenic syncope.

28. C: Recent recommendations suggest performing two fasting lipid panel profiles and averaging the results for children ages 2–8 years if they have risk factors such as parents with known dyslipidemia or first-degree relatives with early heart disease. Limiting saturated fat intake to less than 7% is the second stage of dietary modifications after a 6-month trial of less stringent fat limitations. Statin therapy is not recommended for children younger than 10 years.

☐ BIBLIOGRAPHY

American Heart Association Atherosclerosis, Hypertension, and Obesity in Youth Committee, Council of Cardiovascular Disease in the Young, & Council on Cardiovascular Nursing. (2007). Drug therapy of high-risk lipid abnormalities in children and adolescents: A scientific statement. *Circulation, 115*(14), 1948–1967.

Balakrishnan, P. L. (2014). Identification of obesity and cardiovascular risk factors in childhood and adolescence. *Pediatric Clinics of North America, 61*, 153–171.

Berul, C. I., Seslar, S. P., Zimetbaum, P. J., & Josephon, M. E. (2014). Acquired long QT syndrome. *UpToDate.* Retrieved from http://www.uptodate.com/contents /acquired-long-qt-syndrome

Blake, J. M. (2014). A teen with chest pain. *Pediatric Clinics of North America, 61*(1), 17–28.

Canter, C. E., & Simpson, K. P. (2014). Diagnosis and treatment of myocarditis in children in the current era. *Circulation, 129*, 115–128.

Council on Quality of Care and Outcomes Research. (2009). Prevention of rheumatic fever and diagnosis and treatment of acute streptococcal pharyngitis. *Circulation, 119*(11), 1541–1551.

Dajani, A. S., Ayoub, E., Bierman, F. Z., Bisno, A. L., Denny, F. W., Durack, D. T., . . . Wilson, W. (1993). Guidelines for the diagnosis of rheumatic fever: Jones criteria, updated 1992. *Circulation, 87*(1), 302–307.

Daniels, S. R., Arnett, D. K., Eckel, R. H., Gidding, S. S., Hayman, L. L., . . . Williams, C. L. (2005). Overweight in children and adolescents: Pathophysiology, consequences, prevention, and treatment. *Circulation, 111*, 1999–2012.

Daniels, S. R., Greer, F. R., & the Committee on Nutrition. (2008). Lipid screening and cardiovascular health in childhood. *Pediatrics, 122*(1), 198–208.

deFerranti, S., & Washington, R. L. (2012). NHLBI guidelines on cholesterol in kids: What's new and how does this change practice? *AAP News, 33*(2), 1.

Eleftheriou, D., Levin, M., Shingadia, D., Tulloh, R., Klein, N. J., & Brogan, P. A. (2014). Management of Kawasaki disease. *Archives of Disease in Childhood, 99*, 74–83.

Evangelista, J. K. (2007). Assessment of pediatric heart sounds. *American Journal for Nurse Practitioners, 11*(3), 15–28.

Ferrieri, P. (2002). Proceedings of the Jones criteria workshop. *Circulation, 106*, 2521–2523.

Fimbres, A. M., & Shulman, S. T. (2008). Kawasaki disease. *Pediatrics in Review, 29*(9), 308–316.

Friedman, K. G., & Alexander, M. E. (2013). Chest pain and syncope in children: A practical approach to the diagnosis of cardiac disease. *Journal of Pediatrics, 163*(3), 896–901.

Gerber, M. A., Baltimore, R. S., Eaton, C. B., Gewitz, M., Rowley, A. H., Shulman, S. T., & Taubert, K. A. (2009). Prevention of rheumatic fever and diagnosis and treatment of acute streptococcal pharyngitis. *Circulation, 119*, 1541–1551.

Gidding, S. S., Dennison, B. A., Birch, L. L., Daniels, S. R., Gilman, M. W., Lichtenstein, A. H., & Van Horn, L. (2006). Dietary recommendations for children and adolescents: A guide for practitioners. *Pediatrics, 117*(2), 544–559.

Go, A. S., Mozaffarian, D., Roger, V. L., Benjamin, E. J., Jarett Berry, D., Borden, W. B., . . . Turner, M. B. (2013). AHA statistical update: Heart disease and stroke statistics—2013 update. A report from the American Heart Association. *Circulation, 127*, e6–e245.

Ingelfinger, J. R. (2014). The child or adolescent with elevated blood pressure. *New England Journal of Medicine, 370*(24), 2316–2325.

Jacobs, D. S., DeMott, W. R., & Oxley, D. K. (2004). *Laboratory test handbook concise: With disease index* (3rd ed.). Hudson, OH: Lexicomp.

Keane, J. F., Lock, J. E., & Fyler, D. C. (Eds.). (2006). *Nadas' pediatric cardiology* (2nd ed.). Philadelphia, PA: Saunders Elsevier.

Kelly, A. S., Barlow, S. E., Roa, G., Inge, T. H., Hayman, L. L., Steinberger, J., . . . Daniels, S. R. (2013). Severe obesity in children and adolescents: Identification, associated health risks, and treatment approaches. *Circulation, 128*, 1689–1712.

Krebs, N. F., & Jacobson, M. S. (2003). Prevention of pediatric overweight and obesity. *Pediatrics, 112*(2), 424–430.

May, L. E. (2008). *Pediatric heart surgery: A ready reference for professionals.* Milwaukee, WI: Maxishare.

Minette, M. S. & Sahn, D. J. (2006). Ventricular septal defects. *Circulation, 114*, 2190–2197.

Naik, R. J., & Shah, N. C. (2014). Teenage heart murmurs. *Pediatric Clinics of North America, 61*(1), 1–16.

National High Blood Pressure Education Program Working Group on High Blood Pressure in Children and Adolescents. (2004). The fourth report on the diagnosis, evaluation, and treatment of high blood pressure in children and adolescents. *Pediatrics, 114*(2), 555–576.

Newburger, J. W., Takahashi, M., Gerber, M. A., Gewitz, M. H., Tani, L. Y., Burns, J. C., … Taubert, K.A. (2004). Diagnosis, treatment, and long-term management of Kawasaki disease: A statement for health professionals. *Pediatrics, 114*(6), 1708–1733.

O'Connor, M., McDaniel, N., & Brady, W. J. (2008). The pediatric electrocardiogram: Part II: Dysryhthmias. *American Journal of Emergency Medicine, 26*(3), 348–358.

Park, N. (2007). *Pediatric cardiology for practitioners* (5th ed.). Philadelphia, PA: Mosby-Elsevier.

Pinna, G. S., Kafetzis, D. A., Tselkas, O. I., & Skevaki, C. L. (2008). Kawasaki disease: An overview. *Current Opinion in Infectious Disease, 21*(3), 263–270.

Schlechte, E. A., Boramanand, N., & Funk, M. (2008). Supraventricular tachycardia in the pediatric primary care setting: Age related presentation, diagnosis, and management. *Journal of Pediatric Health Care, 22*(5), 289–299.

Sedaghat-Yazdi, F., & Koenig, P. R. (2014). The teenager with palpitations. *Pediatric Clinics of North America, 61*(1), 63–79.

Uhl, T. L. (2008). Viral myocarditis in children. *Critical Care Nurse, 28*(1), 42–63.

Wilson, W., Taubert, K. A., Gewitz, M., Lockhart, P. B. Baddour, L. M., Levison, M., … Durack, D. T. (2007). Prevention of infective endocarditis. Guidelines from the American Heart Association. *Circulation, 116*(15), 1736–1754.

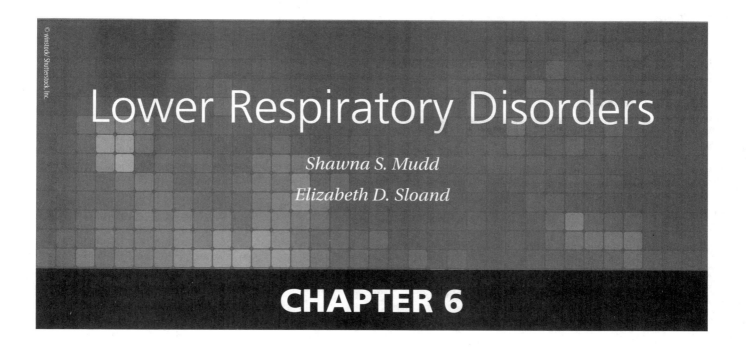

Lower Respiratory Disorders

Shawna S. Mudd

Elizabeth D. Sloand

CHAPTER 6

☐ VIRAL CROUP (LARYNGOTRACHEOBRONCHITIS)

- Definition: An acute inflammatory disease of the upper airway and larynx caused by a viral infection
- Etiology/Incidence: Parainfluenza virus is the most common organism, followed by rhinovirus, enterovirus, respiratory syncytial virus (RSV), and influenza A and B
  1. Most common in children 6 months to 6 years of age; 60% younger than 24 months
  2. Males more often affected than females
  3. Peak incidence during fall and winter
- Signs and Symptoms
  1. Upper respiratory infection (URI) prodrome; rhinitis for 3 to 4 days, sore throat
  2. Rapid onset of characteristic "barky" cough, inspiratory stridor, hoarseness
  3. Fever usually absent or low-grade
  4. Symptoms worse at night; symptoms increase with agitation or crying
  5. Mild when no stridor at rest; moderate if stridor persists when at rest; severe when retractions and cyanosis
- Differential Diagnosis
  1. Bacterial tracheitis
  2. Epiglottitis
  3. Laryngotracheomalacia
  4. Foreign body aspiration
  5. Extrinsic compression of airway from trauma, tumor, abscess, or congenital malformations
  6. Diphtheria
  7. Severe asthma
  8. Retropharyngeal abscess

- Physical Findings
  1. Inspiratory stridor
  2. Brassy, barky cough
  3. Dyspnea; expiratory stridor if severe
  4. Chest sounds are usually clear
  5. Low-grade fever; may be high grade
  6. Usually no involvement of lower respiratory tract
- Diagnostic Tests/Findings
  1. Croup is typically a clinical diagnosis; diagnostic tests usually not done
  2. If severe or atypical presentation:
     a. Pulse oximetry—hypoxia indicates severe disease
     b. Radiographic image of airway—classic tapering of the subglottic trachea ("steeple sign")
     c. White blood cell count—normal or elevated (not usually done)
- Management/Treatment
  1. Mild disease—no dyspnea, hypoxia, or dehydration
     a. Supportive outpatient care—adequate oral hydration, antipyretics, calm nonintrusive care
     b. Family education regarding worsening respiratory distress
     c. There is no evidence to support the use of mist therapy; it is often still used since it is harmless and some parents find it soothing
  2. Moderate to severe disease—stridor at rest, dyspnea, hypoxemia, or dehydration
     a. Airway maintenance is the first priority
     b. Hospitalize for supportive care, oxygen supplementation, medications, and intravenous fluids if indicated
     c. Fewer than 1% of patients require intubation

3. Medications

a. Corticosteroids indicated for all children with croup regardless of severity; lessens the severity and duration of symptoms

(1) Intramuscular dexamethasone in a single dose of 0.6 mg/kg

(2) Oral dexamethasone—a single dose of 0.15 mg/kg for mild to moderate croup

(3) Inhaled budesonide (2-4 mg) may also be effective

b. Moderate to severe croup: Nebulized racemic or L-epinephrine (0.05 mL/kg of 2.25% solution diluted in sterile saline); observe for 3 hours after a dose for rebound respiratory distress

c. Antibiotics are not indicated unless a bacterial infection is present

☐ FOREIGN BODY ASPIRATION

- Definition: Inhalation of a foreign body that lodges in the upper trachea or lower airways, resulting in total or partial airway obstruction with local injury and inflammation
- Etiology/Incidence
  1. Food or objects with pliable, slick, or cylindrical surface; peanuts, other nuts or seeds, hot dogs, candy, grapes and other raw fruits and vegetables, latex balloons, and small toys or toy parts; nuts are the most common
  2. 6 months to 4 years is highest risk; peak incidence is during second year of life
- Signs and Symptoms
  1. Abrupt onset of violent cough with gagging, choking, stridor, wheezing, and possible cyanosis
  2. Later, may be asymptomatic after object lodges and symptoms decrease; this occurs if object is not obstructing or irritating airway
- Differential Diagnosis
  1. Acute phase—laryngotracheitis, epiglottitis, laryngeal edema, pertussis, status asthmaticus, croup, retropharyngeal abscess
  2. Chronic phase—asthma, pneumonia, bronchitis, tuberculosis, and tracheal stenosis
- Physical Findings
  1. Presentation dependent on substance aspirated as well as size and location of foreign body
  2. Unilateral wheezing and localized decreased breath sounds on side of aspiration; may also be bilateral
  3. Persistent cough, voice changes, stridor, dyspnea, sputum production, and emesis may be present
  4. If foreign body persists, bronchiectasis and abscess formation is likely; may present with recurrent pneumonia and/or hemoptysis
- Diagnostic Tests/Findings
  1. Pulse oximetry—decreased O_2 saturations with significant obstruction
  2. Chest radiograph and other imaging studies may be used

3. If high index of suspicion (witnessed choking and/or abnormal films), rigid bronchoscopy is indicated for diagnostic and therapeutic purposes; if diagnosis uncertain, flexible bronchoscopy may aid diagnosis, but rigid bronchoscopy will still be needed if foreign body found

- Management/Treatment
  1. If complete obstruction:
     a. <1 year and awake: Infant face down on rescuer's arm and back blows delivered
     b. >1 year: Give abdominal thrusts (Heimlich)
     c. If unresponsive: Institute cardiopulmonary resuscitation
  2. Do not perform blind finger sweep; if object can be seen with jaw thrust, careful removal can be done
  3. Transport to ER as needed
  4. Refer to an expert pediatric endoscopy team for rigid bronchoscopy evaluation and removal (if convincing history of foreign body aspiration, regardless of radiographic findings)
  5. Humidification, bronchodilators, and anti-inflammatory medications may be useful after removal
  6. Antibiotics if evidence of pneumonia or bronchitis
  7. Prevention with parental education
     a. Remove small items from environment of small child
     b. Sit while eating and provide adult supervision
     c. Cut food in small pieces for young children
     d. Avoid commonly aspirated foods and objects with children younger than 3 years of age

☐ BRONCHITIS

- Definition
  1. Bronchitis is a nonspecific inflammation of the larger lower airways, associated with several childhood conditions; excess mucus is present due to poor clearance or increased production; cough is prominent
  2. Acute bronchitis often follows a URI
  3. Chronic bronchitis symptoms persist for more than 2 weeks; chronic bronchitis is rarely an isolated entity in children, but a symptom of another condition such as asthma, cystic fibrosis, or foreign body aspiration
- Etiology/Incidence
  1. Most commonly viral—parainfluenza, RSV, and rhinovirus
  2. Bacterial causes—*Mycoplasma pneumoniae*, *Bordetella pertussis*, *Chlamydia pneumoniae*, and *Corynebacterium diphtheriae*
  3. Acute bronchitis occurs most frequently in the winter and early spring
- Signs and Symptoms
  1. Initial phase includes symptoms of an upper respiratory illness, such as rhinitis, nasopharyngitis, and conjunctivitis
  2. Cough is the hallmark symptom; is initially dry and brassy but may become productive as illness progresses

3. Sputum may become purulent, which reflects leukocyte migration and not necessarily bacterial involvement
4. Swallowing sputum may result in nausea
5. Retrosternal pain is common as cough persists
- Differential Diagnosis
  1. Pneumonia
  2. Asthma
  3. Allergic disease/posterior nasal drainage
  4. Gastroesophageal reflux and/or aspiration
  5. Exposure to irritants such as cigarette smoke
  6. Cystic fibrosis
  7. Immune deficiency
  8. Chronic sinusitis
  9. Immotile cilia syndrome
  10. Foreign body aspiration
  11. Respiratory tract anomalies
  12. Tobacco or marijuana use in adolescents
- Physical Findings
  1. Brassy cough
  2. Coarse, bronchial breath sounds in periphery of lungs
  3. Fever may be low-grade or absent
- Diagnostic Tests/Findings
  1. Diagnosis primarily based on history and physical
  2. Chest radiograph may be normal or show peribronchial thickening
  3. Pulmonary function tests (PFTs) may be normal or may indicate an obstructive pattern; PFT may or may not improve after bronchodilator
- Management/Treatment
  1. Primarily supportive
  2. Acute bronchitis—increase fluid intake; avoid expectorants, antihistamines, and cough suppressants
  3. Chronic bronchitis is not a distinct entity in children; investigate underlying systemic or pulmonary problem
  4. Bronchodilators if accompanied by wheezing
  5. Inhaled steroids may be indicated for chronic bronchitis
  6. Antibiotics are not usually helpful for viral illnesses; however, antibiotics (with efficacy against *Mycoplasma* and *Chlamydia* species) are useful if bacterial etiology is suspected and cough is >10 to 14 days' duration; children with chronic pulmonary disease other than asthma may benefit from antibiotics for acute exacerbations; consider pertussis if immunizations incomplete
  7. Prevention
     a. Avoidance of irritants
     b. Frequent hand washing with careful disposal of nasal and oral drainage
     c. Avoid overcrowding

❏ BRONCHIOLITIS

- Definition: An acute viral infection of the lower respiratory tract; the most common serious acute respiratory illness of young children and infants; characterized by acute inflammation, edema, and necrosis of epithelial cells of the small airways, increased mucus production, and bronchospasm
- Etiology/Incidence
  1. Primarily caused by RSV (December–March in North America)
  2. Other viral pathogens: Rhinovirus, human metapneumovirus, influenza, adenovirus, parainfluenza
  3. Older family members may be the infection source for young children, with older children and adults having a much milder illness
  4. High risk for hospitalization includes premature or young infants and those with cardiorespiratory disease (especially bronchopulmonary dysplasia) or immunodeficiency
  5. Most commonly occurs in midwinter to early spring
  6. More severe disease in boys, infants who have not been breastfed, and those with lower socioeconomic status
  7. Most common cause of hospitalization in infants 0–1 years old
- Signs and Symptoms
  1. Initial symptoms—rhinorrhea, congestion, cough, decreased appetite, and low-grade fever
  2. Progresses to increased work of breathing, tachypnea, hypoxia, decreased appetite or poor suck; change in level of consciousness or activity level
  3. May have history of exposure to an older child or adult with a mild respiratory illness
  4. May present as apnea, lethargy, irritability, or poor feeding in very young or premature infants
- Differential Diagnosis
  1. Bacterial or chlamydial pneumonia
  2. Aspiration pneumonia
  3. Asthma and allergy
  4. Foreign body aspiration
  5. Cystic fibrosis
  6. Congenital malformations of the respiratory tract
- Physical Findings
  1. Wheezing is the most prominent physical finding; crackles; very faint breath sounds suggest more severe disease with more significant obstruction
  2. Tachypnea with shallow breathing, retractions, nasal flaring, prolonged expiratory phase, paroxysmal wheezy cough
  3. Rhinorrhea, otitis, conjunctivitis, and/or pharyngitis
  4. Afebrile or low-grade fever
  5. Palpable liver and spleen due to hyperinflation of lungs
- Diagnostic Tests/Findings
  1. Diagnosis primarily based on history and physical
     a. Assess risk for severe disease: <12 weeks old, hx of prematurity, underlying conditions of immunodeficiency or cardiopulmonary disease
     b. Laboratory and imaging studies not indicated
  2. Chest radiograph—if done, findings are nonspecific; may include hyperinflation, peribronchial thickening, air trapping, patchy or subsegmental atelectasis

3. Pulse oximetry—hypoxemia with significant disease
4. White blood cell count with differential—may or may not be increased
5. Viral nasal wash with rapid diagnostic techniques—may be positive for RSV

- Management/Treatment
1. Usually outpatient care with fluids, nutritional support, and monitoring
2. Careful monitoring of respiratory status, use oxygen therapy if hypoxemic
3. Bronchodilators (albuterol), epinephrine, and corticosteroids—not recommended
4. Nebulized hypertonic saline may be given to hospitalized infants; not recommended for ER administration
5. Antibiotics not routinely used unless bacterial infection is suspected
6. Prevention
   a. Palivizumab vaccine is indicated for high-risk children in first year of life:
      (1) Infants born at <29 weeks' gestation
      (2) Infants born at >29 weeks' gestation with chronic lung disease (CLD) of prematurity, congenital heart disease (CHD), or other condition
      (3) Dose: 15 mg/kg IM, given in five monthly doses, beginning in November
      (4) For second year of life, strict guidelines for children with CLD and CHD; see American Academy of Pediatrics policy statement (AAP, 2014)
   b. Strict contact precautions (gown, gloves) in hospitalized children
   c. Home measures—decrease exposure to contagious settings, avoid environmental smoke exposure, careful hand washing, avoid touching face, disinfect surfaces, cover coughs and sneezes
   d. An RSV vaccine is currently in development

☐ PNEUMONIA

- Definition: An inflammation of the pulmonary parenchyma
1. Infectious pneumonia—infection that usually involves small airways in children but may also infect the larger airways and/or the alveoli
2. Aspiration pneumonia—caused by the ingestion of food, saliva, gastric contents, or other substances into air passages
- Etiology/Incidence
1. Common viral agents—RSV, parainfluenza, influenza A and B, and human metapneumovirus; usually involves the small airways
2. Neonates: Group B strep, *Enterococcus*, *Listeria monocytogenes*, *Escherichia coli*, *Ureaplasma urealyticum*
3. 1 to 3 months: Most common bacterial causes include *Staphylococcus aureus*, *Streptococcus pneumoniae*, *Haemophilus influenzae* (*H. flu*), *Chlamydia trachomatis*, *Bordetella pertussis*, *Ureaplasma*

4. 4 months to 4 years: *S. pneumoniae*, *S. aureus*, *H. flu*
5. All ages: *Streptococcus pneumoniae* is most common cause of bacterial pneumonia; *Mycoplasma pneumoniae*, *Mycoplasma tuberculosis*
6. Immunocompromised or malnourished children—consider opportunistic organisms, such as *Pneumocystis carinii*, yeasts
7. Many other less common pathogens can be considered
8. Aspiration pneumonia occurs most frequently in children with upper airway abnormalities or neurologic deficits, severe gastroesophageal reflux, and other esophageal problems; may also occur subsequent to the inhalation of smoke or hydrocarbons; following near drowning or ethanol ingestion by adolescents
9. Annual incidence 3% to 5%; highest incidence in children <5 years
10. Incidence of *Haemophilus influenzae* pneumonia and pneumococcal pneumonia have dramatically decreased since introduction of Hib and heptavalent pneumococcal conjugate vaccines, respectively

- Signs and Symptoms
1. Cough occasionally productive or associated with emesis
2. Tachypnea is a key finding; also retractions, expiratory grunting, nasal flaring, cyanosis, and rash
3. Fever
4. Neck or chest pain (upper lobe) or abdominal pain (lower lobe); nausea/vomiting
5. Wheezing (frequent in viral etiology)
6. May have change in level of consciousness, activity, feeding
7. Bacterial pneumonia—usually an abrupt onset of fever, chills, cough, and chest pain
8. Viral pneumonia may be preceded by a URI
9. May have extrapulmonary findings or infection at other sites such as otitis media, sinusitis, and meningitis

- Differential Diagnosis
1. Bronchiolitis, URI, croup
2. Foreign body aspiration
3. Asthma
4. Cystic fibrosis
5. Sepsis, meningitis, pertussis
6. Tuberculosis
7. Immunodeficiency
8. Reflux, swallowing dysfunction

- Physical Findings
1. Fever with bacterial pneumonia
2. Tachypnea is most consistent finding; substernal, supraclavicular, and intercostal retractions; grunting, nasal flaring; pallor/cyanosis/decreased oxygen saturation
3. Rales/crackles, wheezing, crackles, diminished or tubular breath sounds
4. If pleural effusion present, may have decreased breath sounds with dullness to percussion

- Diagnostic Tests/Findings—in an uncomplicated patient who is stable, no diagnostic tests are needed; if not stable or with fever >39°C, chest radiography is advised
  1. Chest radiograph—severity of disease may not directly correlate with radiography findings; not reliable for distinguishing between bacterial and viral disease
     a. Atelectasis—opacification, intrathoracic structures will shift toward the atelectatic area; hemidiaphragm on affected side may be elevated and intercostal spaces on that side may be narrow
     b. Viral pneumonia—may show hyperinflation and bilateral interstitial infiltrates and peribronchial cuffing
     c. Bacterial pneumonias—may show patchy infiltrates in infants; lobar consolidation is most common with *Streptococcus pneumoniae* or *Haemophilus influenzae*; hilar adenopathy is most common with *Haemophilus influenzae* or *Staphylococcus aureus*; pleural effusion may be present
     d. Acute aspiration pneumonia usually develops in portion of lung that is dependent at time of aspiration; otherwise, radiograph typically shows diffuse or localized mottled infiltrates with or without atelectasis
  2. White blood cell (WBC) count—bacterial pneumonia is associated with elevated WBCs (15,000–40,000/mm^3); may or may not be elevated with viral pneumonia
  3. Viral cultures of nasopharyngeal secretions; rapid identification with immunofluorescent assay can confirm diagnosis for high-risk children or for epidemiologic surveillance and control
  4. Blood cultures—if child is toxic, if child is an infant, or if bacterial pneumonia is suspected
  5. Sputum cultures—warranted in older child if cough is productive
  6. Positive cold agglutinin screen or titer: 1:64 is suggestive of *Mycoplasma* pneumonia; positive polymerase chain reaction (PCR) test or seroconversion in an IgG assay can diagnose *Mycoplasma* pneumonia. (Usually not done because of usual clinical diagnosis and effective treatment)
  7. PPD if tuberculosis (TB) is suspected
  8. Pulse oximetry—decreased O$_2$ saturations with severe disease
- Management/Treatment
  1. Most often viral and self-limited
  2. Difficult to distinguish between viral and bacterial since radiographs and WBC counts are not specific
  3. Antimicrobial treatment based on setting of care, etiology, and age of the child
     a. Neonates: Ampicillin + gentamycin for 10–21 days; if *Chlamydia trachomatis* suspected: erythromycin for 14 days
     b. Hospitalized: IV ampicillin ± azithromycin
     c. Outpatient:
        (1) 3 months to 5 years old—amoxicillin 90 mg/kg/day, ± azithromycin for 7–10 days
        (2) 5 years or older—azithromycin or amoxicillin 90 mg/kg/day for 7–10 days or penicillin G
     d. Close follow-up (12 hours–5 days) when treated as outpatient
     e. For infants consider *Bordetella pertussis* if immunizations incomplete or *C. trachomatis* if mother infected
     f. Consider anaerobes if aspiration pneumonia; treat with clindamycin
     g. Bronchodilators and chest physiotherapy may improve airway clearance
     h. Other supportive therapy may include additional fluids and/or oxygen
     i. Pneumonia in immunocompromised hosts or those with underlying cardiac or lung disease can progress rapidly; should be managed in a monitored setting, with aggressive diagnostic measures and appropriate broad-spectrum antimicrobial coverage
     j. Refer to pulmonary specialist if recurrent disease without known cause

☐ CYSTIC FIBROSIS (CF)

- Definition: Autosomal recessive disorder of cystic fibrosis transmembrane regulation (CFTR) that causes defective epithelial ion transport, which results in dehydrated, viscous secretions that obstruct the exocrine ducts (with subsequent destruction and scarring) in the respiratory, hepatobiliary, gastrointestinal, and reproductive tracts
- Etiology/Incidence
  1. Caused by mutations in a single gene on the long arm of chromosome 7, which directs the production of CFTR
     a. CFTR is the principal chloride channel of epithelial cells and controls other ion transport
     b. Defective CFTR results in increased sodium reabsorption, decreased chloride secretion, and dehydrated, highly viscous secretions in all exocrine ducts, which causes disease
     c. There are more than 1500 mutations of the *CFTR* gene causing CF, although the functional importance of only a small number is known
  2. Incidence—most common fatal genetic disorder affecting Caucasian population; less frequent among other racial groups. In the United States, 1:3000 among Caucasians, 1:9200 among Hispanic population; affects more than 100,000 people worldwide
  3. Median life expectancy is 41 years and continues to rise as a result of new treatments; respiratory failure is the leading cause of death
- Signs and Symptoms
  1. Extremely viscid meconium (newborns), with delayed passage

2. Poor growth despite normal to increased appetite; failure to thrive
3. Recurrent and chronic respiratory infections (sinuses and lower airways); dyspnea on exertion that progresses to dyspnea at rest as disease progresses
4. Large, bulky, foul-smelling, greasy stools
5. Frequent flatulence or abdominal pain
6. Chronic cough, varies in character, but usually productive, blood-streaked mucus not uncommon; major hemoptysis can be life-threatening
7. Recurrent or persistent wheezing
8. Salty-tasting skin
9. Distal small bowel obstruction
10. Recurrent pancreatitis
11. CF-related diabetes mellitus (30% of those older than 25 years)
12. Salt loss syndromes
13. Heat prostration with hypernatremia dehydration
14. Male infertility (98% of men sterile) and women have reduced fertility

- Differential Diagnosis
  1. Asthma
  2. Recurrent pneumonia, bronchitis
  3. Immunologic deficiencies, metabolic alkalosis
  4. Celiac disease, protein-losing enteropathy, alpha-1-antitrypsin deficiency (rare)
  5. Airway abnormalities, e.g., airway stenosis, vascular ring
  6. Gastroesophageal reflux, with or without aspiration
  7. Other causes of malabsorption and/or failure to thrive

- Physical Findings
  1. Wheezing and air trapping with increased anteroposterior diameter of the chest (barrel chest) as disease progresses
  2. Crackles
  3. Increased work of breathing with accessory muscle use
  4. Nasal polyps, chronic sinusitis
  5. Failure to thrive from maldigestion and fat malabsorption (90% of patients)
  6. Abdominal pain and distention, unexplained pancreatitis or cirrhosis, hepatosplenomegaly, cholelithiasis
  7. Rectal prolapse
  8. Digital clubbing
  9. Delayed puberty
  10. Meconium ileus (15% of newborns)

- Diagnostic Tests/Findings
  1. Pilocarpine iontophoresis sweat test—two tests with a sweat chloride in excess of 60 mmol/L; test should be performed by a Cystic Fibrosis Foundation–approved laboratory
  2. Genotyping can show two disease-causing mutations
  3. All states in the United States and many countries include genetic analysis in newborn screening; prenatal screening available
  4. Other findings
     a. Elevated immunoreactive trypsin (IRT) in newborn; elevated IRT must be confirmed with sweat test

b. Milder, atypical presentations are being identified by expanded diagnostic criteria
c. Chest radiograph—hyperinflation, increased peribronchial markings, atelectasis, bronchiectasis
d. CT scan—early bronchiectasis
e. Pulmonary function tests—demonstrates obstructive pattern; decreased flow rates and vital capacity as disease progresses
f. Sputum culture—typical CF pathogens: *Staphylococcus aureus*, *Haemophilus influenzae*, *Pseudomonas aeruginosa*, *Burkholderia cepacia*
g. Oximetry—decreased oxygen saturation with exacerbation and worsening disease
h. Hyponatremia, hypoproteinemia, hypochloremic alkalosis
i. Elevated liver enzymes (AST or ALT)
j. Fat-soluble vitamin (A, E, and K) deficiencies
k. Glucose testing
l. Sinus CT—chronic inflammation/disease

- Management/Treatment
  1. Referral to cystic fibrosis care center for long-term care
     Cystic Fibrosis Foundation
     6931 Arlington Road, 2nd floor
     Bethesda, Maryland 20814
     301-951-4422
     Fax: 301-951-6378
     1-800-FIGHT CF (800-344-4823) for list of approved centers
     http://www.cff.org
  2. Interdisciplinary management involving replacement of pancreatic enzymes, nutritional support, airway clearance techniques, prevention and aggressive treatment of infection, intensive education, and psychosocial support
  3. Routinely given medications
     a. Inhaled mucolytic agent
     b. Recombinant human DNase (Pulmozyme [dornase alfa])
     c. For chronic *Pseudomonas aeruginosa*: Inhaled tobramycin or inhaled aztreonam and chronic oral azithromycin. Bronchodilators and anti-inflammatory therapies
  4. Antibiotic therapy based on sputum culture and sensitivity
     a. Given early in course of disease to delay onset of chronic colonization with *P. aeruginosa* (the primary organism found in the airways of CF children and adults; once established, it is nearly impossible to eradicate)
     b. Once colonized, given to slow decline in pulmonary function
     c. Intravenous courses given for pulmonary exacerbations to restore pulmonary function and reduce symptoms
  5. Isolation—standard precautions for all patients; contact and droplet precautions when indicated, minimize contact with other CF patients to avoid spread of

infections (particularly if infected with *Burkholderia cepacia,* a virulent pathogen that has innate antibiotic resistance, causes rapid decline in lung function, and is associated with mortality in CF patients)
6. Role of primary care provider—annual influenza vaccine, aggressive use of antibiotics for respiratory infections, close monitoring for CF complications

☐ ASTHMA

- Definition: Chronic inflammatory disorder characterized by:
  1. Chronic airway inflammation, the underlying pathologic process, which contributes to:
     a. Airway hyperresponsiveness to a variety of stimuli
     b. Variable airway obstruction
     c. Clinical symptoms that can be variable over time
  2. Immunohistopathologic features include:
     a. Inflammatory cell infiltration with neutrophils, eosinophils, lymphocytes
     b. Mast cell activation and epithelial cell injury
  3. Persistent airway inflammation can lead to airway wall remodeling, irreversible changes, and loss of pulmonary function
- Etiology/Incidence
  1. Airway inflammation plays a central role
     a. Inflammation causes airway narrowing and increased airway secretions
     b. Inflammation contributes to airway hyperresponsiveness
     c. Broad variety of factors trigger inflammation
     d. Causes recurrent acute episodes
  2. The most important environmental factors in the development and severity of asthma are:
     a. Airborne allergen sensitization, such as dust mites, cockroaches, mice, pet dander
     b. Viral respiratory infections, such as early RSV, parainfluenza, rhinovirus
  3. Other exposures/risk factors that can precipitate asthma exacerbations
     a. Outdoor pollutants
     b. Tobacco smoke
     c. Formaldehyde/volatile organic compounds
     d. Outdoor allergens—seasonal trees, grasses, weeds, pollens, molds
     e. Weather/humidity changes
     f. Exercise induced
     g. Comorbid conditions such as:
        (1) Gastroesophageal reflux
        (2) Obesity
        (3) Chronic stress
        (4) Obstructive sleep apnea
        (5) Sinusitis/rhinitis
     h. Food allergies—nuts, shellfish, sulfites (shrimp, dried fruit, beer or wine)
     i. Medications—aspirin, beta blockers, nonsteroidal anti-inflammatory drugs

  4. Approximately 8.9% of children, 6.5 million in the United States, affected; incidence and mortality increasing worldwide
     a. Rising incidence in childhood and all age groups, especially among males, lower socioeconomic groups, urban African Americans and Hispanics, and those with family history of asthma or allergies
     b. A leading cause of hospitalization and school absenteeism
  5. Underdiagnosis and inappropriate treatment are major contributors to morbidity and mortality
- Signs and Symptoms
  1. Recurrent episodes of cough, wheezing, mucus production, chest tightness, breathlessness, and decreased endurance
  2. Symptoms often display an initial response (bronchospasm) to a trigger (early-phase asthmatic response), and then a late (inflammatory) phase response approximately 4 to 12 hours after the initial response that is more severe and prolonged than the earlier response and can last hours to several weeks
  3. Symptoms often worse at night, early morning, and during or after exercise
  4. Variability—some may have severe, life-threatening exacerbations separated by long periods of normal lung function and no clinical symptoms
  5. A subset present with chronic (usually nighttime) cough without wheezing or exercise intolerance (cough-variant asthma)
- Differential Diagnosis
  1. Upper or lower respiratory tract infections
  2. Foreign body aspiration
  3. Cystic fibrosis
  4. Cardiac or anatomic defects
  5. Vocal cord dysfunction
  6. Conditions that may coexist with asthma and complicate diagnosis include gastroesophageal reflux and obstructive sleep apnea
- Physical Findings: Clinical exam is normal when asymptomatic; when symptomatic:
  1. Cough and shortness of breath
  2. Diffuse wheezes (initially heard at the end of the expiratory phase) with decreased airflow and prolonged expiratory phase
  3. Respiratory distress, retractions, increased hypoxia, and decreased breath sounds as severity increases
  4. Allergic appearance—allergic "shiners," Dennie's lines, nasal crease, nasal congestion and mouth breathing, and boggy turbinates and nasal edema; nasal polyps (consider CF)
  5. Skin—atopic dermatitis
  6. Concurrent respiratory infection—viral respiratory illness, sinusitis
- Diagnostic Tests/Findings
  1. Thorough history is vital to diagnosis and management, with special emphasis on triggers, severity of previous episodes, pattern and characteristics of

previous episodes, response to medications, and family history of asthma or allergy

2. Pulmonary function testing (spirometry)—the gold standard in diagnosing asthma in children older than 4 to 5 years; demonstrates obstruction and assesses reversibility
   a. Lower airway obstruction indicated by a reduction in the values for both FEV$_1$ (forced expiratory volume in 1 second) and the FEV$_1$/FVC ratio (FEV$_1$ to forced vital capacity [or FEV$_1$/ FEV$_6$]) relative to reference or predicted values
   b. Reversibility—FEV$_1$ increases at least 12% from baseline *or* FEV$_1$ increases at least 10% above predicted after using a short-acting inhaled beta-2 agonist
3. Chest radiograph
   a. Bilateral hyperinflation with peribronchial thickening
   b. Atelectasis (can be misread as pneumonia)
   c. May be normal
   d. May be unnecessary unless uncertain diagnosis or if poor response to treatment
4. Evaluation of other factors contributing to asthma severity
   a. Allergy evaluation and treatment as indicated to improve allergy/asthma control
      (1) Complete blood count (CBC)—eosinophilia
      (2) Immunoglobulin E—elevated, values age dependent
      (3) Radioallergosorbent test (RAST)—serum test that identifies possible allergic responses to various environmental substances
      (4) Skin testing
   b. Nasal and sinus evaluation—identify and treat allergic rhinitis, sinusitis; consider sweat test if CF is suspected
   c. Gastroesophageal reflux assessment
5. Pulse oximetry—evaluate hypoxemia during an acute episode
- Management/Treatment: As recommended by National Heart, Lung, and Blood Institute, *Expert Panel Report 3: Guidelines for the Diagnosis and Management of Asthma. National Asthma Education and Prevention Program (EPR 3)*; asthma treatment should be based on this comprehensive plan and document, available at http://www.nhlbi.nih.gov/health-pro/guidelines/current/asthma-guidelines/full-report.htm
1. Goals in primary care—reduce current impairment and reduce future risk; child should live as normal a life as possible
2. Four components of asthma management in guidelines:
   a. Accurate measures of assessment and monitoring
   b. Pharmacologic therapy
   c. Education of family and child for a partnership in asthma care
   d. Control of environmental factors and comorbid conditions that affect asthma

3. Initially, assess asthma for severity to initiate therapy, and subsequently, assess control for monitoring and adjusting therapy
4. Asthma severity is determined *before* therapy; if already on medications, determined by type of medications needed for control
   a. Classifications divided into four groups: intermittent, mild persistent, moderate persistent, and severe persistent, and consider both impairment (burden of symptoms) and risk (morbidity potential)
   b. Guidelines for assessment and treatment are divided into three age groups: 0 to 4 years old, 5 to 11 years old, and 12 years old and older
   c. Classification based on:
      (1) Frequency and timing of symptoms
      (2) Interference with daily activities
      (3) PFTs
      (4) Need for short-acting medications
   d. If a child's assessment falls between two levels of severity, child should be treated for the highest level (most aggressive)
5. Medication treatment is based on severity and control, using a step-wise approach created by the EPR 3 Guidelines
   a. Ranges from step 1 (intermittent asthma) to step 6 (severe persistent)
   b. Step-wise approach is intended to assist, not substitute for, clinical decision making and individualized care
6. Medications are in two categories: long-term control and quick relief
   a. Long-term control medicines—taken daily
      (1) Inhaled corticosteroids (ICSs) are the preferred medication for all children with mild, moderate, or severe persistent asthma (i.e., beclomethasone, budesonide, flunisolide, fluticasone); delivered by nebulizer or inhaler; dose of drug matched to level of disease severity
      (2) Leukotriene modifiers (montelukast and zafirlukast)
      (3) Long-acting beta-2 agonists (LABAs)—salmeterol and formoterol, inhaled
         (a) Use in combination with ICSs, but only use when ICSs are not effective alone; do not use as monotherapy
         (b) Black box warning due to association with severe asthma attacks and death; close monitoring advised
      (4) Omalizumab, an immunomodulator that prevents binding of IgE to mast cells, used for steps 5 and 6 in controlled clinical settings because of side effects
      (5) Cromolyn sodium or nedocromil (inhaled)—useful for exercise-induced bronchospasm; not preferred treatment of mild persistent asthma
      (6) Methylxanthines—used rarely
      (7) Oral corticosteroids in short courses for control of symptoms; also used as controller with

step 6 severity (if severe, chronic asthma, not to exceed 60 mg/day)

    b. Quick-relief medications—taken as needed to provide prompt reversal of acute airflow obstruction and relief of bronchoconstriction; not for daily long-term use

      (1) Inhaled short-acting beta-2 agonists (albuterol, levalbuterol)

      (2) Anticholinergics (ipratroprium bromide, inhaled)

      (3) Short-course systemic corticosteroids (oral or parenteral)

7. Assess for control and adjust treatment

    a. Close follow-up; return visits scheduled every 1 to 6 months

    b. Step therapy up or down according to level of control and severity

    c. Spirometry can assist in follow-up visits

8. Educate for a partnership in care of child with asthma

    a. Identify and address family's and child's concerns

    b. Establish open lines of communication; be mindful of cultural differences

    c. At every visit, review the written asthma action plan, which has clear instructions of medications, doses, signs/symptoms of problems, and instructions for increasing therapy or contacting provider

    d. Review child's technique with devices: peak flow meter, inhaler, and spacer

9. Control of environmental factors and comorbid conditions

    a. Those with persistent asthma should have skin testing or in vitro testing to identify specific allergens

    b. Identify and reduce child-specific triggers such as house dust mites, cockroaches, pet dander, indoor and outdoor plants and trees, and molds

    c. Employ a broad approach with family to reduce allergen exposure in the environment

    d. Make strong recommendations to eliminate environmental tobacco smoke (ETS)

      (1) Identify all tobacco smokers in child's environment and advise them to quit

      (2) Assist by referral to appropriate smoking cessation programs and advising nicotine replacement therapy

☐ BRONCHOPULMONARY DYSPLASIA (BPD)

- Definition: Any child requiring supplemental oxygen at 36 weeks or greater (postconception age) with radiographic changes of chronic lung disease
- Etiology/Incidence
  1. Disease of infants <1000 g at birth and <32 weeks' gestation
  2. Most have normal lung function at birth but develop respiratory failure within the first weeks of life
  3. Can develop in babies who are oxygen dependent for >28 days after birth
  4. Majority of those who develop BPD do so following respiratory distress syndrome; other causes include persistent pulmonary hypertension, meconium aspiration, severe lower respiratory infection, maternal infection (amnionitis), and chronic aspiration
  5. Leading cause of chronic lung disease in infants
  6. Multifactorial—lung immaturity, oxygen toxicity, barotrauma from mechanical ventilation, infections, malnutrition, fluid overload, prenatal risk factors—intrauterine growth restriction (IUGR), lack of antenatal steroids
  7. Mild to severe disease possible (decreased lung compliance and increased airway resistance)
  8. 5000 to 10,000 infants per year develop BPD in the United States; white male infants at higher risk
- Signs and Symptoms
  1. Acute respiratory distress in first week of life; may have cough and wheeze
  2. Poor growth and poor feeding skills
  3. Fussy with decreased endurance
- Differential Diagnosis
  1. Meconium aspiration syndrome
  2. Congenital infection
  3. Congenital cardiac or pulmonary defects that result in supplemental oxygen requirement
  4. Upper airway obstruction
  5. Lower airway abnormalities (structural/anatomic, extrinsic compression, tracheomalacia)
  6. Pulmonary hypertension
  7. Metabolic disorders
  8. Respiratory infections/immunodeficiency
  9. Chronic gastroesophageal reflux
  10. Chronic or recurrent aspiration
- Physical Findings—vary with severity of disease
  1. Tachypnea with retractions
  2. Diffuse inspiratory or expiratory crackles and/or wheezes
  3. Pale with cyanotic episodes
  4. Findings consistent with cardiac insufficiency or fluid overload
  5. Fluid sensitivity
  6. Associated findings consistent with sequelae of prematurity and/or chronic lung disease
- Diagnostic Tests/Findings
  1. Oximetry on room air—hypoxemia
  2. Growth curve—often failure to thrive (FTT), even after corrected for prematurity
  3. Serum electrolytes
     a. Carbon dioxide retention
     b. Chloride and potassium depletion, metabolic alkalosis—with diuretic use
  4. Arterial blood gases (on room air)—to monitor in acute and chronic stages
  5. Chest radiograph—abnormalities may include hyperinflation, emphysema, cyst formation, fibrosis, cardiovascular (CV) changes
  6. Electrocardiogram and echocardiogram to monitor cardiac status

- Management/Treatment
1. Maintain adequate oxygenation (92% or greater) to prevent cor pulmonale and to promote growth
   a. Provide supplemental oxygen—wean as tolerated, expect gradual improvement with growth
   b. Desaturation commonly occurs during sleeping and feeding
   c. More severe BPD may need long-term mechanical ventilation and tracheotomy
2. Adequate nutrition and fluids
   a. Nutritional supplementation and hypercaloric formulas to provide additional calories; nutrition referral
   b. Occupational therapy intervention for feeding skills
   c. Gastrostomy or supplemental tube feedings as needed
   d. Balance nutrition volume with fluid restriction when fluid sensitive
   e. Treat gastroesophageal reflux as needed
3. Medications
   a. Bronchodilators—inhaled, may decrease airway resistance
   b. Diuretics—as needed for acute fluid overload; avoid chronic use if possible
   c. In older BPD children, inhaled beta agonists with inhaled steroids can be used for symptomatic relief
4. Protective care to avoid lung re-injury
   a. Immunizations, including influenza
   b. Smoke-free environment
   c. RSV prevention—administer palivizumab or RSV intravenous immunoglobulin
   d. Avoid high-density day care settings
   e. Good hand washing and other infection control precautions
   f. Avoid elective procedures, especially during winter months
5. Family education, support, and follow-up
   a. Close follow-up (every 1 to 3 months) to determine adequate oxygenation and growth
   b. Higher incidence of rehospitalization in early years due to exacerbations
6. Monitor for associated findings, manage/refer as needed—airway disorders, hypertension, gastroesophageal reflux, heart failure, neurodevelopmental problems, ophthalmology or renal complications
7. High risk for neurologic, developmental, or academic concerns throughout childhood
8. Referrals
   a. Early intervention for developmental assistance and monitoring
   b. Financial assistance and counseling
   c. Home nursing and equipment companies
   d. Family counseling and support groups
   e. Community rescue services
   f. Case management
9. Prevention—reduce incidence of premature births

☐ APNEA

- Definition: Respiratory pause lasting >20 seconds or associated with cyanosis, bradycardia, marked pallor, or hypotonia; a disorder of respiratory control; may be central, obstructive, or mixed
1. Types
   a. Central apnea—caused by decreased central nervous system (CNS) stimuli to respiratory muscles; cessation of airflow without accompanying respiratory effort
   b. Obstructive sleep apnea (OSA)—most common form of apnea; cessation of airflow despite accompanying respiratory effort due to partial or complete intermittent airway obstruction
   c. Mixed apnea—evidence of both central and obstructive apnea
   d. Apnea of infancy—pathologic apnea in infants that are >37 weeks' gestation at onset; always demands diagnostic evaluation
   e. Apnea of prematurity—periodic breathing with pathologic apnea in a premature infant <37 weeks' gestation; occurs in the absence of identifiable predisposing disease; common and may be due to prematurity or an associated illness
   f. Periodic breathing—three or more respiratory pauses of >3 seconds duration with <20 seconds of respiration between pauses; common and physiologic in preterm infants; pathologic if accompanied by cardiac or respiratory instability
   g. Apparent life-threatening event (ALTE)—an episode that an observer believes is life-threatening; includes some combination of apnea, change in skin color, marked change in muscle tone, choking, or gagging
- Etiology/Incidence
1. Apneas vary significantly depending on underlying etiology
2. Prematurity, hx of multiple ALTEs, child abuse are associated with a higher recurrence risk or adverse outcome
3. ALTE—nearly half of all cases of ALTE are due to gastroesophageal reflux, seizure, and lower respiratory tract infection; more than 50% remain unexplained and then are termed "apnea of infancy"; no causal link with sudden infant death syndrome (SIDS); other more serious causes can exist such as nonaccidental trauma, metabolic disease, medication reactions, cardiac disease, and infections
4. Obstructive sleep apnea syndrome (OSAS)
   a. Prevalence of 1% to 5% in pediatrics
   b. 2 to 8 years peak age (peak age of adenotonsillar hypertrophy)
   c. Increased risk with craniofacial anomalies, obesity, Down syndrome, chronic nasal congestion, gastroesophageal reflux disease (GERD), hypothyroidism

- Signs and Symptoms
  1. During event, partial and/or intermittent complete airway obstruction that interferes with normal sleep and ventilation; respiratory pause accompanied by marked pallor, cyanosis, hypotonia, and bradycardia
  2. OSAS—most common presentation is snoring; typically loud, habitual snoring; apnea followed by gasping, choking, and arousal; restless sleep (frequent awakenings), diaphoresis, unusual sleep positions (hyperextension of neck), nocturnal enuresis
  3. OSAS daytime symptoms—morning headache, behavioral changes, poor school performance, daytime sleepiness, hyperactivity that may mimic attention deficit hyperactivity disorder (ADHD), decreased quality of life
- Differential Diagnosis of ALTE: Very broad range, including:
  1. Gatroesophageal reflux (GER)
  2. Sepsis/meningitis
  3. Respiratory syncytial virus infection
  4. Seizures
  5. Metabolic defects
  6. Cardiac defects
  7. Munchausen syndrome by proxy (MSP)
- Physical Findings
  1. Often normal at time of examination
  2. OSAS—mouth breathing; upper airway narrowed/obstructed from inflammation or structural defects; allergic stigmata; congestive heart failure; obese, normal weight, or failure to thrive; adenotonsillar hypertrophy
  3. Lungs usually clear
  4. May have physical findings of cardiac insufficiency or fluid overload with longstanding, severe obstruction
- Diagnostic Tests/Findings
  1. Complete history—emphasize circumstances surrounding the event (ALTE), medical and family history
  2. Complete physical examination with detailed neuro-developmental assessment
  3. Based on history, examination, and age of child
  4. Arterial blood gas—indicate severity of event and current stability
  5. Pulse oximetry—likely normal, may show hypoxemia
  6. Electroencephalogram—seizure disorder
  7. Viral respiratory panel—RSV infection
  8. Complete blood count, blood culture—indicative of sepsis, polycythemia (chronic hypoxemia), anemia
  9. Electrolytes—elevated bicarbonate level suggests compensation for hypoventilation
  10. Fluid balance profile—metabolic status, elevated bicarbonate (chronic respiratory insufficiency)
  11. Lumbar puncture—meningitis
  12. Electrocardiogram—cardiac arrhythmias
  13. Radiographs—chest to evaluate structure and anatomy, heart size; lateral neck to evaluate size of adenoids

  14. Sleep study (overnight polysomnography)—gold standard to identify significant apneas and differentiate type of apneas
- Management/Treatment: Based on history and physical findings
  1. Institute treatment and referrals based on diagnostic findings, history, and physical examination
  2. If cause unclear, decision is more complex but should include:
     a. Frequent follow-up visits with serial measurements of:
        (1) Height, weight, and head circumference
        (2) Developmental assessment
        (3) Emotional support and parental counseling
  3. ALTE—admit to hospital for close observation and monitoring
  4. Infants—apnea monitor recommendations with a specific clinical indication
     a. Use monitor with an event recorder
     b. Monitor only detects episodes of central apnea
     c. Monitoring does not prevent all deaths
     d. Monitoring is stressful (false alarms, child safety, travel cumbersome, and financial burden)
     e. Requires close supervision and plan for monitor termination
     f. CPR instruction for family and other caregivers
  5. OSAS
     a. Referrals as indicated for adenotonsillectomy (first-line treatment), weight loss, or continuous positive airway pressure device with sleep
     b. Repeat sleep study after adenotonsillectomy (may have persistent obstruction despite resolution of snoring)

❏ TUBERCULOSIS (TB)

- Definition: A chronic and serious granulomatous infection that may cause pulmonary, extrapulmonary, or disseminated disease
- Etiology/Incidence
  1. Caused by *Mycobacterium tuberculosis*
  2. Primary mode of transmission is inhalation of aerosol droplets through person-to-person contact; almost all cases of pediatric TB are acquired through close and prolonged contact with an untreated infected adolescent or adult
  3. Tuberculosis is classified as primary infection or tuberculosis disease
     a. Latent tuberculosis infection (LTBI)—positive tuberculin skin test without clinical or radiographic evidence of disease; children with LTBI serve as a major reservoir and have an increased risk of progression to TB disease than other groups
     b. Tuberculosis disease—when child has signs or symptoms of disease or there is radiographic evidence of disease; incubation period of 3–10 weeks

after exposure; clinical manifestations occur 1 to 6 months after infection

    (1) Pulmonary—the lung is the primary site of infection; involves hilar, subcarinal, or paratracheal adenopathy, usually with chest radiographic findings of patchy infiltrates; chest radiographic evidence may be so subtle that chest CT is needed for diagnosis

    (2) Extrapulmonary—miliary tuberculosis may involve any organ of the body, most frequently seen in lymph nodes and central nervous system, and can include meningitis

4. TB rates for all ages in United States are highest in urban, low-income areas, and in nonwhite and foreign-born groups

5. Increased TB risk associated with:

  a. Contacts of persons with confirmed or suspected infectious TB

  b. Foreign-born persons from high-risk countries in Asia, Africa, China, Haiti, and Eastern Europe; children who travel to these countries; significant contact with persons from these countries

  c. Homeless, migrant, institutionalized, or prison populations

  d. Other—immunodeficiency (HIV) or immunosuppression, IV drug use, diabetes, chronic renal failure, malnourished

- Signs and Symptoms

1. Typically insidious in onset—often attributed to viral URI

2. Cough, wheezing, dyspnea

3. Abdominal pain, diarrhea, poor weight gain or weight loss, anorexia, or poor suck

4. Fever, lethargy, night sweats, chills

5. May present with clinical symptoms of meningitis

6. Late clinical presentations include symptoms of TB of middle ear and mastoid, bones, joints, skin, and kidneys

7. Drug-resistant TB is clinically indistinguishable from drug-susceptible disease

- Differential Diagnosis

1. Histoplasmosis

2. Atypical mycobacteria

3. Pneumonia

4. Lung abscess

5. Foreign body aspiration

6. Sarcoidosis

7. Neoplasm

8. Crohn's disease

9. Meningitis

- Physical Findings

1. Usually asymptomatic—even with abnormal chest x-ray (CXR)

2. Dry, hacking, or brassy, paroxysmal cough

3. Localized wheezing, crackles, rales

4. Lymphadenopathy—cervical or axillary

5. Poor weight gain, possibly growth delay

6. Low-grade fever, night sweats, chills

7. Splenomegaly, hepatomegaly

- Diagnostic Tests/Findings

1. Tuberculin skin test (TST)—Mantoux test recommended; multiple-puncture test lacks adequate specificity and sensitivity

  a. All children should have a routine assessment of their risk of exposure to TB; risk assessment should be done every 6 months until 2 years old; after 2 years, perform annual risk assessment; skin-test all children with increased risk

  b. Skin-test immediately any child identified as a contact of a person with confirmed or suspected infectious TB, any child with clinical or radiographic findings suggestive of TB, any child emigrating from an endemic area including international adoptees, those traveling in endemic areas or having significant contact with persons from endemic areas

  c. Skin-test annually any children with HIV, incarcerated adolescents, children with increased risk of progression of LTBI to tuberculosis disease

  d. Skin-test every 2 to 3 years any child exposed to high-risk persons (refer to Etiology/Incidence)

  e. Skin-test before initiation of immunosuppressive therapy

  f. Culture from gastric aspirates, sputum, bronchial washings, and other body fluids or tissue can establish the diagnosis

  g. Some new identification methods, including nucleic acid amplification tests (NAATs) from the respiratory tract, are available

  h. A positive TST—induration of 15 mm or greater is considered positive in any population; reactions of ≥5 to 14 mm may be considered positive in certain high-risk groups; cannot distinguish between infection, current disease, and past disease

2. Chest radiograph findings vary from normal to lobar or segmental parenchymal lesion, or collapsed consolidation, lymphadenopathy, pleural effusion, or miliary disease (characterized by snowflake appearance)

3. Recent availability of interferon-gamma release assays (IGRAs) that test for the presence of *M. tuberculosis* have become available in the United States in the form of QuantiFERON-TB Gold; IGRA testing is more specific than TST

  a. Recommendation for IGRAs—should generally not replace TST, but act as a complement to TST to improve sensitivity and specificity of diagnosis of TB infection

  b. Positive result from an IGRA indicates possible *M. tuberculosis* infection

  c. Negative result—not necessarily absence of infection

- Management/Treatment
  1. Diagnosing a child with TB infection or disease represents recent transmission of TB in the community; every effort should be made to identify and treat the source case and others infected by the source case; all cases should be reported to local health department; epidemiological investigation, isolation, compliance with therapy, and evaluation of the resolution of disease are crucial in controlling spread of disease; prescribing provider and public health authorities are responsible for treatment completion
  2. Referral to appropriate specialist
  3. Guidelines for chemotherapy vary widely depending on the sensitivity of the organism, the condition of the patient, and the location of disease; refer to most recent edition of American Academy of Pediatrics (AAP) *Red Book* for a complete list of drug dosages and side effects as well as therapeutic regimens; commonly used medications are isoniazid, ethambutol, rifampin, pyrazinamide
  4. For LTBI, 9 months of treatment with isoniazid, once a day, is regimen of choice; prolonged therapy for immunocompromised conditions
  5. For newborns exposed to household contact infected with TB, recommendations vary based on categorization of infection of household contact; refer to most recent edition of AAP *Red Book*
  6. Directly observed therapy and patient-centered case management are recommended for treatment of people with tuberculosis disease; management plan should be tailored to promote adherence to the drug regimen
  7. Children younger than 10 years with primary pulmonary disease are usually not contagious; older children and adults suspected of having TB require TB isolation until proved noncontagious
  8. Bacillus Calmette-Guérin (BCG) vaccine—live vaccine from attenuated strains of *Mycobacterium bovis*; recommended only in limited and select circumstances in United States; recommended internationally by World Health Organization for administration at birth to help prevent disseminated and other life-threatening diseases caused by *Mycobacterium tuberculosis*; indications, adverse reactions, contraindications, and interpretations of Mantoux skin tests in persons who have received BCG described in AAP *Red Book*
  9. Chest radiographs after 2 months of therapy to evaluate medication response

☐ QUESTIONS

Select the best answer.

1. A 4-week-old presents to your office in mid-January with a 1-week history of nasal congestion and occasional cough. On the evening prior to this visit, the infant developed a temperature of 102°F, refused to breastfeed, and had paroxysmal coughing and noisy, labored breathing. On exam, you note an ill-appearing infant who is lethargic with tachypnea, wheezing, and intercostal retractions. The infant does not attend day care but has a 3-year-old sibling who is in day care and who recently had a "cold." Considering the clinical presentation, what is the most likely cause of the infant's illness?
   a. *Mycoplasma* pneumonia
   b. RSV bronchiolitis
   c. Aspiration pneumonia
   d. Streptococcal infection of the pharynx

2. In the scenario of an infant with RSV bronchiolitis, which of the following would be the treatment of choice?
   a. Antihistamine, decongestant, and cough suppressant
   b. Oral antibiotics and follow-up chest radiograph in 2 weeks
   c. Bronchoscopy with lavage, chest physiotherapy, and respiratory isolation
   d. Fluids and nutritional support and close monitoring

3. Of the following children, which one should not have tuberculin skin testing?
   a. A 14-year-old whose uncle was recently granted parole after 5 years in prison and who is currently living with the child's family
   b. A 2-year-old who was infected with RSV 3 months ago and who is currently asymptomatic
   c. A 3-month-old whose family emigrated from Cambodia to the United States 1 month ago
   d. An 18-month-old whose mother is infected with HIV

4. Which of the following clinical presentations least warrants sweat chloride testing?
   a. 10-year-old female sibling of a patient newly diagnosed with cystic fibrosis; sibling is without pulmonary problems and growth parameters are at 50% for age
   b. 2-year-old male with recurrent pneumonia and growth parameters at 5% for age
   c. 4-year-old female with nocturnal cough, which resolves after treatment with bronchodilators and short-term steroids; growth parameters at 10% for age
   d. 7-year-old female with nasal polyps, mildly hyperexpanded lungs; growth parameters at 25% for age

5. What is the most common agent for nonviral pneumonia from school age to young adulthood?
   a. *Mycoplasma pneumoniae*
   b. *Staphylococcus aureus*
   c. *Ureaplasma urealyticum*
   d. *Haemophilus influenzae*

6. Which one of the following diagnoses would not be part of the differential for recurrent lobar pneumonia in a 2-year-old?
   a. Cystic fibrosis
   b. Foreign body aspiration
   c. Atelectasis
   d. Bronchitis

7. The most common clinical presentation of pneumonia includes:
   a. Cough, fever, tachypnea, and abdominal pain
   b. Hemoptysis, putrid breath, and weight loss
   c. Sudden chest pain, cyanosis
   d. Retractions, stridor

8. The classic radiographic finding in croup is:
   a. Hyperinflation
   b. Perihilar lymphadenopathy
   c. Thumb sign
   d. Steeple sign

9. Unilateral wheezing is a finding suggestive of:
   a. Croup
   b. Asthma
   c. Foreign body aspiration
   d. Cystic fibrosis

10. An ex-preemie with bronchopulmonary dysplasia has been discharged to home from the NICU. A potential problem area that requires close monitoring is:
    a. Insufficient caloric intake
    b. Atrophy of abdominal muscles due to abdominal breathing patterns
    c. Lack of tactile stimuli due to restrictions on parental handling
    d. The predisposition to development of nasal polyps

11. A 10-day-old is brought to the clinic because the parent is concerned about his breathing. The parents report that while the baby is feeding, he often stops breathing for periods of about 10 seconds. History reveals that the baby eats well, has never appeared pale or cyanotic, and has never become limp during any of these episodes. Your management plan is based on which of the following?
    a. This is a normal breathing pattern for an infant.
    b. These episodes likely indicate aspiration of formula and should be evaluated.
    c. A variety of pathologic processes are associated with the episodes described.
    d. Neurologic deficits in infants are often manifested by such episodes.

12. A 4-year-old with a history of asthma presents with wheezing and cough that has been persistent over the past day. Physical examination reveals a respiratory rate of 14 breaths per minute. Respirations are shallow without wheezing, and there are no retractions. What is the most likely reason that wheezes are not auscultated?
    a. The child has faked an asthma attack.
    b. The parent needs education regarding the identification of wheezing.

   c. The child's condition has resolved.
   d. Wheezing is not being heard because the breathing is shallow.

13. What is the appropriate management of a child with asthma who presents with acute wheezing and/or coughing?
    a. Administer an inhaled corticosteroid.
    b. Administer a short-acting beta agonist.
    c. Administer an expectorant.
    d. Administer an oral corticosteroid.

14. A 5-month-old is brought to the clinic because he has been coughing and has had clear rhinorrhea for the last 2 days. His mother tells you that he has never been sick before. Family history is positive for allergies, and you hear generalized wheezing. You may conclude that:
    a. The infant has familial asthma.
    b. The infant has asthma exacerbated by a viral infection.
    c. The infant should be referred for allergy testing.
    d. Asthma should not be diagnosed at this stage.

15. In mild to moderate attacks of acute asthma, albuterol should be given every 4–6 hours prn and routine medications should be:
    a. Continued as usual
    b. Discontinued until albuterol treatments are deemed unnecessary
    c. Given only if the albuterol is ineffective
    d. Decreased to the minimum recommended dose

16. A 4-year-old stays with her great aunt during the day while her mother works. The child's mother has brought her to the clinic because the great aunt has just been diagnosed with TB. The child's Mantoux skin test is positive, but there is no clinical or radiographic evidence of disease. Appropriate management includes:
    a. Reassuring the mother that no treatment is needed
    b. Administering another skin test in 3 months
    c. Oral penicillin therapy
    d. Oral preventive isoniazid therapy

17. In addition to airway hyperresponsiveness and reversible airway obstruction, asthma is a chronic lung disease characterized by:
    a. Bronchiectasis
    b. Inflammation
    c. Pleural effusion
    d. Pulmonary edema

18. The most common trigger for an acute asthma episode in the very young child is:
    a. Respiratory infections
    b. Exercise
    c. Tobacco smoke
    d. Outdoor allergens

19. A child has mild persistent asthma. Appropriate daily medication should include:
    a. An inhaled low-dose corticosteroid
    b. Short-acting beta-2 agonists

c. An oral systemic corticosteroid

d. A cough suppressant

20. The most typical chest radiographic finding consistent with the diagnosis of asthma is:
    a. Normal chest film
    b. Diffuse airway edema
    c. Right upper lobe infiltrate
    d. Hyperinflation

21. An 8-year-old with moderate persistent asthma presents with a daily cough. At her clinic visit, she reports that three times a day she uses a short-acting inhaled beta-2 agonist and twice daily she uses an inhaled corticosteroid, cromolyn sodium. Your management plan should be altered to include:
    a. Broad-spectrum antibiotics and recheck in 2 weeks
    b. Addition of oral systemic corticosteroids for 5 days
    c. Increased use of the short-acting beta agonist, and replace cromolyn sodium with inhaled corticosteroids
    d. Addition of an inhaled anticholinergic

22. A 10-year-old has recently been diagnosed with mild intermittent asthma. Which of the following is not a routine part of his clinic management?
    a. Spirometry evaluation
    b. Metered-dose inhaler technique demonstration
    c. Environmental triggers and control methods review
    d. School excuse to not participate in physical education activities

23. The most significant major contributor or contributors to asthma morbidity and mortality is/are:
    a. Underdiagnosis and inappropriate treatment
    b. An increase in indoor allergens
    c. Overuse of anti-inflammatory medications
    d. An increase in air pollution

24. The primary treatment for bronchopulmonary dysplasia is:
    a. Pancreatic enzymes
    b. Surgical repair
    c. Adequate oxygenation
    d. Chest physiotherapy

25. Which of the following is the greatest risk factor in the development of bronchopulmonary dysplasia?
    a. Birth weight
    b. Maternal age
    c. Maternal education level
    d. Respiratory infections

26. Which of the following is not characteristic of an apparent life-threatening event (ALTE)?
    a. Change in muscle tone
    b. Fever
    c. Change in skin color
    d. Apnea

27. Following an ALTE, management and treatment are based on findings from:
    a. A thorough history and physical exam
    b. An electroencephalogram

c. A chest radiograph

d. A sleep study

28. The predominant characteristic of a young infant with bronchopulmonary dysplasia is:
    a. Prolonged fevers
    b. Hypoxemia on room air
    c. Recurrent pneumonias
    d. Chronic hypoinflation

☐ ANSWERS AND RATIONALES

1. B: December through March is a typical season for respiratory syncytial virus (RSV), and it is commonly seen in infants 0–12 months of age. This presentation of fever, tachypnea, and wheezing with retractions is classic.

2. D: Bronchiolitis is treated on an outpatient basis unless severe with fluids and observation. Bronchodilators, epinephrine, antibiotics, and steroids are not usually recommended.

3. B: Respiratory syncytial virus (RSV) is not a risk factor for tuberculosis (TB). The other children all have increased risk (exposure to prison population or HIV-affected person or recent immigration), so should be tested.

4. C: The 4-year-old female child with the nocturnal cough appears to have reactive airway disease. The others should be evaluated for cystic fibrosis (CF) with sweat chloride testing because of their symptoms or presentation, which points to possible CF, including a sibling with CF. CF is an inherited condition that is associated with poor growth, frequent respiratory infection, and nasal polyps.

5. A: *M. pneumoniae* is a common pathogen in symptomatic pneumonia for this age group. *H. flu* is a much less common pathogen now that infants are vaccinated with the HIB vaccine. *Ureaplasma* is seen in neonates and young infants with pneumonia. *S. aureus* is also seen in children <4 years old with pneumonia.

6. D: Bronchitis is a nonspecific diagnosis and is usually a symptom of another respiratory condition. The other conditions should be considered in this 2-year-old with recurrent pneumonia.

7. A: Cough, fever, tachypnea, and abdominal pain are typical signs of pneumonia. Retractions and stridor are associated with croup.

8. D: The classic tapering of the subglottic trachea, or steeple sign, is commonly seen in the chest x-ray of a child with croup.

9. C: Unilateral findings in the chest suggest foreign body aspiration because the foreign body lodges in the lower airway on the right or left side. Cystic fibrosis (CF), asthma, and croup all present with bilateral respiratory findings such as wheezing, crackles, or rales.

10. A: The pathophysiology of bronchopulmonary dysplasia (BPD) is similar to chronic obstructive lung disease (COLD). Diuretic use and limitation of fluids are

often part of the management plan. Limitation of fluids may make it difficult to provide adequate caloric intake.

11. A: Brief apnea episodes (less than 15 to 20 seconds) are normal in infants and are most frequent in preterm infants. These normal episodes are not associated with pallor, gagging, cyanosis, or hypotonia.

12. D: A respiratory rate of 14 breaths per minute is slow for a 4-year-old child and is an indicator that there is muscle fatigue or that the child is in extreme respiratory distress. When the wheezing child develops muscle fatigue, a wheeze may not be generated, even in the presence of severe obstruction.

13. B: Short-acting beta agonists (SABAs) are used as a rescue medication during an acute asthma exacerbation. An inhaled corticosteroid (ICS) will not stop an acute attack; oral corticosteroids may be added but in addition to SABAs. Cough medicines are not recommended in children.

14. D: Asthma is not diagnosed during a child's first episode of wheezing but after a documented pattern of recurrent wheezing responsive to bronchodilator therapy. Differential diagnoses should include foreign body aspiration, congenital malformation, and bronchiolitis.

15. A: Routine asthma medications should continue even when albuterol is needed. A review of routine medications may indicate a step up in controller medicines.

16. D: Isoniazid therapy is indicated if a child has a positive tuberculosis (TB) skin test and known exposure to TB even if there is no clinical or radiographic evidence of disease. Referral to a pediatric pulmonary specialist and reporting to the health department are also indicated.

17. B: Asthma is a condition caused by inflammation that can contribute to airway hyperresponsiveness, obstruction, and clinical symptoms.

18. A: Although respiratory infections, exercise, tobacco smoke, and outdoor allergens are potential triggers, viral respiratory infections are the most common trigger in the very young child.

19. A: Based on the National Heart, Lung, and Blood Institute (NHLBI) guidelines, a child with mild persistent asthma should be on an inhaled low-dose corticosteroid. Short-acting beta-2 agonists have no role in preventative treatment. Short-term oral corticosteroids may be needed during an exacerbation but should not be used long term. Cough suppressants are not recommended in children.

20. D: Hyperinflation may be seen on chest x-ray because of air trapping. A normal x-ray does not rule out asthma. Diffuse airway edema and right upper lobe (RUL) infiltrate point to other diagnoses.

21. B: The child's symptoms indicate an exacerbation that warrants oral corticosteroids. Without signs of infection, antibiotics are not warranted. Increased use of the short-acting beta agonist (SABA) may have a role

temporarily, but not without the addition of an oral steroid. An inhaled anticholinergic is not indicated.

22. D: The goal of asthma management is to enable children to have normal functioning. If a child is not able to participate in physical education activities, it is an indication that the asthma is not adequately controlled.

23. A: Whereas indoor allergens and air pollution can contribute to asthma morbidity and mortality, underdiagnosis and inappropriate treatment are the most significant contributors. Underuse of inflammatory medications (ICS) is more common than overuse.

24. C: Adequate oxygenation (>92%) can help promote growth and prevent cor pulmonale. In addition, adequate nutrition balanced with fluid restriction is needed.

25. A: Low birth weight is an important risk factor for the development of bronchopulmonary dysplasia (BPD), along with gestational age, gender, respiratory distress syndrome, and patent ductus arteriosus (PDA), among others.

26. B: Fever would indicate an underlying illness. Change in muscle tone, pallor, and apnea are common presenting symptoms of ALTEs.

27. A: A thorough history and exam should guide the rest of the work-up. Additional work-up would depend on the results of a comprehensive history and exam.

28. B: Hypoxemia on room air is the predominant characteristic of an infant with bronchopulmonary dysplasia (BPD), often <92% on room air.

☐ BIBLIOGRAPHY

American Academy of Pediatrics. (2012). *Red book: 2012 report of the committee on infectious diseases* (29th ed.). Elk Grove Village, IL: Author.

American Academy of Pediatrics. (2014). Updated guidance for palivizumab prophylaxis among infants and young children at increased risk of hospitalization for respiratory syncytial virus infection. *Pediatrics, 134*(2), 415–420. doi:10.1542/peds.2014-1665

Davies, J. C., Ebdon, A., & Orchard, C. (2014). Recent advances in the management of cystic fibrosis. *Archives of Diseases in Childhood, 99*(11), 1133–1136. doi:10.1136/archdischild-2013-304400

Engorn, B., & Flerlage, J. (2014). *The Harriet Lane handbook* (20th ed.). Baltimore, MD: Elsevier Mosby.

Fu, L. Y., & Moon, R. Y. (2012). Apparent life-threatening events: An update. *Pediatrics in Review, 33*(8), 361–369. doi:10.1542/pir.33-8-361

Hay, W., Levin, M., Deterding, R., & Abzug, M. (2014). *Current diagnosis and treatment: Pediatrics* (22nd ed.). New York, NY: McGraw-Hill.

Jain, M., & Goss, C. H. (2014). Update in cystic fibrosis. *American Journal of Respiratory and Critical Care Medicine, 189*(10), 1181–1186. doi:10.1164/rccm.201402-0203UP

Jensen, E. A., & Schmidt, B. (2014). Epidemiology of bronchopulmonary dysplasia. *Clinical and Molecular Teratology, 100*(3), 145–157. doi:10.1002/bdra.23235

Marcus, C. L. Brooks, L. J, Draper, K. A., Gozal, D., Halbower, A. C., Jones, J., ... American Academy of Pediatrics. (2012). Diagnosis and management of childhood obstructive sleep apnea. *Pediatrics, 130*(3), 576–584. doi:10.1542/peds.2012-1671

National Heart, Lung, and Blood Institute. (2007). *Expert panel report 3: Guidelines for the diagnosis and management of asthma. National Asthma Education and Prevention Program.* Retrieved from http://www.nhlbi.nih.gov/health-pro/guidelines/current/asthma-guidelines/full-report.htm

O'Sullivan, B. P., & Freedman, S. D. (2009). Cystic fibrosis. *Lancet, 373*(9678), 1891–1904.

Perez-Velez, C. M. (2012). Pediatric tuberculosis: New guidelines and recommendations. *Current Opinion in Pediatrics, 24*(3), 319–328. doi:10.1097/MOP.0b013e32835357c3

Petrocheilou, A., Tanou, K., Kalampouka, E., Malakasioti, G., Giannios, C., & Kaditis, A. G. (2014). Viral croup: Diagnosis and a treatment algorithm. *Pediatric Pulmonology, 49*(5), 421–429. doi:10.1002/ppul.22993

Sidell, D. R., Kim, I. A., Coker, T. R., Moreno, C., & Shapiro, N. L. (2013). Food choking hazards in children. *International Journal of Pediatric Otorhinolaryngology, 77*(12), 1940–1946. doi:0.1016/j.ijporl.2013.09.005

Taussig, L. M., & Landau, L. I. (Eds.). (2008). *Pediatric emergency medicine* (2nd ed.). Philadelphia, PA: Mosby Elsevier.

Weiss, M., & Owens, J. (2014). Recognizing pediatric sleep apnea. *Nurse Practitioner, 39*(8), 43–48. doi:10.1097/01.NPR.0000451859.08918.70

Zitelli, B. J., McIntire, S. C., & Nowalk, A. J. (2012). *Atlas of pediatric physical diagnosis* (6th ed.). Philadelphia, PA: Mosby Elsevier.

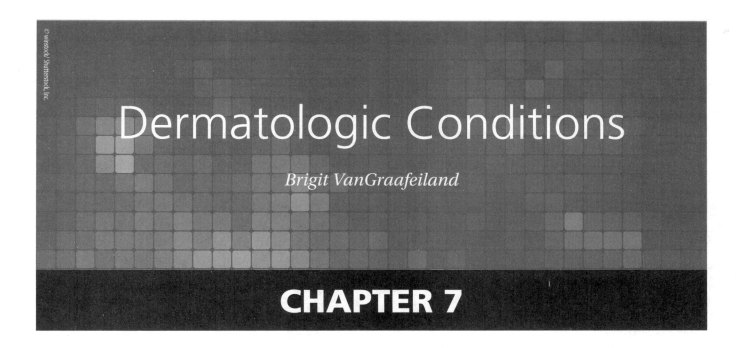

Dermatologic Conditions

Brigit VanGraafeiland

CHAPTER 7

☐ NEWBORN EXANTHEMA

Cutis Marmorata

- Definition: Transient mottling of the neonate's skin with a lacy, bluish appearance
- Etiology/Incidence
  1. Physiologic response of uneven blood flow that results from constriction of small blood vessels while others dilate
  2. Often precipitated by exposure to cold
  3. More common in premature infants
  4. Persistence after neonatal period found in Down syndrome
- Signs and Symptoms: Generalized lacy, reddish-blue appearance to the skin
- Differential Diagnosis
  1. Cutis marmorata telangiectatica congenita
  2. Cyanosis
  3. Erythema toxicum neonatorum
- Physical Findings: Generalized reddish-blue, reticulated pattern to most of body surface
- Diagnostic Tests/Findings: None
  1. 50% of these patients have one or more congenital skin conditions, including glaucoma, hemangiomas, and vascular malformations
- Management/Treatment
  1. Keep neonate at stable temperature
  2. Reduce exposure to cold environment
  3. Do not overdress or keep environment overly warm

Erythema Toxicum Neonatorum

- Definition: Transient, benign, self-limited skin rash with lesions of varied morphology; erythematous macules; wheals, vesicles, and pustules

- Etiology/Incidence:
  1. Unknown cause
  2. Occurs in 50% to 60% of neonates
  3. More common in full-term and postterm neonates
  4. More common in neonates with birth weight >2500 g
  5. Onset usually within first 24 to 48 hours of life, but occasionally present at birth
- Signs and Symptoms
  1. Yellow-white lesions on reddish-pink base; may be blotchy
  2. Extent of rash varies from minimal to most of body surface; palms and soles are usually spared
- Differential Diagnosis
  1. Congenital candidiasis
  2. Incontinentia pigmenti
  3. Miliaria rubra
  4. Sterile transient neonatal pustular melanosis
  5. Urticaria pigmentosa
  6. Bacterial infection
  7. Folliculitis
  8. Herpes simplex
- Physical Findings
  1. Lesions of varied morphology—erythematous macules 2 to 3 cm in diameter appear first, followed by wheals, vesicles, and, rarely, pustules
  2. Lesions usually arise from erythematous base with macular erythema fading within 2 to 3 days
  3. Occurs predominately on the trunk; however, may occur anywhere on body except soles and palms
  4. Number of lesions varies from few to many
  5. Spontaneous resolution in 5 to 7 days
- Diagnostic Tests/Findings: Wright's stained smear of pustules identifies predominance of 90% eosinophils rather than neutrophils, which rules out neonatal pustular melanosis; consider bacterial and fungal cultures

- Management/Treatment
  1. Obtain detailed history of onset, duration, and progression
  2. Describe and monitor lesions in terms of morphology/structure, size, shape, number, color, location, distribution
  3. No treatment necessary
  4. Educate regarding characteristics of condition and expected resolution
  5. Refer to dermatologist for evaluation if condition does not improve

Milia

- Definition: Benign and common condition of small, yellow-white, 1- to 2-mm-sized inclusion cysts filled with cheesy keratinous material on face of newborn
- Etiology/Incidence
  1. Caused by superficial keratinous material accumulated within developing pilosebaceous follicle
  2. Occurs in 50% of newborns
- Signs and Symptoms: Numerous small, yellow-white raised lesions on face of newborn
- Differential Diagnosis
  1. Sebaceous hyperplasia
  2. Calcinosis cutis (especially in Down syndrome infants)
  3. Acne vulgaris
  4. Syringoma
- Physical Findings
  1. Numerous firm, pearly yellow-white, 1- to 2-mm inclusion papular cysts on the cheeks, forehead, and nose; predominately on face; may be found on other body surfaces
  2. Oral counterpart is yellow, papular lesions on hard palate known as Epstein's pearls
  3. Condition resolves spontaneously without treatment within a few weeks as lesions exfoliate
- Diagnostic Tests/Findings: None
- Management/Treatment
  1. Describe and monitor lesions in terms of morphology/structure, size, shape, number, color, location, distribution
  2. No treatment necessary
  3. Educate regarding characteristics of condition and expected resolution

☐ VASCULAR LESIONS

Salmon Patch (Nevus Simplex)

- Definition: Benign, flat, light red to orange vascular birthmark on head and face
- Etiology/Incidence
  1. Caused by overgrowth of blood vessels within dermis skin layer
  2. Seen in approximately 40% to 50% of newborns
  3. More common in girls

- Signs and Symptoms: Flat, light red to orange lesions on face and head of newborn
- Differential Diagnosis
  1. Port-wine stain (nevus flammeus)
  2. Hemangioma
  3. Contact irritation or chronic rubbing
  4. Child maltreatment
- Physical Findings
  1. Single or multiple irregular, light red to orange macular lesions on eyelids, nape of neck, glabella, and/or occiput; vary in size
  2. Lesions gradually fade and disappear spontaneously with time
     a. Eyelid lesions fade first, resolving completely within 3 to 6 months
     b. Nape of neck lesions fade but may persist into adulthood
     c. Other lesions resolve completely by 7 years of age
- Diagnostic Tests/Findings: None
- Management/Treatment
  1. Describe and monitor lesions in terms of morphology/structure, size, shape, number, color, location, distribution
  2. No treatment necessary
  3. Educate regarding characteristics of condition and expected resolution

Port-Wine Stain (Previously Termed Nevus Flammeus)

- Definition: Benign, permanent, flat, dark red to purple vascular lesion, predominantly on head and face
- Etiology/Incidence
  1. Caused by proliferation of dilated capillaries in the dermis
  2. Lesions may be associated with other conditions
     a. Lesions covering entire half of face or bilateral; may be associated with Sturge-Weber syndrome
     b. Lesions on extremities may be associated with hypertrophy of soft tissue and bone
     c. Lesions on the back, especially crossing the midline, may be associated with defects in the spinal cord and vertebrae
  3. Seen in approximately 0.4% of newborns
- Differential Diagnosis
  1. Nevus simplex
  2. Hemangioma
  3. Child maltreatment
- Physical Findings
  1. Irregular dark red or purple macular lesions occurring on any body surface, predominantly on face and head
  2. Size varies from less than 1 cm to more than 20 cm
  3. May initially appear pink in infancy and gradually become darker
  4. Lesion never fades and becomes thickened and raised in adulthood

- Diagnostic Tests/Findings: If there is uncertainty about the diagnosis, pediatric ophthalmology examination and ultrasonography, 5 months old
- Management/Treatment
  1. Describe and monitor lesions in terms of morphology/structure, size, shape, number, color, location, distribution
  2. Refer for dermatologist evaluation to rule out Sturge-Weber syndrome and other associated conditions
  3. Treatment of choice: b, with a and c as adjuncts
     a. Refer for dermatologist evaluation for consideration of pulsed dye laser treatment, which is recommended to start as early as possible in infancy, definitely before 1 year of age
     b. May be camouflaged later in childhood with water-resistant cosmetics
     c. Counseling as needed for related psychological concerns
  4. Educate regarding characteristics of condition

Capillary Hemangioma (Strawberry Nevus)

- Definition: Bright red or blue-red nodular tumors of varying sizes and shape with a rubbery and rough surface predominately on head and face
- Etiology/Incidence
  1. Caused by proliferation of capillary endothelial cells, which may be superficial or deep
  2. Seen in approximately 2.5% of newborns, although may not be present at birth
  3. More common in girls
  4. More common in light-skinned and premature infants
- Signs and Symptoms: Red or blue-red lesions on skin surface
- Differential Diagnosis
  1. Venous malformation
  2. Cystic hygroma
  3. Neonatal hemangiomatosis
  4. Blue rubber bleb nevus syndrome
- Physical Findings
  1. Often is not present at birth; however, area of eventual lesion is blanched or slightly colored
  2. Size varies from less than 1 cm to over 4 cm
  3. Pattern of growth and resolution
     a. Grows quickly within 2 to 4 weeks to a red or blue-red, protuberant, rubbery nodule or plaque
     b. Most growth the first 6 months
     c. Gradual reduction in proliferation usually begins between 9 and 12 months with gray areas developing, followed by flattening from center to periphery
     d. A flat or involuted area of hyperpigmentation often remains following dissolution of the lesion
  4. Complications may occur resulting from location and depth of lesion (size does not determine risk of complication)

  a. Lesions involving eye area and orbit may cause visual disturbances
  b. Lesions of head and neck may be associated with subglottic hemangiomas causing airway obstruction
  c. Lesions may cause cardiovascular disturbances through compression
  d. Lesions may ulcerate as they involute
  5. Complication of thrombocytopenia may occur resulting from trapped platelets within lesion
  6. Lesions resolve spontaneously and completely disappear with age
     a. 50% are cleared by 5 years of age
     b. 90% are cleared by 10 years of age
     c. Remainder clear during adolescence
- Diagnostic Tests/Findings: None
- Management/Treatment
  1. Describe and monitor lesions in terms of morphology/structure, size, shape, number, color, location, distribution
  2. Refer for dermatologist evaluation to rule out involvement with vital organs
  3. Treatment depends on location and complications; if ulcerates, pulsed dye laser may be needed; oral prednisone was the treatment of choice until recently, with oral propranolol protocols being established to replace oral steroids; surgical intervention is rarely indicated
  4. Educate regarding characteristics of condition and expected resolution

□ MELANOCYTE CELL AND PIGMENTATION CONDITIONS

Café au Lait Spots

- Definition: Light to medium brown pigmented macular lesions of varying sizes and shapes found anywhere on the body; the color of coffee with milk, from which the name is derived
- Etiology/Incidence
  1. Caused by increased pigmentation activity of melanocyte cells
  2. Overall incidence is higher in dark-skinned populations than in light-skinned
  3. Lesions larger than 1.5 cm occur in 10% of light-skinned population and in 20% of darker-skinned populations
  4. Lesions are usually present at birth; however, may develop at any age
  5. Lesions are present throughout life; however, color intensity may fade
  6. Six or more lesions and/or lesions larger than 1.5 cm in diameter may be associated with neurofibromatosis or Albright syndrome
- Signs and Symptoms: Flat, light brown lesions on skin; may be deeper in color in dark-skinned populations
- Differential Diagnosis: None

- Physical Findings
  1. Macular light to medium brown lesions on any skin surface
  2. Size varies from less than 0.5 cm to 20 cm in diameter
  3. May be single or multiple
  4. Vary in shape, frequently oval
  5. Six or more lesions and/or lesions larger than 1.5 cm may be associated with neurofibromatosis or Albright syndrome
- Diagnostic Tests/Findings: None
- Management/Treatment
  1. Describe and monitor lesions in terms of morphology/structure, size, shape, number, color, location, distribution
  2. If suspected that lesions may be associated with any other condition, refer to dermatologist for further evaluation
  3. No treatment necessary
  4. Educate regarding characteristics of condition

Mongolian Spots

- Definition: Blue-black and gray macular lesions of irregular shape and varying sizes; usually on sacrococcygeal region, buttocks, and lumbar areas but may also involve extremities, upper back, and shoulders
- Etiology/Incidence
  1. Lesions consist of migrating spindle-shaped pigmented/melanocyte cells deep within dermis layer
  2. Occurs in 90% of darker-skinned infants; 5% of light-skinned infants
- Signs and Symptoms: Blue-black or gray lesions of irregular shape and varying size on lower aspect of back
- Differential Diagnosis: Child maltreatment
- Physical Findings
  1. Blue-black or gray macular lesions of irregular shapes
  2. Vary in size from <2 cm to >10 cm
  3. Located on dorsal body surface, predominately on sacrococcygeal area of buttocks and lumbar areas, but also on upper back, shoulders, and extremities
  4. Lesions not seen on palms or soles
  5. Lesions resolve spontaneously without treatment
     a. Most fade completely during childhood and adolescence
     b. Some may still be evident in adulthood
- Diagnostic Tests/Findings: None
- Management/Treatment
  1. Describe and monitor lesions in terms of morphology/structure, size, shape, number, color, location, and distribution
  2. No treatment necessary
  3. Educate regarding characteristics of condition and expected resolution

Malignant Melanoma

- Definition: Lethal form of skin cancer involving melanocyte cells; may occur on any skin surface

- Etiology/Incidence
  1. Caused by abnormal growth within melanocyte cells
  2. Severe sunburn or excessive exposure to the sun before the age of 10 years predisposes developing melanoma later in childhood or in adult life
     a. Sun-damaged skin cells may be dormant for years
     b. Melanocyte cells provide mechanism to activate malignant process
  3. Melanoma cells spread through the lymphatic system and invade other skin surfaces and organs
     a. 90% survival rate with localized condition
     b. 20% survival with metastasis
  4. Increasing incidence in general population
  5. In the United States it is more common in females from birth to 40 years of age and light-skinned individuals
  6. Increased incidence with family history
  7. More lethal and faster growing than basal cell or squamous cell cancers
- Signs and Symptoms
  1. Localized change in skin color or increase in size of existing nevus
  2. May have itching with bleeding and tenderness
- Differential Diagnosis: Other skin cancers
- Physical Findings
  1. Asymmetrical lesion with irregular, ragged, and blurred borders
  2. Uneven color with shades of blue, black, brown, tan, and red; all colors may exist within same lesion
  3. More common on arms and lower legs of females and on chest of males
  4. Single or multiple lesions (clusters) may be found in distant areas with metastasis
  5. Bleeding and ulceration—usually late signs
- Diagnostic Tests/Findings: Skin biopsy confirms diagnosis
- Management/Treatment
  1. Obtain detailed history of onset, duration, and progression
  2. Refer to dermatologist for evaluation immediately if suspected; surgical excision is indicated
  3. Educate regarding characteristics of condition, treatment, and expected prognosis
  4. Educate regarding specific preventive measures
     a. Protect skin from exposure to sunlight
        (1) Cover-up clothing and hats
        (2) Sunglasses
        (3) Water-resistant sunblocks that protect against UVB and UVA ultraviolet light with sun protection factor (SPF) of 30
     b. Avoid exposure to sunlight especially from 10 a.m. to 3 p.m.
     c. Avoid sun lamps and tanning booths
     d. Teach the ABCDEs of pigmented lesions: asymmetry, borders, color, diameter, and evolution of lesions, along with checking for the "ugly duckling" lesion that doesn't resemble any other pigmented skin lesions; recommend monthly mole checks at home for high-risk individuals

Albinism

- Definition: Inherited congenital defect of total or partial lack of pigmentation in which affected body parts lack normal color; condition is present at birth; there are two main types:
  1. Total form (type 1)—affects entire skin, hair, and retina
  2. Partial or localized forms (type 2)—confined to specific area of skin (2), hair (forelock of hair) (3), or eyes (pupil or retina) (4)
- Etiology/Incidence
  1. Metabolic process within melanocyte cells required for melanin production is impaired—melanin, giving skin its distinctive color, is not secreted
  2. Incidence equal between males and females with type 2 more common in African American population and type 1 only confirmed in African Americans
- Signs and Symptoms
  1. Milky-white skin (localized or generalized)
  2. Light sensitivity
- Differential Diagnosis
  1. Homocystinuria
  2. Phenylketonuria
- Physical Findings
  1. Skin is milky-white, hair is white or yellow, iris is usually blue, pupil usually appears red and becomes darker in adulthood
  2. Skin is sensitive to light and sunburns easily
  3. Other symptoms not involving skin include decreased visual acuity, photosensitivity
- Diagnostic Tests/Findings: None
- Management/Treatment
  1. Describe skin and areas of hypopigmentation and monitor routinely for any skin changes that may occur, including development of lesions
  2. Educate regarding need to protect from exposure to sunlight
     a. Cover-up clothing and hats
     b. Sunglasses
     c. Water-resistant sunblocks that protect against UVB and UVA ultraviolet light with SPF 30
  3. Educate regarding characteristics and prognosis of condition
  4. Counsel as indicated regarding:
     a. Related psychological effects
     b. Genetic counseling related to potential inheritance factors
  5. Refer to dermatologist for evaluation if skin changes occur
  6. Refer to ophthalmologist for evaluation of vision and eye involvement

Vitiligo

- Definition: Acquired autoimmune condition involving patches of depigmentation on skin surfaces and in mouth and genitalia

  1. Segmented form—unilateral involving two dermatones
  2. Generalized form—involves more than two dermatones, often has bilateral distribution
- Etiology/Incidence
  1. Unknown cause
     a. Affected areas of hypopigmentation have loss or destruction of melanocyte cells
     b. May be associated with autoimmune conditions—diabetes mellitus, Addison's disease, or thyroiditis
  2. Occurs in approximately 4% of all ethnic populations
  3. Onset is usually before 20 years of age
- Signs and Symptoms: Milky-white patches on skin
- Differential Diagnosis
  1. Postinflammatory hypopigmentation
  2. Pityriasis alba
  3. Idiopathic guttate hypomelanosis
  4. Pityriasis versicolor
  5. Nevus anemicus
- Physical Findings
  1. Milky-white macular patches of depigmentation with sharply demarcated borders occur in unilateral or bilateral pattern on skin of normal texture
  2. Shape varies from round, oval to irregular
  3. Size varies from less than 2 cm to well over 20 cm
  4. Varies in number from one to many
  5. Condition is often permanent without repigmentation
- Diagnostic Tests/Findings: None
- Management/Treatment
  1. Obtain detailed history of onset, duration, severity, progression, and possible precipitating factors
  2. Describe skin and areas of depigmentation and monitor for any skin changes that may occur, including development of lesions
  3. Protect skin from exposure to sunlight especially from 10 a.m. to 3 p.m.
     a. Use cover-up clothing, hats, and sunglasses
     b. Apply water-resistant sunblocks that protect against UVB and UVA ultraviolet light with SPF >30
  4. Refer for dermatologist evaluation and treatment to stimulate repigmentation
     a. Topical steroid applications and controlled ultraviolet light exposure
     b. Repigmentation efforts have varying degrees of success especially for involved areas on extremities
     c. Excimer laser FDA approved for treatment of vitiligo
  5. Educate regarding characteristics and expected prognoses
  6. Recommend camouflage with water-resistant cosmetics for adolescents
  7. Counsel regarding:
     a. Related psychological impact of condition
     b. Serious need for protection to reduce risk for skin cancer and sunburn
  8. Refer for dermatologist evaluation if complications develop

☐ PITYRIASIS ALBA

- Definition: Acquired condition of hypopigmented, finely scaled macular lesions of varying sizes and shapes with indistinct borders occurring predominately on cheeks
- Etiology/Incidence
  1. Unknown cause
  2. May be associated with overdrying of skin causing inflammation and hypopigmentation
  3. Occurs most often in children ages 3 to 12 years
  4. More apparent in dark-skinned populations
- Signs and Symptoms
  1. Finely scaled white patches most commonly seen on cheeks
  2. May be pruritic
  3. May appear mildly erythematous
- Differential Diagnosis
  1. Psoriasis
  2. Tinea corporis
  3. Vitiligo
- Physical Findings
  1. Scaly hypopigmented lesions of varying sizes or shapes with nondistinct borders occurring predominately on cheeks, less commonly on other skin surfaces
  2. Some lesions may be slightly erythematous
  3. Number of lesions varies from one to many
  4. Exposure to sunlight may exacerbate lesions, making them more pronounced
  5. Repigmentation occurs as condition resolves spontaneously in 3 to 4 months
- Diagnostic Tests/Findings: Potassium hydroxide (KOH) preparation to rule out tinea corporis
- Management/Treatment
  1. Obtain detailed history of onset, duration, severity, and progression of symptoms and possible precipitating factors
  2. Describe and monitor lesions in terms of morphology/structure, size, shape, number, color, location, distribution
  3. Educate child and parents regarding need to protect skin from exposure to sunlight, especially from 10 a.m. to 3 p.m.
     a. Use cover-up clothing, hats, and sunglasses
     b. Apply water-resistant sunblocks that protect against UVB and UVA ultraviolet light with SPF >30
  4. Use bland moisturizer to reduce overdrying
  5. Educate regarding characteristics and expected prognoses
  6. Recommend camouflage with water-resistant cosmetics for adolescents
  7. Refer for dermatologist evaluation if condition does not improve

☐ PAPULOSQUAMOUS CONDITIONS

Pityriasis Rosea

- Definition: Acquired common mild inflammatory condition characterized by scaly, hypopigmented, and hyperpigmented lesions predominately on the trunk, upper arms, and upper thighs
- Etiology/Incidence
  1. Unknown cause
  2. Possible viral association
  3. Occurs more often in fall and spring months
  4. Occurs especially in older children of all ethnic groups
- Signs and Symptoms
  1. Scaly pink marks on skin in light-skinned individuals; appears hyperpigmented on darker skin
  2. Periodic pruritus of varying degrees of severity especially at onset
  3. Possible prodrome of malaise and low-grade fever before onset of rash
- Differential Diagnosis
  1. Pityriasis alba
  2. Seborrheic dermatitis
  3. Secondary syphilis
  4. Tinea corporis
  5. Guttate psoriasis
- Physical Findings
  1. Scaly, hyperpigmented pink to salmon to violaceous lesions with progressive pattern
     a. "Herald" patch of 1 cm to 5 cm on trunk or buttocks, usually occurs 5 to 10 days before generalized rash
     b. Round and oval scaly, macular lesions develop over 2-week period on skin lines and in parallel fashion suggestive of a Christmas tree pattern
     c. Individual lesions clear in central to peripheral pattern
  2. On darker-skinned populations, lesions are more predominant on neck, axillary, and inguinal regions
  3. Condition is self-limiting and resolves spontaneously in 3 to 4 months
- Diagnostic Tests/Findings
  1. KOH test to rule out tinea corporis
  2. VDRL (Venereal Disease Research Laboratory test) to rule out secondary syphilis, especially in sexually active individuals
- Management/Treatment
  1. Obtain detailed history of onset, duration, severity, and progression of symptoms and possible precipitating factors
  2. Describe and monitor lesions in terms of morphology/structure, size, shape, number, color, location, distribution
  3. Educate regarding characteristics of condition and prognosis
  4. Use symptomatic treatment for pruritus
     a. Topical calamine lotion on lesions
     b. Oral antipruritic agents for severe pruritus, e.g., diphenhydramine
     c. Cool bath or compresses on lesions
     d. Low-potency steroid creams
  5. Educate regarding medication dosage, signs of irritation, sensitivity
  6. Use controlled and limited sunlight exposure to shorten resolution time

7. Refer for dermatologist evaluation if condition worsens or does not resolve

Psoriasis

- Definition: Acquired chronic, relapsing inflammatory condition characterized by erythematous plaques with silver-gray-white scales
  1. Psoriasis vulgaris—large plaques occurring predominately on elbows and knees
  2. Psoriasis guttate—small patches occurring predominately on trunk, upper arms, and thighs
- Etiology/Incidence
  1. Specific cause is unknown
  2. Associated with overproduction and too rapid migration of epithelial cells to skin surface; cells migrate in 3 to 4 days in comparison to usual 28 days
     a. Psoriasis vulgaris—often associated with constant rubbing, or with trauma to the affected area known as Koebner's response
     b. Psoriasis guttate—often follows streptococcal infection
  3. Occurs in more than 33% of children
  4. Up to 20% of people with psoriasis have psoriatic arthritis
  5. More common in light-skinned than dark-skinned populations
  6. Positive family history in approximately one third of cases strongly suggestive of a genetic connection
- Signs and Symptoms
  1. Silvery, gray-white scaling of skin, mainly on trunk or extremities, especially elbows and knees; less commonly on scalp and face
  2. Bleeding may occur if scales are picked at or removed
  3. Nails may be dystrophic with thickening with pits and ridges
- Differential Diagnosis
  1. Atopic dermatitis
  2. Drug eruptions
  3. Pityriasis rosea
  4. Seborrhea
  5. Secondary syphilis
  6. Tinea corporis
- Physical Findings
  1. Psoriasis vulgaris—large 5- to 10-cm plaques with thick silvery-white scales located on elbows and knees
  2. Psoriasis guttate—small 3- to 10-mm multiple teardrop, round or oval papules and patches that become covered by a silvery-gray-white scale on trunk and proximal extremities
  3. Bleeding occurs when scale is removed
  4. Nail plates may be thicker and show signs of pits, ridges, "oil spots," which are yellow discolorations of the nail plate; onycholysis: not all nail plates are involved
- Diagnostic Tests/Findings
  1. VDRL to rule out secondary syphilis
  2. KOH to rule out fungal infections

- Management/Treatment
  1. Obtain detailed history of onset, duration, severity, and progression of symptoms and possible precipitating factors
  2. Describe and monitor lesions in terms of morphology/structure, size, shape, number, color, location, distribution
  3. Reduce hypertrophy of lesion
     a. Use controlled and limited sunlight exposure
     b. Apply topical steroids, e.g., hydrocortisone, triamcinolone
     c. Apply mineral oil and moisturizers at least BID to decrease drying
  4. Educate regarding medication dosage, signs of irritation, sensitivity
  5. Educate regarding characteristics of condition and prognosis
  6. Refer for dermatologist evaluation if condition does not improve

☐ DERMATITIS CONDITIONS
Atopic Dermatitis

- Definition: Common skin disorder with lesions of varied morphology commonly known as eczema; it is called "the itch that rashes"
  1. Acute form—occurs predominately in infants
  2. Chronic form—occurs predominately in children and adolescents
- Etiology/Incidence
  1. Specific cause is unknown
  2. May be associated with a disorder of immunity in some cases due to elevated levels of IgE; it is primarily a disease with an altered skin barrier function
  3. Positive family history may be predisposing factor in some cases
  4. Occurs in approximately 10% to 15% of children
  5. Up to 50% of affected infants develop asthma and/or other respiratory manifestations, e.g., allergic rhinitis, hay fever, and progress to chronic form
  6. Up to 25% of children and adolescents continue to have symptoms throughout adulthood
- Signs and Symptoms
  1. Skin changes are acute and chronic with xerosis (dry skin)
     a. Infant—erythematous, itchy, easily irritated scaly patches
     b. Older children—more focal pruritic patches in the antecubital and popliteal creases
     c. Chronic skin changes include hyperpigmentation and lichenification
  2. Pruritus for both, worsens with sweating and temperature extremes
- Differential Diagnosis
  1. Contact dermatitis
  2. Psoriasis
  3. Seborrheic dermatitis

4. Scabies
5. Tinea corporis
6. Impetigo or other secondary bacterial infection
- Physical Findings
1. Acute form in infants usually develops between ages 2 weeks and 6 months with 50% of cases resolving by 3 years and remainder progressing to chronic form
   a. Lesions appear as erythematous, scaly patches of skin on face, head, trunk, and extensor surfaces
   b. Lesions of varied morphology, e.g., xerotic, scaly, erythematous papules, sometimes with excoriations; oozing and crusting are present in various locations
2. Chronic form develops with poor skin management and personal and family history of atopy; may continue into adulthood
   a. Skin is hyperpigmented, leathery, and lichenified in the flexor surfaces of the neck, antecubital areas, wrists, popliteal area, ankle, fingers, and toes
   b. Scratch marks on affected areas
3. Other findings include:
   a. Circles under eyes: "allergic shiners"
   b. Facial pallor
   c. Nasal crease on top of nose from frequent rubbing
   d. Dry scalp
   e. Prominent Dennie's creases
4. Pustules may be present as sign of secondary bacterial infection
- Diagnostic Tests/Findings
1. No specific test confirms diagnosis—serum level of IgE may support diagnosis in some cases
2. Skin scraping to rule out scabies
- Management/Treatment
1. Obtain detailed history of onset, duration, severity/ progression of symptoms, and possible precipitating factors
2. Describe and monitor lesions in terms of morphology/structure, size, shape, number, color, location, distribution
3. Treat secondary infections if present
   a. Oral antibiotics, e.g., Bactrim, cefadroxil, cephalexin, clindamycin
   b. Topical antibiotics for localized infection—mupirocin or Altabax (retapamulin); others may lead to sensitivity reactions
4. Reduce and prevent nocturnal pruritus with oral antipruritics, e.g., hydroxyzine, diphenhydramine; nonsedating antihistamines during the day only if comorbid environmental or seasonal allergies suspected
5. Use topical steroids to reduce inflammation, immune response, and pruritus, e.g., hydrocortisone, triamcinolone
6. Rehydrate skin with daily lukewarm baths
   a. Wet compresses applied over bland emollients helpful to manage chronic eczema or during eczema flares
   b. Avoid skin-drying agents such as harsh soaps, perfumes, lotions

   c. Apply cream emollients and lubricants at least BID, e.g., petroleum jelly
7. Educate regarding medication dosage, signs of irritation, sensitivity
8. Use mild soaps for general bathing and hygiene habits
9. Eliminate exposure to all substances and agents that may dry or irritate the skin and exacerbate condition; individually determined
   a. Soaps, perfumes, hand and body lotions, makeup, household cleaning agents, bleach, chlorine, turpentine
   b. Materials and fabrics such as wool, feathers, polyesters, stuffed animals and other fabric toys
   c. If there is a positive family history or correlation with increased skin symptoms, eliminate suspected food products such as cow's milk, eggs, nuts, citrus fruits
   d. If there is a positive family history of correlation with increased skin symptoms, minimize exposure to pets and other animals
   e. Dust and dust mites
10. Monitor environment
    a. Maintain cool temperature to reduce sweating
    b. Increase humidity during cold winter months
11. Educate regarding characteristics of condition and expected prognosis
12. Refer for dermatologist evaluation if condition does not resolve

Contact Dermatitis (Allergic Contact Dermatitis)

- Definition: Allergic response to local contact with an allergen manifested by development of skin eruptions at site of contact
- Etiology/Incidence
1. Caused by hypersensitivity to an allergen
   a. Initial contact—allergic response usually delayed for several days
   b. Reexposure—allergic response usually occurs within 24 hours due to prior sensitization
2. Numerous substances are associated with producing hypersensitivity reactions in sensitive individuals, with the most common including:
   a. Perfumes, soaps, cosmetics, fabric dyes
   b. Topical medications, e.g., neomycin
   c. Animal products—animal dander, feathers, fur, wool, leather
   d. Plastics, synthetics—latex, rubber
   e. Plants—poison sumac/ivy/oak
   f. Metals—jewelry, clothing snaps, and belt buckles; especially nickel
- Signs and Symptoms
1. Erythema and edema at site of contact
2. Pruritus with varying degrees of intensity
3. Vesicle and bulla formation
- Differential Diagnosis
1. Bacterial infection
2. Candida

3. Diaper dermatitis
4. Seborrhea dermatitis
5. Impetigo
6. Herpes simplex

- Physical Findings
  1. Erythema and edema with development of lesions of varying morphology—papules, vesicles, and denudation
  2. Lesions confined to area of direct contact with allergen
  3. Pruritus with varying degrees of intensity
  4. Excoriation/scratch marks and bleeding
  5. Chronic exposure may produce areas of hyperpigmentation and lichenification

- Diagnostic Tests/Findings: Skin testing to determine allergen hypersensitivities after acute stage

- Management/Treatment
  1. Obtain detailed history of onset, duration, severity, and progression of symptoms and possible precipitating factors
  2. Describe and monitor lesions in terms of morphology/structure, size, shape, number, color, location, distribution
  3. Avoid contact with allergen if sensitivity is known; if unknown, consider skin testing after acute phase to determine allergen
  4. Cool compresses of Burrow's solution to affected areas
  5. Steroids to reduce inflammation, immune response, and pruritus
     a. Apply topical steroids to affected areas, e.g., hydrocortisone, triamcinolone
     b. Oral steroids for severe cases, e.g., hydrocortisone
  6. Oral antihistamines for pruritus, e.g., hydroxyzine, diphenhydramine
  7. Oral antibiotics if secondary infection present, e.g., cephalexin, Bactrim (sulfamethoxazole and trimethoprim)
  8. Educate regarding medication dosage, signs of irritation, sensitivity
  9. Educate regarding characteristics of condition and expected resolution
  10. Refer to dermatologist for:
     a. Evaluation if condition does not show improvement in 2 days
     b. Consideration of skin testing for hypersensitivities after acute episode to identify specific allergens

Contact Irritant Dermatitis (Diaper Dermatitis)

- Definition: Common disorder of genital-perineal area due to skin breakdown; characterized by erythema, scale, and other skin lesions such as vesicles
- Etiology/Incidence
  1. Breakdown of skin associated with:
     a. Exposure to chemical irritants in soaps, bleach, water softeners, skin lotions, diaper cleansing tissues

     b. Excessive contact with urine, feces; lax hygiene habits (primary irritant)
  2. Occurs in more than 95% of all infants
  3. Peak incidence is 9 to 12 months of age
  4. Monilial rash caused by *Candida albicans*
  5. May persist until completion of toilet training

- Signs and Symptoms
  1. Redness, sores in diaper area, blisters
  2. Fiery red rash with satellite lesions on lower abdomen or upper thighs
  3. May have general irritability and/or crying, especially after elimination

- Differential Diagnosis
  1. Atopic dermatitis
  2. Seborrheic dermatitis
  3. Intertrigo
  4. Allergic/contact dermatitis
  5. Psoriasis
  6. Secondary bacterial infection
  7. Child maltreatment

- Physical Findings
  1. Erythema with varying degrees of severity that may be generalized to entire area or localized to small area
  2. Lesions of varied morphology may develop—papules, vesicles, crusts, erosions, and ulcerations
  3. Pustules may be present, signaling secondary bacterial infection
  4. Monilial rash—fiery red papular lesions within folds and on genitals; may also be pustular; may have associated oral thrush
  5. Poor genital hygiene may be present in some children

- Diagnostic Tests/Findings: No specific test confirms diagnosis

- Management/Treatment
  1. Obtain detailed history of onset, duration, severity, and progression of symptoms and possible precipitating factors
  2. Describe and monitor lesions in terms of morphology/structure, size, shape, number, color, location, distribution
  3. Treat secondary bacterial infection if present with topical antibiotics, e.g., mupirocin
  4. Treat present diaper dermatitis
     a. Mild erythema—emollients to affected areas with each diaper change, e.g., petroleum jelly, zinc oxide
     b. Erythema with papules—topical steroids, e.g., hydrocortisone
     c. Severe erythema and edema with papules, vesicles, and ulcerations—wet dressings may be soothing, e.g., Burrow's compresses; topical antibiotics may be indicated
     d. Monilial rash—topical nystatin, clotrimazole, ketoconazole; oral nystatin for thrush
     e. Avoid occlusive diapers and plastic pants
     f. Expose diaper area to air as often as possible
     g. Use appropriate preventive measures

5. Educate regarding medication dosage, signs of irritation, sensitivity
6. Preventive measures
   a. Expose diaper area to air several times each day
   b. Increase oral fluids to make urine less irritating
      (1) Water for infant younger than 12 months
      (2) Cranberry juice for older child
   c. Change diaper immediately after soiling
   d. Wash diaper area with nonirritating agents after each diaper change, e.g., mild soap and water
   e. Avoid occlusive diapers and plastic pants
   f. Diaper selection and care
      (1) Home laundry—mild soap and double rinse using 1 ounce of vinegar per gallon of water in last rinse
      (2) Disposable diapers—select alternate brand if sensitivity occurs
   g. "Diaper-wipes" may need to be avoided because of irritation or sensitivity
   h. Use lubricating ointment on diaper area skin at each diaper change, e.g., petroleum jelly
7. Refer for dermatologist evaluation if no improvement within 2 to 3 days or if condition worsens

Seborrhea Dermatitis

- Definition: Inflammatory condition usually on sebum-rich areas such as the scalp and face
  1. Newborn and young infant—cradle cap
  2. Adolescents—dandruff
- Etiology/Incidence
  1. Associated with overproduction of sebum in areas abundant with sebaceous glands
  2. Increase in sebaceous gland activity may be connected with hormonal stimulation at times when hormonal influence is highest
  3. Occurs more often in spring and summer months
- Signs and Symptoms
  1. Newborns and infants—areas of erythema under yellow crusts and greasy scales on scalp, face, neck folds, postauricular, and axillary creases
  2. Adolescents—white flakes and greasy scaling on scalp, forehead, eyebrows, and face; often pruritic
- Differential Diagnosis
  1. Atopic dermatitis
  2. Bacterial infection
  3. Candidiasis
  4. Irritant contact dermatitis
  5. Psoriasis
- Physical Findings
  1. Newborns and infants—areas of underlying erythema with yellow crusts and greasy scaling on scalp and face; in more severe cases lesions may be present on trunk and in diaper area
  2. Adolescents—white flakes and greasy scaling on scalp, forehead, eyebrows, and face; severity varies from simple dandruff to extensive, giving appearance

of psoriasis; mild underlying erythema may be present
- Diagnostic Tests/Findings: No tests necessary to confirm diagnosis
- Management/Treatment
  1. Obtain detailed history of onset, duration, severity, and progression of symptoms and possible precipitating factors
  2. Describe and monitor lesions in terms of morphology/structure, size, shape, number, color, location, distribution
  3. Treat existing condition
     a. For infants, shampoo and wash affected areas with a nonperfumed baby shampoo or baby wash; for adolescents, use antiseborrheic soaps and shampoos
     b. Mineral oil with brushing to loosen crusts prior to washing
     c. Topical steroid lotions for extreme cases to reduce inflammation, e.g., hydrocortisone
  4. Educate regarding medication dosage, signs of irritation, sensitivity
  5. Educate regarding characteristics of condition and expected prognosis
  6. Refer for dermatologist evaluation if condition persists without improvement

☐ BURN CONDITIONS

Burns

- Definition: Injury of skin from exposure to hot surfaces and agents
  1. Classified according to depth of injury to skin layers
     a. First-degree/superficial burns—involve epidermis layer only
     b. Second-degree/partial thickness burns—involve epidermis and part of dermis, which may be superficial dermis or deep dermis
     c. Third-degree/full-thickness burns—involve epidermis, dermis, and dermal appendages
  2. Classified also according to extent of affected area
     a. Minor burns—less than 10% of body surface if burn is superficial and less than 2% if burn is partial or full thickness
     b. Major burns—10% or more of body surface if burn is superficial and 2% or more if burn is partial or full thickness
     c. Major burns—hands, feet, face, eyes, ears, and perineal burns are always considered major burns, regardless of extent of body surface affected
- Etiology/Incidence
  1. Caused by external exposure to hot chemicals, electrical and thermal substances, and materials, including the sun, electrical cords and outlets, irons, flames, fireworks, hot water and foods, cigarettes, light bulbs
  2. Affected cells in epidermis, dermis, or subcutaneous skin layers are injured and no longer capable of

providing protective, electrolyte storage, sensory, and other functions of normal skin cells
   3. Third leading cause of death in children and adolescents
      a. More common in toddlers and males
      b. Commonly occurs in kitchen in late afternoon during dinner preparation
      c. Approximately 10% of burns are thought to be intentional in infant, toddler, and young child
- Signs and Symptoms: According to degree, appearance, and healing time
   1. Superficial—red, swollen, and dry areas with tenderness
   2. Partial-thickness and superficial burns—red, swollen, moist, and blistered areas with tenderness
   3. Partial-thickness and deep burns—white, dry areas with loss of sensation
   4. Full-thickness burns—white, brown, black, swollen dry areas with loss of sensation
- Differential Diagnosis
   1. Child maltreatment
   2. Staphylococcal scalded skin syndrome
- Physical Findings
   1. Superficial burns—erythema, mild edema, dryness, tenderness, and general discomfort of affected areas
   2. Partial-thickness and superficial burns—erythema, edema, moist, few vesicles/blisters may develop, sensitive to touch and air
   3. Partial-thickness and deep burns—white, dry, decreased sensitivity to touch, pain, temperature, and may blanch with pressure
   4. Full-thickness burns—white, brown, to black; swollen, dry; lack full touch, pain, temperature sensitivity
   5. Physical findings associated with secondary bacterial infection may be present
- Diagnostic Tests/Findings
   1. Electrolyte studies especially if burn is extensive
   2. Culture to determine causal agent if secondary bacterial infection is present
- Management/Treatment
   1. Obtain detailed history of onset, duration, severity, and progression of symptoms
   2. Describe and monitor burn area in terms of morphology/structure, extent of burn area, location, distribution
   3. Inpatient hospital management for all children with major burns, suspected abuse, esophageal and airway burns, and/or injuries such as fractures
   4. Outpatient management for children in stable environment with minor burns
      a. Partial-thickness burn if ≤10% of body surface area (BSA) or full-thickness burn if ≤2% BSA
      b. Monitor daily healing process by documenting changes
      c. Cool compresses to affected areas
      d. Medication for pain control, e.g., acetaminophen, ibuprofen
      e. Topical antimicrobial agents to prevent infection on open blistered areas, e.g., silver sulfadiazine (except on face because of potential for hyperpigmentation), mupirocin
      f. Do not excise vesicles/blisters
      g. Fluids to reduce possibility of dehydration, e.g., water, juices
      h. Topical emollients to repair and maintain skin barrier, e.g., petroleum jelly
   5. Educate regarding need to protect skin from exposure to sunlight especially from 10 a.m. to 3 p.m.
      a. Cover-up clothing, hats, and sunglasses
      b. Water-resistant sunblocks that protect against UVB and UVA ultraviolet light with SPF >30
      c. Educate regarding myths about getting a "base tan"
   6. Educate regarding medication dosage, signs of irritation, sensitivity
   7. Educate regarding characteristics of condition and prognosis
   8. Educate regarding measures to prevent further burn episodes and injuries
   9. Refer for dermatologist evaluation if condition does not show improvement

Sunburns

- Definition: Thermal burn due to excessive sunlight exposure
- Etiology/Incidence
   1. Exposed skin results in altered cell function and properties
      a. Inflammatory skin response with increased blood flow
      b. Increased melanin production
   2. Fair-skinned populations are most sensitive
   3. Other factors involving sensitivity include high altitude, nearness to equator, and exposure to sun during hours of 10 a.m. to 3 p.m. when UVB waves are strongest
- Signs and Symptoms
   1. Redness, swelling, blisters, and tenderness of sun-exposed areas
   2. Fatigue, chills, and headache after sun exposure
- Differential Diagnosis
   1. Child maltreatment
   2. Photosensitivity from medications
   3. Systemic viral exanthema
   4. Systemic drug reaction
- Physical Findings
   1. Dependent on degree of exposure and injury; develops within several minutes to several hours after exposure
      a. First-degree burns—erythema and tenderness
      b. Second-degree burns—increased intensity of erythema and tenderness with edema, some vesicles/blisters
      c. Third-degree burns—increased intensity of erythema, tenderness, edema, and vesicles/blisters

2. Systemic symptoms of malaise, fever, headache may be evident especially in younger child with second- and third-degree burns
3. Epidermis cells scale and desquamate within 3 to 7 days after injury
4. Exposed areas may become hyperpigmented with development of freckles and moles
- Diagnostic Tests/Findings: None used to confirm diagnosis
- Management/Treatment
  1. Obtain detailed history of onset, duration, severity, and progression of symptoms and precipitating factors
  2. Describe and monitor location, color, degree of burn, and symptoms
  3. Treat existing condition
     a. Remove from sunlight exposure
     b. Cool water or saline compresses to affected areas
     c. Do not use warm or hot showers/baths
     d. Increase oral fluids to prevent dehydration
     e. Oral pain medications, e.g., acetaminophen, ibuprofen
     f. Topical emollients for dry skin, e.g., petroleum jelly
  4. Educate regarding medication dosage, signs of irritation, sensitivity
  5. Educate regarding measures of prevention
     a. Risk factors of sun exposure
        (1) Teach early signs of skin cancer
        (2) Teach regarding individuals most vulnerable to sun exposure
     b. Use sun screens and blocks with SPF 30 or greater
        (1) Apply at least 20 minutes before exposure
        (2) Apply frequently if sustained exposure—every hour
        (3) Use waterproof agents when in water
        (4) Discontinue if sensitivity is suspected
        (5) Avoid use in infants <6 months
     c. Use cover-up clothing and hats designed to block UVB waves
  6. Refer for dermatologist evaluation if condition does not improve or becomes worse

☐ BACTERIAL CONDITIONS

Cellulitis

- Definition: Localized acute infection often precipitated by an insect bite (spider, mosquito, flea) or trauma that penetrates the protective skin barrier
- Etiology/Incidence: Caused when surface streptococci, *Haemophilus influenzae*, or *Staphylococcus aureus* bacteria invade all skin layers—epidermis, dermis, and subcutis—after a break in the skin has occurred
- Signs and Symptoms
  1. Irregular-shaped areas of skin with redness, swelling
  2. Warm and tender to touch
  3. Fever, chills, and malaise may be present

- Differential Diagnosis
  1. Impetigo
  2. Furuncle
  3. Pyoderma gangrenosum
- Physical Findings
  1. Erythema and edema with ill-defined, irregular borders
  2. Tenderness and warmth
  3. Regional lymphadenopathy may be present
  4. Fever, chills, and malaise indicates systemic involvement
  5. Facial, periorbital, or orbital involvement is vulnerable to development of more severe conditions
- Diagnostic Tests/Findings: Blood culture to confirm causal agent
- Management/Treatment
  1. Detailed history of onset, duration, severity, and progression of symptoms and precipitating factors
  2. Describe and monitor:
     a. Affected skin areas in terms of morphology/structure, size, shape, color, location, distribution
     b. Systemic signs and symptoms of fever, chills, and malaise
  3. Hospitalization for severe cases and those involving face and eyes
  4. Treat with intramuscular, intravenous, and/or oral antibiotics according to severity of condition, organism, and site of involvement
     a. If *Streptococcus* suspected—cefazolin, amoxicillin, nafcillin
     b. If *Haemophilus influenzae* suspected—augmentin
     c. If *Staphylococcus aureus* suspected—dicloxacillin
     d. If methicillin-resistant *Staphylococcus aureus* (MRSA)—Bactrim or clindamycin
  5. Educate regarding medication dosage, signs of irritation, sensitivity
  6. Educate regarding characteristics of condition and expected prognosis
  7. Refer for dermatologist evaluation if condition shows no improvement

Impetigo

- Definition: Localized bacterial infection of skin often precipitated by insect bites (spider, mosquito, flea) or other trauma that breaks protective skin barrier; predominately involves face and less commonly other body surfaces, including perineum
- Etiology/Incidence
  1. *Staphylococcus aureus* and streptococci bacteria invade epidermis after break in skin
  2. Children <6 years old have a higher incidence than adults
  3. Bullous impetigo most common in neonates and infants; nonbullous impetigo most common in 2- to 5-year-olds
  4. Highly communicable with incubation period of 1 to 10 days
  5. Autoinoculable

- Signs and Symptoms
  1. Itching and tenderness may be present
  2. Areas of erythematous swollen skin, blisters, and/or moist, honey-colored crusts
- Differential Diagnosis
  1. Eczema
  2. Herpes simplex
  3. Scabies
- Physical Findings
  1. Two major forms
     a. Nonbullous—underlying erythema with vesicles that erupt, resulting in honey-colored/serous crusts with erosion of epidermis
     b. Bullous—underlying erythema with pustules and vesicles that erupt, resulting in smooth, shiny appearance
  2. Regional adenopathy with tenderness
- Diagnostic Tests/Findings: Culture will confirm diagnosis and causative organism
- Management/Treatment
  1. Obtain detailed history of onset, duration, severity, and progression of symptoms and precipitating factors
  2. Describe and monitor lesions in terms of morphology/structure, size, location, distribution
  3. Apply compresses of Burrow's solution several times daily to aid in cleaning and removing crusts
  4. Apply topical antibiotics to areas of involvement, e.g., mupirocin
  5. Prescribe oral antibiotics according to specific bacterial cause
     a. For staphylococci—cephalexin, dicloxacillin
     b. For streptococci—amoxicillin or erythromycin
     c. For MRSA—Bactrim or clindamycin
  6. Educate regarding medication dosage, signs of irritation, sensitivity
  7. Educate regarding characteristics of condition, treatment regime, prognosis, and good hygiene for prevention
  8. Exclude from school and other public programs until treated for 48 hours because of high communicability
  9. Refer for dermatologist evaluation if condition does not improve

Staphylococcal Scalded Skin Syndrome

- Definition: Toxin-mediated systemic bacterial infection with skin manifestations
- Etiology/Incidence
  1. Caused by effects of toxin produced by *Staphylococcus aureus* bacteria
  2. Occurs any season
  3. More common in neonates and infants than in older children
  4. Incubation is variable, commonly 3 to 10 days
- Signs and Symptoms
  1. May present with abrupt onset of fever, irritability, and general malaise

  2. Bright, red, painful rash; more pronounced around eyes, mouth, neck, underarms, elbow, groin, and knees
  3. Pain on pressure
  4. Blistering and/or scaling of skin
- Differential Diagnosis
  1. Streptococcal scarlet fever
  2. Kawasaki disease
  3. Stevens-Johnson syndrome
  4. Toxic epidermal necrolysis
  5. Burns
  6. Child maltreatment
  7. Drug toxicity
- Physical Findings
  1. Abrupt onset of fever and general malaise
  2. General exanthema with erythema and swelling; more pronounced in perioral, periorbital areas; flexure surfaces of neck, axilla, antecubital, groin, and popliteal areas
  3. Light pressure causes extreme pain and exfoliation of top epidermal layers
  4. After peeling, skin appears glistening and scalded
  5. Vesicles/bullae may occur in more toxic cases
- Diagnostic Tests/Findings
  1. Blood culture to confirm *Staphylococcus aureus*
  2. Culture secretions to confirm *Staphylococcus aureus*
- Management/Treatment
  1. Obtain detailed history of onset, duration, severity, and progression of symptoms and precipitating factors
  2. Describe and monitor in terms of morphology/structure, size, shape, number, color, location, distribution
  3. Hospitalization is indicated for all neonates; treat more severe cases with IV antibiotics and monitor fluid and electrolytes
  4. Outpatient management may be considered with less toxic cases if environment is stable
     a. Oral antistaphylococcal antibiotics, e.g., cefazolin, dicloxacillin
     b. Oral antipyretics and analgesics for fever and pain control, e.g., acetaminophen, ibuprofen
     c. Increase fluids to maintain hydration and prevent dehydration, e.g., water, juices
  5. Educate regarding medication dosage, signs of irritation, sensitivity
  6. Educate regarding characteristics of condition, treatment, and prognosis
  7. Refer for dermatologist evaluation if condition does not improve

☐ BACTERIAL CONDITIONS INVOLVING PILOSEBACEOUS UNIT

Acne Vulgaris

- Definition: Common, inflammatory, chronic skin disorder involving the pilosebaceous follicle unit
  1. Occurs predominately on the face, neck, chest, and upper-back skin surfaces; less commonly in other areas

2. Often occurs in cyclic periods of exacerbation and remission
- Etiology/Incidence
  1. Specific cause is unknown
     a. Associated with breakdown of follicle wall
     b. Cells combine with sebum and plug follicle
     c. Enzymes from *Corynebacterium acnes* mix with trapped debris, causing edema and irritation
  2. Proven factors that may contribute to acne development:
     a. Increased androgenic hormonal influence
     b. Positive family history
     c. Stress
  3. Unproven factors with questionable and unsubstantiated contribution:
     a. Food—nuts, eggs, cheese, chocolate, milk
     b. Poor hygiene
  4. Affects more than 70% of adolescents with varying degrees of severity
     a. Onset parallels puberty
     b. More common in females
     c. More males develop severe acne
     d. More females experience continuation of acne into adult years
- Signs and Symptoms
  1. Open and closed comedones ("blackheads" and "whiteheads")
  2. Soreness at site of lesions
  3. Postinflammatory hyperpigmentation and scars at site of previous lesions
- Differential Diagnosis
  1. Folliculitis
  2. Rosacea
  3. Tuberous sclerosis
  4. Perioral dermatitis
  5. Contact dermatitis
  6. Urticaria
  7. Allergic drug reaction
- Physical Findings
  1. Lesions of varying morphology
     a. Mild acne—lesions are scattered, covering small areas
        (1) Open comedones/blackheads—lesions filled with dry, oxidized sebum; brown in color
        (2) Closed comedones/whiteheads—lesions filled with follicle cells and sebum
     b. Moderate acne—lesions are more numerous, covering large areas
        (1) All lesions of mild acne
        (2) Pustules—lesions filled with follicle cells, sebum, and white blood cells
     c. Severe acne—lesions are much more numerous, covering larger areas
        (1) All lesions of mild and moderate acne
        (2) Erythema with papules and pustules
        (3) Nodules and cysts—deep dermal lesions filled with follicle debris, often with communicating tracks to other cysts
  2. Increased oiliness of hair and skin

3. Scarring especially when:
   a. Lesions at any stage have been manipulated and squeezed
   b. Cysts have erupted deep within the dermis
4. Signs of related psychological distress/depression may be present
- Diagnostic Tests/Findings: None; clinically determined diagnosis
- Management/Treatment
  1. Obtain detailed history of onset, duration, severity, and progression of symptoms and possible precipitating factors
  2. Describe in terms of morphology/structure, size, shape, number, color, location, distribution
  3. Wash and dry face and affected areas with mild, non-oil-based soap
  4. Use topical exfoliates and comedolytic preparations
     a. Mild acne—topical benzoyl peroxide
     b. Moderate acne—topical tretinoin, topical benzoyl peroxide
     c. Severe acne—topical tretinoin, topical or oral antibiotics, oral tretinoin
  5. Use topical antibiotics for moderate to severe acne, e.g., clindamycin
  6. Add oral antibiotics for persistent and unresponsive cases of moderate and severe acne
     a. Tetracycline, doxycycline, minocycline, tetracycline
     b. Oral clindamycin contraindicated because of adverse gastrointestinal (GI) side effects
  7. Consider using isotretinoin for unresponsive, persistent severe acne
     a. Contraindicated in pregnancy; teratogenic
     b. For sexually active females, birth control measures required
     c. Federally mandated enrollment in iPLEDGE program requires informed, signed consent, monthly laboratory studies, and monthly office visits
  8. Educate regarding medication dosage, signs of irritation, sensitivity
  9. Consider counseling for signs of psychological distress and depression
  10. Educate regarding characteristics of condition, treatment regime, and expected prognosis
      a. Condition may become worse with treatment before improvement
      b. Treatment will improve, but not cure most cases; may take months
      c. Treatment must be consistent to be effective
  11. Monitor progress every 4 to 6 weeks initially; less often as indicated when improvement is evident
  12. Refer for dermatologist evaluation if condition does not meet prognostic expectations and/or considering need for isotretinoin

Folliculitis and Furuncles

- Definition: Infectious condition involving pilosebaceous follicle occurring on any skin surface where hair follicles are present but predominately on face, neck, scalp, and buttocks

1. Folliculitis—superficial involvement of upper follicle
2. Furuncle or boil—deeper involvement of follicle and dermal appendages

- Etiology/Incidence
  1. Caused most often by *Staphylococcus aureus*; less commonly by *Streptococcus* bacteria
  2. Also seen with some tinea infections
  3. More common in males
- Signs and Symptoms
  1. Areas of tenderness, erythema, and swelling
  2. Nodules may be present with deep-seated furuncles
  3. Tenderness and warmth at site
- Differential Diagnosis
  1. *Candida*
  2. Impetigo
- Physical Findings
  1. Localized areas of erythema and edema with papular or pustular lesions on face, scalp, neck, buttocks, and other areas
  2. Nodules are present with deep-seated furuncles
  3. Tenderness and warmth may be present
  4. Regional adenopathy may be present
- Diagnostic Tests/Findings: Culture confirms specific bacterial agent
- Management/Treatment
  1. Obtain detailed history of onset, duration, severity, and progression of symptoms and possible precipitating factors
  2. Describe and monitor lesions in terms of morphology/structure, size, shape, number, color, location, distribution
  3. Wash with antimicrobial soap and apply warm, moist compresses to affected areas
  4. Topical antibiotics, e.g., mupirocin
  5. Oral antibiotics
     a. For staphylococci—use dicloxacillin or cephalexin
     b. For streptococci infection—penicillin or cephalosporin; erythromycin for penicillin-allergic patients
     c. For MRSA—Bactrim or clindamycin
  6. Educate regarding medication dosage, signs of irritation, sensitivity
  7. Educate regarding characteristics of condition, treatment regime, prognosis, and good hygiene measures
  8. Refer for dermatologist evaluation if condition does not follow prognostic expectation

☐ VIRAL CONDITIONS

Herpes Simplex/Common Cold Sore

- Definition: Contagious infection, predominately of lips and oral mucosa, commonly known as fever blisters
  1. Initial infectious state—more severe, lasts longer, and is more painful
  2. Dormant state—virus lives on ending of selected nerves, asymptomatic
  3. Secondary infectious state—activated at times of increased stress, illness, fatigue, sun exposure, menses, dental procedures
- Etiology/Incidence
  1. Herpes simplex virus type 1—most common cause
  2. Herpes simplex virus type 2—considered in situations of oral sex
  3. Incubation varies, commonly 2 to 12 days
- Signs and Symptoms
  1. Erythema with grouped vesicles and crusting on lips
  2. Erythema and swelling with painful white ulcerated patches inside mouth
  3. Fever, generalized malaise, and sore throat may occur
  4. Mild itching, tingling, pain, and burning may precede blisters
- Differential Diagnosis
  1. Erythema multiforme
  2. Hand-foot-mouth disease
  3. Candidiasis
  4. Localized bacterial infection
  5. Sexual abuse
- Physical Findings
  1. Lip lesions—grouped or singular vesicles on an erythematous base erupt and form crusts; usually can be found on mucocutaneous border of lips
  2. Oral cavity lesions—erythema and edema of mucous membranes with singular or multiple vesicles and white ulcerations; may include tongue, palate, and gums
  3. Regional adenopathy may be present
  4. Halitosis may be present with oral lesions
  5. Lesions are present 10 to 14 days, gradually resolving
  6. Secondary infection may be present—most caused by *Staphylococcus* bacteria
- Diagnostic Tests/Findings
  1. Tzanck smear confirms presence of multinuclear giant cells indicative of herpes
  2. Culture to confirm causal agent
- Management/Treatment
  1. Obtain detailed history of onset, duration, severity, and progression of symptoms and precipitating factors
  2. Describe and monitor lesions in terms of morphology/structure, size, shape, number, color, location, distribution
  3. Treat lip lesions
     a. Burrow's compresses to alleviate discomfort
     b. Topical antiviral applications, e.g., acyclovir, for recurrent disease
  4. Treat oral lesions
     a. Avoid spicy and acid foods
     b. Cool, bland fluids, especially when lesions are most painful
     c. Anesthetic mouth rinses, e.g., lidocaine (with caution) or diphenhydramine
  5. Oral antiviral medication with recurrent disease at first sign of prodrome (skin tingling), e.g., acyclovir, famciclovir, valacyclovir

6. Oral antibiotic to treat secondary bacterial infection, e.g., dicloxacillin, cefadroxil, cephalexin
7. Educate regarding medication dosage, signs of irritation, sensitivity
8. Educate regarding cause, characteristics of condition, communicability, and prognosis
9. Educate regarding preventive measures
   a. Avoid direct exposure of others to lesions (kissing)
   b. Wash hands before and after applying topical medications or touching lesions
   c. Avoid sharing personal items—cosmetics, cups, eating utensils
10. Refer for dermatologist evaluation if condition does not improve

Molluscum Contagiosum

- Definition: Common infectious, self-limiting skin condition characterized by waxy, firm papules that may occur on any skin surface; predominately on face, axillae, abdomen, and arms
- Etiology/Incidence
  1. Caused by a poxvirus
  2. Most common in children and adolescents
  3. Common in children with atopic dermatitis, HIV, or AIDS
  4. Incubation is usually 2 to 8 weeks but may be up to 6 months
  5. Period of communicability uncertain
     a. May persist as long as lesions are present
     b. Spread by direct contact and through autoinoculation
- Signs and Symptoms
  1. Mild itching may be present
  2. Few or multiple small, firm, raised, pinkish-white or skin-colored lesions
- Differential Diagnosis
  1. Warts
  2. Closed comedones
  3. Milia
  4. Juvenile xanthogranuloma
  5. Condylomata acuminata
- Physical Findings
  1. Papular pink-white or skin-colored lesions of 1 to 5 mm in size, usually on face, neck, axillae, abdomen, and arms
  2. Occasionally, lesions grow to 1 to 2 cm
  3. Secondary bacterial infection may be present
  4. Lesions may become umbilicated (central pitting, dimpled, or depressed)
  5. Lesions are self-limiting but may be present for 2 to 3 years if left untreated
  6. May occur in genital area in sexually active and sexually abused; more typically they are transmitted by a caregiver
- Diagnostic Tests/Findings
  1. Usually not necessary

2. Wright or Giemsa stain of papule core will show characteristic intracytoplasmic inclusions
- Management/Treatment
  1. Obtain a detailed history of onset, duration, severity, and progression of symptoms and precipitating factors
  2. Describe and monitor lesions in terms of morphology/structure, size, shape, number, color, location, distribution
  3. Rule out child maltreatment if lesions in genital area
  4. Treatment options—with the exception of observation, none are cures
     a. In otherwise healthy individuals, lesions typically resolve spontaneously without treatment over time
     b. Curettage removal of lesions provides more expedient resolution as this is one method of stimulating an immune response; not recommended for facial lesions because of potential scarring
     c. Topical application of keratolytics; not recommended for lesions near eyes
        (1) Tretinoin cream
        (2) Cantharidin
     d. Topical antibiotics for secondary bacterial infection, e.g., mupirocin
  5. Education regarding medication dosages, signs of irritation, sensitivity
  6. Education regarding cause, characteristics of lesions, communicability, and prognosis
  7. Education regarding preventive measures
     a. Avoid direct exposure of others to lesions
     b. Wash hands before and after application of topical medications and/or touching lesions
     c. Avoid sharing personal items—cosmetics, towels, cups, eating utensils—and siblings sharing baths if one of them has molluscum lesions
  8. Refer for dermatologist evaluation if condition does not resolve with selected treatment

Verruca Vulgaris (Warts)

- Definition: Common self-limiting skin lesions characterized by firm, well-circumscribed, smooth to irregular, singular or multiple hyperkeratotic papules; predominately on fingers, palms, and soles of feet; commonly known as warts
- Etiology/Incidence
  1. Human papillomaviruses, with more than 50 identified types
  2. Virus enters skin through minor trauma
  3. Occurs in 10% of children and adolescents, with school-age children having the highest incidence
  4. Incidence may be increased with ongoing exposure to moisture
  5. Period of incubation varies widely, and estimated from 2 months to 2 years
  6. Period of communicability unknown
     a. May persist as long as lesions are present

b. Spread by direct and indirect contact and through autoinoculation

- Signs and Symptoms
  1. Raised gray, brownish to skin-colored, smooth to rough, singular or multiple lesions on hands
  2. Painful flat ingrown lesions on soles
  3. Bleeding may occur with trauma or picking
- Differential Diagnosis
  1. Molluscum contagiosum
  2. Calluses
- Physical Findings
  1. Common verruca—gray, brown, or skin-colored; rough, singular, or multiple papular lesions; most common on hands and fingers
  2. Flat verruca—skin-colored, smooth, round, multiple lesions, slightly elevated; most common on the face and extremities
  3. Plantar verruca—skin-colored, irregular, single or multiple lesions that appear flush with sole of foot and grow inward
  4. May occur in genital area of sexually active and sexually abused
  5. Lesions are self-limiting, usually 6 to 9 months, but because of reinfection through autoinoculation, condition may persist for several years
- Diagnostic Tests/Findings: Excision and histologic examination may confirm diagnosis
- Management/Treatment
  1. Obtain a detailed history of onset, duration, severity, and progression of symptoms and possible precipitating factors
  2. Describe and monitor lesions in terms of morphology/structure, size, shape, number, color, location, distribution
  3. Rule out child abuse if genital lesions are present
  4. Consider treatment options, knowing that, with the exception of observation, none of the treatment options are cures; some of the treatment options are painful and some can scar
     a. No treatment is usually necessary because of self-limiting condition
        (1) Ideal treatment has not been established
        (2) Frequently recur regardless of treatment choice until individual immune system creates immunity to the virus
     b. Topical applications of keratolytics, e.g., over-the-counter (OTC) wart preparations, cantharidin, tretinoin
     c. Applications of waterproof plastic tapes treated with keratolytics
     d. Excision of lesions except those on face because of potential scarring
  5. Topical antibiotics to treat secondary bacterial infection, e.g., mupirocin
  6. Educate regarding medication dosages, signs of irritation, sensitivity
  7. Educate regarding cause, characteristics of condition, communicability, and prognosis
  8. Consider congenital or acquired immunodeficiency if no resolution and/or widespread
  9. Refer for dermatologist evaluation if condition does not improve or bleeds with light trauma

☐ FUNGAL INFECTIONS

Tinea Capitis (Ringworm of the Scalp)

- Definition: Superficial dermatophyte fungal skin infection of the scalp
- Etiology/Incidence
  1. Caused predominately by *Trichophyton tonsurans* (90%); also by *Microsporum canis*, *Microsporum audouinii*, and *Trichophyton mentagrophytes* (less common)
  2. Dermatophytes attach to epidermis skin layer of host's scalp and multiply within stratum corneum; do not involve lower layers of epidermis or dermis
  3. Spreads through direct and indirect contact with infected individuals, animals, caps, combs, brushes, glasses, and other personal articles
  4. *Microsporum canis* may be transmitted through contact with infected dogs or cats
  5. Occurs more often in hot, humid climates
  6. More common in darker-skinned individuals; boys more than girls
  7. Incubation period is unknown, possibly 10 to 14 days
  8. Communicability occurs as long as lesions with dermatophytes are present
- Signs and Symptoms
  1. Itching with varying degrees of severity
  2. Slightly raised round or angular scaly areas
  3. Sometimes yellow honeycomb crusts
  4. Broken hairs and alopecia may be present
- Differential Diagnosis
  1. Impetigo
  2. Eczema
  3. Seborrhea dermatitis
  4. Psoriasis
  5. Trichotillomania
  6. Alopecia areata
- Physical Findings
  1. Several presentations may occur singularly or at the same time
     a. Scaly patches of varying sizes with or without alopecia and pruritus
     b. Pustules, papules with areas of honeycomb crusts
     c. Tender erythematous areas with broken hairs at scalp level leaving a "black-dot" appearance
  2. Regional adenopathy may be present, especially occipital nodes
- Diagnostic Tests/Findings
  1. Wood's lamp will fluoresce *Microsporum canis* only and is of limited use in confirming tinea capitis

2. KOH scraping from the areas of scalp with alopecia, "black dots," or broken hairs will confirm hyphae and spores of dermatophytes

- Management/Treatment
1. Obtain detailed history of onset, duration, severity, and progression of symptoms and precipitating factors
2. Describe and monitor lesions in terms of morphology/structure, size, shape, number, color, location, and distribution
3. Treat with oral antifungal medication
   a. Griseofulvin; ultramicrosize formulation has best absorption
   b. Treat for 8 weeks
   c. Topical antifungal medications are ineffective
4. Shampoo 2 to 3 times weekly with selenium sulfide or ketoconazole to reduce spore count and infectivity
5. Although condition is communicable, exclusion from school and other groups is not indicated unless treatment is refused or not followed
6. Educate regarding medication dosage, signs of irritation, sensitivity
7. Educate regarding characteristics of condition, treatment regime, and prognosis
8. Educate regarding communicability and prevention
   a. Avoid sharing personal items such as caps, combs, brushes, towels, pillows, glasses, razors; wash these items frequently
   b. Wash hair immediately after barbershop or salon haircut
   c. Maintain personal hygiene, wash hands before/after treatment
   d. Avoid touching or scratching affected areas
9. Refer for dermatologist evaluation if condition does not improve

Tinea Corporis (Ringworm of the Body)

- Definition: Superficial dermatophyte fungal skin infection of less-hairy surfaces of body and face; commonly known as "ringworm" because of pattern of healing centrally while spreading peripherally
- Etiology/Incidence
1. Primary source—*Trichophyton rubrum*, *Trichophyton mentagrophytes*, as well as *Microsporum canis* and *Epidermophyton floccosum*
2. Dermatophytes attach to epidermis skin layer of host and multiply within stratum corneum; do not involve lower layers of the epidermis or dermis
3. Spreads through direct and indirect contact with infected individuals, animals, shower stalls, benches, and other articles
4. *Microsporum canis* may be transmitted through contact with infected dogs or cats
5. Occurs more often in hot, humid climates
6. Incubation period is unknown, possibly 4 to 14 days
7. Communicability occurs as long as lesions with dermatophytes are present

- Signs and Symptoms
1. Mild itching at site of affected areas
2. Slightly raised, round or angular scaly areas with pink borders
- Differential Diagnosis
1. Contact dermatitis
2. Nummular eczema
3. Psoriasis
4. Pityriasis rosea
5. Pityriasis versicolor
6. Granuloma annulare
- Physical Findings
1. Typical lesions are scaly plaques of varying sizes from less than 5 mm to more than 3 cm with mild erythematous active borders
2. Lesions spread peripherally as they heal centrally
3. Lesions may be singular or several; numerous lesions are uncommon
- Diagnostic Tests/Findings
1. Wood's lamp will fluoresce *Microsporum canis*
2. KOH scraping of lesion border—confirms hyphae and spores
3. Dermatophyte test medium (DTM)—confirms diagnosis
- Management/Treatment
1. Obtain a detailed history of onset, duration, severity, and progression of symptoms and precipitating factors
2. Describe and monitor lesions in terms of morphology/structure, size, shape, number, color, location, and distribution
3. Treat with topical antifungal medications
   a. Clotrimazole, miconazole, econazole, terbinafine, tolnaftate, naftifine, ciclopirox, ketoconazole
   b. May require treatment up to 8 weeks before resolution
4. Treat with oral antifungal medication for extensive, recurrent, and unresponsive conditions, e.g., griseofulvin
5. Educate regarding medication dosage, signs of irritation, sensitivity
6. Educate regarding characteristics of condition, treatment regime, and prognosis
7. Educate regarding communicability and prevention
   a. Avoid sharing personal items of clothing, towels, pillows, razors, and wash these items frequently
   b. Maintain personal hygiene and wash hands before and after applying treatment
   c. Avoid touching or scratching affected areas
   d. Avoid or shower after using public pools
   e. Wash clothing touching affected areas after each use
8. Refer for dermatologist evaluation if condition does not improve

Tinea Cruris (Jock Itch)

- Definition: Superficial dermatophyte fungal skin infection of the groin, upper thighs, and/or inguinal folds; commonly called "jock itch"

- Etiology/Incidence
  1. Caused by *Epidermophyton floccosum, Trichophyton rubrum,* and *Trichophyton mentagrophytes*
  2. Dermatophytes attach to epidermis skin layer of host and multiply within stratum corneum; lower layers of epidermis or dermis are not involved
  3. Occurs more often during hot, humid weather with increased sweating
  4. More common in adolescents, athletes, obese children, and males
  5. Spreads through direct and indirect contact with infected individuals, including sexual contact
  6. Incubation period is unknown, possibly 4 to 14 days
  7. Communicability occurs as long as lesions with dermatophytes are present
- Signs and Symptoms
  1. Pain and tenderness with varying degrees of severity
  2. Itching with varying degrees of severity reported, especially during healing
  3. Erythematous, hyperpigmented, slightly raised scaly patches with defined borders
  4. Blisters may also be present
- Differential Diagnosis
  1. Contact dermatitis
  2. Eczema
  3. Intertrigo
  4. Psoriasis
  5. Seborrheic dermatitis
  6. Acanthosis nigricans
- Physical Findings
  1. Erythematous, scaly red to brown lesions of varying sizes with well-defined raised borders
     a. Small vesicles, central clearing, and peripheral spreading may or may not be present
     b. Affected areas may be singular or multiple
     c. In chronic cases, lichenification may be present
  2. All areas of the groin may be affected, including scrotum, gluteal folds, buttocks, inner aspect of thighs
  3. Painful to touch and with movement
  4. Often concurrent with tinea pedis
- Diagnostic Tests/Findings
  1. KOH scraping of lesion border—confirms hyphae and spores
  2. DTM—confirms diagnosis
- Management/Treatment
  1. Obtain a detailed history of onset, duration, severity, and progression of symptoms and precipitating factors
  2. Describe and monitor lesions in terms of morphology/structure, size, shape, number, color, location, and distribution
  3. Treat with topical antifungal medications
     a. Clotrimazole, haloprogin, miconazole, terbinafine, tolnaftate, ciclopirox, econazole, ketoconazole, naftifine, oxiconazole, sulconazole
     b. May require treatment up to 4 to 6 weeks before resolution

  4. Treat with oral antifungal medication for extensive, recurrent, and/or unresponsive conditions, e.g., griseofulvin
  5. Educate regarding medication dosage, signs of irritation, sensitivity
  6. Educate regarding characteristics of condition, treatment regime, and prognosis
  7. Educate regarding communicability and prevention
     a. Avoid sharing undergarments—pants, jock straps
     b. Wash personal undergarments frequently
     c. Maintain good daily personal hygiene and dry well after bathing
     d. Wash hands before and after applying topical treatment
     e. Avoid touching or scratching affected areas
     f. Avoid or shower after using public pools
     g. Launder clothing touching affected areas after each use
     h. Do not wear tight clothes next to affected area, including jeans and undergarments
     i. Use cotton undergarments and change daily
  8. Refer for dermatologist evaluation if condition does not improve

Tinea Pedis (Athlete's Foot or Ringworm of the Feet)

- Definition: Superficial dermatophyte fungal skin infection of toes and feet
- Etiology/Incidence
  1. Caused by *Trichophyton rubrum, Trichophyton mentagrophytes,* and *Epidermophyton floccosum* fungal dermatophytes
  2. Dermatophytes attach to epidermis skin layer of host and multiply within stratum corneum; do not involve lower layers of epidermis or dermis
  3. Occurs more often during hot, humid weather with increased sweating
  4. Occurs worldwide; more common in adolescents, athletes, and males
  5. Spreads through direct and indirect contact with infected individuals, public baths, swimming pools, and locker rooms
  6. Incubation period is unknown
  7. Communicability occurs as long as lesions with dermatophytes are present
- Signs and Symptoms
  1. Pruritus of affected areas
  2. Erythematous, scaly, and occasionally blistered areas anywhere on foot; cracks and scaling between toes
  3. Stinging or pain if cracks between toes
- Differential Diagnosis
  1. Atopic dermatitis
  2. Contact dermatitis
  3. Candidiasis
  4. Eczema

- Physical Findings
  1. Erythematous scaly patches of varying sizes
     a. Small vesicles, central clearing, and peripheral spreading may or may not be present
     b. Affected areas may be anywhere on foot, most commonly on lateral and plantar portions
  2. Lesions on or between toes are scaly with mild erythema
     a. Interdigital fissures are present
     b. One or multiple toes may be involved, most commonly between third and fourth toes
  3. Dystrophy of toenails may be present with yellow discoloration of the nail matrix and periungual debris
- Diagnostic Tests/Findings
  1. KOH scraping of lesion border confirms hyphae and spores
  2. DTM of skin scraping or nail clippings confirms diagnosis
- Management/Treatment
  1. Obtain a detailed history of onset, duration, severity, and progression of symptoms and precipitating factors
  2. Describe and monitor lesions in terms of morphology/structure, size, shape, number, color, location, and distribution
  3. Treat with topical antifungal medications
     a. Clotrimazole, haloprogin, miconazole, econazole, ciclopirox, terbinafine, tolnaftate, ketoconazole, naftifine, oxiconazole, sulconazole
     b. May require treatment of 8 to 12 weeks before resolution
  4. Treat vesicular and fissured lesions with compresses of Burrow's solution
  5. Use absorbent antifungal powder
  6. Treat with oral antifungal medication for extensive, recurrent, and unresponsive conditions, e.g., griseofulvin
  7. Educate regarding medication dosage and signs of irritation and sensitivity
  8. Educate regarding characteristics of condition, treatment regime, and prognosis
  9. Educate regarding communicability and prevention
     a. Avoid sharing personal items of shoes, socks, and towels
     b. Wash personal items frequently
     c. Maintain good daily personal hygiene and dry well after bathing
     d. Wash hands before and after applying topical treatment
     e. Avoid touching or scratching affected areas
     f. Avoid using public pools or shower after each use
     g. Launder clothing touching affected areas after each use
     h. Do not wear tight and closed shoes
     i. Use cotton socks instead of nylon or polyester
  10. Refer for dermatologist evaluation if condition does not improve

☐ INSECT CONDITIONS

Common Insect Bites

- Definition: Wound inflicted by bite of a blood-sucking arthropod
- Etiology/Incidence
  1. Caused when mosquitoes, fleas, chiggers, and bedbugs feed on human blood
     a. Are attracted to host's moisture, odor, and warmth
     b. Serve as vectors for diseases such as malaria
  2. Pet dogs and cats act as hosts for some fleas that are also attracted to humans
  3. More bites occur:
     a. In warm and humid weather
     b. Around stagnant water
     c. In outside grassy and sandy areas
     d. On uncovered body areas
  4. Itching caused by sensitivity to insect's saliva
- Signs and Symptoms
  1. Itching is major symptom—may persist 5 to 7 days after exposure
  2. Pain—variable
  3. Single or multiple pink/red raised lesions on legs, abdomen, and exposed areas of upper body
- Differential Diagnosis
  1. Folliculitis
  2. Insect sting
  3. Spider bite
  4. Scabies
- Physical Findings
  1. Single or multiple erythematous papules and wheals on lower extremities, abdomen, and exposed upper body parts
  2. Lesions from bed bug and chigger bites are smaller, more erythematous, and more numerous
  3. Vesicles may develop, signaling greater sensitivity
  4. Excoriation may be present with intense pruritus
  5. Pustules may develop, indicating secondary bacterial infection
- Diagnostic Tests/Findings: Culture of pustules confirms causal organism of secondary infection
- Management/Treatment
  1. Obtain detailed history of bite, progression of symptoms, and precipitating factors
  2. Describe and monitor lesions in terms of morphology/structure, size, shape, number, color, location, and distribution
  3. Provide symptomatic treatment of pruritus
     a. Cool compresses
     b. Topical histamines, e.g., hydroxyzine, diphenhydramine
     c. Oral antihistamines if topical treatment is ineffective, e.g., hydroxyzine, diphenhydramine
  4. Topical steroids to reduce inflammation and immune response, e.g., hydrocortisone, triamcinolone

5. Treat secondary bacterial infection
   a. Use topical antibiotics, e.g., mupirocin
   b. Treat with oral antibiotics if extensive, recurrent, or unresponsive, e.g., cefadroxil, cephalexin
6. Educate regarding characteristics of condition, treatment regime, and prognosis
7. Educate regarding medication dosage, signs of irritation, sensitivity
8. Educate regarding prevention
   a. Outside environmental controls—clearing areas, pesticide spraying, removing stagnant water
   b. Inside environmental controls—routine cleaning, vacuuming
   c. Bathe flea-infested pets
   d. Wear cover-up clothing
   e. Wear insect repellants
   f. Avoid wearing fragrances that may attract
   g. Avoid scratching to prevent infection
9. Refer for dermatologist evaluation if condition does not resolve

Spider Bites

- Definition: Wound inflicted by spider, characterized by both local and systemic manifestations
- Etiology/Incidence
  1. Most spider bites are harmless, causing small, localized reaction at site of bite
  2. In United States, bites from two nonaggressive venomous spiders produce severe toxic reactions in some individuals
     a. Black widow
        (1) Mature female is shiny, black, gray, or brown with an orange hourglass marking on the ventral surface
        (2) Overall size is 2.5 to 4.5 cm including legs
        (3) Male is smaller with fangs that cannot penetrate human skin
        (4) Most common in Ohio, South, Southwest, and West Coast
        (5) Likes dry, warm, dark areas; found in grass, wood piles, gardens, sheds, basements, closets, and trunks
        (6) Spin irregular asymmetrical web to catch flies and other prey
     b. Brown recluse
        (1) Mature spider is gray, or varying shades of red to pale brown, with a violin-shaped marking on cephalothorax
        (2) Overall size is 1.5 to 2.5 cm, including legs
        (3) Most common in the Midwest and South
        (4) Likes trunks, carpets, old shoes, old clothes, closets, crates, shelves
  3. Most bites are in self-defense when spider feels threatened
  4. Most bites occur in warmer months

5. Infants and small children are most vulnerable to developing serious reactions
- Signs and Symptoms
  1. Black widow
     a. Initial sensation of pinch or sting is often unnoticed
     b. Later within 1 hour of the bite
        (1) Dull burning or pain at site of bite
        (2) Two red puncture marks surrounded by white area with bluish-red border
        (3) Muscle cramps and sweating
        (4) Muscle spasms can spread to rest of body
        (5) In severe cases can progress to shock, coma, and death
  2. Brown recluse
     a. Initial sensation of bite is most often unnoticed or moderately painful
     b. Later within 2 to 7 hours:
        (1) Mild localized tingling
        (2) Redness or blanching
     c. After 48 to 72 hours:
        (1) Blister surrounded by blue-gray area
        (2) Flu-like symptoms may be experienced
  3. Reactions from bites of both spiders may become more intense and last for days with more serious life-threatening signs/symptoms developing in a few cases
- Differential Diagnosis—black widow and brown recluse
  1. Other insect bites (both)
  2. Tetanus (black widow)
  3. Appendicitis (black widow)
  4. Diabetic ulcers (brown recluse)
  5. Stevens-Johnson syndrome (brown recluse)
- Physical Findings—specifics vary by type of spider
  1. Black widow spider bite
     a. Symptoms begin within 1 hour
     b. Dull burning or pain at site
     c. Two red puncture marks surrounded by a blanched area with bluish erythematous border
     d. Muscle spasms, hypertension, tachycardia, diaphoresis
  2. Brown recluse spider bite
     a. Initial symptoms begin within 2 to 7 hours
        (1) Mild, localized tingling
        (2) Erythema or blanching at site
     b. Delayed symptoms after 48 to 72 hours
        (1) Hemorrhagic vesicle surrounded by bluish, gray areas of developing necrosis
        (2) Flu-like symptoms
  3. Both (black widow and brown recluse)
     a. Reactions may last for days to weeks
     b. Potential to become serious and life-threatening with major renal, respiratory, cardiovascular, and neurologic system involvement
- Diagnostic Tests/Findings
  1. No tests confirm specific diagnosis
  2. Dead spider specimen may help to confirm specific species

- Management/Treatment
  1. Obtain detailed history of onset, duration, severity, progression of symptoms, and precipitating factors
  2. Describe and monitor symptoms and lesions in terms of morphology/structure, size, shape, number, color, location, and distribution
  3. If bite from black widow or brown recluse spider is suspected:
     a. Apply cold compresses to site of bite
     b. Refer immediately for dermatologist evaluation and hospitalization due to potential risk of severe reaction
  4. If bite from another less harmful spider is suspected:
     a. Apply cool compresses to site of bite
     b. Use oral antihistamines to reduce severe pruritus, e.g., hydroxyzine, diphenhydramine
     c. Monitor for hypersensitivity reaction
  5. Educate regarding characteristics of condition, treatment regime, and prognosis
  6. Educate regarding medication dosage, signs of irritation, sensitivity
  7. Educate regarding prevention
     a. Outside environmental controls—clearing areas, pesticide spraying
     b. Inside environmental controls—routine cleaning, vacuuming
     c. Avoid and/or be observant around areas of natural habitat
     d. Wear protective clothing and hats
     e. Wear gloves when cleaning closets and trunks
     f. Inspect clothing and shoes prior to wearing

Insect Stings

- Definition: Wound inflicted by sting of an insect, characterized by systemic and/or local manifestations
- Etiology/Incidence
  1. Caused by bees, hornets, wasps, yellow jackets, and fire ants
  2. Hypersensitivity to venom develops after initial exposure with more severe reactions upon subsequent exposures
     a. Mild reactions occur in 90% of children
     b. Anaphylaxis occurs in approximately 7% of general population
  3. Most stings occur in self-defense when insect feels threatened
  4. Most stings occur in warmer months
  5. Multiple stings may occur when around nests or swarms of insects
- Signs and Symptoms
  1. Usual reaction after initial exposure lasts up to 24 hours
     a. Pain with varying degrees of severity
     b. Redness and swelling at site of sting
  2. More pronounced reaction after reexposure
     a. Nausea and abdominal pain
     b. Sneezing and coughing
     c. Itching
     d. Larger area of redness and swelling
  3. Anaphylactic reaction may occur after initial or reexposure
     a. Early signs within minutes of exposure
        (1) Dizziness
        (2) Swelling of lips and throat
        (3) Difficulty breathing
        (4) Difficulty swallowing
     b. Later signs
        (1) Weakness and collapse
        (2) Confusion
        (3) Coma
- Differential Diagnosis
  1. Spider bites
  2. Other insect bites
- Physical Findings
  1. Usual reaction after initial exposure may last up to 24 hours
     a. Pain with varying degrees of severity
     b. Erythema and edema surrounding central punctum at site of sting
  2. Thin white to gray stinger may project from center
  3. More pronounced reaction may last several days especially after reexposure
     a. Nausea, abdominal pain
     b. Sneezing, coughing
     c. Pruritus
     d. Larger area of redness, swelling
  4. Anaphylactic reaction may occur after initial or reexposure
     a. Could result in ultimate collapse and death
     b. Early signs within minutes of exposure
        (1) Dizziness
        (2) Swelling of lips and throat
        (3) Difficulty breathing
        (4) Difficulty swallowing
     c. Later signs
        (1) Weakness and collapse
        (2) Confusion
        (3) Coma
        (4) Stridor
- Diagnostic Tests/Findings: None
- Management/Treatment
  1. Obtain detailed history of onset, duration, severity, and progression of symptoms
  2. Describe and monitor area in terms of size, color, and location
  3. If known sensitivity, life-threatening and/or severe reaction:
     a. Administer epinephrine as indicated
     b. Apply cool compresses
     c. Refer immediately for dermatologist evaluation and hospitalization
  4. If mild reaction:
     a. Remove stinger by flicking off; do not squeeze
     b. Apply cool compresses to site of sting

c. Use oral antihistamines to reduce severe pruritus, e.g., hydroxyzine, diphenhydramine

d. Monitor for hypersensitivity reaction

5. Provide emotional support as needed to child and family

6. Educate regarding characteristics of condition, treatment regime, and prognosis

7. Educate regarding medication dosage, signs of irritation, sensitivity

8. Educate regarding prevention

a. Outside environmental controls—clearing areas, pesticide spraying

b. Inside environmental controls—routine cleaning, vacuuming

c. Avoid and/or be observant around areas of natural habitat

d. Wear protective clothing, hats, and gloves

e. Avoid wearing bright clothing when hiking around natural habitat

f. Avoid wearing perfumes when around natural habitat

g. If known sensitivity, wear medical alert tag and carry epinephrine kit

☐ INSECT INFESTATIONS

Scabies Infestation

- Definition: Highly contagious condition caused by parasitic mite infestation
- Etiology/Incidence
  1. Caused by the *Sarcoptes scabiei* (itch mite); gravid female mite burrows into stratum corneum to lay ova, which hatch in 4 to 14 days
  2. Incubation period of 4 to 6 weeks with initial exposure; 1 to 5 days with reexposure causing intense itching
  3. Worldwide distribution in all population groups regardless of hygiene
  4. Major infestations have occurred in cyclic patterns of every 15 to 30 years
  5. Spreads through direct contact with infected person or indirect contact with clothing, bed linens, and other personal items
  6. Communicability is present until all mites, larvae, and ova are destroyed on body surface and in surrounding environment
- Signs and Symptoms
  1. Irritability in infants
  2. Intense pruritus, especially at night in older children and adolescents
  3. Red bumps, blisters, pustules, and small burrow marks, which may be obliterated by scratch marks
- Differential Diagnosis
  1. Insect bites
  2. Impetigo
  3. Secondary bacterial infection

- Physical Findings
  1. Intense itching
  2. Fine gray- to skin-colored superficial 2- to 8-mm linear curved burrows with small papule at proximal end; burrows may be obliterated by scratch and excoriation marks due to scratching
  3. Infants—typically have red-brown papular, vesicular lesions on head, neck, palms, and soles
  4. Older children and adolescents—typically have red papular lesions on webs of fingers and folds of wrists, elbows, axillae, waist, buttocks, groin, umbilicus, abdomen, knees, ankles
  5. Pustules indicate secondary bacterial infection
  6. Regional adenopathy may be present
- Diagnostic Tests/Findings
  1. Skin scrapings of burrow or papule material and microscopic examination for body parts of mite, ova, or feces
  2. Culture of pustule will confirm agent of secondary infection
- Management/Treatment
  1. Obtain a detailed history of onset, duration, severity, and progression of symptoms
  2. Describe and monitor lesions in terms of morphology/structure, size, shape, number, color, location, and distribution
  3. Bathe and dry skin, and then treat with topical medication
     a. Infants and young children—permethrin 5% (drug of choice)
     b. Older children and adolescents—permethrin 5%; lindane, crotamiton 10%; sulfur in petrolatum
     c. Since 2004, lindane has had an FDA-mandated boxed warning about not using this product on children weighing <110 pounds
  4. Use topical steroids to reduce inflammation, immune response, and pruritus, e.g., hydrocortisone, triamcinolone
  5. Use oral antihistamines to reduce pruritus, e.g., hydroxyzine, diphenhydramine
  6. Treat secondary bacterial infection
     a. Use topical antibiotics, e.g., mupirocin
     b. Use oral antibiotics if extensive, recurrent, or unresponsive, e.g., dicloxacillin, cefadroxil, cephalexin
  7. Educate regarding medication dosage, signs of irritation, sensitivity
  8. Treat household and other close contacts
  9. Wash clothes, bed linens, towels, and hats with hot water and dry in hot dryer
  10. Store nonwashable items in plastic bags for 1 week; do not use
  11. Educate regarding characteristics of condition, treatment regime, and prognosis. Residual pruritus and skin irritation can persist for weeks after successful treatment
  12. Educate regarding medication dosage and signs of irritation and sensitivity

13. Educate regarding communicability and prevention
    a. Avoid sharing personal items of clothes, linens, towels, and wash these items frequently
    b. Maintain good daily personal hygiene and dry well after bathing
    c. Wash hands before and after applying topical treatment
    d. Avoid touching or scratching affected areas
14. Refer for dermatologist evaluation if condition does not improve

Pediculosis Infestation (Lice)

- Definition: Highly contagious parasitic louse infestation affecting hairy body surfaces
- Etiology/Incidence
  1. Caused by several species of lice
     a. *Pediculus capitis*—affects scalp
     b. *Pediculus humanus*—affects less hairy body surfaces
     c. *Phthirus pubis*—affects pubic and axilla areas, eyelashes, eyebrows
  2. Worldwide distribution in all population groups regardless of hygiene practices
  3. More common in school-age children and adolescents as a result of sharing of personal items
  4. More common in Caucasians, less common in African Americans
  5. Spreads through direct contact with infected person or indirect contact with clothing, bed linens, and other personal items
  6. Lice do not fly or jump
  7. Incubation of 6 to 10 days from laying of eggs to hatching; hatched lice mature in 2 to 3 weeks
  8. Communicability present until all lice, neophytes, and ova are destroyed on body surface and in environment
- Signs and Symptoms
  1. Pruritus; however, this may not be present until 4 to 6 weeks after initial infestation
  2. Tenacious white "flakes" on hair (nits); however, these egg casings may be empty (already hatched)
  3. Erythematous blotches and bumps (rare)
- Differential Diagnosis
  1. Bites from other insects
  2. Bacterial infection
  3. Dandruff
  4. Impetigo
  5. Scabies
- Physical Findings
  1. The only definitive way to diagnose an active infestation is to identify a live louse
  2. Small white nits (eggs) on hair strands—inch from skin surface; difficult to remove; the nits must be close to the scalp for a blood meal
     a. Head lice most common on back of head, behind ears

b. Body lice most common in seams of clothing
3. Macular, papular lesions with mild erythema and excoriation
4. Pustules secondary to scratching (secondary bacterial infection)
5. Regional adenopathy may be present
- Diagnostic Tests/Findings
  1. Clinical examination of hair shaft for ova is usually sufficient to confirm diagnosis
  2. Microscopic examination of ova may confirm questionable diagnosis
- Management/Treatment
  1. Obtain detailed history of onset, duration, severity, and progression of symptoms
  2. Describe and monitor lesions in terms of morphology/structure, size, shape, number, color, location, and distribution
  3. Treat infestation with topical antiparasitics to destroy louse and ova, e.g., permethrin, pyrethrins, malathion, ivermectin
  4. Resistance to antiparasitics is increasing; permethrin only has 70% efficacy
  5. Since 2004, lindane has had an FDA-mandated boxed warning about not using this product on children weighing <110 pounds
  6. Two treatments of medication of choice recommended
  7. Educate regarding medication dosage, signs of irritation, sensitivity
  8. Remove ova/nits after topical treatment
     a. Head lice—manually with fine-tooth comb
     b. Vinegar and water preparation may help soften cement
     c. Eyelashes—may coat with petroleum jelly for several days
  9. Use topical antibiotics to treat secondary bacterial infection, e.g., mupirocin
  10. Only treat other infested family members; you do not need to automatically treat every household contact
  11. Remove infestation from surrounding environment
      a. Wash clothes, bed linens, towels, and hats with hot water and dry in hot dryer
      b. Wash personal items such as combs and brushes with pediculicide
      c. Lice can live only 24 hours away from a human host, so you do not need to vacuum drapes, rugs, floors, and furniture
  12. Educate regarding characteristics of condition and prognosis. Residual pruritus and skin irritation can persist for weeks after successful treatment
  13. Educate regarding communicability and prevention
      a. Avoid sharing personal items of towels, hats, hair brushes, combs; wash these items frequently
      b. Maintain personal hygiene, wash hands before/after treatments
      c. Avoid touching or scratching affected areas
      d. Avoid promoting a "no nit" return-to-school policy

14. Refer for dermatologist evaluation if condition does not resolve

☐ MISCELLANEOUS CONDITIONS OF HYPERSENSITIVITY

Drug Eruptions

- Definition: Acute condition of the skin involving an allergic hypersensitivity reaction to a drug characterized predominately by a morbilliform generalized rash
- Etiology/Incidence
  1. Caused by release of histamine in reaction to immune system's response to drug allergen
  2. Most common drugs
     a. Sulfates
     b. Penicillins
     c. Barbiturates
     d. Dilantin
  3. Onset usually occurs within first week of exposure; may be delayed for more than 2 weeks and/or after drug has been discontinued
  4. Recurrences are frequent with reexposures—response varies depending on antigen exposure
- Signs and Symptoms
  1. Intense generalized and localized pruritus
  2. Generalized erythematous lesions beginning on trunk and progressing to extremities
- Differential Diagnosis
  1. Syphilis
  2. Contact dermatitis
  3. Erythema multiforme
  4. Rubeola
  5. Urticaria
  6. Gianotti-Crosti syndrome
  7. Erythema nodosum
- Physical Findings
  1. Generalized and localized pruritus
  2. Generalized morbilliform erythematous rash occurring first on trunk and progressing to extremities; initially macular, becoming papular and confluent
  3. Wheals are less typical and less frequent
- Diagnostic Tests/Findings: None
- Management/Treatment
  1. Obtain detailed history of onset, duration, severity, and progression of symptoms and possible precipitating factors
  2. Describe and monitor lesions in terms of morphology/structure, size, shape, number, color, location, distribution
  3. Discontinue contact with drug/medication allergen if known sensitivity
  4. Oral steroids to reduce inflammation and immune response in severe and extensive cases, e.g., prednisone
  5. Oral antihistamines for nocturnal pruritus, e.g., hydroxyzine, diphenhydramine; nonsedating oral antihistamines for daytime pruritus, e.g., OTC loratadine, cetirizine
  6. Educate regarding medication dosage, signs of irritation, sensitivity
  7. Educate regarding characteristics of condition, cause, treatment prognosis, and recurrence
  8. Refer to dermatologist for evaluation if condition does not improve in 2 days or if becomes more severe at any time

Erythema Multiforme Minor

- Definition: Acute condition of the skin involving hypersensitivity reaction characterized by multimorphology skin and mucous membrane eruptions; lasts approximately 2 to 3 weeks with spontaneous resolution
- Etiology/Incidence
  1. Hypersensitivity caused by exposure to variety of substances
     a. Infectious organisms—most common are enteroviruses, *Mycoplasma pneumoniae*, and herpes simplex, especially in recurrent conditions
     b. Drugs—most common are barbiturates, sulfa and penicillin drugs
     c. Other substances—food reactions
  2. More common in adults; however, approximately 20% of cases are in children and adolescents
  3. Recurrent episodes occur in approximately one third of cases
- Signs and Symptoms
  1. Itching may be present
  2. Pain, especially in mouth
  3. Redness and swelling may present with blisters and/or ulcers on hands, elbows, knees, ankles, feet, eyes, lips, mouth
  4. Develop in crops over period of 1 to 2 weeks with each crop lasting 1 week
- Differential Diagnosis
  1. Allergic vasculitis
  2. Kawasaki disease
  3. Urticaria
  4. Varicella or other viral infections
- Physical Findings
  1. Pruritus and pain may be present at site of lesions, especially those in oral cavity
  2. Erythema and edema with lesions progressing from macules to papules, vesicles, bullae, and petechiae
  3. Lesions occur on bilateral exposed areas predominately—includes hands, elbows, knees, ankles, feet, eyes, lips, oral mucous membranes, tongue, oral cavity, and less commonly on chest and trunk
  4. Lesions develop in crops over period of 1 to 2 weeks with each crop lasting 1 week
  5. Targetoid or "bull's-eye" lesions may be present, which have three distinct characteristics—a necrotic or vesicular center, a pale middle macular ring, and an outer erythematous peripheral ring

6. Lasts from 2 to 3 weeks with spontaneous resolution
- Diagnostic Tests/Findings
  1. Chest radiograph to rule out *Mycoplasma pneumoniae*
  2. Tzanck test to rule out herpes simplex
- Management/Treatment
  1. Obtain detailed history of onset, duration, severity, and progression of symptoms and possible precipitating factors
  2. Describe and monitor lesions in terms of morphology/structure, size, shape, number, color, location, distribution
  3. Cool compresses for pain and pruritus
  4. Antihistamines for nocturnal pruritus, e.g., hydroxyzine, diphenhydramine; nonsedating antihistamines for daytime pruritus, e.g., OTC loratadine and cetirizine
  5. Oral analgesics for generalized pain, e.g., acetaminophen
  6. Topical anesthetics and mouthwashes for oral lesions, e.g., lidocaine
  7. Maintain hydration with cool fluids, e.g., water, nonacidic juices
  8. Determine underlying trigger and remove or treat as indicated
  9. Educate regarding medication dosages, signs of irritation, sensitivity
  10. Educate regarding characteristics of condition, cause, prognosis, and recurrence
  11. Refer for dermatologist evaluation if:
      a. Condition does not improve
      b. Systemic symptoms of fever and malaise develop

Erythema Multiforme Major (Stevens-Johnson Syndrome)

- Definition: Skin condition involving hypersensitivity reaction characterized by multimorphology mucous membrane and skin eruptions with associated systemic involvement; also known as Stevens-Johnson syndrome
- Etiology/Incidence
  1. Hypersensitivity caused by exposure to a variety of substances
     a. Infectious organisms—most common are enteroviruses, *Mycoplasma pneumoniae*, and herpes simplex, especially in recurrent conditions
     b. Drugs—most common are barbiturates, sulfa, and penicillin
     c. Other substances—food reactions
  2. More common in adults; however, approximately 20% of cases are in children and adolescents
  3. Recurrent episodes occur in approximately one third of the cases
  4. Can be life-threatening; approximately 5% mortality of diagnosed cases
- Signs and Symptoms
  1. Fever, fatigue, sore throat, headache, nausea, vomiting, diarrhea, muscle pain, and/or joint pain

2. Skin rash develops in 2 to 3 days after generalized symptoms
   a. Areas of erythema and edema
   b. Variety of skin reactions on hands, elbows, knees, ankles, feet, eyes, lips, mouth, chest, and/or trunk
3. Pruritus may be present
4. Pain, especially in mouth
- Differential Diagnosis
  1. Gingivostomatitis
  2. Pemphigus
  3. Toxic epidermal necrolysis
  4. Urticaria
  5. Varicella
  6. Staphylococcal scalded skin syndrome
- Physical Findings
  1. Sudden onset of prodromal state—high temperature, malaise, weakness
  2. Multimorphology rash develops in progressive pattern
     a. Macular erythematous with edematous areas
     b. Progress to papules, vesicles, erosions, and petechiae
  3. Pruritus and pain, especially lesions in oral cavity
  4. Lesions occur on bilateral exposed areas predominately—includes hands, elbows, knees, ankles, feet, eyes, lips, oral mucous membranes, tongue; less common on chest and trunk
  5. Targetoid or herald lesions may be present, which have three distinct characteristics—necrotic or vesicular center, pale middle macular ring, and an outer erythematous peripheral ring
  6. Lesions develop in crops over period of 1 to 2 weeks with each crop lasting 1 week
  7. Condition may progress to more severe stage involving the respiratory, renal, and gastrointestinal systems
- Diagnostic Tests/Findings
  1. Chest radiograph to rule out *Mycoplasma pneumoniae*
  2. Tzanck to rule out herpes simplex
  3. Skin biopsy to confirm diagnosis
- Management/Treatment
  1. Obtain detailed history of onset, duration, severity, and progression of symptoms and possible precipitating factors
  2. Describe and monitor lesions in terms of morphology/structure, size, shape, number, color, location, distribution
  3. Immediate dermatologist referral for evaluation and hospitalization due to potential life-threatening situation
  4. Educate regarding characteristics of condition, cause, and prognosis

Urticaria (Hives)

- Definition: Acute or chronic condition of the skin involving an allergic hypersensitivity reaction characterized by transient pale or skin-colored skin lesions

- Etiology/Incidence
  1. Caused by release of histamine as reaction to immune system's response to an allergen
     a. Foods
     b. Temperature changes of heat and cold
     c. Viral infections
     d. Vibrations and scratching
     e. Emotional elation or stress
     f. Insect bites
     g. Materials and fabrics
  2. Symptoms may last for minutes or for up to 24 hours after initial exposure to antigen
  3. Recurrences are frequent with reexposure to allergen; response is varied and may become chronic
- Signs and Symptoms
  1. Intense generalized and localized pruritus
  2. Mild erythema and edema of irregular-shaped wheals—may involve eyelids, lips, hands, feet, mouth, and genitalia
- Differential Diagnosis
  1. Atopic dermatitis
  2. Contact dermatitis
  3. Erythema multiforme
- Physical Findings
  1. Intense generalized and localized pruritus at site of lesions
  2. Mild erythema and swelling with irregular-shaped wheals on any skin surface
     a. May have edema of eyelids, lips, hands, feet, and genitalia
     b. May have edema and erythema of mucous membranes
  3. Individual lesions range in size from under 1 cm to over 15 cm
  4. Distribution pattern is generalized and scattered
  5. Become more pronounced with heat
  6. Will blanch with pressure
  7. Excoriation due to scratching secondary to severe pruritus
- Diagnostic Tests/Findings: No tests confirm condition
- Management/Treatment
  1. Obtain detailed history of onset, duration, severity, and progression of symptoms and possible precipitating factors
  2. Describe and monitor lesions in terms of morphology/structure, size, shape, number, color, location, distribution
  3. Discontinue contact with allergen if known sensitivity
  4. Cool compresses of Burrow's solution for comfort
  5. Topical steroids to reduce immune response and pruritus, e.g., hydrocortisone, triamcinolone
  6. Oral steroids for severe and extensive reactions, e.g., prednisone
  7. Sedating oral antihistamines for nocturnal pruritus, e.g., hydroxyzine, diphenhydramine; OTC nonsedating antihistamines for daytime pruritus, e.g., cetirizine or loratadine
  8. Educate regarding characteristics of condition
  9. Educate regarding medication dosages, signs of irritation, sensitivity
  10. Teach measures for prevention, e.g., avoid known allergens and overheating
  11. Refer to dermatologist for evaluation
      a. If acute episode does not improve
      b. Consideration of skin testing for hypersensitivities after acute episode resolves

☐ QUESTIONS

Select the best answer.

1. J. D. is a postterm infant with lesions of varying morphology, including wheals, vesicles, and pustules, on her trunk. You suspect J. D. has:
   a. Cutis marmorata
   b. Erythema toxicum neonatorum
   c. Milia
   d. Contact dermatitis

2. In order to confirm your diagnosis of J. D., you order a Wright's stained smear. If your diagnosis is correct, what are the expected results of the smear?
   a. Presence of eosinophils
   b. Presence of neutrophils
   c. Presence of keratinous material
   d. Presence of *Staphylococcus* bacteria

3. In addition to monitoring the skin for any changes, what is the best management for J. D.?
   a. Topical antibiotics on lesions
   b. Topical steroids on lesions
   c. A moisturizer on lesions
   d. No treatment necessary since J. D.'s condition will resolve spontaneously in 5 to 7 days

4. You examine C. C., a newborn, and observe numerous white papular lesions on the cheeks, forehead, and nose. You suspect either milia or neonatal acne. Which physical finding helps to confirm a diagnosis of milia?
   a. Papular lesions are intermixed with pale yellow macules
   b. Papular lesions have an erythematous circular ring at the base
   c. Papular lesions are surrounded by lacy-blue area with erythematous mottling
   d. Papular lesions, yellow in color, are observed on the hard palate

5. Newborn W. R. has a vascular lesion that will not fade as she gets older. What is your diagnosis?
   a. Salmon patch
   b. Capillary hemangioma
   c. Café au lait spot
   d. Port-wine stain (nevus flammeus)

6. W. R.'s parents are concerned about her appearance and the psychological effect on their daughter as she becomes aware of her condition. In educating the parents, you tell them about several options. Which

of the following is not an appropriate management or treatment consideration for W. R.?

 a. Application of topical steroids to the affected area to prevent pruritus
 b. Camouflage of affected area with cosmetics
 c. Pulsed laser treatment of affected area
 d. Counseling for psychological concerns

7. Which condition is thought to be more apparent in darker-skinned individuals or during the summer months?

 a. Tinea corporis
 b. Psoriasis
 c. Pityriasis alba
 d. Pityriasis rosea

8. J. R., an 8-year-old boy, has scaly, hyperpigmented lesions in a "fir tree" distribution, predominately on his trunk. One lesion on the buttocks is larger than all the other lesions and measures 4 cm in diameter. What is your likely diagnosis?

 a. Psoriasis
 b. Eczema
 c. Pityriasis alba
 d. Pityriasis rosea

9. What symptom is commonly experienced in J. R.'s condition?

 a. Pruritus
 b. Pain at site of lesions
 c. Nausea
 d. Headache

10. What management would you not recommend for J. R. with his condition?

 a. Cool bath or cool compresses to lesions
 b. Topical steroids to lesions
 c. Oral antibiotics
 d. Monitored and controlled daily sunlight exposure

11. You have diagnosed D. L. with acute atopic dermatitis. Which of the following is not correct regarding the incidence of this condition?

 a. D. L. is most likely an infant
 b. D. L. has a greater chance of developing asthma later in childhood than the average individual
 c. D. L. has a greater chance of developing malignant melanoma in adulthood than the average individual
 d. D. L. has a condition associated with familial predisposition

12. Which of the following management measures or treatments would you not recommend for D. L.?

 a. Topical steroids to affected areas
 b. Wet compresses to affected skin areas
 c. Maintain a dry, warm environment
 d. Eliminate all substances that dry the skin

13. In addition to having atopic dermatitis, you have diagnosed D. L. with a secondary bacterial infection at the site of several lesions. What is the best management for the infection?

 a. Topical antibiotics to affected areas
 b. Oral antibiotics

 c. Hot compresses to affected areas
 d. Monitored and controlled daily sun exposure until lesions resolve

14. You see B. D. for the first time at age 6 weeks. B. D. has a bright red, raised, rubbery lesion of irregular shape and 2 cm in diameter on the occiput. What condition do you suspect B. D. has?

 a. Malignant melanoma
 b. Port-wine stain
 c. Capillary hemangioma
 d. Burn

15. Which of the following is not characteristic of the lesion B. D. has?

 a. It was not present at birth; however, B. D.'s mother noticed the site was blanched.
 b. It will continue to grow for the first 9 to 12 months of B. D.'s life.
 c. It will begin to gradually resolve when B. D. is between 12 and 15 months of age.
 d. It is expected to completely resolve by the time B. D. is 10 years old.

16. You notice 10 macular tan lesions of varying sizes on D. D. and refer him for a medical evaluation to rule out neurofibromatosis or Albright syndrome. What kind of lesion does D. D. have?

 a. Malignant melanoma
 b. Café au lait spots
 c. Mongolian spots
 d. Vitiligo

17. What is characteristic of the lesion that D. D. has?

 a. They are more common in Caucasians than in dark-skinned individuals.
 b. They are more common in males than in females.
 c. Lesions can be present at birth; however, more lesions may develop at any age.
 d. Lesions usually fade spontaneously and completely resolve in adult life.

18. A. F. was diagnosed with pityriasis alba. Which of the following is proper management of A. F.'s condition?

 a. Bland moisturizers to reduce overdrying
 b. Topical steroids to the affected areas
 c. Exposure of affected areas to short periods of sunlight each day
 d. Burrow's wet compresses to affected areas

19. Patient education is a major part of the PNP's role. What would you teach A. F. and her parent regarding the progress and prognosis of pityriasis alba?

 a. A. F. will continue to develop lesions for the rest of her life.
 b. A. F.'s condition should fade appreciably in 3 to 4 months.
 c. A. F.'s condition is permanent, and affected areas will not repigment.
 d. A. F.'s condition will resolve completely; however, the affected areas can become slightly reddened when exposed to sunlight.

20. Malignant melanoma is a form of much dreaded skin cancer. Which of the following is not characteristic of this condition?
    a. Occurs in all ethnic groups but more commonly in light-skinned individuals
    b. Severe sunburn or excessive exposure to sunlight before the age of 10 years predisposes developing melanoma later in childhood or in adult life
    c. Spreads through the lymphatic system and invades other distant skin surfaces and organs
    d. Spreads primarily by invading skin surfaces that surround the major lesion

21. Which of the following does not characterize the lesion of malignant melanoma?
    a. Irregular, asymmetrical nodule with blurred borders
    b. Raised with distinct, symmetrical borders
    c. Uneven coloring in which blue, black, brown, tan, and red may all be present in the same lesion
    d. Bleeding, ulceration in later stages

22. Patient education regarding prevention of malignant melanoma is essential. Which of the following is not considered best prevention education?
    a. Avoid sunlight, especially during the hours of 9:00 a.m. to 1:00 p.m.
    b. Avoid sun tanning lamps
    c. Use cover-up clothing, hats, and sunglasses
    d. Use sunblocks that protect against ultraviolet exposure with SPF 30

23. You suspect M. N. has chronic psoriasis. Which of the following is characteristic of her lesions if she has psoriasis vulgaris?
    a. Scaly erythematous patches and plaques 3 to 10 mm in diameter
    b. Round or oval in shape
    c. Large scaly silver-white plaque 5 to 10 cm in diameter
    d. Located mainly on her trunk

24. M. N.'s condition of psoriasis is common in approximately 33% of children. Which of the following is not correct regarding the etiology or incidence of this condition?
    a. Occurs more commonly in dark-skinned ethnic individuals
    b. Associated with constant rubbing or trauma to exposed affected areas such as elbows
    c. Associated with overproduction of epithelial cells
    d. Associated with epithelial cells that migrate to the skin surface much more quickly than normal

25. What would you not advise regarding the management or treatment of M. N.'s condition?
    a. Excise lesions
    b. Apply topical steroids
    c. Apply mineral oil and moisturizers
    d. Expose to monitored short periods of sunlight

26. You have diagnosed Jale as having contact dermatitis. Which symptom is most characteristic of his condition?
    a. Headache
    b. Difficulty breathing

c. Pruritus at site of affected areas
    d. Pain at site of affected areas

27. Which of the following is not characteristic of Jale's condition?
    a. He has hypersensitivity to a substance within his environment when direct contact is made.
    b. He may experience a delayed reaction of several days with reexposure to an allergen.
    c. His dermatitis may be caused by direct contact with topical medications, soaps, cosmetics, fabrics, and plants.
    d. Typical response is redness and edema at the site of contact, which may progress to papules and vesicles.

28. What would you not recommend as management and treatment of Jale's condition?
    a. Skin testing during the acute episode to determine whether Jale has an allergy
    b. Cool compresses of Burrow's solution to affected areas
    c. Topical steroids to affected areas for 5 days
    d. Oral antihistamines

29. Seborrhea dermatitis is common in both infants and adolescents. Which of the following is not correct of this condition?
    a. Can cause irritating pigment changes to include hyperpigmentation and hypopigmentation
    b. Is associated with an overproduction of sebum in areas abundant with sebaceous glands
    c. The condition in infants is known as "cradle cap" in which lesions have erythematous base with yellow crusted areas and greasy scales
    d. The condition in adolescents is known as acne with comedones and papular and pustular lesions

30. What is the best treatment of seborrhea in the infant?
    a. Mineral oil to loosen crusts prior to washing affected areas with a nonperfumed baby shampoo
    b. Topical antibiotics
    c. Oral antibiotics for severe cases
    d. Oral steroids for severe cases

31. You are evaluating F. P., age 3 years, who acutely sustained a burn when she pulled a pan of boiling water onto herself within the past hour. Since burns are classified according to the depth of injury to the skin layers and the amount of area involved, how would you rate the burn if 5% of her body surface is burned and the burned area involves the epidermis and upper part of the dermis?
    a. She has minor first- and second-degree burns
    b. She has a major second-degree burn
    c. She has a major full-thickness burn
    d. She has major first- and second-degree burns

32. F. P.'s burn should appear:
    a. Dry, with mild edema and erythema
    b. As dry whitish areas that blanch with pressure
    c. As dry whitish to brownish areas with edema
    d. Moist with edema, erythema, and a few vesicles

33. What is the best treatment for F. P.'s burn?
    a. Warm compresses to affected areas and mild analgesic for discomfort
    b. Topical emollients to affected areas
    c. Topical steroids to affected areas
    d. Refer for urgent treatment in an ED
34. Jerry has been diagnosed as having folliculitis, an inflammatory condition involving the pilosebaceous follicle. What is the most common cause of this condition?
    a. *Microsporum canis* tinea
    b. Poxvirus
    c. *Staphylococcus aureus*
    d. *Streptococcus* group A
35. Jerry has a condition that most commonly occurs on which body surface?
    a. Neck and scalp
    b. Upper arms
    c. Chest and abdomen
    d. Legs
36. You order a culture and the results confirm that Jerry's condition is caused by the most common organism for this condition. What treatment do you prescribe?
    a. Oral penicillin
    b. Dicloxacillin
    c. Tinactin
    d. Tretinoin
37. Sandra, age 12 years, has several vesicles and honey-colored crusted lesions on her face above the right nares. She has a history of having had a scratch in the same area several days ago. What condition do you suspect?
    a. Acne
    b. Impetigo
    c. Herpes simplex
    d. Eczema
38. Judy, age 15 years, has been diagnosed as having acne. Which of the following is not true of this condition?
    a. Poor hygiene is the primary cause of acne.
    b. Acne is associated with increased androgenic hormonal activity.
    c. Females can have a "cyclic" component to their acne.
    d. Severe acne having a later onset in puberty is more common among males.
39. Judy has a history of remission and exacerbation of acne that has followed the pattern of menses for 2 years. However, the condition over the last 6 months has worsened to a moderate degree of severity and has been chronic and persistent. You prescribe antibiotic therapy. Which of the following antibiotics would you not consider?
    a. Topical clindamycin
    b. Oral erythromycin
    c. Oral minocycline
    d. Oral tetracycline
40. K. C., age 13 years, has several firm, small (2-mm), white or skin-colored umbilicated papules on her neck. The lesions have been present for 3 months and have increased in number. What is your diagnosis?
    a. Acne
    b. Molluscum contagiosum
    c. Warts
    d. Cellulitis
41. What is the cause of K. C.'s condition?
    a. *Microsporum canis* tinea
    b. Poxvirus
    c. *Staphylococcus aureus*
    d. *Streptococcus* group A
42. Which treatment would you not recommend for K. C.'s condition?
    a. Curettage lesions
    b. Oral antibiotics
    c. Observation
    d. Topical imiquimod
43. Paul has four superficial lesions on his anterior lower abdomen of 1 week duration. The lesions are 4 cm in diameter, scaly, irregular-shaped plaques with skin-colored centers and erythematous borders. The affected areas are slightly pruritic. What condition do you suspect Paul has?
    a. Psoriasis
    b. Eczema
    c. Tinea corporis
    d. Pityriasis rosea
44. You see Paul after 8 weeks of treatment with a topical antifungal preparation. The original lesions have almost resolved; however, the condition has worsened with the development of several other larger lesions on the abdomen and groin area. Which of the following would you not consider?
    a. Oral antifungal medication, griseofulvin
    b. Topical antibiotic preparation
    c. Continuing with the topical antifungal applications
    d. Educating again regarding not sharing personal items
45. Dale, age 7 years, is complaining of pain and burning on his right leg, where you observe two small red puncture marks surrounded by a blanched area with an erythematous border. He had been playing with his dog all morning outside in a grassy wooded area near his home and was wearing shorts. You suspect he has been bitten by which insect?
    a. Mosquito
    b. Bee
    c. Brown recluse spider
    d. Black widow spider
46. Which of the following is not true of insect stings from bees, wasps, and fire ants?
    a. Greater reaction of hypersensitivity occurs most often with the initial exposure than with subsequent exposures.
    b. For mild reactions, applying cool compresses to the site of injury is the usual management.
    c. Insect stings occur more often during the spring and summer months.
    d. Most stings occur in self-defense when the nonaggressive insect feels threatened or irritated.

47. You diagnose W. A. with scabies. Which of the following is not characteristic of this condition?
    a. He has several erythematous papular, pustular, and crusted lesions on his face.
    b. He has several excoriated scratched areas around the umbilicus and waist area.
    c. He has several curved lines approximately 4 mm in length with a papule at the proximal end.
    d. He complains of severe pruritus that is worse at night.

48. Which of the following is not recommended as a management and treatment strategy for W. A.?
    a. Put nonwashable items in a plastic bag and store for 1 week.
    b. Prescribe topical antifungal applications.
    c. Prescribe topical antiparasitics.
    d. Prescribe topical steroids and/or oral antihistamines for pruritus.

49. Pediculosis is a highly communicable, common condition in children. Which of the following is not correct of *Pediculus humanus*?
    a. An insect that does not fly or jump
    b. Gravid females lay ova in seams of clothing
    c. Likes hairy areas of the body better than the nonhairy body surfaces
    d. Same medication used for scabies may be used to effectively eradicate this species

50. Hypersensitivity may occur to a variety of substances, causing a variety of reactions. It is important to determine whether the body's hypersensitivity reaction will cause erythema multiforme condition. Which of the following is not typical of the erythema multiforme reaction?
    a. Target "bulls-eye" lesion with a necrotic center surrounded by a pale macular middle area and then by an erythematous peripheral ring
    b. Itching at site of affected skin areas
    c. Pain at site of affected areas, especially in the oral cavity
    d. Lesions that all have the same morphology on the trunk

51. You see D. Y. in your clinic and suspect she has a form of erythema multiforme. Erythema multiforme minor must be differentiated from erythema multiforme major. Which of the following is the most important confirming evidence for making a diagnosis of erythema multiforme major?
    a. Presence of deeper lesions within the dermis
    b. Presence of lesions on the exposed areas of the body
    c. Presence of pustules, indicating a secondary infectious process
    d. Occurrence of prodromal systemic symptoms of fever, malaise, sore throat, headache, nausea, and/or vomiting

52. You suspect D. Y. has erythema multiforme major. What treatment or management is most indicated?
    a. Prescribe topical antibiotics because of secondary infection
    b. Prescribe topical steroids applied to lesions for pruritus
    c. Refer for medical evaluation
    d. No treatment is indicated because the condition will resolve spontaneously in 1 week

53. Urticaria is a hypersensitivity allergic reaction to a variety of substances and agents. You suspect W. P. has urticaria because of the typical morphology of lesions on her trunk and arms, which are:
    a. Erythematous papules
    b. Vesicles
    c. Pustules
    d. Wheals

54. During W. P.'s acute episode of urticaria, which of the following is not considered an appropriate management or treatment measure?
    a. Oral antibiotics to prevent secondary infection
    b. Oral antihistamines for pruritus
    c. Topical steroids to affected areas to reduce the immune response
    d. Cool compresses to affected areas

55. A 7-year-old African American female presents with several hyperkeratotic raised, periungual lesions on the two middle fingers of her left hand. She has a history of nail biting. The most likely diagnosis is:
    a. Impetigo
    b. Molluscum contagiosum
    c. Verruca vulgaris
    d. Herpetic whitlow

56. Which of the following secondary skin changes is not associated with atopic dermatitis?
    a. Lichenification
    b. Striae
    c. Pigment changes
    d. Excoriations

57. In infants, the lesions associated with atopic dermatitis are most likely to be distributed on the:
    a. Cheeks and forehead
    b. Wrists and ankles
    c. Antecubital and popliteal fossae
    d. Flexural surfaces

58. During your newborn examination of K. L., you note a generalized lacy reticulated blue discoloration. This clinical presentation describes:
    a. Harlequin color change
    b. Mongolian spots
    c. Blue nevus
    d. Cutis marmorata

59. Mrs. Franklin is concerned about a light pink lesion on the back of 2-month-old Aaron's neck that darkens with crying. This description is consistent with:
    a. Sturge-Weber disease
    b. Salmon patch

c. Port-wine stain

d. Hemangioma

60. D. M., 7 months old, presents with a beefy red macular-papular rash in the diaper area with satellite lesions on the abdomen. The appropriate treatment would be:

a. Clotrimazole

b. A & D ointment

c. Gentian violet 1% to 2%

d. Cornstarch

Questions 61 and 62 refer to the following scenario.

The mother of 4-month-old T. W. states that the infant has been irritable and has not been sleeping well. During the physical examination, you note papular lesions on his feet and erythematous papules over his back.

61. To confirm your suspicion of scabies, you would order a:

a. Wood's lamp examination

b. Microscopic skin scraping

c. KOH preparation of skin scraping

d. Skin culture

62. Having confirmed the diagnosis of scabies in T. W., the treatment of choice would be:

a. Permethrin 5%

b. Lindane 1%

c. Sulfur ointment 6%

d. Crotamiton 10%

63. Which of the following statements regarding treatment of pediculosis capitis is true?

a. Carpeting and furniture must be shampooed and sprayed with a pediculicide.

b. Nonwashable items that have come into contact with an infected person should be sealed in plastic bags for 2 to 4 weeks.

c. Hair must be trimmed close to the scalp to ensure elimination of nits.

d. Frequent shampooing with permethrin 1% will prevent reinfestation.

64. Mrs. J. brings her 6-year-old son in because of "hives" that she describes as a red, raised rash. Which finding would support a diagnosis of erythema multiforme rather than urticaria?

a. Lesions that blanch with pressure

b. Eyelid edema

c. Lesions that are present for more than 24 hours

d. Intense pruritus

65. When examining 7-month-old R. V., you note red scaly plaques in his diaper area, particularly in the inguinal folds, with satellite lesions on his abdomen. The appropriate treatment would be:

a. Petrolatum/lanolin ointment

b. Petroleum jelly

c. Zinc oxide

d. Nystatin

Questions 66, 67, and 68 refer to the following scenario.

During 15-year-old N. M.'s routine physical examination, she complains of getting pimples all the time. You note open and closed comedones over her forehead and chin. There are more than 15 papules and pustules, but no cysts.

66. N. M.'s clinical presentation is consistent with:

a. Comedonal acne

b. Mild acne

c. Moderate acne

d. Severe acne

67. Which medication is the appropriate choice?

a. Antiandrogens

b. Isotretinoin

c. Minocycline

d. Corticosteroids

68. Which of the following statements is not consistent with an appropriate management plan for acne?

a. Improvement with use of keratolytic agents should occur within 4 to 6 weeks.

b. Facial scrubs are recommended before applying topical antibiotics.

c. Noncomedogenic moisturizers and cosmetics may be used.

d. Sunscreens should always be used in conjunction with retinoic acid.

69. H. B. is 2 days old. Her mother calls and reports a rash consisting of redness with yellow-white "bumps" all over her body except for the palms and soles. The infant most likely has:

a. Erythema toxicum

b. Transient neonatal pustular melanosis

c. Molluscum contagiosum

d. Milia

70. D. J. is a 4-year-old African American child with a depigmented macular lesion on his forehead. The lesion has sharp borders. No scales are present. The most appropriate treatment would be:

a. 1% hydrocortisone

b. Alpha hydroxy acid

c. Ketoconazole

d. Silver sulfadiazine

71. While examining 7-year-old S. R.'s scalp, you note three small patches of hair loss. Broken hair is present, as is erythema and scaling. On the basis of this information, which of the following diagnoses is most likely?

a. Tinea capitis

b. Traction alopecia

c. Trichotillomania

d. Alopecia areata

☐ ANSWERS AND RATIONALES

1. B: Transient, benign, self-limited skin rash with lesions of varied morphology; erythematous macules; wheals, vesicles, and pustules in 50–60% of all newborns. Lesions usually arise from erythematous base, with macular erythema fading within 2 to 3 days. Occurs predominately on the trunk; however, may occur anywhere on body except soles and palms.

2. A: Wright's stained smear of pustules identifies predominance of 90% eosinophils rather than neutrophils, which rules out neonatal pustular melanosis.

3. D: No treatment is necessary because this is benign and self-limiting.

4. D: In milia there is an oral counterpart of yellow, papular lesions on hard palate known as Epstein's pearls, which does not occur in neonatal acne.

5. D: Port-wine stains are irregular dark red or purple macular lesions occurring on any body surface, predominately on face and head, that never fade and become thickened and raised in adulthood.

6. A: Management consists of referral for dermatologist evaluation for consideration of pulsed dye laser treatment, which is recommended to start as early as possible in infancy and definitely before 1 year of age. The area may be camouflaged later in childhood with water-resistant cosmetics. Using a steroid cream is not indicated.

7. C: Pityriasis alba is more apparent in darker-skinned populations and occurs in warmer months.

8. D: Pityriasis rosea is an acquired common mild inflammatory condition characterized by scaly, hypopigmented, and hyperpigmented lesions predominately on the trunk, upper arms, and upper thighs. Also has a "herald" patch of 1 cm to 5 cm on trunk or buttocks.

9. A: The most common symptom is periodic pruritus of varying degrees of severity especially at onset.

10. C: Management does not consist of antibiotics but rather topical calamine lotion on lesions, oral antipruritic agents for severe pruritus (for example, diphenhydramine), cool bath or compresses on lesions, and low-potency steroid creams.

11. C: Infants, children, and adolescents with atopic dermatitis are not more likely to develop malignant melanoma as adults.

12. C: Atopic dermatitis worsens with sweating and temperature extremes, so a dry and warm environment makes symptoms worse.

13. B: For secondary infections, if present, treat with oral antibiotics, for example, Bactrim, cefadroxil, cephalexin, and clindamycin.

14. C: Capillary hemangiomas are bright red or blue-red nodular tumors of varying sizes and shapes with a rubbery and rough surface that occur predominately on the head and face.

15. B: Capillary hemangiomas often are not present at birth; however, the area of eventual lesion is blanched or slightly colored. They grow quickly within 2 to 4 weeks to a red or blue-red, protuberant, rubbery nodule or plaque, with the most growth in the first 6 months. There is a gradual reduction in proliferation usually beginning between 9 and 12 months.

16. B: Café au lait spots are light to medium brown pigmented macular lesions of varying sizes and shapes found anywhere on the body; they are the color of coffee with milk, from which the name is derived. If there are six or more lesions, this condition may be associated with neurofibromatosis or Albright syndrome.

17. C: Café au lait spots are usually present at birth; however, they may develop at any age. Twenty percent of darker-skinned populations have these lesions.

18. A: The treatment for pityriasis alba is the use of bland moisturizer to reduce overdrying.

19. B: Pityriasis alba resolves spontaneously in 3 to 4 months. You can also educate the parent regarding characteristics and expected prognoses.

20. D: Malignant melanoma is characterized by being more common in females from birth to 40 years of age and in light-skinned individuals. Severe sunburn or excessive exposure to the sun before the age of 10 years predisposes developing melanoma later in childhood or in adult life. Malignant melanoma is spread through the lymphatic system and invades other skin surfaces and organs. It is not spread by invading skin surfaces that surround the major lesion.

21. B: Malignant melanoma is not characterized by having raised distinct, symmetrical borders. They can be irregular, asymmetrical, with uneven coloring and may bleed.

22. A: Avoiding sunlight is not the best prevention. Avoiding tanning beds and using cover-ups, hats, sunglasses, and sunscreen are the best prevention.

23. C: Chronic psoriasis is characterized by erythematous plaques with silver-gray-white scaly plaques occurring predominately on the elbows and knees.

24. A: Psoriasis is more common in light-skinned than in dark-skinned populations. It also occurs in those with a positive family history: approximately one third of cases is strongly suggestive of a genetic connection.

25. A: Management does not consist of excising the lesions. The use of topical steroids, mineral oil, and moisturizers may help with lesions. Decreasing exposure to direct sunlight also is part of the management.

26. C: The most common characteristic of contact dermatitis is pruritus with varying degrees of intensity.

27. B: Contact dermatitis is caused by hypersensitivity to an allergen with reexposure—allergic response usually occurs within 24 hours due to prior sensitization. However, numerous substances are associated with producing hypersensitivity reactions in sensitive individuals, with the most common including perfumes, soaps, cosmetics, and fabric dyes.

28. A: Treatment for contact dermatitis consists of cool compresses with Burrow's solution, oral antihistamines, and topical steroids. Skin testing during an acute episode is not recommended.

29. D: Seborrhea dermatitis in newborns and infants is characterized by areas of underlying erythema with yellow crusts and greasy scaling on scalp and face; in more severe cases lesions may be present on trunk and in diaper area. Adolescent will have white flakes

and greasy scaling on scalp, forehead, eyebrows, and face.

30. A: For infants, shampoo and wash affected areas with a nonperfumed baby shampoo or baby wash and use mineral oil with brushing to loosen crusts prior to washing.

31. D: Burns are classified according to depth of injury to skin layers. First-degree/superficial burns involve the epidermis layer only. Second-degree/partial-thickness burns involve the epidermis and part of the dermis, which may be superficial dermis or deep dermis.

32. D: First- and second-degree burns are red, swollen, moist, and blistered areas with tenderness.

33. D: For second-degree burns, evaluation at a tertiary care center is the recommendation.

34. C: The most common cause of folliculitis is *Staphylococcus aureus*; less commonly it is caused by *Streptococcus* bacteria.

35. A: Folliculitis most commonly occurs on localized areas of erythema and edema with papular or pustular lesions on face, scalp, neck, buttocks, and other areas.

36. B: Treatment for folliculitis caused by staph infection is with dicloxacillin.

37. B: Impetigo is caused by a localized bacterial infection of skin often precipitated by insect bites (spider, mosquito, flea) or other trauma that breaks protective skin barrier; it predominately involves face and less commonly other body surfaces, including perineum. Vesicles that erupt result in honey-colored serous crusts with erosion of the epidermis.

38. A: Proven factors that may contribute to acne development are increased androgenic hormonal influence, positive family history, and stress. Unproven factors with questionable and unsubstantiated contribution are food—nuts, eggs, cheese, chocolate, milk—and poor hygiene.

39. B: In moderate chronic acne, oral antibiotics may be recommended. The choice of antibiotics is tetracycline, doxycycline, or minocycline.

40. B: Molluscum contagiosum is characterized by a self-limiting skin condition characterized by waxy, firm papules that may occur on any skin surface but predominately on the face, axillae, abdomen, and arms.

41. B: Molluscum contagiosum is caused by a poxvirus.

42. B: Molluscum contagiosum treatment does not consist of antibiotics but, with observation, at times consists of curettage of the lesions or topical imiquimod.

43. C: Tinea corporis lesions are characterized as scaly plaques of varying sizes from less than 5 mm to more than 3 cm with mild erythematous active borders. Lesions spread peripherally as they heal centrally and may be singular or several; numerous lesions are uncommon.

44. B: Treatment consists of topical antifungal medications, clotrimazole, miconazole, econazole, terbinafine, tolnaftate, naftifine, ciclopirox, or ketoconazole. Antibiotics are not indicated.

45. D: Spider bites are characterized by a dull burning or pain at site of bite with two red puncture marks surrounded by white area with bluish-red border.

46. A: With insect stings, hypersensitivity to venom develops after initial exposure, with more severe reactions upon subsequent exposures.

47. A: Scabies is characterized by intense pruritus—especially at night in older children and adolescents—red bumps, blisters, pustules, and small burrow marks that may be obliterated by scratch marks. The burrows are superficial, 2 to 8 mm long, linear, and curved with small papules at the proximal end; burrows may be obliterated by scratch and excoriation marks resulting from scratching.

48. B: Topical antifungal applications are not recommended for treatment of scabies. Treatment is using topical antiparasitics, antihistamines, or topical steroids along with storing nonwashables in a plastic bag for a week.

49. C: *Pediculus humanus* prefers less-hairy body surfaces.

50. D: Target or "bull's-eye" lesions may be present, which have three distinct characteristics—a necrotic or vesicular center, a pale middle macular ring, and an outer erythematous peripheral ring. Itching may be present, and pain may occur in the mouth. Lesions are not all the same size and morphology.

51. D: The key distinction between erythema multiforme (EM) major and EM minor is the occurrence of prodromal systemic symptoms of fever, malaise, sore throat, headache, nausea, and vomiting.

52. C: Patients with erythema multiforme (EM) major need immediate attention at a hospital for a full medical evaluation.

53. D: Urticarial lesions are consistent with wheals as their typical morphology.

54. A: Treatment for urticaria consists of oral antihistamines, topical steroids, and cool compresses. Oral antibiotics are not indicated for the treatment of urticaria.

55. C: Common warts are found most usually on fingers, hands, and feet in children and are often preceded by trauma such as nail biting or picking at cuticles.

56. B: Striae are skin areas that have been stretched, whereas the skin in atopic dermatitis is thickened, crusted, and hyperpigmented.

57. A: The infantile phase of atopic dermatitis follows a different distribution pattern than that associated with the childhood phase and may include the face, trunk, and extensor surfaces.

58. D: Mongolian spots and blue nevus have a bluish discoloration. Cutis marmorata is the only condition that is generalized. Harlequin color change is more red than pale.

59. B: A salmon patch is a flat, light pink to light red mark seen on the eyelid, glabella, or nape of neck that intensifies with crying.

60. A: The rash described is *Candida albicans* and should be treated with an antifungal agent.

61. B: Microscopic skin scrapings of burrows will reveal the mite, eggs, or feces if scabies are present. Although skin scrapings are not routinely done, they are definitive if there is any doubt of the diagnosis.

62. A: Permethrin is the only safe choice in this case. Lindane is contraindicated in infants younger than 6 months of age. Sulfur ointment and crotamiton are not as effective and are difficult to use.

63. B: Objects that cannot be washed should be sealed in plastic bags. Since eggs mature in 7 to 10 days, 2 to 4 weeks should be sufficient to prevent reinfestation. Frequent shampooing and close haircuts are unnecessary and may contribute to a feeling of shame and embarrassment. Environmental cleaning includes vacuuming, although sprays are not recommended.

64. C: Urticarial lesions tend to be pruritic and blanch with pressure but generally fade within a few hours. Due to the large number of mast cells present in the eyelids, edema is common with urticaria. The lesions of erythema multiforme are fixed and present for up to 2 to 3 weeks.

65. D: Petrolatum/lanolin ointment, petroleum jelly, and zinc oxide are all ointments that act as barriers to irritants such as urine and feces. The presence of satellite lesions indicates a *Candida* rash requiring an antifungal such as nystatin.

66. C: Mild acne is characterized by open and closed comedones and occasional pustules, whereas comedonal acne is limited to open and closed comedones only. Open and closed comedones, papules, and pustules characterize moderate acne. Severe acne, in addition to the lesions described above, also involves cysts.

67. C: Moderate acne includes open and closed comedones, papules, and pustules. Oral antibiotics are used to control moderate papulopustular acne in addition to topical keratolytics. Antiandrogens are not recommended. Corticosteroids may be used for more severe forms or the flare-ups associated with isotretinoin therapy.

68. B: Facial scrubs are not recommended and may exacerbate acne.

69. A: The location (all over the body) and type of lesion (papule as opposed to vesicle) are consistent with the rash seen in erythema toxicum.

70. A: The most likely diagnosis is vitiligo, an area of depigmented skin more common in African Americans. It responds to steroids 30% to 50% of the time. Antifungals, antibiotics, or keratolytics would be of no value.

71. A: Erythema, scaling, and broken hair are characteristic findings associated with tinea capitis. Traction alopecia may have associated erythema, but not scaling. Whereas neither trichotillomania nor alopecia areata are associated with erythema or scaling, only alopecia areata is noted for total hair loss.

☐ REFERENCE MATERIALS

■ Dermatology Terminology

Primary	Secondary
Macule	Scale
Nonpalpable	Crust ("scabbed")
Papule	Can be hemorrhagic
Palpable	Can be moist
<1 cm in diameter	Excoriation (scratched, rubbed)
Pustule	
Pus-filled papule	Oozing
Open comedone ("blackhead")	Erosion
	Ulceration
Closed comedone ("whitehead")	
Nodule	
Raised, palpable	
Deep; in dermis	
Tumor	
A large nodule	
Wheal	
Edematous	
Slightly raised	
Plaque	
Raised, flat topped	
>1 cm in diameter	
Vesicle	
Fluid-filled papule	
Cyst	
Raised	
Fluid-filled sac	
Bulla	
A cyst >1 cm in size	

DermAtlas. Adapted from Cohen, B.A., & Lehmann, C.U. (2009). *DermAtlas*. Retrieved from http://www.dermatlas.com/derm/

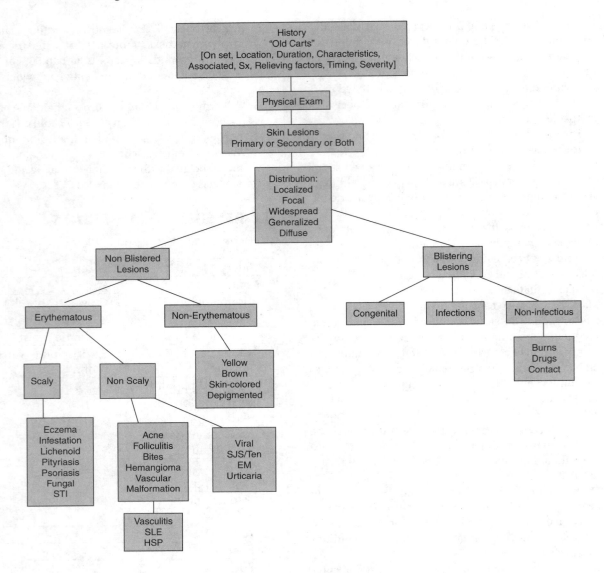

◻ BIBLIOGRAPHY

American Academy of Pediatrics. (2012). *Red book: 2012 report of the committee on infectious diseases* (29th ed.). Elk Grove Village, IL: Author.

Burns, C. E., Dunn, A. M., Brady, M. A., Starr, N. B., & Blosser, C. (2012). *Pediatric primary care: A handbook for nurse practitioners* (5th ed.) Philadelphia, PA: W. B. Saunders.

Cohen, B. A. (2013). *Pediatric dermatology* (4th ed.). Philadelphia, PA: Mosby Yearbook.

Cohen, B. A., & Lehmann, C. U. (2009). *DermAtlas.* Retrieved from http://www.dermatlas.com/derm/

Crowson, A. N., Magro, C. M., & Mihm, M. C. (2001). *The melanocytic proliferation: A comprehensive textbook of pigmented lesions.* New York, NY: Wiley.

Fitzpatrick, T., Johnson, R. A., Wolff, K., & Suurmond, D. (2013). *Color atlas and synopsis of clinical dermatology* (7th ed.). St. Louis, MO: McGraw-Hill.

Hay, W., Levin, M., Deterding, R., & Sondheimer, J. (2012). *Current diagnosis and treatment: Pediatric* (21st ed.). New York, NY: Lange Medical Books/McGraw-Hill.

Morrell, D. S., & Burkhart, D. N. (2009). Dermatologic therapies, part I. *Pediatric Annals, 38*(6), 300.

Morrell, D. S., & Burkhart, D. N. (2009). Dermatologic therapies, part II. *Pediatric Annals, 38*(7), 368–395.

Pomerantz, A. J., & O'Brien, T. (2007). *Nelson's instructions for pediatric patients.* St. Louis, MO: Elsevier.

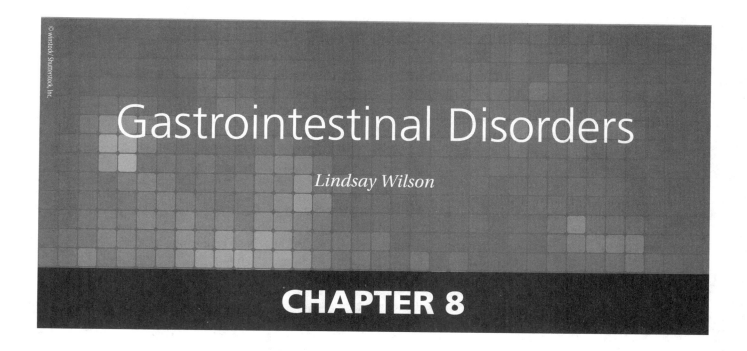

Gastrointestinal Disorders

Lindsay Wilson

CHAPTER 8

☐ GASTROESOPHAGEAL REFLUX (GER) IN INFANCY

- Definition: Reflux of gastric contents into esophagus as a result of immaturity of lower esophageal sphincter; normal physiologic process that occurs throughout the day in healthy infants, children, and adults; GER occurs during periods of transient relaxation of the lower esophageal sphincter
- Etiology/Incidence
  1. Etiology multifactorial
     a. Occurs in 50% of infants in first 3 months of life, 67% of 4-month-old infants, and 5% of 10- to 12-month-old infants
     b. Resolves as child becomes more upright and starts solids
     c. Often caused by overfeeding or incomplete burping
     d. Childhood diagnoses with higher incidence of gastroesophageal reflux disease (GERD) include neurologic impairment and delay, esophageal atresia, hiatal hernia, bronchopulmonary dysplasia, asthma, and cystic fibrosis
- Signs and Symptoms
  1. Physiologic GER
     a. Effortless, painless spitting up of varying amounts, often within 40 minutes of eating
     b. No choking or color changes
     c. Normal growth—growth chart is key
     d. Feeding history may indicate excessive intake; burp heard during vomiting may indicate incomplete burping

  2. Gastroesophageal reflux disease (GERD)
     a. Reflux may cause other physical complications, such as:
        (1) Failure to thrive (FTT)—caused by long-term, forceful regurgitation
        (2) Esophagitis—causing irritability, anemia, and guaiac-positive stools or hematemesis; dysphagia
        (3) Aspiration—pneumonia, wheezing, apnea
        (4) Sandifer syndrome—abnormal posturing of head and neck
     b. May be "silent GER"—no overt vomiting, but complications may be presenting symptom
     c. 60% show improvement by 16 months; 30% may remain symptomatic up to 4 years
- Differential Diagnosis
  1. Pyloric stenosis
  2. (Partial) anatomic obstruction
  3. Formula intolerance (cow's milk protein or soy allergy)
  4. Eosinophilic esophagitis
  5. Gastroenteritis
  6. Infections—urinary tract infection (UTI); otitis media (OM); pneumonia
  7. Increased intracranial pressure (ICP)/neurologic disorder
- Physical Findings
  1. May have wheezing or respiratory symptoms with aspiration
  2. Abdominal examination normal—no masses, olive, or peristaltic waves

3. Neurologic examination normal—no signs of increased ICP
- Diagnostic Tests/Findings
1. Diagnosis often made by observation and history; testing only to determine whether reflux is causing problems since vomiting indicates reflux
2. Upper gastrointestinal (UGI) to ligament of Treitz—only evaluates anatomy, not sensitive or specific for GER: use to rule out anomalies of the gastrointestinal (GI) tract such as malrotation
3. pH probe/impedance—indicates amount of reflux occurring; does not confirm diagnosis; can determine association of reflux with recurring symptoms. Impedance catheter measures pH as well as the type and direction of the flow of the esophageal contents. It can distinguish between acid and nonacid reflux
4. Upper endoscopy—assesses presence and degree of esophagitis, can diagnose other disorders such as eosinophilic infiltration associated with allergy (eosinophilic esophagitis), and infectious esophagitis
5. Scintigraphy—"Milk scan"; evaluates for slow gastric emptying and aspiration; lack of standardized techniques and age-specific norms limit usefulness of test
6. Guaiac stool/emesis—positive for occult blood if abnormal
7. Empiric medical therapy—trial of medication to relieve specific symptoms. If symptom is relieved with medication, then GER can be determined to be the cause
- Management/Treatment
1. Conservative therapy
   a. Positioning—(most important) postprandial, prone position for 1 to 2 hours if infant can be observed; infant seats/swings worsen by increasing intra-abdominal pressure; caution with diapering/playing postfeeding
   b. Breastfeeding or predominately whey formula
   c. A 1- to 2-week trial of hypoallergenic formula may be warranted if vomiting or other symptoms severe enough to consider drug treatment
   d. Thickening agents such as rice cereal have not been proven to decrease reflux but may decrease vomiting
   e. Avoid overfeeding—offer small, frequent feedings with frequent burping
   f. Reassure parents with growth charts
   g. Decrease anxiety in mother–infant interaction
   h. Monitor for problems—aspiration/esophagitis
   i. Since the risk of sudden infant death syndrome (SIDS) is greater than the risk of aspiration from birth to 12 months, nonprone position (preferably supine) during sleep to prevent SIDS is the recommendation of the American Academy of Pediatrics (AAP) except in very severe cases of GER
2. Medications: (if conservative therapy has failed)
   a. H$_2$ blockers (first line), protein pump inhibitors (second line), and antacids (short term) if irritable

from esophagitis (aluminum-containing antacids increase plasma aluminum levels in infants; there are no studies on safety of magnesium or calcium carbonate preparations; antacids should not be used long term)
   b. Metoclopramide may be cautiously considered for severe reflux under the supervision of a physician or gastroenterologist—"black box" warning from FDA; can cause tardive dyskinesia, a serious irreversible movement disorder
   c. Erythromycin 2 mg/kg up to four times prior to meals can promote gastric emptying (motilin agonist), should only be used in infants older than 4 weeks of age because of increased incidence of pyloric stenosis when given in first few weeks of life
3. Surgery—Nissen fundoplication only as last resort in an infant with GERD

☐ PYLORIC STENOSIS

- Definition: Obstruction due to thickening of circular muscle of the pylorus
- Etiology/Incidence
1. Unknown cause, genetic disposition, environmental factors
2. Young infants exposed to erythromycin in the first few weeks of life are at increased risk for developing pyloric stenosis
3. Occurs in 3:1000 infants; male > female; more likely in first-born males
4. Familial predisposition—25% chance if mother had pyloric stenosis, 15% chance if other family member, 22% if identical twin
5. More common in Caucasians than in African Americans or Asians
6. Symptoms occur later in breastfed infants; greater muscle thickness required to obstruct smaller-sized breastmilk curd
7. Delayed timing in premature infants
- Signs and Symptoms
1. Not present at birth; may occur in first week; average age of presentation from 3 to 6 weeks through 3 to 4 months of age
2. Vigorous, nonbilious vomiting after eating; with time becomes projectile with brownish color
3. "Hungry" after emesis; progressing to lethargy and irritability
4. Weight loss or poor weight gain
5. Constipation
6. Dehydration, metabolic alkalosis, malnutrition, and gastritis can occur with prolonged symptoms
- Differential Diagnosis
1. Overfeeding
2. Gastroesophageal reflux
3. Milk protein allergy
4. Gastroenteritis
5. Malrotation/volvulus if bilious emesis

- Physical Findings
  1. Visible peristaltic waves progressing from left to right across abdomen—darken room, shine bright light on abdomen of naked, supine baby; feed bottle of sugar water; peristaltic waves visible
  2. Palpable pyloric "olive" after vomiting—palpate epigastrium in right upper quadrant (RUQ) deep under liver edge; need very relaxed abdomen; hard, smooth, mobile, nontender mass may be palpable
  3. Dehydration as obstruction increases
- Diagnostic Tests/Findings
  1. Abdominal ultrasound to determine size of pylorus—preferred test
  2. Upper GI—avoid due to risk of barium aspiration; shows "string sign"; elongated pyloric channel and delayed gastric emptying
  3. Electrolytes to determine dehydration status
- Management/Treatment
  1. Surgical treatment after correction of fluid and electrolyte deficits
  2. Postoperative monitoring for hypoglycemia
  3. Excellent prognosis

ACUTE INFECTIOUS GASTROENTERITIS

- Definition: Illness of rapid onset, includes diarrhea with possible nausea, vomiting, fever, or abdominal pain
- Etiology/Incidence
  1. 70% to 80% caused by viral agents; 25% by rotavirus
  2. Younger than age 3 years 1.3 to 2.3 episodes/year; higher if in child care facility
  3. Predisposing factors (see **Table 8-1**)
     a. Child care facility
     b. Poor sanitation—improper hand washing, food preparation, or water quality
     c. Recent travel, especially to endemic areas
     d. Ill contacts—animals or humans
     e. Immunocompromised children at risk
     f. Recent antibiotic use
- Signs and Symptoms
  1. *Rotavirus*—nonbloody diarrhea, preceded or accompanied by vomiting and fever; symptoms last 3 to 8 days; dehydration may develop in severe cases

■ **Table 8-1** Most Common Causative Agents in the United States

Agent	Source/Transmission	Risk Factors	Incubation	Duration
Virus				
Rotavirus	Infected persons; contaminated toys; hard surfaces	<3 years; child care; low SES*; winter	2–4 days	3–8 days
Adenovirus	Infected person; contaminated toys; hard surfaces	<4 years; child care; not seasonal	3–10 days	5–12 days
Norwalk	Infected persons; contaminated food or water	Older children and adults	12 hours–4 days	12–48 hours
Bacteria				
Shigella	Infected persons; contaminated food, water, objects; houseflies	1–4 years; child care; crowding; poor sanitation; summer/fall months, need very few organisms for transmission	1–7 days	48–72 hours, even without treatment
Salmonella (nontyphoidal)	Contaminated foods (poultry, red meat, eggs, milk, fruits); contaminated water; infected persons or animals, pet snakes, turtles	<5 years; especially first year	6–72 hours	2–7 days
Salmonella typhi (typhoid fever)	Infected persons; rare in U.S., may be acquired during international travel	All ages	7–14 days	2–21 days
Campylobacter jejuni	Contaminated poultry; unpasteurized milk; pets	All ages; summer months	1–7 days	5–7 days

(continues)

■ **Table 8-1** Most Common Causative Agents in the United States (*continued*)

Agent	Source/Transmission	Risk Factors	Incubation	Duration
Parasitic				
Giardia lamblia	Infected persons, animals; contaminated food or water	Child care, institutions; campers	1–4 weeks	May be long term
Cryptosporidium	Infected persons, animals; contaminated water supplies	Parasite is chlorine resistant	2–14 days	1–20 days
Entamoeba histolytica	Mebic cysts; contaminated food and water	Tropical areas; crowding; poor sanitation	1–4 weeks	May be long term
Toxin				
Staphylococcus aureus	Ingestion of contaminated food products: ham, poultry, salads (egg and potato), cream-filled pastries	Inadequate cooking, refrigeration	>5–6 hours	1–2 days
Escherichia coli (0157:H7)	Infected persons or carriers; contaminated foods (undercooked ground beef, apple cider, raw vegetables, salami, yogurt, water)	Child care; poor sanitation; inadequate cooking; poor hand washing; travel to developing countries	3–4 days, up to 8 days	Varies
Clostridium difficile	Infected persons or hospital environment	Hospitals, child care, normal intestinal flora altered—antibiotics; repeated enemas, prolonged NG tube; intestinal surgery, inflammatory bowel disease; *C. diff* disease rare <12 months	Unknown	May improve with discontinuation of antibiotic if cause

Note: NG, nasogastric; SES, socioeconomic status.

Millonig, V. L., & Mobley, C. (Eds.). (2004). *Pediatric nurse practitioner certification review guide* (4th ed.). Sudbury, MA: Health Leadership Associates.

2. *Adenovirus*—upper respiratory tract infection most common; children younger than 4 years are susceptible to enteric infection; symptoms similar to *Rotavirus* but last longer

3. Norwalk—nausea, fever, abdominal cramps, headache, malaise, myalgia; vomiting more frequent than diarrhea

4. *Shigella*—high fever, headache, abdominal pain and tenderness; large, watery stools in which blood and mucus may be seen; can lead to dehydration

5. *Salmonella*—fever, abdominal pain and cramps; watery, mucoid, or bloody stools

6. *Campylobacter jejuni*—fever, malaise, abdominal pain, can mimic appendicitis or intussusception, bloody stools

7. *Giardia lamblia*—flatulence, abdominal pain, failure to thrive, anorexia, range of stools, e.g., asymptomatic carrier to foul, steatorrhea, consider in persistent diarrhea (>7 days)

8. *Cryptosporidium parvum*—frequent watery stools most common symptom with abdominal pain, anorexia and weight loss, fever, vomiting common; consider in persistent diarrhea (>7 days)

9. *Entamoeba histolytica*—asymptomatic, mild symptoms, e.g., abdominal distention, constipation, occasionally loose stools; or severe abdominal pain with increasingly severe bloody and mucoid diarrhea, weight loss, fever in approximately one third of patients

10. *Staphylococcus aureus* food poisoning—abrupt onset of nausea, vomiting, abdominal pain, watery stools

11. *Escherichia coli* (EHEC 0157:H7)—fever, less than one third of cases, severe abdominal pain, cramping, watery diarrhea, stools usually progress to grossly bloody or occult; hemolytic uremic syndrome (HUS) can occur 1 week or more after diarrhea

12. *Clostridium difficile*—abdominal pain and cramps; pseudomembranous colitis, stools bloody with leukocytes, mucus, pus; symptom-free carrier state common, 1 year

- Signs and Symptoms
  1. Nocturnal anal itching
  2. Vaginal itching (pinworm crawls into vagina)
  3. Insomnia (itching)
  4. Wormlike "threads"—seen in toilet or on underwear
- Differential Diagnosis
  1. Vulvovaginitis secondary to local irritation
  2. Poor hygiene
- Physical Findings
  1. Excoriation of perianal and perineal area
  2. Threadlike worms will be seen on visualization of anus (early morning using flashlight)
- Diagnostic Tests/Findings: Adhesive cellophane tape "paddle" with kits available for parental use; or can be made with clear Scotch tape and glass slide; prior to arising and bathing, paddle is pressed against anus and then examined for eggs
- Management/Treatment
  1. Medication (older than age 2 and nonpregnant)
     a. Pyrantel pamoate 11 mg/kg one dose (maximum dose 1 g)
     b. Albendazole 400 mg orally as a single dose; repeat in 2 weeks (same dose for all ages and weights)
  2. Reassure parents ubiquitous nature of organism; reinfection likely
  3. Test other family members and treat at same time if infected
  4. Prevention
     a. Keep nails clean and short
     b. Bathing will remove eggs from skin and decrease pruritus
     c. Excellent hand washing

☐ INFLAMMATORY BOWEL DISEASE (IBD)

- Definition: Chronic intestinal inflammation with two specific entities of ulcerative colitis (UC) and Crohn's disease (CD); may have extraintestinal symptoms and acute or insidious onset
  1. Location of inflammation in GI tract—CD occurs in any part of GI tract, terminal ileum typical, inflammation extends through entire thickness of intestinal wall, and strictures and fistulae may develop; UC affects only the lining of the colon
  2. Pattern of inflammation—CD skip pattern; discrete areas of inflammation interspersed with normal mucosa; UC mucosal and submucosal inflammation, diffuse and continuous
- Etiology/Incidence (for both types of IBD)
  1. Etiology—genetic disposition, environmental factors, and alteration in intestinal flora
  2. Genetic link—30% of children with IBD have a positive family history
  3. Occurs more often in Caucasians than in African Americans and Asians; highest in descendants of Ashkenazic Jews

  4. Age of onset—25% of cases diagnosed before 20 years of age; IBD can begin in infancy, but most commonly diagnosed in children between 10 and 20 years of age
- Signs and Symptoms
  1. Symptoms may be acute or unrecognized for years, dependent on location of lesions; more variability with CD since any part of GI tract can be involved
  2. Diarrhea
     a. CD—loose with blood if colon involved, or can have pain but no diarrhea
     b. UC—mild to profuse bloody diarrhea
  3. Weight loss/delayed pubertal maturation—often due to inadequate food intake because eating causes cramps, bloating, diarrhea
     a. Growth failure may be only presenting problem, especially in CD
     b. Weight loss and delayed puberty more common with CD
  4. Abdominal pain
     a. CD—located in right lower quadrant sometimes as fullness or mass; food related
     b. UC—left lower abdomen
  5. Severe cramps, low-grade fevers, anorexia
- Differential Diagnosis (based on area of bowel involved)
  1. Ulcerative colitis
     a. Enteric infection (particularly those involving bloody diarrhea)
  2. CD (particularly if manifested as extraintestinal symptoms)
     a. Rheumatoid arthritis
     b. Acute appendicitis
     c. Lupus erythematosus
     d. Lactose intolerance
     e. Celiac disease
     f. Infection—tuberculosis, *C. difficile*, *Yersinia*, *Campylobacter*
     g. Irritable bowel syndrome (IBS)
- Physical Findings (common to both UC and CD unless noted)
  1. Weight deceleration or poor growth
  2. Diffuse abdominal pain or no tenderness
  3. Extraintestinal symptoms
     a. Fever of unknown origin (FUO)
     b. Short stature
     c. Uveitis/iritis
     d. Aphthous stomatitis
     e. Arthritis/arthralgias
     f. Inflammatory lesions of skin
     g. Liver disease
     h. Perianal fissures/tags/abscesses with CD
- Diagnostic Tests/Findings
  1. Blood studies—CBC with differential shows microcytic anemia, increased white blood cells (WBCs); sedimentation rate (ESR), C-reactive protein (CRP) elevated; chemistry panel shows low serum total protein and albumin; findings suggest IBD and indicate the need for further studies for both CD and UC

2. Stool studies—infectious agents that cause bloody diarrhea for both CD and UC. Stool for fecal calprotectin (is an indicator of neutrophilic presence in the stool). Calprotectin is a substance that is released into the intestinal lumen when there is inflammation of the intestinal lining
3. Endoscopy and colonoscopy with biopsy—for diagnosis and to differentiate Crohn's from UC
4. Upper GI with small bowel—shows IBD changes and extent of disease in small intestine in areas not accessible by endoscopy

- Management/Treatment
  1. Refer to pediatric gastroenterologist
  2. Nutritional therapy to ensure adequate growth and pubertal development; total parenteral nutrition (TPN) or elemental formula may be necessary and can improve clinical symptoms; in milder cases, high-protein, high-carbohydrate, normal fat diet providing 75 to 90 kcal/kg/day; avoid overly restrictive diets
  3. Anti-inflammatory agents
     a. Induction of remission—corticosteroids, biologic agents
     b. Maintenance—mesalamine, immunosuppressants (6-mercaptopurine, azathioprine); biologics—infliximab, adalimumab
  4. Long-term patients may require surgery, often ileocecectomy in CD and colectomy/ostomy; curative for UC
  5. At higher risk for colorectal cancer
  6. Need emotional support to deal with chronic illness with reassurance that emotional factors are not primary cause

☐ CHRONIC DIARRHEA

- Definition: Gradual or acute increase in the number and volume of stools that are liquid/watery
  1. Noninfectious causes
     a. Antibiotic therapy—caused by alteration or eradication of usual intestinal flora, diarrhea usually watery, not associated with systemic symptoms, probiotics may help in its resolution; *C. difficile* infection occurs in 0.2% to 10% of patients treated with antibiotics
  2. Extraintestinal infections—infections of urinary tract and upper respiratory tract (otitis media) are sometimes associated with diarrhea
  3. Allergy to whole cow's milk or other foods
  4. Functional or nonspecific diarrhea—daily painless, recurrent passage of 3 or more large, unformed stools for 4 or more weeks; most common cause of diarrhea in young children; assess for overfeeding, excessive fruit juice or sorbitol consumption, excessive carbohydrate ingestion with low fat intake; older children may have diarrhea associated with irritable bowel syndrome
  5. Malabsorption (see below)

6. Secretory diarrhea—very watery, voluminous stools that do not resolve when child is fasting; due to rare disorders, including malignancies (neuroblastoma and GI neuroendocrine tumors), autoimmune enteropathy, microvillus inclusion disease

☐ MALABSORPTION

- Definition: Impaired intestinal absorption of nutrients and electrolytes
- Etiology/Incidence: Many causes—classified according to stage of digestion affected
  1. Intraluminal phase—exocrine pancreatic deficiency; cystic fibrosis most common cause of pancreatic deficiency in children
  2. Intestinal phase—abnormalities of mucosal surface area; absorption (celiac disease); inflammation, infections can damage mucosa
     a. Lactose malabsorption—most common cause of malabsorption in children, results in gas, pain, and diarrhea, but growth normal; can be temporary following gastrointestinal infection; lactose intolerance less common < age 4, but occurs in 80% Asian, African American adults; primary lactase deficiency very rare
     b. Infectious—bacterial, viral, parasites, e.g., *Giardia lamblia*
     c. Celiac disease—immune-mediated systemic disease due to intestinal intolerance to gluten; rate in population 1:1000; more common in children with Irish, Swedish heritage, but increasingly diagnosed in all ethnic groups; more common in children with type 1 diabetes, Down syndrome
     d. Crohn's disease
     e. Food allergy
  3. Decreased conjugated bile acids
     a. Biliary atresia
     b. Hepatitis
     c. Short bowel syndrome
- Signs and Symptoms
  1. Failure to thrive
  2. Adequate or increased intake per dietary history
  3. Severe, chronic diarrhea
  4. Bulky, foul, pale, steatorrhea stools
  5. Abdominal distention
- Differential Diagnosis
  1. Renal disease
  2. Poor dietary intake
  3. Failure to thrive
- Physical Findings: Disease-specific findings
  1. Lactose intolerance—persistent diarrhea after infectious diarrhea with normal growth
  2. Cystic fibrosis—recurrent pulmonary infection, "salty" taste to skin; nasal polyps; rectal prolapse; failure to thrive
  3. Celiac disease—vomiting, abdominal pain, irritability, anorexia, pallor; protuberant abdomen; failure to

thrive often noted around 6 months of age with the introduction of solids

- Diagnostic Tests/Findings
  1. Stool—(most important) inspection, culture, microscopic examination
     a. Hemoccult test—intestinal mucosa damage
     b. Ova and parasite; *Giardia* antigen to test for *Giardia* and other parasites
     c. pH-reducing substances—to rule out carbohydrate malabsorption
     d. Sudan stain for fat (microscopic examination of stool for fat)
     e. 3-day quantitative fecal fat (quantitates amount of fat losses in stool)
     f. Stool for pancreatic elastase (The determination of enzyme concentration in feces reflects the exocrine secretory capacity of the pancreas.) Can be used to aid in the diagnosis of pancreatic insufficiency
  2. Urinalysis/culture
  3. CBC, comprehensive metabolic panel, ESR, CRP
  4. Celiac screen—serum IgA (have to screen for IgA deficiency to ensure accuracy of test); tissue transglutaminase (most sensitive and specific test)
  5. Sweat test >60 mEq/L chloride—cystic fibrosis
  6. Hydrogen breath test—increased with lactose intolerance
- Management/Treatment
  1. Refer to gastroenterologist
  2. Lactose intolerance—avoid lactose-containing foods
  3. Celiac disease—gluten-free diet; no wheat, oats, rye, barley
  4. Cystic fibrosis—pancreatic enzyme replacement

☐ ACUTE ABDOMINAL PAIN

Intussusception

- Definition: Acute episode of prolapse of one portion of intestine into the lumen of the adjoining part, usually ileocolic
- Etiology/Incidence
  1. Unknown cause—85% idiopathic; may be caused by polyps, adenovirus, or *Rotavirus* with Peyer patch (lymphoid) hypertrophy, Henoch-Schönlein purpura, celiac disease, cystic fibrosis (CF); Meckel diverticulum of small intestine; lymphoma primary cause in children >6 years; intermittent intussusception is a rare cause of abdominal pain
  2. Greater incidence in males than in females
  3. 60% occurs before first birthday; 80% by 2 years
- Signs and Symptoms
  1. Healthy infant/child presents with sudden cycle of inconsolable screaming, flexing of leg, colicky abdominal pain
  2. 90% have nonbilious vomiting after pain
  3. Periods of quietness or sleepiness between episodes; lethargy if intussusception not reduced

  4. Eventually shock-like state develops
  5. Within 12 hours of onset, "currant jelly" (blood with mucus) stool is passed; late presentation
- Differential Diagnosis
  1. Gastroenteritis
  2. Incarcerated hernia
  3. Volvulus/obstruction
- Physical Findings
  1. Abdomen soft between episodes; may palpate sausage-shaped mass RUQ or upper-mid abdomen
  2. Distention and tenderness increased as obstruction increases
  3. Guaiac-positive or grossly bloody stool
  4. If not reduced, develops perforation and peritonitis leading to fever and shock
- Diagnostic Tests/Findings
  1. Radiography only to clarify diagnosis—no gas RLQ, air fluid levels consistent with obstruction
  2. Contrast enema done with air alone (safer and uses less radiation) or barium enema—diagnostic and therapeutic. Results in reduction in 90% of cases
  3. CBC and electrolytes—dehydration and anemia
  4. Ultrasound—tubular mass longitudinal image, doughnut on transverse view
- Management/Treatment
  1. Reduction via barium/air enema; air becoming more common
  2. Emergency surgery if unsuccessful
  3. Can recur usually within 24 hours, child observed for 24–36 hours; fatal if untreated

Appendicitis

- Definition: Acute inflammation of the appendix
- Etiology/Incidence
  1. Cause—obstruction of lumen by fecaliths or lymphocytic hyperplasia
  2. Most common in children between 6 and 14 years of age with peak incidence at ages 9–11 years
  3. Incidence in males greater than in females
  4. Seasonal distribution—autumn and spring
  5. Increased incidence following gastrointestinal infection
  6. Most common cause of pediatric abdominal surgery
- Signs and Symptoms
  1. Young child may not appear ill or have severe pain, particularly in early phase
  2. Abdominal pain—earliest symptom
     a. Vague, possibly midline, constant pain for several hours
     b. Pain eventually localized in RLQ; in some, pain may begin in RLQ
     c. Can wake at night over time with increasing severity of pain
     d. Pain on ambulation
     e. Pain precedes vomiting
  3. Anorexia, nausea, and vomiting

4. Variable changes in bowel patterns—constipation or diarrhea may be noted
5. Afebrile to very low-grade fever in early phase
- Differential Diagnosis
  1. Gastroenteritis—especially if fever (early stage) and/ or diarrhea
  2. Mittelschmerz
  3. Ovary cyst/ovary torsion/ruptured follicle
  4. Lower lobe pneumonia
  5. Pelvic inflammatory disease (PID)
  6. Constipation
  7. UTI/pyelonephritis
  8. Ruptured ectopic pregnancy
  9. Inflammatory bowel disease
  10. Intussusception
  11. Perforated peptic ulcer
- Physical Findings: Depends upon the stage of appendicitis
  1. Observe child—may be motionless, with legs flexed
  2. Tenderness localized to RLQ; intense at McBurney's point, halfway between umbilicus and anterior superior iliac crest
  3. Rebound tenderness
  4. Rovsing's sign—pain RLQ with left-side pressure; highly indicative of appendicitis in children
  5. Local, right-sided tenderness or mass on rectal examination
  6. Won't jump/difficulty ambulating
  7. Obturator sign—rotating thigh may produce pain in RLQ
  8. Complete examination to rule out other causes of abdominal pain, especially throat, chest, testicles
  9. Perforation and peritonitis within 24 to 48 hours
     a. Rigidity
     b. Higher fever
     c. Pain improves
     d. Generalized tenderness
     e. Increased vomiting
     f. 40% incidence in young children
- Diagnostic Tests/Findings
  1. Diagnosis based on history and physical; tests often not helpful in diagnosing appendicitis, but can rule out other sources of pain
  2. CBC with differential—may have a mild leukocytosis with left shift
  3. CT—most sensitive and specific; useful, especially in early stages of diagnosis; better to identify other diagnoses; ultrasound (US) versus CT often depends upon institution; some will do US because it is quicker and to minimize radiation exposure, and if equivocal proceed to CT scan
  4. Ultrasound—if ovarian condition part of differential or findings unclear
  5. Radiography of abdomen to rule out constipation
  6. UA to rule out UTI—UA can be abnormal in appendicitis
- Management/Treatment: Immediate surgical referral

☐ FUNCTIONAL GASTROINTESTINAL DISORDERS

Functional GI disorders include functional abdominal pain, functional dyspepsia, abdominal migraine, and irritable bowel syndrome. A thorough history and physical examination will often be sufficient to lead to the diagnosis of most common disorders.

Once any underlying organic disease is eliminated, it is the primary care provider's role to reassure the child and family and to encourage participation in normal activities, including school attendance. Work-up is similar for each functional disorder.

Functional Abdominal Pain (Also Called Chronic Abdominal Pain, Recurrent Abdominal Pain)

- Definition: Episodic or continuous abdominal pain that occurs at least weekly for at least 2 months where there is no evidence of an inflammatory, anatomic, metabolic, or oncological process to explain the child's symptoms
- Etiology/Incidence
  1. Unclear mechanism of pain; multifactorial, altered brain–gut interaction
  2. Multifaceted problem that includes predisposition aggravated by early life events or personality
  3. Most common cause of chronic pain in school-aged and young adolescent; incidence unknown, accounts for 2% to 4% of pediatric office visits; 13% to 17% of all adolescents have had chronic abdominal pain
  4. Most common between ages 8 and 15 years, uncommon younger than 4 years of age
  5. Greater incidence in girls than in boys; average age for females 9 to 10 years, males 10 to 11 years
  6. Family history of GI complaints and somatization disorders, e.g., migraines, peptic ulcers
  7. Differential diagnosis
     a. Organic—approximately 10%
        (1) Peptic ulcer disease
        (2) *Helicobacter pylori*
        (3) GER
        (4) Eosinophilic gastroenteritis
        (5) Pancreatitis—more common if positive family history; corticosteroid use
        (6) Cholecystitis—rare <9 years of age; increased with obesity; positive family history of gall stones; birth control pills
        (7) Inflammatory bowel disease
        (8) Celiac disease
        (9) Constipation
        (10) Malabsorption/lactose intolerance
        (11) Parasites (especially *Giardia*)
        (12) Gynecological disorders
        (13) Urinary tract infection
        (14) Sexual abuse

- Signs and Symptoms
  1. Certain personality traits (maladaptive coping skills, anxiety, internalization of feelings) and family characteristics (protective parents) more frequent; often adversely affects school performance as child frequently absent due to pain (red flag) and child's quality of life
  2. Nature of pain
     a. Onset of crampy or dull ache; no radiation of pain
     b. Pain usually periumbilical
     c. Nothing relieves pain
     d. Interferes with activities, but no night wakening
     e. Unrelated to meals
- Physical Findings: Indicate nonorganic cause
  1. Normal weight
  2. Afebrile
  3. Abdomen may have diffuse tenderness, but no guarding
  4. Normal findings on complete examination
- Diagnostic Tests/Findings: Diagnosis of exclusion
  1. Excellent history and physical examination key to diagnosis; special attention to growth parameters
  2. Exacerbating factors (foods, stress, time of day) and relieving (acid suppression, diet/food avoidance) factors
  3. Family history—peptic ulcer disease, IBD
  4. Guaiac stool—negative; rule out inflammatory bowel disease
  5. Blood tests—CBC with differential; ESR, CRP to rule out infection/inflammation
  6. Urinalysis/culture—rule out UTI
  7. Ova and parasites; *Giardia* antigen
  8. Additional/selected studies may be warranted depending on symptoms
     a. Pelvic examination of adolescent female
     b. Endoscopy for esophagitis, peptic ulcer—dysphagia, chest pain, weight loss present
     c. Upper gastrointestinal (UGI) with small bowel—if recurrent vomiting, stool blood to rule out obstructive lesions, Crohn's disease
     d. Hydrogen breath test—increased with lactose intolerance
     e. Pregnancy test
     f. Endoscopy or stool for *H. pylori* antigen (preferred test to serology)—rule out *Helicobacter pylori*
     g. Abdominal ultrasound—rule out cholecystitis
     h. Amylase/lipase—increased with pancreatitis
- Management/Treatment
  1. Emphasize to child and family—pain is real, even though no organic cause can be found; work-up should reassure them child is healthy
  2. Reinforce normal behavior; go to school, don't allow secondary gain; may go to school nurse briefly if symptoms severe; if too sick to attend school, follow-up with provider required
  3. Decrease hectic lifestyle and hurried meals
  4. Limited evidence-based knowledge on the use of medications and functional abdominal pain
  5. Try to identify source of stress in patient and/or family; stress reduction techniques may help, such as biofeedback and relaxation techniques; may need referral to behavior psychologist
  6. Keep pain diary to identify situations associated with symptoms
  7. Treat identified organic disease

Functional Dyspepsia

- Definition: Persistent or recurrent pain in the upper abdomen above the umbilicus. No evidence, including upper endoscopy, of organic disease. No evidence that dyspepsia is relieved by defecation. Acid suppression can be useful in relief of symptoms.

Abdominal Migraine

- Definition: Three or more paroxysmal episodes of acute, midline, abdominal pain lasting for 2 hours to several days with intervening symptom-free episodes. No evidence of organic disease, including CNS. And at least two of the following: headache during episodes, photophobia during episodes, family history of migraines, headache confined to one side only and aura. Pizotifen (serotonergic agent) has been found to improve symptoms

Irritable Bowel Syndrome

- Definition: Chronic disorder with a range of symptoms, including abdominal pain, altered bowel habits (diarrhea or constipation), bloating, fecal urgency, and a feeling of incomplete evacuation
- Treatment
  1. Diarrhea predominant—consider fructose and lactose elimination from diet for 2 to 3 weeks; antidiarrheal agents and antispasmodic agents may be helpful
  2. Constipation predominant—increased dietary soluble fiber (5 + age in years = daily dose in grams); stool softener such as polyethylene glycol 3350

☐ CONSTIPATION

- Definition: Alteration in frequency, passage, size, or consistency of stool
- Etiology/Incidence
  1. Functional—less than 5% of pediatric constipation has an organic cause; constipation most commonly due to voluntary withholding of stool following the passage of a painful bowel movement; painful stools can be caused by many factors, including change in diet, toilet training, stressful events, intercurrent illness, delayed defecation due to play or lack of available toilets; stool holding leads to increased stool mass, stools become hard as fluids are reabsorbed into the colon; a cycle of stool holding and painful stools occurs,

resulting in constipation, which if untreated leads to impaction and encopresis

2. Encopresis (involuntary fecal soiling)—chronic withholding leads to impaction and soiling; eventually loses urge to stool and results in megacolon; psychological problem not primary cause

3. Anatomic abnormalities—anal or rectal abnormalities; problems often seen in immediate newborn period

4. Intrinsic motor disorder—Hirschsprung disease (most common), congenital absence of ganglion in segments of colon; 1:5000 births; 4:1 male-to-female ratio; increased with positive family history or Down syndrome

5. Metabolic, e.g., hypothyroidism

6. Neurologic, e.g., tumors, spinal injury, myelomeningocele

- Signs and Symptoms
  1. Onset
     a. Functional—during infancy, particularly after change from breastmilk to formula or starting solids; 1 to 3 years of age after life change, e.g., new sibling, home, introduction of toilet training
     b. Encopresis—4 to 7 years, male > female
     c. Hirschsprung disease—less than 10% of infants with Hirschsprung disease will pass meconium in first 24 hours; history of failure to have bowel movement without aid of laxative or enema; short-segment Hirschsprung may manifest itself beyond the newborn period
  2. Stools
     a. Functional—hard, dry stools, "pellets"; occasionally stool caliber very large/wide; may be dark or have strong odor
     b. Encopresis—soiled underwear, may appear to be diarrhea; may occur daily
     c. Hirschsprung—small, ribbon-like stools; no leakage
  3. Complaints
     a. Functional—abdominal pain, blood-streaked stools, straining or "dancing around" indicates withholding
     b. Hirschsprung—no stooling
- Differential Diagnosis
  1. Tumor, sacral teratoma
  2. Anatomic defect
  3. Metabolic and gastrointestinal disorders—celiac disease, cystic fibrosis
  4. Infantile botulism—(recent onset)
  5. Tethered spinal cord and other neuropathic disorders
  6. Drugs
  7. Heavy metal ingestion (lead)
  8. Cow's milk protein intolerance
- Physical Findings
  1. Functional—rectal examination may show fissure, ampulla full of stool, normal tone; may have no palpable abdominal mass; may have abdominal pain

or cramping, but no distention; normal growth and development

2. Encopresis—may have impacted stool and/or large, dilated rectal vault, normal tone; abdominal distention with sausage-shaped mass in left pelvis or midline

3. Hirschsprung—tight, empty rectum in presence of palpable abdominal stool mass, may be explosion of stool on withdrawal of examining finger; stool may be guaiac positive; abnormal bowel sounds; abdominal distention; failure to thrive

4. Anal wink, neurologic examination, muscle strength, and tone should be normal

5. Spinal dimple may indicate underlying spinal abnormality

- Diagnostic Tests/Findings
  1. Radiograph of abdomen to examine for stool can be helpful especially in older children
  2. Unprepped barium enema—rule out Hirschsprung disease
- Management/Treatment:
  1. Emphasize to parents the definition of constipation; straining with soft stool in infancy is normal
  2. Ensure proper preparation of formula
  3. Infants >6 months of age—prune juice; malt soup extract to 3 teaspoons twice per day for maximum of 3 days
  4. Constipation causing abdominal pain or encopresis requires more aggressive treatment; withheld stool causes intestinal muscle stretching; multifaceted treatment involves emptying intestines, leading to a return of sensation; preventing recurrence of painful stools; and bowel training
  5. Plan for otherwise healthy child
     a. If impacted—day 1 mineral enema to soften stool
     b. No impaction or day 2—sodium phosphate enema one time per day for 2 to 3 days
     c. May choose oral medications for disimpaction, polyethylene glycol 3350, 1 to 1.5 g/kg/day for 3 days
     d. After intestines emptied, keep stool soft to prevent recurrence of withholding cycle—polyethylene glycol 3350, 1 g/kg/day
     e. Prevent pain cycle—emphasize to child that medicine will prevent painful stools
     f. Bowel retraining—child should sit on toilet for 1 minute per year of age twice per day; don't expect bowel movement every sitting. Institute reward system for positive reinforcement
     g. Goal—soft bowel movement every day or every other day without encopresis
  6. Hirschsprung—GI/surgery referral

☐ HEPATITIS

- Definition: Inflammation of the liver
- Etiology/Incidence

1. Hepatitis A virus (HAV)
   a. Most common form of viral hepatitis in children
   b. Highest rates of symptomatic infection 5 to 14 years; less than 10% of infected children younger than 6 years are symptomatic
   c. Transmission—fecal/oral, raw shellfish, contaminated water; in United States, HAV shed from asymptomatic, infected children to adults
   d. Incubation—15 to 50 days, average 25 to 30 days; can infect others up to 2 weeks before onset of illness and 1 week after
   e. High-risk populations—Native Americans, Alaska Natives, homosexuals, IV drug users; some Hasidic, Hispanic communities; travelers to developing countries; children in day care

2. Hepatitis B virus (HBV)
   a. Most common form of hepatitis in world
   b. Transmission—blood or body fluids; virus can survive more than 1 week on inanimate objects
   c. Incubation—45 to 160 days, average 120 days
   d. 5% to 10% of infected people become chronic carriers; inverse relationship between age of infection and carrier state; majority of perinatally infected infants become carriers
   e. High-risk populations—sexually active; institutionalized; IV drug users; patients with clotting disorders; household contacts of HBV carriers; hemodialysis patients; infants of Alaska Natives or Pacific Islanders; travelers to China, Southeast Asia

3. Hepatitis C virus (HCV)
   a. Very low rates in children younger than 12 years of age
   b. Transmission—blood and blood products, occasionally blood transfusion; maternal-fetal transmission 5%. The duration of presence of passive maternal antibody in infants can be as long as 18 months. Therefore, testing for anti-HCV should not be performed until after 18 months of age
   c. Incubation—6 to 7 weeks, range of 2 weeks to 6 months

4. Hepatitis D (HDV)
   a. Only causes infection in persons infected with HBV. Can lead to increased severity of HBV infection
   b. Transmission—blood or blood products, IV drug use, sexual contact
   c. Incubation—2 to 8 weeks, if simultaneous with HBV, average is 120 days

5. Hepatitis E (HEV)
   a. Endemic to Asia, Africa, Mexico; U.S. travelers to those areas at risk
   b. Transmission—fecal-oral route, especially contaminated water
   c. Incubation—40 days, range 15 to 60 days
   d. More common in adults than in children

- Signs and Symptoms
1. HAV
   a. Infants and young children—asymptomatic or nonspecific symptoms, e.g., nausea, vomiting, diarrhea; no jaundice; misdiagnosed as gastroenteritis
   b. Adults—fever, malaise, anorexia, nausea, abdominal pain, jaundice; later pruritus
   c. Self-limiting disease—several weeks to occasionally 6 months; no chronic or carrier state

2. HBV and HDV
   a. Children often asymptomatic—mild to severe disease; macular rash and arthritis (early sign); anorexia, nausea, malaise, arthralgia
   b. Up to 90% of perinatally infected infants can develop carrier state
   c. Chronic carrier state can lead to chronic liver disease or cancer

3. HCV
   a. Children often asymptomatic; those with symptoms have mild disease; <25% become icteric; gradual onset of headache, fever, nausea, fatigue, anorexia
   b. 50% to 85% become chronic carriers; can lead to chronic liver disease or cancer

4. HEV
   a. Acute illness with arthralgia, abdominal pain, jaundice, malaise, anorexia, and fever
   b. No carrier state

- Differential Diagnosis
1. Viral gastroenteritis
2. Hemolytic uremic syndrome
3. Reye syndrome
4. Cytomegalovirus illness
5. Toxin/medication exposure
6. Fitz-Hugh Curtis syndrome with gonorrheal PID

- Physical Findings
1. Possible hepatosplenomegaly; RUQ tenderness
2. If jaundiced, may develop dark urine and light stools, scleral icterus

- Diagnostic Tests/Findings
1. Nonspecific findings
   a. Elevated liver enzymes—AST, ALT
   b. Elevated serum bilirubin
   c. Elevated erythrocyte sedimentation rate (HAV)
2. Specific serologic antigen/antibody testing
   a. Hepatitis A (HAV)
      (1) Anti-HAV IgM—current or recent infection; usually disappears within 4 months
      (2) Anti-HAV IgG—resolved infection and immune status; may last for years following infection; 40% to 45% general population carry anti-HAV IgG
   b. Hepatitis B (HBV)
      (1) HBsAg (surface antigen)—detected in high levels in acute or chronic hepatitis B infection, earliest marker of acute infection; persistence beyond 6 months indicates carrier status. Positivity indicates that patient is infectious
      (2) Anti-HBc (core antibody)—appears at the onset of symptoms in acute hepatitis B and persists for life

(3) IgM anti-HBc—presence indicates recent infection of ≤6 months

(4) Anti-HBs—immune status following resolved infection or immunization (Heptavax)

c. Hepatitis C (HCV)

(1) Oraquick HCV Rapid Antibody test (OraSure Technologies) or HCV antibody

(2) If antibody positive, obtain HCV RNA. Positive result confirms current infection

d. Hepatitis D (HDV)—anti-HDV from reference laboratory. Available through Centers for Disease Control and Prevention (CDC)

e. Hepatitis E (HEV)—no tests for HEV have been approved by the FDA for use in the United States, but some commercial labs use tests approved in other countries and serologic and polymerase chain reaction assays are available experimentally; diagnosis by exclusion of acute hepatitis A, B, C, D, and other causes of viral hepatitis

- Management/Treatment
1. Treatment is supportive, good nutrition, decreased activity, monitor hydration and chronic state
2. HAV—immunoglobulin (IG) available for decreasing course of disease in early stages or prevention in exposed individuals; not recommended for HCV or HEV; defer measles or MMR immunization for 3 months following administration of immune globulin
3. Treatment for HBV
   a. Interferon a-2B treatment for chronic HBV; limited improvement (30% to 40% HBV; 10% to 20% HCV)
   b. Expensive
   c. Side effects
   d. Lamivudine 3 mg/kg/day may be used if interferon fails
   e. Entecavir 0.5 mg daily approved for use in children >2 years
   f. Adefovir 10 mg/day can be used in children >12 years of age
4. Treatment of HCV—interferon a-2B, three times per week, plus oral ribavirin; pegylated interferon weekly, plus oral ribavirin, for children >3 years of age. New treatments have been approved for adults and are likely to be approved for pediatric patients in the near future
5. Report to state health department
6. Prevention
   a. HAV—two inactive HAV vaccines recommended for children > age 12 months; hepatitis A vaccine should be given to previously unvaccinated individuals prior to travel to affected areas; HAV vaccine can also be given as postexposure prophylaxis; for children age <12 months, immunocompromised persons, persons with chronic liver disease, and persons who are allergic to the vaccine or a vaccine component, HAV IG should be used
   b. HBV—vaccine available and highly recommended for all newborns and adolescents

c. Cautious intake of food and water when traveling to endemic areas

d. Avoid unprotected sex and drug use

☐ HERNIA

- Definition: Abnormal protrusion of abdominal tissue/structures through umbilical ring in umbilical hernia or external inguinal ring in inguinal hernia
- Etiology/Incidence
1. Umbilical—due to imperfect closure or weakness of umbilical ring; common in infancy, reported in up to 60% of African American infants; many umbilical hernias resolve by age 2, but in the African American population closure can occur as late as 11 years of age; generally, if not closed by 4 to 5 years of age, the patient should be referred to a surgeon
2. Inguinal—failed closure of processus vaginalis
   a. Congenital defect—can be noticeable at birth
   b. Nine times more frequent in males
   c. Greater risk with premature births
   d. Hydrocele can increase risk; indicates opening present
- Signs and Symptoms
1. Intermittent or constant bulge of abdominal wall or inguinal region that may worsen with crying or straining
2. Uncomplicated hernias—asymptomatic
3. Umbilical—incarceration or strangulation extremely rare
4. Inguinal
   a. Incarcerated—cranky, anorexia, nausea, vomiting, groin discomfort, constipation
   b. Strangulated—area becomes tender, swollen, and progressively reddened in addition to above symptoms, possible fever
- Differential Diagnosis
1. Hydrocele
2. Lymphadenopathy
3. Undescended testes
- Physical Findings
1. Umbilical hernia—size of defect varies from 1 to 5 cm in diameter
2. Inguinal hernia
   a. Maneuvers that increase intra-abdominal pressure (sitting up, crying, coughing) will increase visibility of hernia
   b. May be bilateral; if unilateral, right side more common
   c. "Silk" sign can be diagnostic; elicited by palpation of the spermatic cord over the pubic tubercle, the layers of the peritoneum rubbing together will have a "silky feel"
   d. Transillumination of scrotal sac will highlight the presence of bowel
- Diagnostic Tests/Findings: None may be needed; ultrasound if unclear

- Management/Treatment:
  1. Monitor umbilical hernias; reassure parents
  2. Refer inguinal for surgical correction
  3. Emergency referral if incarcerated/strangulated

☐ QUESTIONS

Select the best answer.

1. A 10-month-old child has been diagnosed with gastroenteritis. He attends a child care facility. What is the most likely cause of his illness?
   a. *Clostridium difficile*
   b. *Rotavirus*
   c. *Salmonella*
   d. *Cryptosporidium*

2. In a healthy, 8-month-old with diarrhea but no dehydration, what would be the most appropriate advice to give parents?
   a. Encourage strength formula for 12 hours
   b. Give oral rehydration solution (ORT) for 12 hours
   c. Give only fluids until stools return to normal
   d. Give bananas and cereal as tolerated

3. When evaluating a child with abdominal pain, what symptom would lead to a likely organic etiology?
   a. Night waking
   b. Pallor
   c. Suprapubic pain
   d. Sweating

4. Vomiting in infancy has a long list of differential diagnoses. Which accompanying symptom would most likely point to pyloric stenosis?
   a. Diarrhea
   b. Appropriate growth
   c. Acts hungry after vomiting
   d. Sausage-shaped mass in abdomen

5. Which of the following is the appropriate regimen for pinworm medication?
   a. Daily times 7 days, repeat as needed
   b. Three times a day for 10 days, repeat as needed
   c. Twice daily for 3 days, repeat in 2 weeks
   d. 1 dose/1 time, repeat in 2 weeks if needed

6. Mrs. Doyle is upset. Two-month-old John's frequent vomiting has her convinced that "something is seriously wrong." Which of the following is most suggestive of GER (gastroesophageal reflux)?
   a. He's gained 5 ounces this month.
   b. He has a slight wheeze today.
   c. He eats hungrily after vomiting.
   d. He drinks 7 to 8 ounces every 3 to 4 hours.

7. You see Jack, a 20-month-old toddler with normal growth and development, in your office for diarrhea. His mother tells you that he is passing up to three loose stools a day and that he drinks 20 ounces of apple juice a day. What is the most likely diagnosis?
   a. Crohn's disease
   b. *Giardia lamblia*
   c. Celiac disease
   d. Nonspecific "toddler" diarrhea

8. Baby Sally was in your office last week for her 6-month checkup. Her weight was 7 kg. Today she presents with diarrhea and vomiting for 4 days. Today her weight is 6.5 kg. What is her percentage of dehydration?
   a. 5%
   b. 7%
   c. 10%
   d. <1%

9. What clinical signs would you expect to see in Sally on your examination?
   a. Normal capillary refill
   b. Normal fontanel
   c. Cool, mottled skin
   d. Dry mucous membranes

10. Sally's vomiting and diarrhea have stopped. If she needs oral replacement therapy (ORT) today, what would be the appropriate amount to recommend?
    a. 325–350 cc over 4 hours
    b. 600–700 cc over 4 hours
    c. 600–700 cc over 12 hours
    d. 325–350 cc over 8 hours

11. Pinworms can cause which of the following?
    a. Constipation
    b. Anal itching
    c. Abdominal pain
    d. Diarrhea

12. In evaluating Billy, a child with bloody diarrhea, which of the following would not be an appropriate first action?
    a. Check growth chart
    b. Stool culture
    c. Upper GI
    d. Hemoccult test stools

13. Billy's family eats at fast-food restaurants four to five times each week. If you suspect the diarrhea is infectious in nature, what is a likely causative organism?
    a. Adenovirus
    b. *E. coli*
    c. *Giardia lamblia*
    d. *S. aureus*

14. Which of the following conditions would be most likely to occur in a 4-year-old boy?
    a. Pyloric stenosis
    b. Recurrent abdominal pain
    c. Intussusception
    d. *Giardia* infection

15. Which of the following findings could be expected to occur in a baby with intussusception?
    a. Inconsolable screaming
    b. Olive-shaped mass
    c. Left-to-right peristaltic waves
    d. Weight loss

16. Which of the following may occur with suspected appendicitis?
    a. Pain not relieved with ambulation
    b. Young children appear very ill in the early phase
    c. Fever is 102°F to 103°F
    d. Leukopenia with left shift

17. In the United States, parasitic gastroenteritis is most commonly caused by which organism?
    a. *Enterobius vermicularis*
    b. *Entamoeba histolytica*
    c. *Cryptosporidium parvum*
    d. *Giardia lamblia*

18. Which of the following serological findings indicates chronic HBV infection?
    a. HBsAg negative for 6 months
    b. Anti-HBc positive and HBsAg positive
    c. IgM anti-HBc positive
    d. Anti-HBs positive

19. Children in child care facilities are at greater risk of being exposed to which of the following infections?
    a. HAV
    b. HBV
    c. HCV
    d. HDV

20. Infant immunization for hepatitis B often raises many parental questions about the disease. Which of the following is not true about hepatitis B virus?
    a. It can survive for more than 1 week on fomites.
    b. It is the most common form of hepatitis in the world.
    c. Contaminated water and shellfish are the major sources.
    d. Perinatally infected infants are likely to become carriers.

21. Two-day-old baby Jamie is in the hospital nursery and still has not passed meconium. This is a red flag for which condition?
    a. Intussusception
    b. Hemolytic uremic syndrome
    c. Pyloric stenosis
    d. Hirschsprung disease

22. Consistent with the condition in question 21, Jamie's findings on rectal examination would be which of the following?
    a. Tight anal canal with no stool in vault
    b. Impacted stool with fissure
    c. Large, dilated rectum
    d. Soft stool, normal tone

23. What treatment would be appropriate for Jamie's condition?
    a. Emulsified mineral oil, tablespoon per day
    b. Referral to gastroenterologist/surgeon
    c. Malt soup extract, 2 teaspoons for 3 days
    d. Rectal dilatation with thermometer

24. When evaluating a child with suspected IBD, which of the following diagnostic tests would not be helpful?
    a. Amylase and lipase
    b. ESR

25. Your patient has inflammatory bowel disease. Which finding is most consistent with ulcerative colitis?
    a. Occult blood
    b. Perirectal abscess
    c. Aphthous ulcers
    d. Left-sided abdominal pain

26. Antimicrobials will improve the condition of a 4-year-old child with diarrhea caused by which of the following organisms?
    a. *Salmonella*
    b. *Rotavirus*
    c. *Shigella*
    d. *E. coli* (0157:H7)

27. Katie has functional abdominal pain. When counseling her family on management of painful episodes, you would recommend which of the following?
    a. Take ibuprofen 200 mg for pain
    b. Stay home from school during episode
    c. Decrease milk products
    d. Go to school during episode

28. Which of the following would not be consistent with a diagnosis of functional constipation in an infant?
    a. Vomiting
    b. Anal fissure
    c. Straining
    d. Starting solids

29. A child has developed her second perirectal abscess in 6 months. She should be evaluated for which condition?
    a. *Giardia lamblia*
    b. Crohn's disease
    c. Ulcerative colitis
    d. Enterobiasis

30. Which of the following symptoms are most common in the early phase of appendicitis in children?
    a. Abdominal pain after eating
    b. Fever and diarrhea
    c. Severe localized RLQ pain with pallor and sweating
    d. Anorexia and vague, diffuse pain

31. Steatorrhea is not consistent with which of the following conditions?
    a. *C. difficile* infection
    b. *Giardia lamblia* infection
    c. Celiac disease
    d. Cystic fibrosis

32. Jamil has had diarrhea for 3 days. His mother calls concerned. Which of the following would not be helpful advice?
    a. Monitor stool for blood or mucus
    b. Encourage solid food
    c. Avoid milk products
    d. Monitor for urination at least every 6 hours

33. Of the following advice, which would be most helpful for the parents of a baby with gastroesophageal reflux?
    a. Most babies continue to vomit until they are walking, at around 1 year of age.

b. Lying prone after eating will decrease the amount of vomiting.

c. Increase the interval between feedings to a minimum of 4 hours.

d. Medications are generally necessary to prevent further problems.

34. Which of the following foods would be appropriate for a child with celiac disease?

a. Oatmeal for breakfast

b. Boiled rice with butter

c. Commercially baked bread

d. Cream of wheat

35. A parent requests that her 6-month-old child receive immunoglobulin (IG) as protection against hepatitis A prior to international travel. Which of the following does this parent need to know?

a. After IG administration, a 3-month interval is needed prior to the administration of measles vaccine.

b. There is no impact on future immunizations.

c. No immunizations can be given for 1 year.

d. Since children do not have symptoms with hepatitis A, IG is not necessary.

❏ ANSWERS AND RATIONALES

1. B: *Rotavirus* is the most common pathogen that causes gastroenteritis. It affects the small intestine, resulting in the passage of large amounts of watery stool. In the United States, it affects mainly infants between 3 and 15 months of age. It is transmitted by the fecal–oral route and can survive for days on hands and hard surfaces.

2. D: Starvation depresses digestive function and prolongs diarrhea. ORT is only given if dehydration is present.

3. A: Nighttime awakening with abdominal pain usually does not occur with functional disorders.

4. C: In pyloric stenosis, projectile vomiting usually starts between 1 and 2 months of age, and the infant will be very hungry after vomiting. Other symptoms of pyloric stenosis include constipation, fussiness, and weight loss.

5. D: Albendazole 400 mg orally as a single dose repeated in 2 weeks is used to treat pinworms.

6. D: John is being overfed, which predisposes infants to GER. A more appropriate intake for a 2-month-old is 4–5 oz every 3–4 hours.

7. D: Toddler diarrhea is caused by carbohydrate malabsorption and will resolve if juice is removed from the diet. Crohn's disease is rare in children <2 years. Celiac disease may cause failure to thrive. *Giardia* causes intermittent diarrhea.

8. B: % dehydration = pre-illness weight – illness weight ÷ pre-illness weight × 100. 7 kg – 6.5 kg = 500 g, and 0.5 ÷ 7 = 0.07 × 100 = 7% dehydration.

9. D: Dehydration of 7% causes dry mucous membranes, normal or sunken fontanel, and increased heart rate. Capillary refill is prolonged.

10. B: 100 mL/kg of ORT is given over 4 hours for moderate dehydration.

11. B: Anal itching is the most common symptom of pinworm infestation. The female lays eggs in the child's perianal area. Scratching and then putting the hands in the mouth lead to the eggs being swallowed. They hatch in the duodenum and then make their way to the colon, and the cycle begins again. Symptoms such as grinding of teeth at night, weight loss, and enuresis have been attributed to pinworm infections, but proof of a causal relationship has not been established.

12. C: An upper GI study is useful for assessing for any anatomic abnormalities. In a child with bloody diarrhea, stool cultures should be obtained to look for an infectious agent. Hemoccult can be done to prove the presence of blood. Suboptimal growth may point to inflammatory bowel disease.

13. B: Undercooked ground beef and leafy greens contaminated with *E. coli* 0157:H7 cause bloody diarrhea. *S. aureus* causes vomiting and diarrhea, but there is no bleeding. *Giardia* is generally contracted from contaminated water, for example, lakes and streams. Adenovirus is found on hard surfaces and usually affects children <3 years old in day care settings.

14. D: The highest incidence of *Giardia* is in children 1 to 9 years of age. Pyloric stenosis occurs in the first few months of life, intussusception mostly in the first 2 years of life. Functional abdominal pain is uncommon in children younger than 4 years of age and mostly occurs between 8 and 15 years of age.

15. A: Intussusception causes abdominal pain. Olive-shaped mass, left-to-right peristaltic waves, and weight loss are all symptoms of pyloric stenosis.

16. A: Children with appendicitis have difficulty ambulating and will not jump. Young children may not appear very ill in the early phases. Fever is absent or low grade. There may be a leukocytosis with left shift.

17. D: *Giardia* is the most common intestinal parasitic infection of humans in the United States. *Enterobius vermicularis* (pinworms) do not cause gastroenteritis.

18. B: HBsAg (hepatitis B surface antigen) is the earliest marker of acute infection, and persistence for >6 months indicates chronic infection. Total anti-HBc (total hepatitis B core antibody) appears in acute infection and persists for life. Its presence indicates prior or ongoing HBV infection. Positive IGM anti-HBc indicates acute infection. Positive anti-HBs indicates positive immune status after vaccination.

19. A: Hepatitis A is the most common form of viral hepatitis in children. It is transmitted by the fecal–oral route and by contaminated shellfish and water.

20. C: Contaminated shellfish and water are the major sources of hepatitis A.

21. D: Hirschsprung disease is the congenital absence of ganglion cells in the colon. The length of bowel affected varies. The other conditions are not present at birth.

22. A: The absence of ganglion cells in the rectum prevents the bowel from relaxing to allow the passage of stool. Impacted stool with fissure and a large, dilated rectum indicate constipation. Soft stool and normal tone are normal.

23. B: Once confirmed, the treatment for Hirschsprung disease is surgical resection of the affected bowel segment.

24. A: Amylase and lipase are raised in pancreatitis. Irritable bowel disease (IBD) may lead to anemia, hypoalbuminemia, and elevation of the erythrocyte sedimentation rate (ESR).

25. D: Ulcerative colitis causes left-sided pain and bloody diarrhea. Perirectal abscesses are seen in Crohn's disease. Aphthous ulcers may be found in Crohn's disease and celiac disease.

26. C: *Shigella* infection is generally self-limited, but antibiotics will shorten the course and decrease the shedding of organisms. *Rotavirus, Salmonella,* and *E. coli* do not require treatment in a 4-year-old.

27. D: In functional disorders, it is important to reinforce normal behaviors and routines.

28. A: Functional constipation does not cause vomiting. Straining and anal fissure may be seen with hard stools that are difficult to pass. Changes in diet can lead to constipation.

29. B: She should be evaluated for Crohn's disease. *Giardia lamblia*, ulcerative colitis, and enterobiasis do not cause perirectal abscesses.

30. D: Anorexia and vague, diffuse pain are seen in early appendicitis. Abdominal pain after eating usually is related to constipation. Severe right lower quadrant (RLQ) pain is seen in the late stages of appendicitis.

31. A: *C. difficile* causes loose stools that may be bloody. *Giardia* infection, celiac disease, and cystic fibrosis may lead to fat malabsorption resulting in steatorrhea.

32. C: In children with diarrhea, but no dehydration, an age-appropriate diet should be offered. Milk should not be restricted. The patient should be monitored for temporary lactose intolerance that occurs in about 20% of children after gastroenteritis.

33. B: Lying prone, if the infant can be observed, can decrease vomiting. Reflux usually improves around 6 months of age when the baby begins to sit up. Smaller, more frequent feeds are recommended for reflux. Medications are not indicated for uncomplicated GER.

34. B: Celiac disease is a systemic disease caused by an immune-mediated intolerance of gluten. Oats, wheat, barley, and rye are not permitted on a gluten-free diet.

35. A: A 3-month waiting period is required prior to the administration of a measles vaccine after receiving hepatitis IG. Ig is recommended as protection against Hepatitis A prior to international travel for children <12 months of age. Children >12 months should receive hepatitis A vaccine.

☐ BIBLIOGRAPHY

American Academy of Pediatrics. (2006). *Red book: 2006 report of the Committee on Infectious Diseases* (28th ed.). Elk Grove Village, IL: Author.

American Academy of Pediatrics. (2009). Red book online. Retrieved from http://aapredbook.aappublications.org/

American Academy of Pediatrics & North American Society for Pediatric Gastroenterology, Hepatology and Nutrition. (2005). Technical report: Chronic abdominal pain in children. *Journal of Pediatric Gastroenterology and Nutrition, 40*(3), 249–261.

Baker, S. S., Liptak, G. S., Colletti, R. B., Croffie, J. M., DiLorenzo, C., Ector, W., & Nurko, S. (2006). Clinical practice guideline: Evaluation and treatment of constipation in infants and children: Recommendations of the North American Society for Pediatric Gastroenterology, Hepatology and Nutrition. *Journal of Pediatric Gastroenterology and Nutrition, 43*(3), e1–e13.

Carroll, A. E., Garrison, M. M., & Christakis, P. H. (2002). A systematic review of nonpharmacological and nonsurgical therapies for gastroesophageal reflux in infants. *Archives of Pediatric and Adolescent Medicine, 156*(2), 109–113.

Centers for Disease Control and Prevention. (2015). What is viral hepatitis. Retrieved from http://www.cdc.gov/hepatitis/ABC/

Garcia-Peña, B. M., Taylor, G. A., Fishman, S. J., & Mandi, K. D. (2000). Costs and effectiveness of ultrasonography and limited computed tomography for diagnosing appendicitis in children. *Pediatrics, 106*(4), 672–676.

Maheshwai, N. (2007). Are young infants treated with erythromycin at risk for developing hypertrophic pyloric stenosis? *Archives of Diseases of Childhood, 92*, 271–273.

McCollough, M., & Sharieff, G. Q. (2003). Abdominal surgical emergencies in infants and young children. *Emergency Medical Clinics of North America, 21*(4), 909–935.

Naik-Mathuria, B., & Olutoye, O. (2006). Foregut abnormalities. *Surgical Clinics of North America, 86*(2), 261–284.

Rudolph, C. D., Mazur, L. J., Liptak, G. S., Baker, R. D., Boyle, J. T., Colletti, R. B., Werlin, S. L. (2001). Pediatric gastroesophageal reflux clinical practice guidelines: Guidelines for evaluation and treatment of gastroesophageal reflux in infants and children. *Journal of Pediatric Gastroenterology & Nutrition, 32*(Suppl. 2), S1–S31.

Scholl, J., & Allen, P. J. (2007). A primary care approach to functional abdominal pain. *Pediatric Nursing, 33*(3), 247–259.

Sondheimer, J. (2003). Gastrointestinal tract. In W. W. Hay, Jr., M. J. Levin, J. M. Sondheimer, & R. R. Deterding (Eds.), *Current pediatric diagnosis and treatment* (pp. 614–643). New York, NY: Lange Medical Books/McGraw-Hill.

Yacob, D., & Dilorenzo, C. (2009). Functional abdominal pain: All roads lead to Rome (criteria). *Pediatric Annals, 38*(5), 253–258.

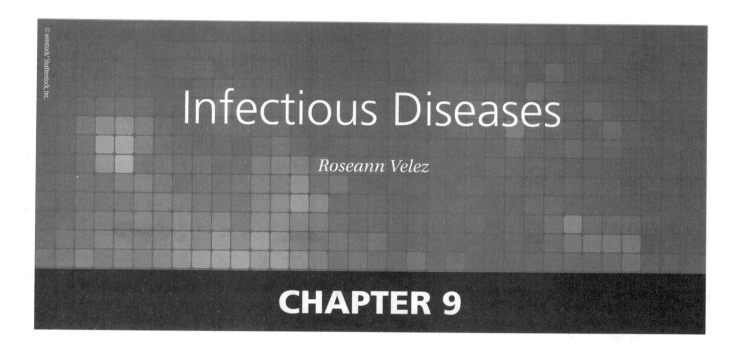

Infectious Diseases

Roseann Velez

CHAPTER 9

Infection is caused by a pathogen and may be suspected or proven by culture, tissue stain, or polymerase chain reaction test. Clinical syndromes may be associated with a high probability of infection.

☐ SEPTICEMIA (SEPSIS)

- Definition: Definitions for sepsis and organ dysfunction were developed by the International Consensus Conference on Pediatric Sepsis. Clinical suspicion for sepsis may occur even though all components of the consensus criteria are not present.
  1. Sepsis: The systemic inflammatory response syndrome (SIRS) in the presence of suspected or proven infection. Sepsis is defined in terms of severity and response to therapy.
     a. SIRS is defined as a widespread inflammatory response. The presence of two or more of the following criteria defines SIRS:
        (1) Temperature >38.5°C or <36°C
        (2) Tachycardia, defined as a mean heart rate more than two standard deviations above normal or age, or for children younger than 1 year of age
        (3) Leukocyte count elevated or depressed for age
     b. SIRS is present if two of these criteria are met; one of the criteria must be abnormal temperature or leukocyte count
  2. Neonates are most susceptible to sepsis because of their immature immune system
- Etiology/Incidence: Caused by bacterial, viral, fungal, parasitic, and rickettsial infection

  1. Bacteria:
     a. Gram positive
        (1) *Escherichia coli*, Group B *Streptococcus, Staphylococcus aureus, Streptococcus pneumoniae*
     b. Gram negative
        (1) *Pseudomonas aeruginosa, Escherichia coli, Klebsiella, Enterobacter, Citrobacter,* and *Acinetobacter*
        (2) Methicillin-resistant *Staphylococcus aureus* (MRSA) and multidrug-resistant Gram-negative bacteria such as *Pseudomonas aeruginosa* are isolated
        (3) Hospital-acquired bacterial infections such as catheter-associated blood stream infections; coagulase-negative staph is most common
  2. Viruses: Respiratory: Influenza, parainfluenza, adenovirus, respiratory syncytial virus (RSV), Epstein-Barr virus (EBV), cytomegalovirus (CMV), herpes simplex virus (HSV)
  3. Fungi: *Candida*
  4. Other: Malaria, Rocky Mountain spotted fever (RMSF)
  5. Culture-negative sepsis: 30–75% of children with sepsis have no infectious etiology
     a. Etiologic agents vary by age, immunologic status, and mechanism of transmission
        (1) Newborn (3 days) placental transfer of pathogens from infected maternal blood stream or from vaginal mucosa during birth
           (a) Group B *Streptococcus* (GBS) high mortality
           (b) *E. coli* most common Gram-negative organism
           (c) *Listeria monocytogenes*

(2) Neonates, 28 days—cross-contamination in nurseries or other crowded conditions; poor hand washing and housekeeping
   (a) *Staphylococcus aureus* most common
   (b) *Klebsiella*
   (c) Enterococci
   (d) *Pseudomonas*

(3) Older infants in the community can be at increased risk for sepsis due to inadequate immunization status—*Haemophilus influenzae* type B

(4) Hospitalized immunosuppressed children at risk for nosocomial sepsis—cancer, postoperative, and patients with HIV/AIDS

b. Leading cause of morbidity and mortality among hospitalized patients due to associated hemodynamic changes affecting tissue perfusion and oxygenation; if not treated, may lead to septic shock

c. Increased risk of septicemia
   (1) High risk, premature infants
   (2) Males > females
   (3) Invasive procedures—IV, intubation
   (4) Bottle feeding—breastmilk may be protective
   (5) Immunocompromised children and adolescents

- Signs and Symptoms: Significant change in vital signs (VS) and white blood cell (WBC) count indicating SIRS in the presence of clinical or lab findings of infection. May progress to shock and organ dysfunction
  1. Neonates—symptoms may be vague and nonspecific, e.g., poor feeding, color changes (pallor, mottling), changes in muscle tone, apnea, cyanosis, low temperature, or fever
  2. Other immunosuppressed children—fever may be only sign; reports by caregiver that child "isn't him- or herself"
  3. Older children (rarer) with normal immune function—fever, irritability, anorexia, general toxic appearance

- Differential Diagnosis
  1. Viral sepsis
  2. Fungal infection
  3. Rocky Mountain spotted fever
  4. Toxic shock syndrome
  5. Noninfectious causes—hemorrhagic, anaphylactic, or neurogenic shock
  6. UTI
  7. Pneumonia
  8. Early bacterial meningitis
  9. Child abuse
  10. Hypoglycemia
  11. Environmental hyperthermia
  12. Seizures
  13. Congenital heart disease
  14. Inborn errors of metabolism
  15. Congenital adrenal hyperplasia
  16. Malrotation with volvulus
  17. Intussusception
  18. Pyloric stenosis
  19. Gastroenteritis
  20. Water intoxication
  21. Exposure to toxins
  22. Encephalopathy due to bilirubin
  23. Differential diagnosis in older children
      a. Heat stroke
      b. Serotonin syndrome
      c. Neuroleptic malignant syndrome
      d. Malignant hyperthermia
      e. Overdose
      f. Kawasaki disease

- Physical Findings
  1. Neonates—hyper- or hypothermia; bradycardia or tachycardia; hepatosplenomegaly, jaundice
  2. Older children—irritability, stiff neck
  3. Later phase—lethargy, delayed capillary refill, hypotension, and subsequent septic shock
  4. 20% of infants and young children have fever without an apparent source
  5. Other physical findings
     a. Toxic appearance
     b. Dehydration (sunken fontanelles or eyes, decreased urine output and skin turgor)
     c. Rigors
     d. Mental status changes
     e. Seizures
     f. Meningismus
     g. Respiratory distress
     h. Distended abdomen
     i. Costovertebral angle (CVA) tenderness
     j. Skin cellulitis or abscess
     k. Peripheral edema
     l. Petechiae or purpura
     m. Multiple nodules

- Diagnostic Tests/Findings (for children with suspected sepsis)
  1. Complete blood count (CBC) with differential—WBC >15,000 with increased neutrophils
  2. Blood cultures—preferably before starting antibiotics (abx)
  3. Urinalysis—bacteria, nitrites, or pyuria suggests urinary tract infection (UTI)
  4. Urine culture—UTI is common source of infection in children with sepsis
  5. Cerebral spinal fluid (CSF), pleocytosis, decreased glucose, increased protein, positive culture
  6. Prothrombin time (PT), partial thromboplastin time (PTT), international normalized ratio (INR) elevation suggests disseminated intravascular coagulation (DIC)
  7. Rapid blood glucose
  8. Arterial blood gas (ABG)
  9. Blood lactate
  10. Serum electrolytes
  11. Blood urea nitrogen (BUN) and serum creatinine
  12. Serum calcium
  13. Serum total bilirubin and alanin anminotransferase

14. Fibrinogen and D-dimer
15. Other cultures as needed
16. Imaging—chest radiograph for children with rales, wheezing, hypoxemia, or WBC >20,000
17. Diagnosis—diagnosed by clinical findings

- Management/Treatment
  1. Medical referral for hospitalization
  2. Close observation, monitoring, and supportive care
  3. IV fluids to maintain hemodynamics space
  4. Broad spectrum parenteral antibiotics for Gram-positive and -negative organisms pending culture and sensitivities
  5. Vasoactive medication if septic shock ensues
  6. Close follow-up, often seen outpatient within 24 hours after discharge from hospital

☐ DIPHTHERIA

- Definition: Infectious disease caused by Gram-positive bacillus *Corynebacterium diphtheriae*; it is a contagious acute infection of the upper respiratory tract and may lead to cutaneous disease. Affected patients may be asymptomatic as carriers
- Etiology/Incidence
  1. There are at least four biotypes of *Corynebacterium diphtheriae*
  2. The primary modes of spread consist of transmission through direct contact with infected person, carrier, or contaminated food/objects; transmission by respiratory droplets or by contact with discharges from mucous membranes or cutaneous lesions
  3. The rate of clinical disease is low because of immunization of DTaP/dT
  4. Increased risk among unimmunized children living in crowded conditions
  5. Fall/winter incidence most common
  6. Incubation period is 2 to 7 days
- Signs and Symptoms
  1. Respiratory diphtheria
     a. Sore throat
     b. Low-grade fever
     c. Nasal discharge (nasal diphtheria)
     d. Bloody nose
     e. Hoarseness or cough
     f. Difficulty breathing (severe cases)
     g. Malaise
     h. Cervical lymphadenopathy
     i. Gray and white tonsillar exudates
  2. Systemic manifestations
     a. Cardiac dysfunction
     b. Neurologic toxicity
     c. Renal failure
  3. Cutaneous diphtheria—chronic, nonhealing sores or shallow ulcers with dirty gray membrane
- Differential Diagnosis
  1. Acute streptococcal pharyngitis
  2. Nasal foreign body

3. Mononucleosis
4. Viral croup
5. Epiglottitis
6. Posttonsillectomy faucial membrane
7. Viral pharyngitis
8. Severe oral candidiasis

- Physical Findings
  1. Grayish-white pseudomembrane found at location of infection—nasopharynx, pharynx, or trachea
  2. Other findings vary by location of membrane
  3. Toxin-related severe complications include severe neck swelling (bull neck), myocarditis, Guillain-Barré-type neuritis, and paralysis
- Diagnostic Tests/Findings
  1. Positive culture of *C. diphtheriae* from nose or throat or any lesion
  2. CBC—normal or slight leukocytosis and thrombocytopenia
- Management/Treatment
  1. Hospitalization with respiratory isolation for respiratory tract disease and contact precautions for cutaneous disease. Isolation until two consecutive diagnoses (dx) taken at least 24 hours apart are negative
  2. Nasal and pharyngeal cultures
  3. Toxin detection via serum
  4. Report to state health department
  5. Evaluation of sensitivity to horse serum; if negative, single dose of equine antitoxin for severe cases
  6. Erythromycin or penicillin G; antimicrobial treatment is not a substitute for antitoxin; erythromycin (EES) parenterally or orally for 14 days at 40 to 50 mg/kg/day divided by 6 hours; or penicillin G benzathine for 14 days (25,000 to 50, 000 units/kg to a maximum of 1.2 million units IV every 12 hours until the child can take oral medicine) followed by Pen VK 250 mg four times daily for a total treatment course of 14 days. EES has been favored over PCN because of its greater efficacy
  7. Identification of contacts for follow-up care, immunization, and treatment according to current American Academy of Pediatrics *Red Book* recommendations. Cultures should be obtained from close contacts and antibiotic therapy should be initiated. If culture-positive, they should have their cultures repeated after finishing antimicrobial therapy and should be retreated for a further 10 days
  8. Prevention through universal immunization; disease may not confer immunity

☐ PERTUSSIS (WHOOPING COUGH)

- Definition: Highly contagious acute respiratory illness caused by *Bordetella pertussis*. It is characterized by prolonged coughing episodes ending in an inspiratory "whoop"; clinical decision is a cough illness lasting 2 weeks without an apparent cause with paroxysms of coughing, inspiratory whoop, or posttussive emesis

- Etiology/Incidence
  1. Caused by Gram-negative coccobacillus *Bordetella pertussis*, a strict human pathogen. There are eight additional *Bordetella* species, and three of those species can cause illness in humans
  2. Infection occurs following person-to-person contact via aerosolized droplets from respiratory tract
  3. Pertussis is most common and most severe in infants younger than 6 months of age, especially in premature infants and those not immunized because these children have the highest mortality. In adolescents, infection may result in a protracted cough and the morbidity may be substantial
  4. Incubation period is 5 to 21 days, usually 7 to 10 days
  5. Infectivity is highest in catarrhal stage and the first 2 weeks after onset of cough; patients are considered infectious until they have completed 5 days of antibiotic treatment
  6. No lifelong immunity is conferred by disease or immunity. Protective immunity decreases after 5 to 10 years; therefore, booster vaccination is recommended for adolescents
  7. The cause for the rising incidence of pertussis is not fully understood but is attributed to increased rates of infection in adolescents and adults
- Signs and Symptoms: Less severe in adolescents than in infants and children
  1. Catarrhal stage—mild upper respiratory infection (URI) symptoms with mild cough for approximately 2 weeks, low-grade fever, malaise, rhinorrhea, excessive lacrimation, and conjunctival injection
  2. Paroxysmal stage—second week of illness, hallmark is paroxysmal cough night and day, and if untreated leads to convalescent phase: vomiting, sucking, or crying precipitates coughing episodes, and poor feeding and poor weight gain, especially in infants
  3. Convalescent stage—symptoms, mostly coughing, gradually subside over several weeks to months
  4. Infants <6 months of age may present with atypical early signs—short catarrhal stage, gagging, gasping, apnea spells possibly with cyanosis, absence of whoop, unexpected death, followed by prolonged convalescence, and, in some cases, may result in unexpected death. Case-fatality rates are approximately 1% in infants younger than 2 months of age and less than 0.5% in infants 2 through 11 months of age. (Red Book 2012)
- Differential Diagnosis: Depends on the duration of the cough
  1. Pneumonia (bacterial, viral, chlamydial, mycoplasma)
  2. Acute bronchitis
  3. Croup
  4. Upper respiratory infection
  5. Foreign body aspiration
  6. Cystic fibrosis
  7. Asthma
  8. Cold

- Physical Findings
  1. Similar to those found with an upper respiratory infection including rhinorrhea, excessive lacrimation, and conjunctival injection, especially during the catarrhal stage
- Diagnostic Tests/Findings
  1. Both culture and polymerase chain reaction (PCR) for patients with less than 2 weeks of cough and clinical concern
  2. For patients with 2 to 4 weeks of cough, chest x-ray (CX) and PCR
  3. For patients with more than 4 weeks of cough, only serology
  4. Patients with discordant test results should be presumed to have pertussis
  5. Specimens must be by swab or aspiration from the posterior nasopharynx
  6. Culture is the standard for diagnosis
  7. Chest radiograph may reveal thickened bronchi and evidence of atelectasis and bronchopneumonia
  8. WBC count reveals marked leukocytosis—usually presents during paroxysmal period and persists for 3 to 4 weeks, more often in infants and young children
- Management/Treatment
  1. Medical referral is necessary and treatment is most effective when administered within 2 weeks of paroxysmal cough
  2. For infants from birth to six months, if the infection is life threatening or the risk of developing an infection is high, the neythromycin (40 mg/kg/day in 4 divided doses for 7–14 days [maximum 1–2 g/day], or azithromycin; 10 mg/kg/day orally once daily for 5 days; is recommended. For infants 1–5 months clariomycin is an alternative 15 mg/kg per day in 2 divided doses for 7 days. After completing the course of macrolide antibiotic infants must be monitored for one month for infantile hypertrophic pyloric stenosis. Trimethoprim-sulfamethoxazole (TMP/SMX) is the alternative for patients over 2 months of age unable to tolerate macrolides or who may have a macrolide-resistant strain. The recommended dose of TMP/SMX is 8–10 mg/kg/day, twice a day for 14 days
  3. Hospitalized children should remain in isolation until they have received 5 days of erythromycin
  4. Children receiving oral erythromycin at home should not attend child care or school until they have received 5 days of therapy
  5. Supportive treatment for children who cannot tolerate oral intake due to paroxysmal coughing episodes—intravenous hydration, oxygen supplementation, ventilatory support
  6. Report cases of pertussis to state health department
  7. Complication for infants—pneumonia, seizures, encephalopathy, death
  8. Complications for adolescents and adults—syncope, sleep disturbances, incontinence, rib fractures, pneumonia

9. Prevention
   a. Appropriate pertussis immunization according to schedule
   b. Children younger than 7 years of age, with close contact with infected individual, who are unimmunized or who have received fewer than four doses of pertussis vaccine should complete the series with the minimal intervals
   c. If the third dose of vaccine was received 6 months or more prior to the exposure, should be given a fourth dose at time of exposure
   d. Children who have not received a vaccine within past 3 years or those ≥6 years of age should receive a booster dose of pertussis vaccine at time of exposure; this can be given as Tdap
   e. Chemoprophylaxis—erythromycin (40 to 50 mg/kg/day divided four times a day for 14 days; maximum 2 g/day) is recommended for all household contacts and other close contacts, regardless of vaccination status

☐ INFLUENZA

- Definition: Highly contagious, acute respiratory tract viral illness characterized by sudden onset of fever, chills, malaise, headache, myalgia, and dry cough
- Etiology/Incidence
  1. Epidemic influenza caused by types A and B; recent subtypes have included H1N1, H1N2, and H3N2 viruses. Seasonal influenza virus is a member of the Orthomyxoviridae family
  2. Transmission occurs by direct person-to-person contact, via airborne droplet, or by articles contaminated with nasopharyngeal secretions
  3. During outbreak, school-aged children are most frequently infected and infect household contacts
  4. Period of highest infectivity 24 hours prior to onset of symptoms and while symptoms are most severe; viral shedding peaks first 3 days of illness with direct correlation to height of fever
  5. Incubation period 1 to 4 days, mean of 2 days
  6. Influenza season mid-October through mid-February
- Signs and Symptoms (upper and lower respiratory tract)
  1. Fever
  2. Chills
  3. Malaise
  4. Headache, myalgia
  5. Dry cough
  6. Anorexia
  7. Rhinorrhea
  8. Sore throat
  9. Less frequently—conjunctivitis, abdominal pain, nausea, vomiting, diarrhea
- Differential Diagnosis
  1. Upper respiratory infections (RSV)
  2. Bacterial pneumonia

- Physical Findings
  1. Listlessness
  2. Nonproductive cough
  3. Rhinorrhea
  4. Rigors
  5. Fever with cough
  6. Conjunctivitis
  7. Pharyngitis
- Diagnostic Tests/Findings
  1. Nasopharyngeal cultures obtained within first 72 hours of illness may reveal influenza; or if using a rapid antigen test for influenza, it can designate the virus as type A or B
  2. Diagnosis is usually made based on clinical signs and available prevalence data
- Management/Treatment
  1. Management of influenza is primarily supportive
  2. Efficacy has not been established if treatment is initiated >40 hours after symptom onset
  3. Less than 30 hours after first symptoms
     a. Acetaminophen 15 mg/kg orally every 4–6 hours prn, maximum 90 mg/kg/day, or ibuprofen 5–10 mg/kg orally every 4–6 hours prn, maximum 40 mg/kg/day for fever (avoid aspirin-containing products in children younger than 16 years of age due to risk of developing Reye syndrome)
     b. Adequate hydration
  4. Antiviral therapy such as osteltamivir or zanamivir may be given within 48 hours of symptoms to decrease the severity and length of symptoms
     a. <15 kg: 2 mg/kg (maximum 30 mg) orally twice daily
     b. 16–23 kg: 45 mg orally twice daily
     c. 24–40 kg: 60 mg orally twice daily
     d. 40 kg or >12 years of age: 75 mg orally twice daily
  5. Zanamivir >7 years of age 10 mg (two inhalations) twice daily
     a. Zanamivir can be used when treatment of seasonal influenza is indicated
     b. Treatment should be given for 5 days
  6. Children <1 year with influenza symptoms should be treated with oseltamivir
  7. Complications of influenza
     a. Bacterial pneumonia; sepsis-like picture in infants; febrile seizures; encephalopathy; myocarditis; sudden death, even in previously healthy children
  8. American Academy of Pediatrics (AAP) and Centers for Disease Control and Prevention (CDC) recommendations at time of publication are for annual vaccinations in all children 6 to 59 months of age, for household contacts and out-of-home caregivers of children 0 to 59 months of age, and for children and adolescents in high-risk groups
  9. High-risk children include asthma, cystic fibrosis, other chronic pulmonary disease, significant cardiac disease, immunosuppressive disorders and treatment, HIV, sickle cell anemia, other hemoglobinopathies,

medical conditions requiring long-term salicylate medication such as juvenile rheumatoid arthritis (JRA) or Kawasaki disease, chronic renal or metabolic (diabetes) diseases, or any cognitive dysfunction, spinal cord injury, or neuromuscular diseases that compromise respiratory functioning

10. There are two forms of influenza vaccine—inactivated trivalent influenza vaccine (TIVA) and live-attenuated influenza vaccine (LAIVA); LAIVA is only for healthy children with no known risk factors and approved for ages 5 to 49 years; also do not give to children with a history of anaphylactic reaction to egg protein or a history of Guillain-Barré syndrome; TIVA is given to all other infants and children and for close contacts of severely immunocompromised individuals

11. Children younger than 9 years who are getting an influenza vaccine for the first time need to receive two doses of TIVA or LAIVA at least 1 month apart, preferably finishing the two-dose regimen by December; this boosts antibody response; in subsequent years, children <9 years old who had one or two doses of vaccine need only one dose per year; children >9 years old require just one dose per year

12. The CDC and state health departments will post recommendations for prevention and treatment guidelines each year and periodically as warranted

13. Exposure to infected individuals in at-risk population may receive prophylactic antiviral therapy with oseltamivir (based on child's weight) and zanamivir (children >5 years of age)

☐ RUBELLA (GERMAN MEASLES)

- Definition: An acute, mild, contagious, viral disease characterized by an erythematous, maculopapular rash, lymphadenopathy, conjunctivitis, and/or arthralgias or arthritis. Up to half of all cases are asymptomatic. The most important consequence of rubella infection is congenital rubella syndrome. Maternal infection in pregnancy can cause spontaneous abortion, death, or congenital deformities
- Etiology/Incidence
  1. Caused by an RNA virus, a *Rubivirus* in the Togaviridae family
  2. Postnatal transmission occurs via contact from nasopharyngeal secretions
  3. Incubation period ranges from 14 to 23 days
  4. Peak incidence is late winter and early spring
  5. Preventable by active immunization
  6. Clinical case definition: Acute onset of a generalized maculopapular rash, fever >99°F, arthralgia/arthritis, lymphadenopathy, or conjunctivitis
- Signs and Symptoms
  1. History of inadequate immunization
  2. Rash starts on forehead and face and spreads over trunk and extremities during the 1st day; facial exanthem fades by 2nd day, disappears by 3rd day

3. Associated signs and symptoms
   a. Malaise, low-grade fever
   b. Transient joint pain, polyarthralgia or polyarthritis rare in children, but more commonly seen in adolescents and adults, particularly in females
   c. Bruising (rare)
- Differential Diagnosis
  1. Rubeola
  2. Scarlet fever
  3. Erythema infectiosum
  4. Adenovirus
  5. Rocky Mountain spotted fever
  6. Roseola
  7. Drug eruption
  8. West Nile virus
  9. Secondary syphilis
  10. Infectious mononucleosis (Epstein-Barr virus)
  11. Kawasaki syndrome
  12. JRA
- Physical Findings
  1. Generalized erythematous, maculopapular discrete rash—usually first indication of illness
  2. Listlessness
  3. Postauricular, suboccipital, and posterior cervical lymphadenopathy—usually precedes rash
  4. Petechiae on soft palate and uvula (Forchheimer sign)
  5. Purpura/petechiae (rare)
  6. Meningeal signs (rare)
  7. Fever
  8. Conjunctivitis
  9. Rash usually 3–4 days
- Diagnostic Tests/Findings
  1. A positive antirubella IgM in acute serum or a significant rise in serum rubella IgG titers between acute and convalescent phases as measured by any standard serologic assay
  2. Presence of rubella-specific IgM antibody indicates recent postnatal infection or congenital infection in newborn
  3. Refer to current AAP *Red Book* for further information on available assays for detecting rubella infection
- Management/Treatment
  1. Management of uncomplicated infection is primarily supportive—includes fever and pain; control with acetaminophen or ibuprofen
  2. Determine contacts, who may require immunization
  3. Infected children should limit contact with susceptible persons, including women of childbearing age; out of school for 5 days after onset of rash
  4. Educate adolescent females regarding teratogenic nature of rubella in pregnancy, resulting in congenital rubella syndrome—multiple congenital anomalies affecting eyes, heart, auditory with hearing loss, and neurologic systems
  5. Educate caretakers regarding complications of arthritis and, rarely, thrombocytopenia and encephalitis

☐ RUBEOLA (RED MEASLES)

- Definition: A highly infectious disease caused by the measles virus, characterized by a maculopapular rash, cough, coryza, conjunctivitis, and a pathognomonic exanthem (Koplik spots) with an incubation period of about 10 days. Rubeola is characterized by a prodrome of upper respiratory symptoms followed by generalized maculopapular eruptions
- Etiology/Incidence
  1. Caused by a spherical RNA virus of the genus *Morbillivirus* and family Paramyxoviridae
  2. Transmitted by direct contact with infected secretions or via airborne droplets through sneezing or coughing
  3. Incubation period is 7 to 18 days
  4. Infected individuals are contagious 3 to 5 days before appearance of rash to 4 days after appearance of rash
  5. Increased incidence during late winter and spring
  6. Preventable by active immunization
- Signs and Symptoms
  1. History of inadequate immunization
  2. Acute onset of fever, coryza, cough, conjunctivitis, Koplik spots, maculopapular rash
  3. Confluent, erythematous, maculopapular rash 3 to 4 days after initial symptoms; progresses in caudal direction, beginning behind the ears and at the hairline
- Differential Diagnosis
  1. Roseola
  2. Viral infections (e.g., echovirus, coxsackievirus, adenovirus)
  3. Infectious mononucleosis
  4. Scarlet fever
  5. Rickettsial diseases
  6. Serum sickness
  7. Morbilliform drug eruption
  8. Secondary syphilis
  9. Rubella
- Physical Findings
  1. Confluent, erythematous maculopapular rash; after 3 to 4 days, rash assumes a brownish appearance
  2. Profuse coryza
  3. Conjunctivitis, photophobia, periorbital edema in prodrome
  4. Pulmonary findings (crackles, rhonchi), a hacking, bark-like cough
  5. Koplik spots (red eruptions with white centers on buccal mucosa) prior to appearance of rash
  6. Generalized lymphadenopathy
- Diagnostic Tests/Findings
  1. Measles-specific IgM and IgG serology (ELISA)
  2. Presence of measles-specific IgM antibody suggests recent infection
- Management/Treatment
  1. Medical referral necessary
  2. No specific antiviral therapy available; World Health Organization (WHO) recommends vitamin A to any child 6 months–2 years, children who are hospitalized with measles, have complications of measles, have immunodeficiency, have clinical evidence of vitamin A deficiency, have impaired intestinal absorption and malnutrition (those who may have a vitamin A deficiency, especially in developing countries)
  3. Management of uncomplicated measles is primarily supportive—bed rest, adequate hydration, acetaminophen or ibuprofen for fever, antitussive therapy
  4. Otitis media is most common complication of measles infection—treated with same antibiotics as in standard otitis media
  5. Educate caretakers regarding complications, including otitis media, diarrhea, encephalitis, croup, and pneumonia

☐ ROSEOLA (EXANTHEM SUBITUM)

- Definition: An acute, common, contagious febrile illness of early childhood characterized by high fever and appearance of a rash with simultaneous decrease in fever
- Etiology/Incidence
  1. Caused by human herpesvirus 6 (HHV-6) or HHV-7
  2. Mode of transmission not known
  3. Incubation period is 5 to 15 days
  4. Period of infectivity is thought to be during the febrile episode, prior to appearance of the rash
  5. Most commonly occurs in children 6 to 24 months of age
  6. Most cases occur in spring and summer
  7. One attack confers lifelong immunity
- Signs and Symptoms
  1. Abrupt onset of high fever (102°F to 105°F) lasting 3 to 5 days
  2. Appearance of a rash (discrete 3- to 5-mm pink-red macules and papules commonly found on the truck) follows resolution of fever
  3. Associated symptoms include irritability and swelling of eyelids
  4. Tympanic membrane (TM) inflammation
  5. Febrile seizure is the most common complication
- Differential Diagnosis
  1. Rubeola
  2. Scarlet fever
  3. Rubella
  4. Erythema infectiosum
  5. Other viral exanthems
  6. Meningococcemia
- Physical Findings
  1. Generalized erythematous, maculopapular rash; starts on trunk and spreads to arms and neck with less involvement of face and legs; generally a well-appearing infant
  2. Irritability
  3. Diarrhea/vomiting
  4. Pharynx, tonsils, and TMs may be infected
  5. Cervical lymphadenopathy

- Diagnostic Tests/Findings: Roseola is almost always diagnosed on the basis of classic presentation of a previously healthy infant, usually 9–12 months of age, with a sudden onset of high fever for 3–4 days, followed by truncal red macules and papules. Labs are seldom necessary
- Management/Treatment
  1. Symptomatic treatment during the febrile phase of the illness
  2. Acetylsalicylic acid (ASA) is avoided
  3. Oral hydration
  4. Acetaminophen or ibuprofen as needed for fever; tepid baths; fluids
  5. Medical referral if meningeal signs appear or if fever persists
  6. Education
     a. Potential for febrile seizures
     b. Reassurance that appearance of rash is sign of recovery

FIFTH DISEASE (ERYTHEMA INFECTIOSUM)

- Definition: A viral exanthematous illness commonly known as "fifth disease" since it was the fifth childhood exanthem described after measles, rubella, scarlet fever, and roseola. Erythema infectiosum (EI) is self-limited and resolves without sequelae in the majority of cases
- Etiology/Incidence
  1. Human parvovirus B19 via direct contact and respiratory droplets
  2. Typically seen in 5- to 14-year-old children
  3. Outbreaks occur most often during late winter and spring months
  4. Incubation period between 4 and 14 days, up to 21 days
  5. Mode of transmission includes respiratory secretions and blood
  6. Most infectious prior to rash
  7. About 60% of adults are immune
- Signs and Symptoms
  1. May have prodromal symptoms of a mild URI for 2 to 3 days, preceding the rash by 7 to 10 days; low-grade fever, headache, chills, malaise, myalgia, pharyngitis, conjunctivitis, arthralgias, arthritis
  2. Rash
     a. Begins as bilateral erythema on cheeks with circumoral pallor ("slapped cheek" appearance)
     b. Spreads to upper arms, legs, trunk, buttocks, hands, and feet
     c. Palms and soles are spared
     d. Lacy-reticular exanthem, slightly raised, appears as facial erythema, begins to diminish
     e. May reappear when skin is exposed to sunlight, temperature extremes, or friction
     f. Rash lasts from 2 to 39 days, average 11 days
  3. Less common symptoms—mild URI with no rash, rubelliform rash, papulopurpuric glove-and-socks

syndrome (painful and pruritic papules, petechiae, purpura of hands and feet)
  4. Can cause aplastic crises in young children, patients with hemolytic diseases, or patients who are immunocompromised
  5. Arthralgias and arthritis are more common in adolescents and adults
- Differential Diagnosis
  1. Drug reactions
  2. Rubella, atypical measles
  3. Enteroviral diseases
  4. Systemic lupus erythematosus
  5. Juvenile rheumatoid arthritis
  6. Roseola infantum
- Physical Findings
  1. Early—bilateral erythema on cheeks ("slapped cheek" appearance)
  2. Late—erythematous, lacy-reticular rash appears as facial erythema begins to diminish and is seen on upper arms and legs, trunk, hands, and feet; palms and soles are spared
- Diagnostic Tests/Findings: The most common tool in dx is the clinical appearance of the classic "slapped cheek" rash with a lacy-reticular exanthem on the extremities and torso. There may be a history (hx) of low-grade fever and nonspecific influenza or respiratory symptoms occurring prior to the onset of the exanthem
  1. Parvovirus B19 IgM antibody confirms current infection or infection within past several months
  2. Parvovirus B19 IgG antibody indicates previous infection and immunity
- Management/Treatment
  1. Symptomatic for fever/arthralgias
  2. Reassure parent of benign nature of disease
  3. Avoid sunlight as exposure may exacerbate the condition
  4. Period of high infectivity in persons with EI is prior to onset of symptoms; unlikely to be infectious after rash develops; conversely, patients with aplastic crises are highly contagious prior to the onset of symptoms and through week of onset or longer
  5. Can result in spontaneous abortion or stillbirth; complications to a developing fetus can occur, including hydrops fetalis and possible fetal death, with the greatest risk in the first half of the pregnancy, but Parvo B19 has not been proven to cause congenital anomalies; the risk of fetal death is 2–6%; pregnant women exposed to the Parvo virus should discuss the implications with their OB/GYN provider

VARICELLA-ZOSTER VIRUS (VZV) (CHICKENPOX)

- Definition: Varicella is one of the childhood exanthems, caused by the human alpha herpes virus, varicella zoster. Varicella-zoster virus is an acute infectious disease characterized by a short or absent prodrome and usually a widespread vesicular and pruritic rash primarily on the torso and face

- Etiology/Incidence
  1. VZV occurs in a nonimmune host
  2. Transmission occurs by direct contact with varicella lesions or by airborne droplet infection
  3. Susceptible individuals can contract chickenpox from patients with varicella zoster (shingles)
  4. Incubation period between 10 and 21 days, most commonly 14 to 16 days
  5. Infected individual contagious for 24 to 48 hours prior to outbreak of lesions, until all lesions have crusted over
  6. Most cases occur in children younger than 10 years old
  7. VZV occurs commonly in late winter and early spring
  8. Primary infection generally confers lifelong immunity
  9. There is a latent phase in which the virus resides in the dorsal root ganglia and may be reactivated at a later time as eruptions of "shingles"
  10. If children received only one dose of the two series varicella vaccines, there can be a second episode of varicella (neonates are a high risk of complication)
- Signs and Symptoms
  1. Early lesions appear as faint erythematous macules that progress to papules, followed by appearance of vesicles primarily on trunk, scalp, face; lesions eventually crust over
  2. Lesions continue to erupt for 3 to 4 days and may be present in various stages
  3. Associated symptoms of a prodrome may include fever, headache, pruritus, malaise, general aches and pains, anorexia, joint pain fatigue, sore throat, tachycardia, hx of exposure
- Differential Diagnosis
  1. Herpes zoster
  2. Stevens Johnson syndrome/toxic epidermal necrolysis
  3. Monkeypox
  4. Disseminated herpes simplex virus
  5. Smallpox
- Physical Findings
  1. Crops of skin lesions that may appear as maculopapular (early), vesicular, pustular with eventual crusts; many maculopapular lesions may progress to vesicular stage and resolve without crusting
  2. Rash usually present on scalp, face, trunk, and extremities; most lesions on face and trunk, with anywhere from a few to several hundred lesions; all stages of lesions are often seen simultaneously; vesicles become umbilicated and progress to pustules and crusts within 8 to 12 hours; vesicles are watery yellow, pustules have white pus, crusts are brownish-red and fall off in 1 to 3 weeks, leaving pink, often punched-out permanent scars
  3. Hepatomegaly (rare)
  4. Meningeal signs (rare)
  5. Pulmonary findings—crackles, wheezes (rare)

- Diagnostic Tests/Findings: Clinical diagnosis is usually sufficient
- Management/Treatment
  1. VZV is a self-limited disease lasting 7 to 10 days
  2. Supportive treatment
     a. Control of pruritus with oatmeal baths, diphenhydramine, calamine lotion
     b. Acetaminophen for fever (avoid aspirin-containing products due to risk of developing Reye syndrome)
  3. Oral acyclovir is beneficial in reducing duration of new lesion formation and total number of lesions (20 mg/kg/dose, four times a day; maximum 800 mg, four times a day); should be started within 24 hours of onset for maximum benefit
  4. Oral acyclovir not usually recommended in healthy children with uncomplicated varicella
  5. Varicella-zoster immune globulin (VZIG) should be given to immune-suppressed contacts to provide passive protection
  6. Medical referral necessary for immune-suppressed children, who are at risk for severe disease, such as pneumonia, encephalitis, glomerulonephritis, and hepatitis
  7. Education
     a. Avoid contact with elderly persons, pregnant women, neonates, and immunocompromised children
     b. Children may return to school when all lesions are crusted, or in immunized children without crusts when the lesions appear to be resolving
     c. Live-attenuated varicella vaccine is available in the United States, and two doses are now recommended for all healthy children at age 12 months and age 4 to 6 years; adolescents past their 13th birthday who lack a reliable history of varicella should be given two doses of varicella vaccine spaced 4 weeks apart
     d. Signs and symptoms of complicated varicella infection—meningeal signs, respiratory distress, dehydration, ocular involvement, secondary bacterial infection, thrombocytopenia, pneumonia
     e. Signs and symptoms of Reye syndrome—persistent vomiting, lethargy, agitation, disorientation, combativeness, coma

MUMPS

- Definition: A systemic, viral infectious disease characterized by swelling of the parotid glands. Involvement of other salivary glands, meninges, gonads, and pancreas is also common
- Etiology/Incidence
  1. Caused by a RNA paramyxovirus virus
  2. Spread by direct contact via respiratory airborne droplet and fomites contaminated with infected saliva
  3. Incubation period between 12 and 25 days after exposure, usually 16–18 days

4. Infected individual is contagious for as many as 7 days prior to and as long as 9 days after onset of symptoms
5. Infection occurs throughout childhood; rarely during adulthood
6. More common in late winter and spring
- Signs and Symptoms
    1. History of inadequate immunization
    2. Parotitis
    3. Malaise, fever
    4. Orchitis, rare cases of sterility
    5. Aseptic meningitis
    6. Oophoritis
- Differential Diagnosis
    1. Submandibular or preauricular lymphadenitis
    2. Salivary duct obstruction
    3. Infectious mononucleosis
    4. Epididymitis
    5. Parainfluenza
    6. Coxsackievirus
    7. Acute HIV infection
    8. EBV
    9. Influenza
    10. Acute suppurative parotitis
    11. Parotid duct obstruction
- Physical Findings
    1. Swelling of salivary glands (specifically parotid gland)
    2. Listlessness
    3. Scrotal swelling and pain
- Diagnostic Tests/Findings: Serum for complement fixation (CF)—positive test for complement-fixing antibody against mumps virus suggests recent infection (salivary mumps IgM)
- Management/Treatment: Isolation plus supportive care and symptom relief
    1. Acetaminophen for pain and fever
    2. Warm compresses for salivary gland swelling
    3. Soft or liquid diet
    4. Education
        a. Complications include pancreatitis, oophoritis, meningitis, orchitis
        b. May return to child care or school when all symptoms have resolved or 9 days after onset of symptoms
    5. Report cases to state health department

☐ CAT SCRATCH DISEASE (CSD)

- Definition: A benign, self-limited form of lymphadenitis in an otherwise healthy person following contact with an infected cat as a result of a cat bite or scratch or contact with cat saliva on broken skin or the conjunctiva of the eye
- Etiology/Incidence
    1. Most cases are caused by *Bartonella henselae*
    2. Cats are common reservoir for human disease; no human-to-human transmission
    3. More common in children, peak incidence 5 to 14 years of age

4. Late fall, winter, early spring; July and August in warmer climates
5. Often multiple cases in the same family
- Signs and Symptoms: Mild systemic symptoms
    1. History of cat exposure, usually a kitten, 6 months old (almost invariably healthy)
    2. Usually do not appear ill
    3. Swollen lymph nodes (usually resolves in 2 months)
    4. May have low-grade fever, general malaise, headache, nausea, chills, general aching
    5. Anorexia
    6. May have rash
- Differential Diagnosis
    1. Bacterial lymphadenitis (pyogenic)
    2. Lymphoma
    3. Tularemia
    4. Lymphogranuloma venereum
    5. Atypical mycobacteria
    6. Infectious mononucleosis
    7. Toxoplasmosis
- Physical Findings
    1. Papule or pustule at site of cat scratch or bite 7 to 12 days after cat contact, followed in 1 to 4 weeks by enlargement of an associated regional lymph node
    2. Lesion may be present for several days to several months
    3. May be erythematous, hot, firm, and tender to touch
    4. Most common on the head, neck, or extremities
    5. Conjunctivitis—if portal of entry is the conjunctiva, a granuloma on the palpebral conjunctiva with associated tender preauricular and/or cervical lymphadenopathy is present
    6. Involved node, usually single, draining the site of inoculation
- Diagnostic Tests/Findings
    1. May have elevated erythrocyte sedimentation rate (ESR)
    2. Immunofluorescence assay (IFA) detects antibody to CSD (performed by CDC)
    3. Warthin-Starry silver stain used to identify CSD in lymph node, skin, or conjunctival tissue
- Management/Treatment
    1. CSD is a self-limited disease lasting 2 to 4 months
    2. Supportive treatment, may be unresponsive to antibiotics
        a. Analgesics for discomfort and fever, warm compresses
        b. Limited activity per comfort level
        c. Needle aspiration of painful, suppurative nodes questionable; may result in chronic draining sinus tract; incision and drainage (I & D) not recommended; rarely is surgical removal of nodes necessary; no treatment required for animal that transmitted CSD; no declawing is needed, nor is removal of cat from home necessary, depending on the case

☐ ROCKY MOUNTAIN SPOTTED FEVER (RMSF)

- Definition: A systemic vasculitis with characteristic petechial or purpuric rash known as the most commonly fatal tickborne infection in the United States
- Etiology/Incidence
  1. Caused by infection with the obligately intracellular aerobic bacterium *Rickettsia rickettsii*, a Gram-negative bacterium
  2. Transmitted to humans via tick bites
  3. White people account for 88% of cases
  4. Usually occurs in persons younger than 15 years of age
  5. Occurs only in the Western Hemisphere; most common from April to September; however, cases do occur in winter months
  6. Incubation period ranges from 2 to 14 days
- Signs and Symptoms
  1. Triad of fever, rash, and hx of tick exposure (45–67% of patients)
  2. Triad of fever, rash, and headache (h/a) (44–58% of patients)
  3. Fever
  4. Fever, myalgia, severe headache, anorexia, nausea, and vomiting precede appearance of rash; abdominal pain, diarrhea, uncommon sudden shaking rigor, photophobia, and prostration may also be present
  5. Erythematous, macular rash (usually appearing before the 6th day of illness), on wrists, ankles, spreading within hours to the trunk, and the palms and soles are often involved; macules become papular in 1 to 3 days
  6. In some cases rash fails to develop or develops late in the illness
  7. Disease can last 3 weeks with multisystem involvement and significant long-term sequelae (e.g., central nervous system, cardiac, pulmonary, gastrointestinal, renal, DIC)
- Differential Diagnosis
  1. Rubeola
  2. Rubella
  3. Lyme disease
  4. Septicemia
  5. Meningococcemia
  6. Ehrlichiosis and other rickettsial diseases
  7. Drug reaction
  8. Immune-complex-mediated vasculitis
  9. Toxic shock syndrome
  10. Scarlet fever
- Physical Findings
  1. Characteristic petechial, erythematous, maculopapular rash (palms, soles, and extremities)
  2. Neurologic deficits, altered consciousness, transient deafness
  3. Photophobia
  4. Vomiting/diarrhea

  5. Decreased urine output
  6. Jaundice, hepatomegaly, splenomegaly uncommon
- Diagnostic Tests/Findings
  1. Blood cultures
  2. Renal failure
  3. WBC typically is normal, leukopenia, anemia, thrombocytopenia, hyponatremia; elevated liver enzymes
  4. CBC, serum electrolytes, liver function tests (LFTs), IFA
  5. Increase in antibody titer as established by serologic testing; indirect hemagglutination (IHA) and micro-immunofluorescence (micro-IF) are most sensitive
- Management/Treatment
  1. Medical referral
  2. Doxycycline is the drug of choice and is initiated based on clinical picture before lab results are available; it is given until patient is afebrile for 3 days and is showing signs of clinical improvement; the usual duration is 7 to 10 days; treatment by day 5 of illness provides the best chance for a good outcome
  3. Tetracyclines are not routinely given to children younger than 8 years of age, but doxycycline is still the drug of choice to be used at any age; doxycycline has less tooth enamel staining than tetracycline and is effective against ehrlichiosis, which can mimic RMSF
  4. Continue abs until CX and clinical course exclude pyogenic bacterial infection
  5. Untreated RMSF has a mortality rate as high as 20%; with adequate treatment, the mortality rate is lowered to 3%; early diagnosis and treatment have the best outcome
  6. Education includes preventive measures such as use of tick repellent and protective clothing in tick-infested areas; checking for ticks after spending time outdoors and removing them promptly
  7. Patients with multisystem organ involvement may require rehabilitative services
  8. Report cases to state health department

☐ LYME DISEASE

- Definition: A zoonotic infection that is transmitted between vertebrate animals and humans that has an immune-mediated, inflammatory response; affects multiple organ systems and is transmitted primarily via the deer tick. Lyme disease is the most common vector-borne infection and one of the most common notifiable diseases in the United States
- Etiology/Incidence
  1. Caused by a spirochete *Borrelia burgdorferi*; is most often transmitted via the deer tick; bacterial transmission usually occurs after the tick is embedded and feeding for 36 hours. In the United States, Lyme disease is transmitted by the ticks *Ixodes scapularis* and *I. pacificus*. Ticks become infected by feeding on an infected animal
  2. Most often seen in temperate regions in the Northern Hemisphere, in the Northeast from Massachusetts to Maryland; the Midwest, primarily Wisconsin

and Minnesota; and California; primarily in heavily wooded areas with nearby tall grass areas

3. Persons of all ages and both sexes are affected, but the incidence in the United States is highest among children ages 10–19 years and adults 50–59 years

4. Most cases occur from April to October with >50% of cases during June and July

5. Incubation period is between 1 and 55 days, with an average of 11 days

- Signs and Symptoms: In three stages
1. Early localized stage
   a. Appearance of well-circumscribed, erythematous, annular rash with central clearing rash known as erythema migrans (EM) at site of recent tick bite; an expanding macule that is painless and not pruritic, usually flat except at the central bite mark, and may have partial central clearing
   b. Accompanied by fever, malaise, headache, arthralgia, conjunctivitis, or mild neck stiffness, myalgia
   c. May initially present as the above flu-like illness if erythema migrans does not occur or is not recognized
2. Early disseminated stage
   a. Multiple EM occurring several weeks after the known or unknown tick bite
   b. Accompanied by systemic symptoms such as arthralgia, myalgia, headache, and fatigue; carditis is rare in children
3. Late disease stage (weeks to months later)
   a. Migratory pain in joints, muscles, and bones
   b. Transient, but severe headaches and stiff neck
   c. Poor memory, mood changes, somnolence
   d. Muscle weakness and poor coordination
   e. Chest pain, cardiac abnormalities
   f. Dizziness/fainting
   g. Facial palsies, peripheral neuropathies
   h. Joint stiffness, recurrent arthritis that is pauciarticular affecting large joints, especially the knees

- Differential Diagnosis
1. Tinea corporis (ringworm)
2. Herald patch of pityriasis rosea
3. Insect bite
4. Cellulitis
5. Urticaria
6. Acute rheumatic fever
7. Influenza
8. Aseptic meningitis
9. Juvenile rheumatoid arthritis
10. Henoch-Schönlein purpura
11. Tick bite allergy
12. Erythema multiforme
13. Rickettiosis
14. Tickborne encephalitis
15. Chronic fatigue syndrome

- Physical Findings
1. Typical rash that occurs 1–2 weeks after a tick bite (can range from 1–36 days). Central clearing is classic, but not necessary for dx

2. Heart block (late)
3. Neurologic findings—seventh cranial nerve palsy
4. Fever, h/a, myalgias, fatigue, or arthralgias

- Diagnostic Tests/Findings
1. Enzyme-linked immunosorbent assay (ELISA)—detects antibodies against *B. burgdorferi*
2. Western blot—used to validate a positive or equivocal ELISA
3. Serum immunoglobulins—IgM, IgG elevated, but not until after the first few weeks, and if treatment is begun based on characteristic rash, seroconversion is blocked by antibiotic use
4. Other tests to consider
   a. Skin biopsy culture
   b. Culture of erythema migrans lesion—expensive, time to isolation may take 4 weeks
   c. PCR
   d. Electrocardiogram (ECG)

- Management
1. Treatment
   a. Medical referral is necessary for late disease or chronic symptoms
   b. Known tick bite
      (1) Single dose abx prophylaxis with doxycycline: children >8 years of age: 4 mg/kg/day orally as a single does
      (2) Postexposure prophylaxis with a single dose of doxycycline may be used for a significant exposure meeting all of the following criteria:
         (1) An engorged *Ixodes scapularis* tick is removed before at least an estimated 36 hours of attachment
         (2) Prophylaxis is started within 72 hours of tick removal

2. Early disease
   a. Children >8 years of age—doxycycline, which is the drug of choice, 2 mg/kg/dose orally twice daily; or amoxicillin; doxycycline 100 mg twice a day for 14 to 21 days
   b. Children ≤8 years of age—amoxicillin, 20–50 mg/kg/day tid for 14 to 21 days
   c. Cefuroxime 15–30 mg/kg/day orally given in two divided doses
   d. Secondary options (not recommended as first-line treatment)
      (1) Azithromycin: Children 10 mg/kg/day orally once daily
      (2) Erythromycin base: Children 30–50 mg/kg/day orally given in four divided doses
      (3) Clarithromycin: Children 15 mg/kg/day orally given in two divided doses
   e. Oral abx are recommended for patients with Lyme disease (local or disseminated) with EM, in the absence of CV or neurologic manifestations

3. Early disseminated disease
   a. Multiple EM is treated the same as for early localized disease, but for 21 days

b. Isolated facial palsy is the same for 21 to 28 days

c. Arthritis is the same for 28 days

4. Late disease for persistent arthritis, carditis, neurologic disease—parenteral ceftriaxone or penicillin G, referral to infectious specialist or Lyme specialist

5. Education/prevention

a. Ticks that carry Lyme disease are 4 to 5 mm in diameter; nymphs are smaller

b. Avoidance of tick-infested areas; prompt removal of ticks from the skin and use of tick repellent decrease the incidence of Lyme disease

c. Use blunt-end tweezers to grasp tick as close to skin surface as possible and gently and steadily pull it straight off; wear rubber gloves; look on the head, neck, behind the ears, the axilla, belt line, and groin

d. Disinfect skin where tick bite occurred

e. Early intervention leads to improved prognosis

f. Wear protective clothing in heavily wooded areas, light-colored clothing is better to see ticks, long-sleeved shirts tucked into pants, long pants tucked into socks, wear a hat, spray clothes with a permethrin; apply DEET insect repellents to exposed areas of skin with cautious use on young children; check skin closely after outdoor activities, daily if live near woods where deer and mice live or if live in an endemic part of the country

g. Keep pets tick free with daily inspection and prompt removal of any ticks

h. Report cases of Lyme disease to state health department

❑ INFECTIOUS MONONUCLEOSIS (IM)

- Definition: A clinical syndrome characterized by fever, exudative pharyngitis, lymphadenopathy, hepatosplenomegaly, and atypical lymphocytosis in a patient with Epstein-Barr virus (EBV)
- Etiology/Incidence
  1. EBV, also known as human herpes virus 4, is the causative agent in about 80–90% of cases of IM
  2. Contact with infected secretions or blood is required for transmission; virus is viable in saliva for several hours outside the body; fomite transmission is unknown
  3. Incubation period is 30 to 50 days
  4. Commonly diagnosed in adolescents and young adults
  5. No seasonal pattern
  6. Viral shedding occurs many months after acute infection and intermittently lifelong; asymptomatic carriage is common (over 90% of humans are infected by the time they are adults)
  7. Range of illness is wide, from asymptomatic to fatal infections
- Signs and Symptoms
  1. Fever (101–104°F), malaise, fatigue, headache, rhinitis, cough
  2. Abdominal pain, anorexia, nausea, vomiting
  3. Severe sore throat, difficulty swallowing, possibly to the point of dehydration
  4. Rash, especially with administration of ampicillin derivatives
  5. Tender, enlarged lymph nodes, including posterior cervical chain
  6. Generally begins as URI signs and symptoms, with increasing sore throat and enlarged tonsils and lymph nodes, along with increasing fatigue
  7. Hepatosplenomegaly
- Differential Diagnosis
  1. Group A streptococcal pharyngitis
  2. Hepatitis A
  3. Adenovirus
  4. Human herpes virus 6
  5. Herpes simplex virus 1
  6. Influenza or viral illness
  7. Cytomegalovirus
  8. HIV
- Physical Findings
  1. Exudative tonsillitis with patchy white or gray exudates
  2. Inflamed pharynx; possibly petechiae at junction of hard and soft palates
  3. May have hepatosplenomegaly
  4. Tender, enlarged anterior and posterior cervical nodes
  5. May have jaundice
  6. May have erythematous, macular, papular rash
  7. Periorbital edema
- Diagnostic Tests/Findings
  1. Positive monospot after 7 to 10 days; or positive Epstein-Barr virus IgM titer with acute illness appears in the first 2 weeks of disease; may need 7 to 10 days to show a positive test. Children younger than 4 years of age more often have negative initial testing
  2. Positive IgG reveals postacute or past infection
  3. WBC count reveals leukocytosis, 10,000 to 20,000 cells/mm^3, with ≥60% lymphocytes and 20% to 40% atypical lymphocytes
  4. Liver function tests may be elevated with hepatomegaly and/or jaundice
  5. Rapid strep test and throat culture—identify presence of beta-hemolytic streptococcal infection if present
  6. EBV-specific antibodies
  7. Real-time PCR
- Management/Treatment
  1. IM is a self-limited disease lasting 2 to 3 weeks
  2. Supportive treatment
     a. Rest and liquids during acute phase
     b. Antipyretics for fever and analgesics for pharyngitis and lymphadenitis
     c. Saline gargles for sore throat
     d. Isolation is unnecessary
     e. May return to school or work when completely recovered

f. Avoid strenuous exercise and contact sports until child is fully recovered, which can be 3 to 4 weeks or up to 2 months status post (sp) from illness onset and when the spleen is no longer palpable; splenic ultrasound may be necessary to show resolution prior to return to sports, particularly contact sports such as football, hockey, soccer, and lacrosse

g. Antibiotic therapy as needed for pharyngitis—avoid use of ampicillin derivatives such as amoxicillin and other penicillins; may result in a nonallergic morbilliform rash

h. Short-course corticosteroids are not routinely recommended but may be prescribed for patients with marked tonsillar hypertrophy and impending airway obstruction or dehydration, massive splenomegaly, myocarditis, or hemolytic anemia; oral prednisone is prescribed at 1 mg/kg/day for 5 to 7 days with a taper

i. Acyclovir or other antivirals are not needed for immunocompetent patients

☐ INFANT BOTULISM

- Definition: A neuroparalytic disorder affecting young infants (<6 months) resulting from ingestion of *Clostridium botulinum* spores with release of toxins as organism colonizes gastrointestinal tract. Toxin ingestion leads to a clinical syndrome characterized by cranial nerve (CN) palsies and descending, symmetrical flaccid paralysis
- Etiology/Incidence: Spores of *Clostridium botulinum* are ubiquitous, with 80–100 pediatric cases in the United States each year. Routes of colonization are foodborne, wound iatrogenic, and inhalational
  1. Etiologic agent is *Clostridium botulinum*; disease is caused by toxins produced by this anaerobic bacillus
  2. Toxin inhibits acetylcholine release at myoneural junction, resulting in impaired motor activity
  3. *C. botulinum* spores have been associated with honey; reported association with corn syrup not substantiated
  4. Rural, farm environments associated with increased incidence
  5. May occur in breastfed infants when first introducing nonhuman milk
  6. Incubation period about 3 to 30 days from time of ingestion
- Signs and Symptoms: Evolving symptomatology
  1. Ingestion of contaminated foods (home-canned vegetables, fruits, and fish products)
  2. Infant botulism is often attributed to honey ingestion, but other sources, including contaminated soil, have emerged
  3. Ingestion of honey and soil in infants are weak risk factors
  4. Paralysis of CN II, IV, and VI (blurred vision, diplopia, impaired accommodation, ptosis)
  5. Oculobulbar weakness (feeding difficulties, weakened cry)

  6. Hypoglossal weakness (CN IX, X, and XII)
  7. Dysarthria (CN IX, X, and XII)
  8. Dysphagia (CN IX, X, and XII)
  9. Symmetrical descending flaccid paralysis
  10. May be asymptomatic or rapidly progressive to apnea and sudden death
  11. Constipation (most common presenting symptom)
  12. Poor or slow feeding
  13. Weak cry
  14. Truncal weakness
  15. Loss of head and neck control, decreased movement
  16. Loss of facial expression
  17. Progressive, descending generalized weakness and hypotonia (floppiness)
- Differential Diagnosis
  1. Sepsis
  2. Benign congenital hypotonia
  3. Benign constipation
  4. Hypothyroidism
  5. Hirschsprung disease
  6. Other neuromuscular disorders
  7. Guillain-Barré syndrome
  8. Tick paralysis
  9. Phosphate or magnesium toxicity
- Physical Findings
  1. Generalized weakness
  2. Diminished deep tendon reflexes
  3. Cranial nerve deficits
  4. Swallowing difficulties
  5. Loss of muscle tone
  6. Diminished gag reflex
  7. Ocular palsies
- Diagnostic Tests/Findings
  1. Stool specimen for toxin assay is test of choice for infant botulism
  2. Stool culture positive for *C. botulinum*
  3. Blood culture—may or may not be positive for *C. botulinum*
  4. Mouse bioassay of food samples
- Management/Treatment: Supportive care is the mainstay of botulism therapy
  1. Human-derived antitoxin (botulism immune globulin intravenous, BabyBIG) is treatment of choice
  2. Equine antitoxin not usually recommended for infant botulism
  3. Hospitalization; possibility of respiratory arrest
  4. Stool softener
  5. Prevention/education regarding honey as potential source of botulism; avoid feeding to infants <12 months of age
  6. Report to state health department

☐ POLIOMYELITIS

Definition: An acute, contagious, viral disease in which 95% of infections are asymptomatic. Polio may manifest as a minor illness, usually gastrointestinal, or as a major illness, characterized by acute flaccid paralysis

- Etiology/Incidence
  1. Caused by enterovirus (EV)
  2. When susceptible person comes in contact with poliovirus, one of three responses occur:
     a. Nonspecific febrile illness (most frequent)—fever, myalgia, sore throat, headache (occurs in 24% of people who become infected)
     b. Aseptic meningitis (nonparalytic poliomyelitis)—headache, stiff neck, spinal rigidity, nausea (occurs in 1% to 5% of patients a few days after the minor illness has resolved)
     c. Paralytic poliomyelitis (least frequent)—flaccid paralysis, loss of reflexes, asymmetrical paralysis, proximal limb muscles and lower extremity muscles are more involved (occurs in fewer than 1% of infections)
  3. Incubation period of asymptomatic or nonparalytic polio is 3 to 6 days; that of paralytic polio to onset of paralysis is 7 to 21 days
  4. Preventable by active immunization—IPV (inactivated poliovirus vaccine) is now used exclusively in the United States since 2000, when the OPV (oral poliovirus vaccine) was discontinued; OPV was known to cause VAPP (vaccine-associated paralytic poliomyelitis)
  5. Spread by fecal-oral routes and respiratory secretions; virus persists in throat for about 1 week and sheds in feces for several weeks
  6. Most contagious shortly before and after onset of clinical signs of disease
  7. Occurs more often in infants and young children
  8. Occurs more commonly in conditions of poor hygiene
- Signs and Symptoms:
  1. History of inadequate immunization or recent immunization
  2. Initially, fever, myalgia, sore throat, and headache for 2–6 days
  3. GI prodrome
  4. Decreased tone and motor function/tendon reflexes of affected limb
  5. In less than 10% of infected children, several symptom-free days are followed by aseptic meningeal signs: headache, stiff neck, spinal rigidity, and nausea
  6. Mild cases resolve completely.
- Differential Diagnosis: Aseptic meningitis due to poliovirus is not distinguishable from other viral causes. Paralysis in the United States is usually due to nonpolio enteroviruses
  1. Guillain-Barré syndrome
  2. Meningitis
  3. Encephalitis
  4. Peripheral neuritis or neuropathy
  5. Botulism
  6. Tick paralysis
- Physical Findings
  1. Meningeal signs
  2. Respiratory compromise
  3. Inability to speak without frequent pauses
  4. Muscle weakness
- Diagnostic Tests/Findings: EV isolated from feces, throat, urine, or CSF in cell culture; isolate is sent to CDC

- Management/Treatment
  1. Medical referral necessary
  2. Supportive management—bed rest, adequate hydration, pain control, acetaminophen or ibuprofen for fever, respiratory support if paralysis ensues, physical therapy for deficits associated with muscle weakness and paralysis
  3. Education—educate family regarding potential complications of possible paralysis, including respiratory compromise and arrest, renal calculi due to immobility, bladder and bowel malfunction
  4. Inform the local health department

☐ TETANUS (LOCKJAW)

- Definition: A neurologic disease characterized by severe muscle spasms and hyperreflexia that can be fatal
- Etiology/Incidence
  1. Caused by the neurotoxin produced by anaerobic bacterium *Clostridium tetani* in contaminated wounds
  2. Occurs throughout the world; neonatal tetanus is common in countries where women are not immunized. The umbilical cord may be a source for entry
  3. Incubation period 2 days to 2 months, usually occurs in 14 days; 5 to 14 days in neonates
  4. More common in warmer climates and warmer months
  5. Has dramatically decreased with advent of tetanus vaccine
  6. *Clostridium tetani* is ubiquitous in the environment, in soil and human and animal intestines
- Signs and Symptoms
  1. Incomplete tetanus immunization series
  2. History of deep puncture wound, laceration
  3. Insidious onset, gradual over 1 to 7 days
  4. Muscle spasms aggravated by stimuli—sound, light, movement
  5. Muscle rigidity
  6. Increased oral secretions
  7. Respiratory compromise
  8. Begins with pain at site of wound, followed by regional muscle spasm, by 48 hours there is difficulty opening the jaw (trismus), followed by generalized tetany
  9. In infants, first sign is irritability and inability to nurse or feed; followed by stiffness of jaw, neck, increasing dysphagia, generalized hyperreflexia with rigidity and spasms of the abdomen and back causing opisthotonus; characteristic facial expression of a grimace; there may be seizures; a high or low temperature is a bad prognostic sign
- Differential Diagnosis
  1. Muscle spasms
  2. Amyotrophic lateral sclerosis (Lou Gehrig's disease)
  3. Hypocalcemic tetany
  4. Neuroleptic malignant syndrome
  5. Strychnine poisoning
  6. Poliomyelitis
  7. Bacterial meningitis

8. Narcotic withdrawal
9. Generalized seizures
- Physical Findings
1. Muscle spasms aggravated by stimuli
2. Muscle rigidity
3. Lockjaw
4. Back pain
5. Dysphagia
6. Hx IV drug habits
7. Increased oral secretions
8. Respiratory compromise
9. Patients are fully conscious
- Diagnostic Tests/Findings: Diagnosis made clinically
- Management/Treatment
1. Medical referral
2. Wounds need to be cleaned and debrided properly
3. Supportive management—treatment of muscle spasms, intravenous fluids, respiratory support
4. Minimize external stimuli (e.g., loud noise, bright light) to prevent aggravating muscle spasms
5. Human tetanus immune globulin (TIG) given to prevent circulating toxin from binding to central nervous system sites
6. Infection with tetanus does not confer immunity; patient should be reimmunized in convalescent period to prevent future infection
7. Education—educate family regarding potential complications from tetanus, including respiratory compromise, inability to speak

☐ MALARIA

- Definition: A parasitic infection primarily acquired via mosquito bite that is characterized by high fever, rigors, sweats, and headache
- Etiology/Incidence
1. Caused by protozoa of the genus *Plasmodium*. It is naturally transmitted to humans through a bite by an infected female *Anopheles* mosquito. Transmission can be congenital; via transfusions or contaminated needles
2. Infection by *Plasmodium falciparum* is most serious and potentially fatal
3. Endemic in tropical areas worldwide; most cases in United States reported annually (approximately 1000) are acquired during foreign travel
- Signs and Symptoms
1. History of recent travel to endemic area
2. Classic paroxysmal symptoms—high fever, rigors, diaphoresis, and headache
3. Fever and other symptoms eventually become synchronized, and depending on the infecting species of *Plasmodium*, fever will occur every other or every third day
4. Associated symptoms—nausea, vomiting, diarrhea, arthralgia, cough, abdominal and back pain, pallor, jaundice

5. Multisystem involvement can develop with *Plasmodium falciparum* infection; may be fatal
   a. Neurologic—seizures, signs of increased intracranial pressure, confusion, stupor, coma, and death
   b. Pulmonary—coarse breath sounds, pulmonary edema
   c. Renal—decreased urine output, oliguria, hematuria
   d. Cardiovascular—absent peripheral pulses, hypotension
   e. Gastrointestinal—diarrhea
   f. Vascular collapse and shock
6. Inadequate or absent chemoprophylaxis
7. Insecticide-treated bed net not used in endemic area
8. Age <5 years
- Differential Diagnosis
1. Influenza
2. Rocky Mountain spotted fever
3. Septicemia
4. Typhoid
5. IM
6. HIV seroconversion
- Physical Findings
1. Early findings—listlessness, rigors, muscle weakness, pallor, jaundice, hepatosplenomegaly
2. Findings seen in *Plasmodium falciparum* infection—neurologic deficits, pneumonia, elevated liver enzymes, renal failure
- Diagnostic Tests/Findings
1. Giemsa-stained thick and thin blood smears
2. Rapid dx tests
3. CBC
4. Clotting profile
5. Serum electrolytes, BUN, and creatinine
6. Diagnosis depends on identification of parasite on stained blood films
- Management/Treatment
1. Medical referral
2. Drug therapy based on the infecting *Plasmodium* species, possible drug resistance, and severity of the disease; refer to the most current AAP *Red Book* for varying treatment regimens
3. Prevention best achieved through prophylactic therapy prior to travel to endemic areas; doses for children are calculated according to weight and should never exceed adult doses; each drug has its own side effects, check the *Red Book* for listing
   a. Use chloroquine for areas in which there is no chloroquine-resistant malaria; begin 1 week before arrival and continue for 4 weeks after departure from area
   b. In areas of chloroquine-resistant malaria, three drugs may be used: atovaquone-proguanil, doxycycline, and mefloquine; one must refer to the *Red Book* for appropriate ages and doses, as well as side effects
4. Control measures include protection against mosquitoes—by use of mosquito nets containing insecticide,

insect repellents containing DEET, and protective clothing; contact the CDC Malaria Hotline at 1-770-488-7788 (or online information) for country-specific risks, drug-resistant strains in that country, and recommendations for travelers
  5. Education should include natural history of the illness and specific follow-up or rehabilitation needed after infection with *Plasmodium falciparum*
  6. Report cases to state health department

☐ METHICILLIN-RESISTANT *STAPHYLOCOCCUS AUREUS* (MRSA)

- Definition: A type of *Staphylococcus aureus* that is resistant to available beta-lactam antibiotics, anti-staphylococcal penicillins (methicillin, oxacillin), and cephalosporins. MRSA can be hospital or community acquired (CA)
- Etiology/Incidence
  1. MRSA is a Gram-positive pathogen that can cause infection in various sites such as the skin, soft tissue, joints, and lungs
  2. Prevalence is increasing globally. Nurses are known to be nasal colonizers of MRSA. Children are more commonly afflicted with CA-MRSA
- Signs and Symptoms
  1. Erythematous skin lesions or pustules, in single or multiple forms
  2. Irritation or pain at indwelling catheter site
  3. Infections unresponsive to PCN
  4. Hx of a presumed spider bite
  5. Abscess formation
  6. Lymphatic streaking
  7. Fever
  8. Fatigue
- Differential Diagnosis
  1. Insect or spider bite
  2. Cellulitis
  3. Folliculitis
  4. Pneumonia not due to MRSA
  5. Bacteremia, UTI, infective endocarditis, joint infections not due to MRSA
- Physical Findings
  1. Erythematous skin lesions or pustules; pt may report the lesion began as a small pimple
  2. Irritation or pain at indwelling catheter site
  3. Infection unresponsive to PCN
  4. Abscess
  5. Lymphatic streaking
  6. Fever
  7. Fatigue
  8. Tachycardia, hypotension
  9. Cough, dyspnea
- Diagnostic Tests/Findings
  1. Culture and sensitivity (C & S) confirms diagnosis
  2. Suspect community-acquired MRSA if abscess formation

- Management/Treatment
  1. Incise and drain (I & D) abscess when appropriate; send culture
  2. Withhold abx therapy in simple uncomplicated cases until cx result obtained
  3. Close follow-up is necessary
  4. Complicated infections (endocarditis, joint infections, pneumonia, and bacteremia) require hospitalization
  5. TMP/SMX is first choice; a tetracycline can be used; clindamycin can be used but a resistant test should be done prior to initiation of clindamycin; clindamycin has more side effects. Linezolid can be bused, but it is expensive
  6. I & D alone (without abx) may be sufficient treatment for small skin and soft tissue abscesses <5 cm
  7. First-line treatment for hospital-acquired MRSA infection is vancomycin

☐ HIV

- Definition: HIV infection is a pandemic caused by a retrovirus that erodes the integrity of the human immune system over time, resulting in immune incompetence and a susceptibility to opportunistic infections and malignancies. AIDS occurs as a result of HIV infection. A strong risk factor is high maternal viral load (mother-to-child transmission)
- Etiology/Incidence: HIV belongs to the genus *Lentivirus* of the family Retroviridae. HIV 1 is responsible for the global epidemic. HIV 2 is less pathogenic and is mostly seen in West Africa
- Signs/Symptoms
  1. Needle sharing with IV drug use
  2. Sexually transmitted diseases (STDs)
  3. Shingles
  4. Medical comorbidities
  5. Recent hospital admissions
  6. Wasting syndrome
  7. High maternal viral load (mother-to-child transmission)
  8. Short of breath (SOB) on exertion, dry cough
  9. Malnutrition
  10. Young age
  11. Crowded or impoverished home environment
  12. Smoking
  13. Substance abuse
  14. Recurrent herpes simplex
- Differential Diagnosis
  1. EBV
  2. CMV
  3. Secondary syphilis
  4. Cold, pharyngitis
  5. Viral hepatitis
  6. Influenza
- Physical Findings
  1. Fever
  2. Night sweats
  3. Weight loss

4. Skin rashes
5. Oral ulcers
6. Diarrhea
7. Generalized lymphadenopathy
8. Genital STDs

• Diagnostic Tests/Findings
1. ELISA test is positive (false negative may occur during window period immediately after infection before AB have developed)
2. Western blot confirms dx

• Management/Treatment
1. Refer to infectious disease (ID) specialist for adequate counseling and advice
2. Highly active antiretroviral therapy (HAART) if indicated (guidelines suggest HIV-1-infected adolescents' primary care should be given by a clinician who is managing at least 20 HIV-positive people)
3. Immunization and prophylaxis should be discussed

❏ QUESTIONS

Select the best answer.

1. Septicemia in the newborn period is most likely caused by which organism?
   a. *Listeria monocytogenes*
   b. *Haemophilus influenzae*
   c. *Neisseria meningitidis*
   d. *Streptococcus* pneumonia

2. Signs and symptoms of bacterial sepsis in children beyond the neonatal period include:
   a. Cough, fever, abdominal pain
   b. Vesicular rash, pruritus, fever
   c. Irritability, fever, lethargy
   d. Abdominal pain, diarrhea, vomiting

3. Which of the following vaccines provides protection against a common type of sepsis/meningitis?
   a. Smallpox vaccination
   b. Hepatitis B vaccine
   c. *Haemophilus influenzae* vaccine
   d. Inactivated polio vaccine

4. Although relatively rare in the United States, diphtheria can occur among underimmunized children. Which of the following clusters of signs, symptoms, and physical findings would suggest diphtheria in a child presenting with upper respiratory complaints?
   a. Low-grade fever, sore throat, nasal discharge, and grayish-white pseudomembrane in his/her throat
   b. Abrupt onset of high fever, severe sore throat, nasal discharge, and grayish-white pseudomembrane in his/her throat space
   c. Low-grade fever, abrupt onset of severe sore throat with difficulty swallowing and drooling
   d. Abrupt onset of high fever, severe sore throat, with difficulty swallowing and drooling

5. Infants younger than 6 months of age with pertussis frequently require hospitalization to manage:
   a. Fever, cough, dehydration
   b. Coughing paroxysms, apnea, cyanosis, feeding difficulties
   c. Coughing paroxysms, dehydration, renal failure
   d. Seizures, fever, pneumonia

6. One of the most appropriate agents used to treat influenza A is:
   a. Acyclovir
   b. Oseltamivir
   c. Erythromycin
   d. Tetracycline

7. Which of the following symptoms are characteristic of rubella?
   a. Vesicular, crusted lesions and high fever
   b. Postauricular lymphadenopathy and low-grade fever
   c. Intense pruritus, usually in finger webs, buttocks, thighs, and ankles
   d. Rough-textured maculopapular rash that blanches with pressure

8. Although uncommon, potential sequelae of rubella may include:
   a. Pneumonia and chronic otitis media
   b. Arthritis, thrombocytopenia, and encephalitis
   c. Oophoritis and infertility
   d. Arthritis, carditis, and neurologic involvement

9. Rubeola is:
   a. Preventable by active immunization
   b. Caused by human herpesvirus 6
   c. Treated with intravenous acyclovir
   d. Not associated with severe complications (e.g., encephalitis, pneumonia)

10. You are examining a child who has fever, coryza, cough, conjunctivitis, malaise, and anorexia. During the oral examination, you observe red eruptions with white centers on the buccal mucosa. What are these eruptions called?
    a. Pastia spots
    b. Rubeola spots
    c. Koplik spots
    d. Strawberry spots

11. Which of the following best describes the treatment for roseola?
    a. Acetaminophen or ibuprofen for fever, parental reassurance
    b. Warm compresses for salivary gland swelling
    c. Oral acyclovir, 20 mg/kg/dose, four times a day
    d. Bed rest, saline gargles for sore throat

12. Fifth disease is usually:
    a. Seen in children ages 5 to 14 year
    b. Transmitted via the deer tick
    c. Treated with oral erythromycin
    d. Characterized by prolonged coughing episodes

13. Which of the following statements is not true regarding the transmission of chickenpox?
    a. Susceptible individuals can contract chickenpox from patients with varicella zoster (shingles).
    b. Children with chickenpox are infectious only during the period of time when skin lesions are present.
    c. Children with chickenpox are no longer infectious once crusting of skin lesions has occurred.

d. Varicella-zoster immune globulin (VZIG) should be administered to susceptible immunocompromised individuals who are exposed to a patient with varicella-zoster infection.

14. A child with chickenpox and temperature of 102°F should receive which medication for fever?
    a. Aspirin
    b. Amoxicillin
    c. Acetaminophen
    d. Acyclovir

15. The most appropriate agent for use in treating varicella-zoster infection in an immunocompromised host is:
    a. Ganciclovir
    b. Acyclovir
    c. Ceftriaxone
    d. Chloramphenicol

16. Varicella-zoster infection is most commonly associated with which of the following skin lesions?
    a. Vesicle
    b. Comedone
    c. Nodule
    d. Macule

17. Which of the following is not a complication of mumps?
    a. Meningitis
    b. Pneumonia
    c. Oophoritis
    d. Pancreatitis

18. What recommendation would you make to a parent whose son has been diagnosed with mumps and who wants to know when the child can return to child care?
    a. He can return once he becomes afebrile and can tolerate eating.
    b. He can return 9 days after onset of symptoms.
    c. He can return when he is well enough to participate in activities.
    d. He can return after a minimum of 5 days of antibiotic therapy.

19. Which of the following are symptoms of cat scratch disease?
    a. Joint pain, conjunctivitis, mild neck stiffness
    b. Irritability, fever, hypotension
    c. Fever, malaise, lymphadenopathy
    d. Severe coughing, vomiting, anorexia

20. The following describes a characteristic rash associated with which disease? Initially erythematous and macular, becoming maculopapular and petechial. The rash first appears on the wrists and ankles and then spreads proximally to the trunk. The palms and soles are often involved.
    a. Lyme disease
    b. Roseola
    c. Rubeola (measles)
    d. Rocky Mountain spotted fever

21. A 10-year-old child manifests symptoms of fever, sore throat, and swollen lymph nodes. Spleen tip is palpable. Throat culture and monospot test results

are negative. The next logical diagnostic test would involve:
    a. Repeat throat culture
    b. Chest radiograph
    c. Bone marrow examination
    d. Epstein-Barr virus titer

22. Which of the following factors is not associated with increased risk for infantile botulism?
    a. Rural environments
    b. Use of honey
    c. Use of corn syrup
    d. Farm families

23. Which of the following interventions would not be appropriate for a 6-month-old infant with a suspected diagnosis of infantile botulism?
    a. Stool and blood cultures
    b. Immediate administration of equine antitoxin
    c. Stool softeners
    d. Supportive care

24. Which of the following are associated with paralytic poliomyelitis?
    a. Lacy, erythematous, pruritic rash
    b. Respiratory compromise, speech disturbances, urinary incontinence
    c. Abdominal swelling, lymphadenopathy, and jaundice
    d. Nonspecific abdominal pain, nausea, and vomiting

25. Muscle spasms associated with tetanus are aggravated by which of the following?
    a. Fever
    b. Tetanus immunoglobulin
    c. External stimuli
    d. NSAIDs

26. Classic symptoms associated with malaria include:
    a. Low-grade fever, upper respiratory congestion, cough
    b. Annular rash, conjunctivitis, headache, arthralgia
    c. High fever, chills, rigors, sweats, headache
    d. High fever, jaundice, lethargy, vomiting

27. Lyme disease is most closely associated with which of the following skin lesions?
    a. Erythema migrans
    b. Nodule
    c. Scale
    d. Pustule

28. Many infectious diseases present with rashes along with general complaints of fever, malaise, and headaches. Which of the following clusters of symptoms would make you consider Lyme disease as a likely diagnosis?
    a. Fever, malaise, headache, arthralgia, and well-circumscribed, erythematous, annular rash with central clearing
    b. Fever, malaise, headache, transient bone pain, and generalized erythematous, maculopapular rash that began on the face and spread to trunk and extremities
    c. Fever, malaise, anorexia, and confluent, erythematous, brownish maculopapular rash
    d. Fever, malaise, anorexia, and erythematous rash beginning on wrists and ankles and then spreading to the trunk

29. Which of the following would be included in patient education regarding Lyme disease?
    a. Educate caretakers regarding complications, including hypertension and renal calculi due to immobility
    b. Educate caretakers to avoid use of aspirin-containing products for fever control due to association with increased risk for Reye syndrome
    c. Educate caretakers regarding use of protective clothing and tick repellent in heavily wooded areas
    d. Educate caretakers regarding natural history of the illness and need for specific follow-up after infection with *Rickettsia rickettsii*

☐ ANSWERS AND RATIONALES

1. A: *Listeria monocytogenes* is the most likely cause of sepsis in the newborn period.
2. C: Irritability, fever, and lethargy are signs and symptoms of sepsis in children beyond the neonatal period.
3. C: *Haemophilus influenzae* vaccine provides protection against sepsis/meningitis.
4. A: Low-grade fever, sore throat, nasal discharge, and grayish-white pharyngeal findings suggests diphtheria.
5. B: Infants younger than 6 months of age require hospitalization to manage the respiratory symptoms of pertussis and maintain adequate nutrition.
6. B: Oseltamivir is recommended to treat influenza A within 2 days of symptom onset.
7. B: The rash in rubella starts on the forehead and face and spreads over trunk and extremities during the 1st day and disappears by 3rd day.
8. B: Complications of rubella include arthritis and, rarely, thrombocytopenia and encephalitis.
9. A: Active immunization can prevent rubeola.
10. C: Koplik spots are red eruptions with white centers on buccal mucosa; they occur prior to appearance of rash.
11. A: Roseola is best managed by controlling fever and reassuring caregivers that appearance of rash is sign of recovery.
12. A: Fifth disease, or erythema infectiosum (EI), is typically seen in older children, and caregivers need reassurance of the benign nature of the disease.
13. B: VZV incubation period is between 10 and 21 days, and infected individuals are contagious for 24–48 hours prior to outbreak of lesions until all lesions have crusted over.
14. C: Aspirin should be avoided in children due to potential for Reye syndrome. Amoxicillin and acyclovir are not indicated for treatment of fever.
15. B: Acyclovir is an antiviral agent that inhibits DNA polymerase; it incorporates into viral DNA. Ganciclovir is indicated for cytomegalovirus (CMV); ceftriaxone is a cephalosporin antibiotic, and chloramphenicol is an antibacterial.
16. A: Vesicles are characteristic lesions of viral infections. Comedones are skin lesions seen in acne. A nodule is a raised lesion, and a macule is a flat lesion; neither are characteristic of varicella-zoster infection.
17. B: Complications of mumps include pancreatitis, oophoritis, meningitis, and orchitis.
18. B: Child may return when all symptoms have resolved or 9 days after onset of symptoms.
19. C: Low-grade fever, general malaise, headache (h/a), nausea, chills, general aching, and swollen lymph nodes are symptoms of CSD.
20. D: RMSF has a characteristic petechial or purpuric rash. Lyme disease rash (EM) has central clearing. Roseola rash is erythematous and maculopapular, starting on the truck and spreading to the arms and neck. Rubeola rash is maculopapular and occurs 3–4 days after initial symptoms.
21. D: An EBV IgM titer may appear in the first 2 weeks of infectious mononucleosis (IM) and may need 7–10 days to show a positive test. A chest x-ray or bone marrow aspiration is not a diagnostic test for IM.
22. C: Rural environments, use of honey, and farm families are risk factors for infantile botulism.
23. B: Equine antitoxin is not usually recommended for infant botulism.
24. B: Physical findings of paralytic poliomyelitis are meningeal signs, respiratory compromise, inability to speak without frequent pauses, and muscle weakness.
25. C: Minimize external stimuli to prevent aggravating muscle spasms.
26. C: High fevers, diaphoresis, rigors, and headache (h/a) are symptoms of malaria. Rash and jaundice are not symptoms of malaria.
27. A: EM is the characteristic rash of Lyme disease. About 70% of patients get the rash of erythema with central clearing.
28. A: The rash in Lyme disease is not maculopapular nor brownish, and it does not spread from the extremities to the trunk. Erythema migrans (EM) rash usually occurs at the site of the tick bite.
29. C: Hypertension (HTN) and renal calculi are not complications of Lyme disease. Aspirin products may be used in adults. The tickborne infection is caused by *Borrelia*.

☐ BIBLIOGRAPHY

Hay, W. W., Levin, M. J., Sondheimer, J. M., & Detarding, R. P. (2011). *Current diagnosis and treatment in pediatrics* (20th ed.). New York, NY: McGraw-Hill.

Kimberlin, D. W., Brady, M. T., Jackson, M. A., & Long, S. S. (Eds.). (2015). *Red Book: 2015 report of the Committee on Infectious Diseases* (30th ed.). Elk Grove Village, IL: American Academy of Pediatrics. Retrieved from http://ebooks.aappublications.org/content/red-book-30th-edition-2015

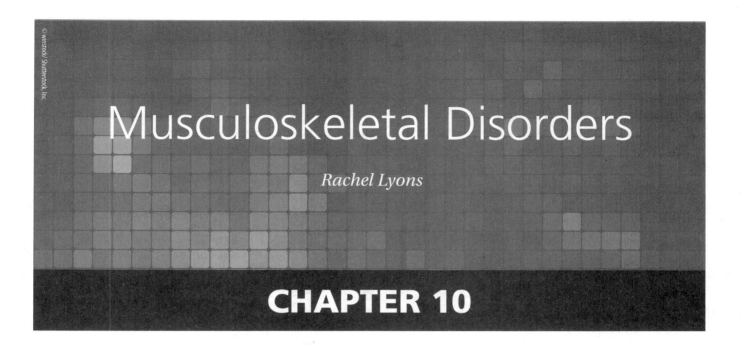

Musculoskeletal Disorders

Rachel Lyons

CHAPTER 10

☐ TORTICOLLIS (WRY NECK)

- Definition: Abnormal position of head and neck, due to unilateral contracture of sternocleidomastoid muscle that may be congenital (most common) or acquired or due to atlantoaxial rotary subluxation, which is a displacement of C1 on C2
- Etiology/Incidence
  1. Cause not well defined but may be due to:
     a. Compartment syndrome due to soft tissue compression of neck at time of delivery
     b. Occlusion of venous outflow of sternocleidomastoid muscle
     c. Uterine crowding
     d. Neurogenic myopathy from trauma or ischemia
     e. Sternocleidomastoid muscle tumor
  2. Neurogenic causes rare
  3. Higher incidence in children with breech presentation and forceps delivery, but occurs with vaginal births or C-sections
  4. 20% have developmental dysplasia of the hip (DDH)
  5. Familial tendency (rare)
  6. 0.4% live births; males more frequently affected
- Signs and Symptoms
  1. Child's head tilted toward side of contracture
  2. Chin rotated away from contracted side (origin of muscle on mastoid process)
- Differential Diagnosis
  1. Central nervous system (CNS) tumors
  2. Syringomyelia
  3. Arnold-Chiari malformation

  4. Ocular dysfunctions
  5. Paroxysmal torticollis of infancy
  6. Klippel-Feil syndrome
- Physical Findings
  1. Contracture of one of sternocleidomastoid muscles
  2. Fusiform, firm mass or "tumor"
     a. In body of contracted muscle
     b. Palpable after 4 weeks of age, then recedes
  3. Plagiocephaly or asymmetry of face/skull development present with progressive deformity
- Diagnostic Tests/Findings
  1. Cervical radiograph
     a. To rule out congenital spine abnormalities, e.g., hemivertebrae
     b. Normal with muscular torticollis
  2. Other imaging (MRI or CT scan) not indicated—abnormalities not detected unless neurogenic pathology (rare) exists
  3. Hip ultrasound or x-ray, depending on age of child, to rule out DDH
- Management/Treatment
  1. Conservative measures—initial treatment
     a. Stretching exercises—guided by physical therapist
     b. Encourage infant stretching by placing toys, mobiles, items of interest in infant's line of vision on the affected side
  2. Surgery recommended when:
     a. Defect persists beyond 1 year of age
     b. Stretching exercises have been unsuccessful
     c. Infant between 1 and 4 years of age; best outcome for surgical release

DEVELOPMENTAL DYSPLASIA OF THE HIP (DDH)

- Definition: Abnormal development dislocation of the hip(s), or ligamentous laxity that is congenital, but may not be recognized until ambulation occurs
- Etiology/Incidence
  1. Multifactorial etiology in an otherwise normal child
     a. Intrauterine mechanical factors
        (1) Breech presentation
        (2) Infants with oligohydramnios
     b. Genetic effects in primary acetabular dysplasia
        (1) Various degrees of joint laxity
        (2) 20% have positive family history
     c. Increased incidence in first-born Caucasian infants; tight uterine muscles limit movement
  2. Left hip involved more commonly than right
  3. Greater incidence in girls (girls more often in breech position); 80% cases
  4. Incidence 1 to 1.5:1000 live births
- Signs and Symptoms
  1. Newborn
     a. Instability without significant fixed deformity
     b. Detected during newborn examination
  2. Sometimes not detected at birth
     a. Untreated dislocation becomes fixed, with less instability, more limitation of movement (abduction)
     b. Limp noticeable at onset of walking
     c. Afebrile, painless, may have ligamentous laxity
- Differential Diagnosis
  1. Leg length discrepancy
  2. Innocent hip "click"—not associated with movement of femoral head
  3. Arthrogryposis
  4. Cerebral palsy
  5. Fracture of femur
- Physical Findings
  1. Galeazzi sign—knee height comparison with infant in supine position with flexed hips/knees
     a. Asymmetry evident in DDH
     b. Shortening of the femoral segment limits abduction and full extension
     c. Not helpful finding for detecting bilateral dislocation
  2. Limited abduction of affected hip in older child
  3. Indicators of hip instability in newborn—test each hip individually
     a. Barlow's sign
        (1) Positive when movement of femoral head can be felt as it slips out onto the posterior lip of acetabulum
        (2) Not diagnostic, but indicates need for surveillance
     b. Ortolani's sign (positive findings)
        (1) Newborn period—sometimes a "click" or "clunk" is heard as femoral head enters or exits acetabulum

(2) After newborn period—"click" is less apparent and decreased abduction of flexed legs (at hip) is more significant
  4. Three degrees of hip dysplasia
     a. Subluxation
        (1) First degree, least severe
        (2) Femoral head rests in acetabulum
        (3) Can be dislocated partially by examination
     b. Dislocatable
        (1) Second degree
        (2) Hip can be dislocated fully with manipulation, but is reducible
     c. Dislocated hips
        (1) Third degree, most severe
        (2) Fixed dislocation
- Diagnostic Tests/Findings
  1. Physical examination is most reliable
  2. Radiographs
     a. Not commonly used before 6 months of age
     b. After 6 months of age assess femoral head/acetabulum relationship
  3. Ultrasonography
     a. Before 6 months of age due to lack of ossification of proximal femoral heads
     b. Assesses hip stability and acetabular development
- Management/Treatment
  1. Identification during newborn period essential for good prognosis
  2. Goal is to restore contact between femoral head and acetabulum
  3. Subluxation in newborn
     a. High incidence of spontaneous improvement in perinatal period
     b. Observe and reexamine 3 to 4 weeks after birth
  4. Dislocated hips
     a. Treat at time of diagnosis
     b. Before 6 months of age
        (1) If unstable, stabilize with an abduction-flexion device (e.g., Pavlik harness); triple diapers not effective
        (2) If device is ineffective, surgery is indicated
     c. If diagnosis made after 6 months of age
        (1) Child usually too large and strong to tolerate brace (failure rate 50% after 6 months old)
        (2) Surgical reduction indicated

TALIPES EQUINOVARUS CONGENITA (CLUBFOOT)

- Definition: Common foot deformity that involves the foot and entire lower leg; classified into three groups, (1) congenital, (2) teratologic, and (3) positional
- Etiology/Incidence
  1. Cause unknown, possible inheritance factors or neuromuscular cause

2. Congenital form—about 75% of all cases
   a. 50% cases are bilateral
   b. 1:1000 live births; more common in males
3. Teratologic form—associated with neuromuscular disorders, e.g., spina bifida, arthrogryposis, multiple congenital, or a syndrome complex
4. Positional form—normal foot that has been held in deformed position in utero
- Signs and Symptoms
  1. Congenital form
     a. Absence of other congenital abnormalities
     b. Variable rigidity of the foot
     c. Mild calf atrophy
     d. Mild hypoplasia of the tibia, fibula, and bones of the foot
  2. Older child—calf and foot atrophy are more obvious than in infant, regardless of how well corrected
- Differential Diagnosis
  1. Internal femoral torsion
  2. Internal tibial torsion
  3. Metatarsus adductus
  4. Neuromuscular disorders
- Physical Findings
  1. Small foot with limited dorsiflexion; usually obvious at birth
  2. Combination of deformities
     a. Results in 90-degree rotation of forefoot in all planes
     b. Leg and foot resemble shape of club
  3. Deep crease on medial border of foot
  4. Calf muscles thin and atrophic (more obvious in older child)
- Diagnostic Tests/Findings: Radiographs
  1. Rule out other conditions
- Management/Treatment
  1. Refer to orthopedist
  2. Serial casting with manipulation begins at birth; usually 3 to 6 months
  3. If further corrections required, surgery to lengthen tendon Achilles indicated

❑ METATARSUS ADDUCTUS/ METATARSUS VARUS

- Definition: Congenital medial deviation of the forefoot on the hind foot
- Etiology/Incidence
  1. Uncertain etiology; often associated with abnormal intrauterine positioning
  2. Most common congenital foot deformity
  3. 1:1000 live births
  4. 10% of children with metatarsus also have developmental dysplasia of the hip
- Signs and Symptoms
  1. Toeing-in; "pigeon-toed" gait in older child
  2. Usually not painful

- Differential Diagnosis
  1. Internal femoral torsion
  2. Internal tibial torsion
  3. Equinovarus
- Physical Findings
  1. Adductus—forefoot adducted only; full range of motion (ROM)
  2. Varus—forefoot adducted and inverted; limited ROM
  3. Ankle joint has normal dorsiflexion and plantar flexion
- Diagnostic Tests/Findings
  1. Physical examination—usually sufficient to establish treatment plan
  2. Radiographs
     a. Usually unnecessary
     b. Used when:
        (1) Underlying congenital anomalies are suspected
        (2) Foot is unusually rigid
        (3) Failure of spontaneous resolution with growth
- Management/Treatment
  1. Supple deformity (adductus)
     a. Parents stretch forefoot in all planes of motion with each diaper change for 4 to 6 months
     b. Observe and follow up
  2. Rigid deformity (varus)
     a. Serial casting or bracing in the first year of life
     b. Then straight-laced/out-flare shoes fitted for daytime until no chance of recurrence
     c. Surgical intervention required for child older than 4 years if significant residual metatarsus adductus persists

❑ TIBIAL TORSION (INTERNAL)

- Definition: Abnormal bowing (internal or external rotation) of the tibia
- Etiology/Incidence
  1. Combination of genetic factors and intrauterine position
  2. Usually not pathological
  3. Internal tibial torsion—12% at birth; usually resolves by 2 years
  4. External tibial torsion—develops after birth or by 2 years
- Signs and Symptoms
  1. Toeing-in appearance of child's legs when walking/ running
  2. Rarely painful
  3. Tripping and falling may be noticed
- Differential Diagnosis
  1. Metatarsus adductus
  2. Femoral neck anteversion
  3. Femoral neck retroversion
  4. Neuromuscular disorders
  5. Equinovarus

- Physical Findings
  1. No obvious deformity
  2. Full ROM
  3. Internal rotation of affected leg, flat feet, increased lumbar lordosis
- Diagnostic Tests/Findings
  1. Observation
  2. Angle measurement
     a. Between foot and thigh
     b. With ankle and knee position at 90-degree angle
     c. With child lying in prone position
- Management/Treatment
  1. Reassure parents that most children have spontaneous correction with growth and need no treatment
  2. Recommend supine sleeping position

☐ GENU VARUM (BOWLEG)

- Definition: Lateral bowing of the tibia
- Etiology/Incidence
  1. Joint laxity may contribute to deformity
  2. Considered normal until 36 months
  3. May be related to intrauterine position
- Signs and Symptoms
  1. Parental concern common regarding appearance of legs
  2. Physiologic bowing of up to 20 degrees is normal in children until 18 to 24 months of age
  3. Bowing does not generally increase after 16 months and usually resolves by age 24 months
- Differential Diagnosis
  1. Hypophosphatemic rickets
  2. Blount disease (tibia vara)
  3. Injury to medial proximal epiphysis of tibia
  4. Osteogenesis imperfecta
  5. Achondroplasia and other skeletal dysplasias
  6. Extreme physiologic bowing
  7. Neoplasms
- Physical Findings
  1. With child standing
     a. Clinically present—space between knees is greater than 5 cm or 2 in. with apposition of medial malleoli (relative, not absolute measurement)
     b. Resolution usually occurs without treatment
  2. Full range of motion throughout lower extremities
- Diagnostic Tests/Findings: Radiographs used for extreme and/or unilateral bowing
- Management/Treatment
  1. Observation to verify resolution
  2. Avoid unnecessary treatment of mild to moderate bowing
  3. Further evaluation with radiographs necessary if:
     a. Genu varum is present after 2 years of age
     b. Progressive after 1 year of age
     c. Unilateral involvement
     d. Appears to be severe
     e. Occurs in a high-risk group, e.g., obese; African American children with early ambulation

☐ GENU VALGUM (KNOCK-KNEE)

- Definition: Deformity in which the knees are abnormally close and space between the ankles is increased
- Etiology/Incidence
  1. A natural shifting occurs from varum to valgus between 30 and 60 months
  2. Normal alignment about 8 years of age
  3. Underlying bone disease can cause marked bilateral valgum
- Signs and Symptoms
  1. Parental concern common regarding appearance of legs
  2. Associated with pronation; more common in overweight children
- Differential Diagnosis
  1. Injury to lateral proximal tibial epiphysis causes unilateral valgum
  2. Hypophosphatemic rickets
  3. Pseudoachondroplasia
- Physical Findings
  1. Knees are together and distance between medial malleoli (ankles) is greater than 3 in. (7.5 cm) when standing (relative, not absolute measurement)
  2. Full range of motion
  3. No pain
  4. Child may walk and run awkwardly
  5. Normal knee alignment usually occurs before 8 years of age
- Diagnostic Tests/Findings: Radiographs used for extreme valgum; standing anteroposterior (AP) and lateral views
- Management
  1. Observation to verify resolution
  2. Further evaluation with radiographs necessary if:
     a. Genu valgum is present after 7 years of age
     b. Unilateral involvement

☐ TRANSIENT (TOXIC) SYNOVITIS OF THE HIP

- Definition: Self-limiting inflammation of hip joint
- Etiology/Incidence
  1. Etiology uncertain; possible immune or viral process
  2. Most common cause of irritable hip
  3. Males affected twice as often as females
  4. Occurs most often in 3- to 12-year-olds
  5. Both hips equally affected
- Signs and Symptoms
  1. Painful limp or hip (groin) pain with acute or insidious onset, usually unilateral, and is often preceded by an upper respiratory infection
  2. Afebrile or low-grade temperature
- Differential Diagnosis
  1. Septic arthritis
  2. Osteomyelitis
  3. Legg-Calvé-Perthes disease
  4. Juvenile monoarthritis

5. Rheumatoid arthritis
6. Slipped capital femoral epiphysis
- Physical Findings
  1. Range of motion of hip causes spasm and pain, particularly with internal rotation
  2. No obvious signs on inspection or with palpation
- Diagnostic Tests/Findings
  1. Radiography normal or slightly widened joint space medially
  2. Ultrasonography is useful in determining effusion
  3. Normal or slightly elevated white blood cell (WBC) count
  4. Joint fluid aspiration—normal
- Management/Treatment
  1. Hospitalize child
     a. If high fever or severe symptoms are present
     b. To differentiate between transient synovitis and septic arthritis
  2. Analgesics (ibuprofen every 6 to 8 hours) for 5 days
  3. Bed rest/non-weight-bearing
  4. Benign, self-limiting illness

LEGG-CALVÉ-PERTHES DISEASE (LCPD)

- Definition: Aseptic or avascular necrosis of the femoral head
- Etiology/Incidence
  1. Unknown etiology; possibly due to vascular interruption, anthropometric abnormalities, transient synovitis, or nutritional deficits
  2. Generally, slightly shorter stature/delayed bone age compared to peers
  3. Most common in Caucasian boys, ages 4 to 9 years
  4. 15% of cases are bilateral
- Signs and Symptoms
  1. Insidious onset of limp with knee pain that is activity-related and resolves with rest
  2. Pain also in groin or lateral hip
  3. Pain less acute and severe than transient synovitis or septic arthritis
  4. Afebrile
- Differential Diagnosis
  1. Transient synovitis
  2. Septic arthritis
  3. Hematogenous osteomyelitis
  4. Various types of hemoglobinopathy
  5. Gaucher's disease
  6. Hypothyroidism
  7. Epiphyseal dysplasias
- Physical Findings
  1. Limited passive internal rotation and abduction of hip joint
  2. May be resisted by mild spasm or guarding
  3. Hip flexion contracture and leg muscle atrophy in long-standing cases
- Diagnostic Tests/Findings
  1. Radiograph studies
     a. Show disease progression and sphericity of femoral head

b. Used initially for definitive diagnosis
     c. Subsequently used to assess reparative process
  2. Other laboratory studies not indicated
- Management/Treatment
  1. Goal—to restore range of motion while maintaining femoral head within acetabulum
  2. Observation only if full ROM preserved
     a. Children <8 years of age
     b. Involvement of less than one-half the femoral head
  3. Aggressive treatment
     a. Indicated when more than one-half femoral head involved and in children older than 8 years
     b. Use of orthosis—rarely used today
     c. Surgical treatment
        (1) Femoral osteotomy
        (2) Shelf arthroplasty
  4. Patient/family education—inform family that LCPD lasts 1 to 3 years and is potentially serious if not treated properly

GROWING PAINS

- Definition: A controversial diagnosis of exclusion for (usually intermittent) lower extremity pain
- Etiology/Incidence
  1. Onset at 3 to 5 years of age or, more commonly, 8 to 12 years of age
  2. Related factors
     a. Rapid growth
     b. Puberty
     c. Fibrositis
     d. Weather
     e. Psychological factors
- Signs and Symptoms: Pain/ache localized to lower extremities; usually intermittent and sometimes nocturnal
- Differential Diagnosis
  1. Trauma
  2. Infection
  3. Hematologic causes—sickle cell, hemophilia
  4. Slipped capital femoral epiphysis
  5. Osgood-Schlatter
  6. Osteochondritis dissecans
- Physical Findings (usually none)
  1. No history of traumatic insult
  2. No loss of ambulation or mobility
  3. No systemic changes
  4. No edema or erythema
  5. Full range of motion
- Diagnostic Tests/Findings
  1. All laboratory studies normal—complete blood count (CBC) with differential, erythrocyte sedimentation rate (ESR), C-reactive protein (CRP)
  2. Radiograph of affected area normal
- Management/Treatment
  1. Prescribe anti-inflammatory medication
  2. Massage and heating pad to area
  3. Rest during painful episodes, activity as tolerated

☐ OSGOOD-SCHLATTER DISEASE

- Definition: Inflammation of tibial tubercle from repetitive stresses in athletes with immature skeletal development
- Etiology/Incidence
  1. Tiny stress fractures in apophysis likely etiology
  2. Associated with a rapid growth spurt
  3. Occurs 10 to 15 years of age when immature cartilage susceptible to repeated trauma
- Signs and Symptoms: Pain and tenderness localized to tibial tubercle in acute phase
- Differential Diagnosis
  1. Osteomyelitis
  2. Osteosarcoma
  3. Patellar tendonitis
- Physical Findings
  1. Point tenderness over tibial tubercle
  2. Prominence/enlargement of tibial tubercle compared with unaffected side after acute phase
  3. 50% have bilateral involvement
- Diagnostic Tests/Findings
  1. Diagnosis accurate by clinical examination
  2. CT and MRI scans rarely indicated
  3. Radiographs
     a. Used to rule out presence of more serious bone pathology
     b. Lateral view
        (1) May demonstrate ossicle between patellar tendon and tibial tubercle
        (2) For pain which persists after skeletal maturity
     c. Rarely useful at follow-up
- Management/Treatment
  1. Self-limiting condition
  2. Conservative and largely symptomatic treatment
  3. Pain resolves with full ossification of tibial tubercle and closure of apophysis
  4. Activity limitations
     a. Complete avoidance of sports activities not recommended
     b. Limit activity to control pain at tibial tubercle
     c. Stretching exercises before activity, icing helpful afterward
     d. Use knee immobilizer
        (1) Pain relief—briefly to avoid muscle atrophy
        (2) In combination with thigh muscle strengthening
  5. Corticosteroid injections—not recommended; may aggravate apophysitis
  6. Surgery
     a. Indicated if tubercle pain persists after skeletal maturity
     b. Excision of ossicle may ameliorate symptoms

☐ SCOLIOSIS (IDIOPATHIC)

- Definition: Lateral curvature of spine
- Etiology/Incidence
  1. Multifactorial etiology
  2. 70% cases idiopathic
  3. Most common occurrence immediately before or during adolescent growth spurt
  4. Female to male ratio of 8:1
  5. Mild curves occur equally between the sexes
  6. Positive family history in about 70% of cases
- Signs and Symptoms (usually asymptomatic)
  1. Infancy to school age—parents may notice alteration in back contour
  2. Adolescence—more likely detected on routine screening
  3. Rarely painful
- Differential Diagnosis
  1. Hip disease
  2. Transient synovitis
  3. Legg-Calvé-Perthes disease
  4. Slipped capital femoral epiphysis
  5. Leg length discrepancy
- Physical Findings: Inspection in standing position
  1. Asymmetry of shoulder height
  2. Uneven hip level
  3. Waistline uneven
  4. Thoracic spinal curve (usually right sided)
  5. Rib asymmetry
  6. Unequal arm length
  7. Asymmetry of scapulae
- Diagnostic Tests/Findings
  1. Adam's forward-bending test
     a. Child bends forward 90 degrees or more, keeping knees straight, feet forward, dropping head with arms hanging downward, elbows extended
     b. Observed from caudal aspect to detect abnormal prominence of thoracic ribs
  2. Radiographs evaluate degree of deformity
- Management/Treatment
  1. If pain occurs, further evaluation required
  2. Treatment mode depends on severity of curve and child's age
     a. Curves of 25 degrees
        (1) No further evaluation/treatment if child skeletally mature
        (2) Follow-up for possible progression if child is still growing
        (3) Bracing treatment
     b. Curves of 40 to 50 degrees
        (1) Likely to increase if curve >50 degrees even after growth complete
        (2) Surgery likely for thoracic curve >50 degrees or lumbar curve >40 degrees
  3. Clinical pulmonary restriction may occur with thoracic curves >75 degrees

☐ SPORTS INJURIES

- Definition: Musculoskeletal injuries occurring as a result of participation in athletic activities; most common include sprains/strains, fractures, or overuse injuries
  1. Head and neck injuries
     a. Common in football and ice hockey
     b. Generally not severe

c. Include brachial plexus injuries

d. Concussions

2. Back injuries—low back pain caused by:

a. Muscle strain

b. Spondylolysis Pars defect—overuse from repetitive hyperextension of back as in gymnastics, most likely in lower lumbar area causes fracture

c. Spondylolisthesis—forward vertebral slippage after spondylolysis

3. Upper extremity injuries

a. Anterior shoulder dislocation, shoulder separation

b. Overuse injuries

(1) Impingement syndrome—"pitcher's shoulder," "swimmer's shoulder," or "tennis shoulder"

(2) Lateral epicondylitis—"tennis elbow"

4. Lower extremity injuries

a. Sprains (common in adolescents, but not in children)

(1) Medial collateral ligament sprain

(2) Anterior cruciate sprain and tear

b. Overuse injuries

(1) Iliac apophysitis

(2) Femoral stress fracture

(3) Chondromalacia (chronic patellar pain "runner's knee")

- Etiology/Incidence

1. Leading causes—trauma, improper training

2. Contributing factors include fatigue and improper nutrition

3. 20 million children participate in organized athletics

4. One out of 14 adolescents treated for athletic injury

5. Highest frequency in adolescent boys; football, soccer, and wrestling cause most injuries

- Signs and Symptoms

1. Fracture

a. Edema

b. Erythema

c. Ecchymosis

d. Pain

e. Obvious angulation

f. Bony point tenderness

2. Sprain

a. Various degrees of pain

b. Swelling

c. Difficulty weight bearing

d. Detectable joint laxity

e. Decreased ROM

3. Overuse—various degrees of pain with or without activity limitations

- Differential Diagnosis: Possible underlying disease process of metabolic, neoplastic, or infectious origins

- Physical Findings

1. Fracture

a. Decreased ROM

b. Pain

c. Obvious deformity

d. Swelling

e. Evidence of injury seen on radiographs at site of injury

f. Localized tenderness

2. Sprains—use subjective grading

a. Grade I

(1) Few fibers torn within ligament; does not compromise ligament's strength

(2) Minimal pain and swelling

(3) Full ROM

(4) No increase in joint laxity

b. Grade II

(1) Tears portion of the ligament

(2) Clinically significant pain and swelling

(3) Impairment of ROM

(4) Detectable increase in joint laxity

c. Grade III

(1) Complete tear of ligament

(2) Marked laxity evident when ligament is stressed

- Diagnostic Tests/Findings

1. Physical examination and accurate history to evaluate injury

2. Radiographs

a. Injured area and contralateral area

b. View open growth plate

c. Rule out fracture or tumor

3. MRI—utilized to evaluate torn ligaments or damage to cartilage

4. Ultrasonography—utilized for visualization of effusion

- Management/Treatment

1. Encourage sports physical examinations prior to participation in athletic events to identify conditions that may interfere/worsen with athletic participation

2. Fractures—immobilization, pain management, ROM exercise

3. Sprain/strain

a. Minimize hematoma and swelling with rest, ice, compression, elevation (RICE)

b. ROM exercise

c. Grade III sprains may require surgery

4. Overuse injuries

a. Usually respond to conservative treatment, rest, ice, and gradual return to athletic activities

b. Nonsteroidal anti-inflammatory drugs (NSAIDs) prescribed to decrease inflammation and pain

5. Refer to orthopedic practitioner

a. Fractures that involve the growth plates are open or displaced

b. If sprain/strain or overuse injuries not resolving with conservative treatment measures

6. Child can return to athletic activity based on functional evaluation of actions required during the activity

☐ SLIPPED CAPITAL FEMORAL EPIPHYSIS (SCFE)

- Definition: Spontaneous dislocation of femoral head (capital epiphysis) posteriorly and usually medially through the physis that typically occurs through adolescent growth spurt

- Etiology/Incidence

1. Etiology unknown—thought to be precipitated by the interplay of hormones related to puberty

2. Generally occurs without severe, sudden force or trauma; sometimes related to trauma
3. Usually occurs during growth spurt (ages 10 to 17) and before menarche in girls
4. Annual incidence is 2 to 13 per 100,000
5. More common in males and African Americans
6. 20% present with bilateral involvement
7. Incidence greater among obese adolescents with sedentary lifestyles

- Signs and Symptoms
  1. Varies with acuity of the process
  2. Most children have limp (if greater than 3 weeks, considered chronic)
  3. Varying degrees of aching or pain (in groin, often referred to thigh/knee)
  4. Some have acute, severe pain, and inability to walk or move hip

- Differential Diagnosis
  1. Knee complaint with no obvious cause
  2. Trauma
  3. Septic arthritis
  4. Transient (toxic) synovitis
  5. Juvenile arthritis
  6. Legg-Calvé-Perthes disease

- Physical Findings
  1. Unable to properly flex hip as femur abducts/rotates externally
  2. May observe limb shortening, resulting from proximal displacement of metaphysic
  3. Loss of internal rotation with hip flexed to 90 degrees

- Diagnostic Tests/Findings
  1. Accurate history combined with knowledge of etiological factors
  2. Radiographs
     a. Confirms diagnosis
     b. Shows degree of slipping between femoral head and neck
  3. Laboratory studies
     a. Depend on findings from physical examination and history
     b. Done to rule out associated causes of infection or inflammation

- Management/Treatment
  1. Immediate referral to orthopedic practitioner
  2. Treatment goal is to prevent further slippage, promote closure of the physis, and avoid chondrolysis or osteonecrosis
  3. No ambulation is allowed on acute/unstable SCFE
  4. Surgery—in situ pin fixation to stabilize upper femur and cause growth plate to close
  5. Monitor other hip for same problem

☐ JUVENILE IDIOPATHIC ARTHRITIS (JIA)

- Definition: Chronic, autoimmune idiopathic arthritis characterized by presence of chronic synovial inflammation with associated swelling, pain, heat, and/or limited ROM

- Etiology/Incidence
  1. Cause unknown; possible etiological factors include infections, autoimmunity, genetic predisposition, or stress and trauma
  2. Most common autoimmune inflammatory disease of childhood
  3. Mean incidence 6–19:100,000; estimated 65,000 to 70,000 children in United States affected
  4. Mean age of onset 1 to 3 years; rarely before 6 months, and again between 8 and 10 years
  5. Females affected twice as often as males; pauciarticular and polyarticular disease occur more frequently in girls, while both sexes are affected with equal frequency in systemic-onset disease

- Signs and Symptoms
  1. Range of severity of disease
     a. May be mild in one joint with no symptoms
     b. May have severe disease in many joints with fever, rash, lymphadenopathy, and organomegaly
  2. Signs of joint inflammation
     a. Swelling with heat
     b. Redness
     c. Pain
     d. Limited ROM
  3. May also exhibit
     a. Morning stiffness, limp, refusal to walk
     b. Irritability, fatigue
  4. Hallmark of systemic disease is high spiking fever with rash

- Differential Diagnosis
  1. Hip disease
  2. Transient synovitis
  3. Legg-Calvé-Perthes disease
  4. Slipped capital femoral epiphysis
  5. Leukemia
  6. Other rheumatic diseases, e.g., Kawasaki, systemic lupus erythematosus (SLE), Lyme, spondyloarthropathy

- Physical Findings
  1. Diagnostic criteria
     a. Age of onset <16 years
     b. Joint involvement
        (1) Arthritis (swelling/effusion) in one or more joints, or
        (2) Presence of two or more of these signs:
           (a) Range of motion limitation
           (b) Tenderness
           (c) Pain with movement
           (d) Increased heat
     c. Duration of disease 6 weeks or longer
     d. Further classified by onset type during first 6 months
     e. Exclusion of other forms of juvenile arthritis
  2. Polyarthritis (polyarticular disease)
     a. 40% to 50% of all cases
     b. Five or more inflamed joints
     c. May be acute or gradual onset
     d. Symmetric pattern

e. Commonly affects large joints, e.g., knees, wrists, elbows, ankles

f. May not complain of pain

3. Oligoarthritis (pauciarticular disease)

a. 50% of cases

b. Four or fewer joints affected (usually larger joints such as knees, ankles, and wrists)

c. Gradual onset

d. Can be painless

e. Hip monoarticular arthritis unusual

f. Usually no systemic signs, except for chronic uveitis

(1) Early onset (5 years of age)

(a) Asymmetric involvement

(b) Large joints commonly affected

(c) Hips and sacroiliac (SI) joint spared

(d) Systemic symptoms usually not present

(2) Late onset

(a) Asymmetric involvement

(b) Hips and SI joint involvement present

(c) Chronic involvement can result in atrophy of extensor muscles in the thigh, tight hamstring ligaments, and knee flexion contractures

4. Systemic

a. 10% to 20% of cases

b. Occurs in late childhood (8 years of age)

c. Systemic onset may precede arthritis appearance by weeks, months, or years

d. High, daily intermittent spiking fevers is hallmark symptom

(1) Temperature elevations occur once or twice/day

(2) To 39°C (102°F) or higher with quick return to baseline temperature or lower

e. Linear evanescent rash present

(1) Salmon-colored nonpruritic macular lesions

(2) Commonly on trunk and proximal extremities

(3) Most characteristic feature is transient nature

f. Painful multiple joint involvement

g. Associated findings

(1) Hepatosplenomegaly

(2) Lymphadenopathy

(3) Visceral disease, e.g., pericarditis, hepatitis

(4) Pulmonary involvement

(5) CNS

h. 50% of cases have chronic, destructive arthritis

5. Associated problems

a. Periarticular soft tissue edema

b. Intra-articular effusion

c. Hypertrophy of synovial membrane

6. Synovitis—painful inflammation of synovial membrane, with fluctuating swelling

a. May develop insidiously, existing months to years without joint destruction

b. May cause joint damage in relatively short time

- Diagnostic Tests/Findings

1. No specific laboratory studies; however, abnormalities may be found

2. Human leukocyte antigen (HLA) B27

3. CBC—characteristics of chronic anemia of inflammation

a. Moderately severe anemia; hemoglobin between 7 and 10 g/dL

b. Leukocytosis

4. Erythrocyte sedimentation rate (ESR)

a. ESR is always elevated in children with systemic JIA

b. Usually elevated in those with polyarticular disease

c. Often within the reference range in those with pauciarticular disease

d. Elevated ESR may be used to monitor success of medical treatment

5. Alanine aminotransferase (ALT) test—obtain ALT levels to exclude the possibility of hepatitis (viral or autoimmune) prior to initiating treatment with NSAIDs, which can cause hepatotoxicity

6. Urinalysis with microscopic examination—perform a urinalysis to exclude the possibility of infection (as a trigger of JIA or transient postinfectious arthritis) and nephritis (observed in individuals with SLE)

7. Synovial fluid WBC count—moderately elevated 10,000/mm^3 to 20,000/mm^3

8. Rheumatoid factor present in:

a. Approximately 15% to 20% of cases

b. Child with later onset or older child

c. Child with prominent symmetric polyarthritis with:

(1) Involvement of small joints

(2) Subcutaneous rheumatoid nodules

(3) Articular erosions

(4) Poor functional outcome

9. Antinuclear antibodies (ANA)—seropositivity for antibodies

a. Present in about 25% of cases

b. Presence correlated significantly with development of chronic uveitis

c. Less commonly found in older boys or in systemic disease

d. Valuable diagnostic measure for JIA

(1) Positive in SLE, scleroderma, transient acute viral disease

10. Anti-double-stranded DNA and anti-Smith (Sm) antibody, anti-cyclic citrullinated peptide (anti-ccp)

11. Radiographs

a. Early changes

(1) Soft tissue swelling

(2) Juxta-articular osteoporosis

(3) Periosteal new bone apposition

b. Development of ossification centers may be age accelerated

c. Stunting of bone growth secondary to premature epiphyseal closure

d. Cervical spine disease characteristic feature

e. Joint disease may be better evaluated with MRI, CT, bone scans

- Management/Treatment

1. Goal is to control clinical manifestations and prevent/minimize deformity

2. Suppress inflammation and fever
   a. Use NSAID (ibuprofen, naproxen) for most children
   b. In severe, progressive disease resistant to therapy
      (1) Methotrexate
         (a) Most successful and safe drug
         (b) 10 to 15 mg/m^2/once a week
         (c) No oncogenic potential or risk of sterility
      (2) Hydroxychloroquine—useful adjunctive agent
         (a) Retinopathy possible adverse reaction
         (b) Low dose, e.g., 5 mg/kg/day
         (c) Frequent ophthalmologic examinations required
      (3) Gold salts—given IM or as oral compound
         (a) Toxicities are hematologic, renal, hepatic
         (b) Must be constantly monitored during treatment
      (4) Glucocorticoid drugs
         (a) Indicated for resistant or life-threatening disease
         (b) Ophthalmic administration for chronic uveitis
         (c) Toxicities, e.g., Cushing syndrome and growth retardation restriction
      (5) Sulfasalazine—sulfa drug 1 salicylate
         (a) Indicated for JIA
         (b) May take 6 weeks to work
      (6) Biologic agents
         (a) Synthetic proteins that block high levels of inflammatory proteins
         (b) Indicated for moderate to severe arthritis that has not responded well to other therapies
3. Maintenance of function and prevention of deformity
   a. Prescriptions for physical and occupational therapies
   b. Balanced program of rest and activity
   c. Selective splinting
   d. Encourage normal play/activity
   e. Avoid high levels of stress on inflamed weight-bearing joints
4. Counsel parents about course of chronic disease with exacerbations
5. Refer to pediatric rheumatologist
6. Counsel regarding corticosteroids and infections/immunizations

☐ SYSTEMIC LUPUS ERYTHEMATOSUS (SLE)

- Definition: Multisystem autoimmune disorder that is characterized by widespread inflammatory involvement of connective tissues with immune complex vasculitis
- Etiology/Incidence
  1. Unknown, but many factors implicated
     a. Excessive sun exposure
     b. Drug reaction
     c. Infection
     d. Hereditary
     e. Immunogenetic
  2. Can develop at any age
     a. Usually after 5 years of age
     b. More common during adolescent years in females
  3. Females affected eight times more often after 5 years of age
- Signs and Symptoms
  1. Fever
  2. Malaise
  3. Weight loss
  4. Malar facial rash
  5. Arthralgias
- Differential Diagnosis
  1. Juvenile rheumatoid arthritis (JRA)
  2. Other forms of acute glomerulonephritis
  3. Hemolytic anemia
  4. Leukemia
  5. Allergic or contact dermatitis
  6. Idiopathic seizure disorder
  7. Mononucleosis
  8. Acute rheumatic fever with carditis
  9. Septicemia
  10. Toxic exposure
- Physical Findings
  1. Onset is usually acute—three-quarters of children usually diagnosed within 6 months of symptoms
  2. Diagnosis delayed for others by 4 to 5 years
  3. Early diagnostic suspicion based on:
     a. Episodic, multisystem constellation of clinical disease
     b. Associated with persistent antinuclear antibody (ANA) seropositivity
  4. Severity of manifestations variable
     a. Rapidly fatal illness
     b. Insidious chronic disability with multisystem exacerbation
  5. Each exacerbation of disease tends to mimic previous episodes
  6. Rash
     a. Characteristic of acute onset or exacerbation
     b. Malar erythematous
     c. Butterfly distribution across bridge of nose and over each cheek
     d. Discoid rash over sun-exposed areas
  7. Arthritis
     a. Affects majority of children
     b. Involves small joints
     c. Transient and migratory
     d. Never erosive
     e. Possible avascular necrosis of bone in 25% children
  8. Pericarditis is most common manifestation of cardiac involvement—murmurs associated with endocarditis
  9. Central and peripheral nervous system manifestations
     a. Recurrent headaches
     b. Seizures

c. Chorea

d. Frank psychosis

10. Kidney involvement in all children

   a. Proteinuria (>500 mg/d) or evidence of nephritis in urinalysis

   b. Hypertension

- Diagnostic Tests/Findings

1. Leukopenia—otherwise unexplained, common at onset

2. ANA, anti-double-stranded DNA, anti-Smith antibody, lupus anticoagulant, and anti-phospholipid antibody panel—positive in most children

3. Coombs test—often positive

4. Rheumatoid factor (RF) and other anti-tissue antibodies—often positive

5. Electrocardiogram (ECG) and chest x-ray

6. MRI/CT of brain

7. Renal ultrasound

8. Tissue biopsy to confirm diagnosis and distinguish disease severity

- Management/Treatment

1. Long-term supportive care

   a. Maintain adequate nutrition

   b. Maintain fluid and electrolyte balance

   c. Early recognition and treatment of infections

   d. Control of hypertension

   e. Exercise is important to maintain bone density

2. Anti-inflammatory drugs useful for minor manifestations, e.g., myalgia and arthralgia

3. Counsel parents and child about chronic nature of disease with repeated exacerbations, remissions often prolonged over many years

☐ OSTEOMYELITIS

- Definition: Inflammation of bone caused by a pyogenic organism

- Etiology/Incidence

1. Causative agents

   a. In all age groups, *Staphylococcus aureus*

   b. Consider also *Streptococcus pneumoniae*, *Haemophilus influenzae*, community-acquired methicillin-resistant *S. aureus* (MRSA), group A hemolytic *Streptococcus*, group B hemolytic *Streptococcus* (neonates), and *Kingella kingae*

2. Peak ages—infancy (less than 1 year) and preadolescence (9 to 11 years)

3. More frequent in males

- Signs and Symptoms

1. May appear well

2. Systemic involvement ranging from malaise to shock

3. Neonates usually afebrile, swollen or motionless limb early sign

4. Earliest symptom in child may be refusal to bear weight or flexion of hip in comfortable position

- Differential Diagnosis

1. Neoplasm

2. Contusion

3. Nondisplaced fracture

4. Sickle cell crisis

5. JIA

6. Transient synovitis

- Physical Findings

1. Early signs

   a. Fever

   b. Local bone tenderness

2. If subperiosteal or soft tissue abscess develops, fluctuant mass present

- Diagnostic Tests/Findings

1. WBC, ESR, and CRP—elevated, but not diagnostic

2. Radiographs—at earliest stage may show soft tissue swelling

3. Technetium-99m scintigraphy

4. MRI

5. Bone scan

   a. May be initially normal

   b. Repeated after 48 hours, may show cold/photopenic areas (indicating avascular sites)

6. Aspiration—always indicated to identify pathogen

- Management/Treatment

1. Refer to physician

2. Delivery of systemic antibiotic

   a. Broad spectrum antibiotic initially

      (1) Most effective against isolated organism

      (2) Least toxic antibiotic

      (3) Used for 4 to 6 weeks

3. Surgery reserved for:

   a. Child with systemic illness

   b. Worsening symptoms under medical treatment

   c. Abscess present

☐ DUCHENNE MUSCULAR DYSTROPHY (DMD)

- Definition: Progressive genetic disorder that affects muscles in lower extremities and eventually muscles of upper extremities, chest wall, and heart

- Etiology/Incidence

1. X-linked recessive genetic disorder that results in absence or severe deficiency of cytoskeletal protein known as dystrophin

2. Most commonly inherited neuromuscular disease in children

3. Affects 1:3500 males; 1:1750 females are carriers

4. Average age of diagnosis is 3 to 5 years of age

- Signs and Symptoms

1. At birth—rarely affected clinically

2. Becomes clinically evident by 3 to 5 years of age

   a. Abnormalities of gait and posture

   b. History of delayed developmental milestones

   c. Large "muscular" looking calves

   d. Inability to keep up with peers when running

3. Progresses over next 2 decades—weakness more evident in proximal muscles

4. Wheelchair dependent by 7 to 12 years of age
   a. Muscles decrease in size
   b. Contractures progress with loss of joint mobility
   c. Kyphoscoliosis develops with respiratory function problems
5. Complications from:
   a. Cardiac involvement
   b. Nervous system involvement
   c. Musculoskeletal deformities
   d. Compromised respiratory function
6. Eventual death from cardiac or respiratory failure

- Differential Diagnosis
  1. Hypothyroidism
  2. Carnitine deficiency
  3. Spinal muscular atrophy
  4. Fascioscapulohumeral dystrophy
  5. Other types of muscular dystrophies of childhood
- Physical Findings
  1. Preschooler—3 to 5 years of age
     a. Increasing lumbar lordosis
     b. Pelvic waddling
     c. Gowers' maneuver
        (1) Child may "walk" hands up legs to attain a standing position when arising from floor
        (2) Indication of pelvic girdle weakness
        (3) Distinctive in DMD, but seen in other conditions as well
     d. Proximal muscle strength and ankle reflexes may be depressed
     e. Calf hypertrophy present and the enlarged muscle tissue is eventually replaced with fat and connective tissue (pseudohypertrophy)
  2. Cardiac involvement in all patients—cardiomyopathy by adolescence
  3. Contractures develop before ambulation is compromised
     a. Iliotibial bands
     b. Hip flexors
     c. Heel cords
- Diagnostic Tests/Findings
  1. Obtain three-generation family history
     a. May be positive history of muscle disorders, weakness, DMD
     b. Carrier females have symptoms of weakness or cramping of muscles
  2. Laboratory studies
     a. Creatine kinase (CK)—will be markedly elevated in affected males (15,000 to 35,000 IU/L)
     b. Electromyogram (EMG)—distinctively myopathic
     c. ECG—changes are distinctive
        (1) Tall right precordial R waves
        (2) Deep Q waves in left precordial and limb leads
     d. Muscle biopsy—histopathologic findings
        (1) Groups of necrotic degenerating fibers most prominent
        (2) Variation in fiber size evident
        (3) Dystrophic immunoreactivity confirms DMD

e. Genetic testing
   (1) Utilizes WBC from blood specimen
   (2) DNA analysis of DMD gene confirms diagnosis
- Management/Treatment
  1. No cure available at present
  2. Goal of treatment is essentially symptomatic, aimed at delay of progression and supportive care
  3. Maintenance of strength and mobility
     a. Exercise
     b. Use of ankle/foot orthoses, bracing, spinal support measures, and wheelchair as needed
  4. Consultation with neuromuscular disease specialty team for diagnosis and for periodic evaluations
  5. Refer family for genetic testing/counseling
  6. Counsel family regarding course of disease
  7. Refer parents
     a. To other families who have children with DMD
     b. To other community resources for support

☐ QUESTIONS

Select the best answer.

1. Which of the following disorders is usually associated with adduction of the forefoot?
   a. Internal femoral torsion
   b. Talipes equinovarus congenita
   c. Genu valgum
   d. Internal tibial torsion
2. The most common rheumatoid disease of childhood is:
   a. Systemic lupus erythematosus
   b. Kawasaki disease
   c. Juvenile idiopathic arthritis
   d. Legg-Calvé-Perthes disease
3. Radiographic findings of disease progression and sphericity of the femoral head is helpful in the diagnosis and follow-up of:
   a. Transient synovitis of the hip
   b. Osgood-Schlatter disease
   c. Legg-Calvé-Perthes disease
   d. Slipped capital femoral epiphysis
4. A 4-year-old boy is brought in by his mother, who is concerned about the sudden onset of a painful limp in his right leg 2 days ago. Today he has a low-grade fever. Which of the following diagnoses is most likely?
   a. Osgood-Schlatter
   b. Juvenile idiopathic arthritis
   c. Osteomyelitis
   d. Transient synovitis of the hip
5. Which of the following would be the most appropriate initial management of a newborn diagnosed with developmental dysplasia of the hip?
   a. Observe and reexamine at 2-week well-child visit
   b. Triple diapering in nursery
   c. Pavlik harness
   d. Surgical reduction

6. A physical finding not usually associated with talipes equinovarus congenita is:
   a. Contracture of the iliotibial bands
   b. Deep crease on medial border of foot
   c. Atrophy of calf muscles
   d. Small foot with limited dorsiflexion
7. A characteristic feature of polyarticular JIA disease is:
   a. The involvement of five or more inflamed joints
   b. Confinement to lower extremity joints, knees, and ankles
   c. Asymmetric involvement
   d. High, daily intermittent spiking fevers
8. ANA seropositivity for antibodies:
   a. Is a valuable diagnostic marker for JIA
   b. Is not positive in any childhood diseases
   c. Is more commonly found in older boys
   d. Has 100% sensitivity and specificity
9. Dislocation in the hip of a child 6 months or older may typically present with:
   a. Asymmetry of skin folds
   b. Atrophied hip muscles
   c. Positive Galeazzi sign
   d. Negative Trendelenburg sign
10. For a newborn, the correct management of hip dislocation should include:
    a. Use of a flexion-abduction device such as a Pavlik harness to stabilize hip
    b. Following and observing closely for 3 to 4 weeks, and then referring to an orthopedist
    c. Surgical reduction
    d. Traction for 6 weeks
11. Duchenne muscular dystrophy is characterized by which of the following signs and symptoms?
    a. At birth, affected infants are notably hypotonic, "floppy" babies.
    b. Earliest symptom is often refusal to bear weight.
    c. Abnormalities of gait and posture become evident during preschool years and during gross motor development.
    d. Children are unable to keep up with peers when running by school age.
12. Most children with Duchenne muscular dystrophy become wheelchair dependent by what age?
    a. 4 to 6 years of age
    b. 10 to 12 years of age
    c. 14 to 16 years of age
    d. Highly variable depending on response to treatment
13. An obese 13-year-old male with 2 days of right knee pain without trauma or illness has an exam of significant pain upon right hip motion, and he maintains his leg in external rotation and adduction. Based on these findings, the most likely diagnosis is:
    a. Osgood-Schlatter disease
    b. Chondromalacia
    c. Spondylolysis
    d. Slipped capital femoral epiphysis

14. Management of scoliosis depends on the severity of curve as well as the age of the child. Which of the following would require surgical intervention?
    a. Curves of 15 degrees in a child who is still growing
    b. Thoracic and/or lumbar curve greater than 25 degrees, even if growth is complete
    c. Thoracic curve greater than 30 degrees or lumbar curve greater than 40 degrees that has not progressed while in brace
    d. Thoracic curve greater than 50 degrees or lumbar curve greater than 40 degrees
15. In a diagnostic work-up and management plan for a child with osteomyelitis, which of the following is not accurate or recommended?
    a. Elevated ESR confirms diagnosis.
    b. Aspiration is usually indicated.
    c. Antibiotic treatment for identified pathogen 4 to 6 weeks is recommended.
    d. Surgery is recommended if abscess is present.
16. A healthy 6-year-old child presents with a limp and knee pain. The PNP finds limited passive internal rotation and abduction of the hip joint on physical examination. The most likely diagnosis is:
    a. Slipped capital femoral epiphysis
    b. Osgood-Schlatter disease
    c. Transient synovitis of the hip
    d. Legg-Calvé-Perthes disease
17. Which of the following statements is true about acute osteomyelitis?
    a. It occurs more frequently in females than in males.
    b. Peak ages are infancy (younger than 1 year) and preadolescence (9 to 11 years).
    c. Most common sites are radius and ulna.
    d. It is a self-limiting disorder.
18. Which of the following statements is not true of slipped capital femoral epiphysis?
    a. It is thought to be precipitated by hormone changes during puberty.
    b. Unilateral involvement is more common than bilateral.
    c. It is more common among males and African Americans.
    d. It is thought to be caused by repetitive stresses in young athletes prior to growth spurt.
19. Genu varum is considered an abnormal condition when:
    a. Extreme knock-knees continues after 7 years of age
    b. Extreme tibial bowing continues after 2 years of age
    c. Parents are concerned about their child's appearance
    d. Tibial bowing is evident before 2 years of age
20. Tibial torsion is commonly associated and can be treated with:
    a. Pain, analgesics
    b. Restricted ROM, braces
    c. Internal rotation of lower extremities, observation
    d. In adolescents 13 to 16 years of age, increasing dietary calcium

21. Which of the following diagnoses is associated with contracture of one of the sternocleidomastoid muscles?
    a. Lordosis
    b. Torticollis
    c. Scoliosis
    d. Kyphosis

22. A 14-year-old diagnosed with JIA is not up-to-date on his immunizations and is currently on methotrexate. Which of the following vaccinations would be cautioned in this case?
    a. Varicella
    b. Influenza
    c. Inactive polio
    d. Tdap

23. Initial treatment of a grade I sprain includes which of the following?
    a. Rest, ice, compression, elevation, and NSAIDs
    b. Heat, ROM exercise, compression, elevation, and NSAIDs
    c. Rest, heat, compression, elevation, and NSAIDs
    d. Rest, ice, ibuprofen, compression, and NSAIDs

24. The most definitive feature or features for a diagnosis of "growing pains" includes:
    a. Exclusion of other causes of lower extremity pain
    b. Pain, swelling, erythema
    c. Loss of ambulation
    d. Decreased ROM

25. Systemic-onset JIA is most commonly associated with:
    a. High, daily intermittent spiking fevers and rash
    b. Single joint involvement
    c. Positive RF factor and iridocyclitis
    d. Painless joint involvement

26. A 14-year-old has pain in the knee. The pain increases with activity and is relieved with rest. The PNP diagnoses Osgood-Schlatter disease and orders:
    a. An x-ray examination, application of hot packs to the knee, and rest
    b. Application of hot packs to the knee, aspirin, and rest
    c. A reduction in activity, application of ice to the knee, and ibuprofen
    d. Application of ice to the knee and continued participation in sports

27. Complications of SLE commonly include which of the following?
    a. Pericarditis, arthritis, nephritis
    b. Encephalitis, nephritis, pericarditis
    c. Nephritis, arthritis, rheumatic fever
    d. Nephritis, hemolytic anemia, contact dermatitis

28. Which of the following children need an orthopedic referral?
    a. A 6-year-old with mild bowing of the lower legs
    b. A 6-month-old with internal tibial torsion
    c. A 3-week-old with equinovarus of feet
    d. A newborn with a positive Pavlik sign

29. Antonio is a newborn, and the PNP notes on physical assessment that both feet turn in with the hind and midfoot in normal neutral position. When attempting range of motion of the forefoot, the PNP finds that both feet move relatively freely past midline in all directions consistent with:
    a. Clubfoot
    b. Syndactyly
    c. Metatarsus adductus
    d. Fracture in his feet

30. Subluxation of the radial head is referred to as "nursemaid's elbow." If the risk for fracture is low or absent, which of the following is recommended?
    a. Supination and flexion of forearm maneuver
    b. Extension and supination
    c. Use of finger traps with weight on the humerus
    d. The hypopronation and extension maneuver

31. In a newborn, a diagnosis of hip dislocation is suspected when:
    a. Positive Galeazzi, Barlow, and Ortolani signs
    b. Wide hip abduction that is symmetric
    c. Flaccidity of the left leg following extension of both legs with return to flexion
    d. Tonic neck reflex in which the left leg is flexed

32. Which of the following statements is true regarding slipped capital femoral epiphysis?
    a. It is more common in females who are underweight.
    b. It generally occurs following severe sudden trauma.
    c. Incidence is more common in athletes.
    d. The goal of treatment is to stabilize or improve the position of the femoral head.

33. The parents of a 5-year-old recently diagnosed with muscular dystrophy want an explanation about the hereditary nature of the disease. The best explanation is:
    a. X-linked recessive gene transmitted by unaffected female carriers
    b. Recessive gene that is known to skip generations between transmission
    c. Dominant sex-linked gene predominantly in white families from Europe
    d. Recessive gene that requires both mother and father to be carriers

34. Which of the following is true for idiopathic scoliosis, which occurs primarily in adolescents?
    a. Mild curves occur equally between the sexes.
    b. Generally, there is no family history.
    c. Back pain is usually associated with curves of 35 degrees or greater.
    d. Bracing is indicated for thoracic curves of 10 to 25 degrees.

35. In Legg-Calvé-Perthes disease, which of the following signs and symptoms are seen?
    a. Insidious onset of limp with knee and groin pain
    b. Sudden onset of limp and pain in lateral hip
    c. Fever and insidious onset of limp
    d. Afebrile and sudden onset of limp

36. Signs and symptoms associated with Duchenne muscular dystrophy are:
    a. History of delayed developmental milestones
    b. Visual-motor disturbance, calf hypertrophy
    c. Delayed motor development, positive Ortolani maneuver
    d. History of "clumsiness," visual-motor disturbance

37. Which of the following is an appropriate goal for a child being treated for osteomyelitis?
    a. Prohibiting activities
    b. Complete course of antibiotic therapy
    c. Encouraging a low-fat diet
    d. Restricting visitors

38. Sports injuries are commonly associated with:
    a. Improper training
    b. Higher frequency in females
    c. Scoliosis
    d. Low socioeconomic status

39. An injury at which of the following sites will most likely result in a bone length discrepancy?
    a. Diaphysis
    b. Epiphysis
    c. Medullary cavity
    d. Metaphysis

40. Growth in muscle length is related to growth in length of:
    a. Underlying bone
    b. Underlying ligament
    c. Underlying tendon
    d. Opposing muscle group

41. Varus between the tibia and femur of up to 15 degrees followed by a progression to a neutral angle, which then progresses to valgus between 7 degrees and 9 degrees, is associated with which of the following?
    a. Blount disease
    b. Internal tibial torsion
    c. Normal developmental growth pattern
    d. Abnormal tibiofemoral growth pattern

42. Tracy, who is 9 years old, complains that she does not like to wear shorts because her knees look funny. Upon examination, you note a genu valgum angle of greater than 15 degrees. You should:
    a. Reevaluate in 1 year if still present
    b. Consult with an orthopedic specialist
    c. Instruct her to avoid the "W" sitting position
    d. Encourage exercise to strengthen quadriceps

43. What is the appropriate treatment for genu varum in a 15-month-old child?
    a. Passive exercise with each diaper change
    b. Denis Browne splint at night
    c. Blount brace at night
    d. No treatment is warranted

44. During examination of 2-week-old J. P., you note irritability when lifted, asymmetrical Moro reflex, and spasm along the right sternocleidomastoid. What does this suggest?
    a. Torticollis
    b. Sprengel deformity

    c. Fractured clavicle
    d. Klippel-Feil syndrome

45. A child with growing pains is most likely to experience:
    a. A mild limp
    b. Bilateral lower extremity pain
    c. Lower extremity pain primarily during the day
    d. Lower extremity pain associated with decreased range of motion

46. C. W., a 20-month-old, presents in the emergency room with a greenstick fracture of his left femur. Physical examination also reveals an enlarged anterior fontanelle and enlarged costochondral junction. What do these clinical findings suggest?
    a. Child abuse
    b. Osteogenesis imperfecta
    c. Osteoporosis
    d. Rickets

47. Which of the following represents appropriate anticipatory guidance for a child diagnosed with slipped capital femoral epiphysis?
    a. Avoid contact sports until pain has resolved
    b. Use crutches to facilitate mobility during acute phase
    c. Apply ice to affected area
    d. Perform range-of-motion and strengthening exercises

48. Which of the following factors most affects outcomes in patients with LCPD?
    a. Age of child
    b. Severity of pain and antalgic gait
    c. Family history of LCPD
    d. Bilateral involvement

49. During physical examination of Jason, a 2.5-year-old, you note large, muscular-looking calves and observe his difficulty rising from a sitting position. The Denver A developmental screening examination reveals delays in the gross motor area. Which of the following laboratory tests would be most beneficial?
    a. Serum calcium
    b. Serum magnesium
    c. Serum phosphorus
    d. Serum creatine kinase

50. The appropriate management of Osgood-Schlatter disease includes:
    a. Local injection of soluble corticosteroid
    b. Decreasing activity, applying ice, and taking prescribing NSAIDs
    c. Program of strengthening and stretching for quadriceps
    d. Casting in adduction for 6 weeks

51. You have been treating a 14-month-old for torticollis since birth. The condition has not resolved and the child still has limited neck rotation. The appropriate management plan would be to:
    a. Refer for surgical consultation
    b. Continue with passive range of motion

c. Provide environmental stimulation opposite the contracture

d. Apply cervical collar at night

52. While completing the hip examination on a newborn infant, you are able to dislocate the infant's right hip. The appropriate management plan would be to:
    a. Triple diaper and reevaluate in 2 weeks
    b. Recommend positioning prone while awake
    c. Refer to orthopedic specialist
    d. Order tight swaddling of the infant

53. Which of the following would not be an appropriate indicator for developmental dysplasia of the hip in a 6-month-old child?
    a. Allis sign
    b. Skinfold symmetry
    c. Galeazzi sign
    d. Ortolani maneuver

54. A 3-year-old presents with a history of fever for the past several days, pain in his left leg, and refusal to bear weight on the left leg. Ten days ago, he fell from a slide and bruised his leg. His WBC count is slightly elevated. You suspect other toxic synovitis or osteomyelitis. Which finding supports a diagnosis of osteomyelitis more so than toxic synovitis?
    a. Recent injury
    b. Leg pain
    c. Non-weight-bearing
    d. Elevated WBCs

55. Which of the following suggests internal tibial torsion rather than internal femoral torsion in a 2-year-old child presenting with an in-toeing gait?
    a. Sitting in "W" position
    b. Knees face forward when walking
    c. Generalized ligament laxity
    d. Limited external rotation of hip

56. A full-term infant in the newborn nursery is noted to have a deformity in her left foot consisting of a convex lateral border and forefoot, which can be abducted past an imaginary line extending from the middle of the heel through the second toe. Which of the following management strategies is most appropriate?
    a. Reverse-last shoes
    b. Out-flare shoes
    c. Stretching exercises
    d. Orthopedic referral

57. A macular, salmon to red-colored rash with irregular borders and central clearing is typical of which of the following?
    a. Systemic juvenile arthritis
    b. Lyme disease
    c. Systemic lupus erythematosus
    d. Rheumatic fever

58. A baseball coach asks for advice on how to prevent Little League elbow in his 8- and 9-year-old players. Which of the following would be incorrect advice?
    a. Have each child pitch only three innings.
    b. Limit or eliminate curve balls.

c. Use ice massage before and after pitching.
d. Conduct slow warm-ups.

❑ ANSWERS AND RATIONALES

1. B: Talipes equinovarus congenita is a congenital birth disorder in which the forefoot is in adducted supination, the hind foot is inverted, and the foot remains in plantar flexion.

2. C: JIA is the most common rheumatologic disease with an autoimmune basis and represents a group of conditions with onset of symptoms in children at or younger than 16 years that causes chronic inflammation of at least one synovial joint for 6 weeks or more (Burns & Dunn, 2012, p. 521).

3. C: Legg-Calvé-Perthes develops from an infarction of the bony epiphysis of the femoral head and often presents as avascular necrosis of the femoral head. Radiographs depict stages of progression and remodeling and are important in diagnosis and management.

4. D: Transient synovitis, also referred to as toxic synovitis, is an inflammatory process that often affects large joint spaces—primarily, the hip. Children ages 3 to 8 are often affected. The typical presentation consists of pain in the affected joint, antalgic gait, refusal to bear weight, and low-grade fever.

5. C: The treatment of choice for subluxation and reducible dislocations identified in the early phase is a Pavlik harness. The harness is applied with hips having greater than 90 degrees of flexion and with adduction of the hip limited to a neutral position (Burns & Dunn, 2012, p. 944).

6. A: Talipes equinovarus has three elements: the ankle is in equinus (the foot is in a pointed-toe position), the sole of the foot is inverted as a result of hind foot varus or inversion deformity of the heel, and the forefoot has the convex shape of metatarsus adductus (MA) (forefoot adduction). The foot cannot be manually corrected to a neutral position with the heel down. Iliotibial bands are not involved with contracture of the foot (Burns & Dunn, 2012, p. 955).

7. A: JIA is the most common rheumatologic disease with an autoimmune basis and represents a group of conditions with onset of symptoms in children at or younger than 16 years that causes chronic inflammation of at least one synovial joint for 6 weeks or more (Burns & Dunn, 2012, p.521).

8. A: Antinuclear antibodies (ANA) consists of immunoglobulins directed against structures within the cell. It is found in various autoimmune diseases and even in children who do not have rheumatologic disorders. The presence of ANA is important in juvenile idiopathic arthritis (JIA) to assess the child's risk of developing uveitis (Reuter-Rice & Bolick, 2012, p. 695).

9. C: The Galeazzi maneuver can depict a leg length discrepancy. The exam is reliable in children with

dislocatable, but not dislocated, hips or in children with bilateral hip dislocation.

10. A: The treatment of choice for subluxation and reducible dislocations identified in the early phase is a Pavlik harness. The harness is applied with hips having greater than 90 degrees of flexion and with adduction of the hip limited to a neutral position (Burns & Dunn, 2012, p. 944).

11. C: DMD typically presents with delayed walking, slower movements, rolling gait, waddle, large calves, and a positive Gower sign (pushing off thighs when changing positions from being seated to standing).

12. B: Many children with DMD begin using a wheelchair sometime between ages 7 and 12 years. Transition to a wheelchair usually is a gradual process; at first, the chair may be required only to conserve the child's energy when covering long distances (Muscular Dystrophy Association, 2014).

13. D: SCFE typically occurs just after the onset of puberty, often in overweight and slightly skeletally immature boys. Pain is typically reported in affected groin, hip, or knee, and there is often a limp.

14. D: Surgery may be required in children with structural problems that cause kyphosis and in adolescents with curvature of the back that exceeds 50 to 60 degrees. Surgery is indicated for children who have progressive spinal deformity that cannot be controlled by nonoperative means, such as bracing, and where there is significant spinal growth remaining

For Cobb angle less than 15 degrees: Observation at 6- to 12-month intervals

For Cobb angle 15 to 20 degrees: Outpatient therapy with a combination of therapist-guided sessions and home exercise program

For Cobb angle 21 to 25 degrees: Outpatient physiotherapy, scoliosis intensive rehabilitation (SIR) program where available. A brace may be indicated

For Cobb angle greater than 25 degrees: Outpatient physical therapy, SIR program, and brace wear. Rationale for surgical intervention (Burns & Dunn, 2012, p. 942)

15. A: Laboratory investigations are helpful but lack specificity for osteomyelitis. Leukocytosis and increased erythrocyte sedimentation rate and C-reactive protein levels may be present.

16. D: LCPD often presents with an intermittent limp (abductor lurch) especially after exertion, with mild or intermittent pain in the anterior part of the thigh. Some children may present with limited range of motion of the affected extremity. The most common symptom is persistent pain that may be referred to the medial aspect of the ipsilateral knee or to the lateral thigh (Burns & Dunn, 2012, p. 945). Slipped capital femoral epiphysis (SCFE) often occurs after age 8 and predominantly in boys who are overweight. Osgood Schlatter does not occur until early adolescence and is often associated with sports. Transient synovitis typically occurs between ages 3 and 8 years, and the child often refuses to bear weight and has a low-grade fever.

17. B: Males are twice as likely as females to be affected. Any bone may be affected, but the femur and tibia are the most common sites. One in 5000 children younger than the age of 13 will develop osteomyelitis, with 50% of those infections occurring in the first 5 years of life (Reuter-Rice & Bollick, 2012, p. 883).

18. D: The etiology of SCFE is unknown but thought to be related to stresses on the physis from rapid growth.

19. B: The typical pattern of normal bowing seen in children is a symmetric lateral bowing of both tibias in the first year followed by bowlegs in the second year. Asymmetric tibial bowing after 18 months is often associated with Blount's or tibia vara.

20. C: Tibial torsion involves the twisting of the long bone along its long axis, resulting in increased internal rotation. Treatment of tibial version (the normal variation in tibial rotation) is observation and monitoring.

21. B: Asymmetric shortening of the sternocleidomastoid muscle results in preferential turning of the head to one side.

22. A: There is risk of developing serious complications of varicella-zoster infection (VZI) in juvenile idiopathic arthritis (JIA) patients receiving disease-modifying antirheumatic drugs (DMARDs), including methotrexate and biologic agents. Varicella zoster (VZ) immune status should therefore be checked in all children before starting such therapy. Seronegative children mostly receive varicella zoster vaccine (VZV).

23. A: Rest, ice, compression, elevation (RICE) for the injured part. Apply ice immediately for 15 to 20 minutes, and then, depending on the severity of the injury, every 2 to 6 hours for the first 24 to 48 hours. Give nonsteroidal anti-inflammatory drugs (NSAIDs) with food. Initially, NSAIDs can be used for 7 to 10 days without affecting muscle healing. Grade II and III sprains should be referred to an orthopedic practitioner.

24. A: Growing pain is a diagnosis of exclusion for (usually intermittent) lower extremity pain. All diagnostic markers are normal.

25. A: Systemic manifestations include fever, erythematous rashes, leukocytosis, serositis, lymphadenopathy, and rheumatoid nodules.

26. C: Osgood-Schlatter disease is a self-limiting condition with symptom management that includes avoiding or modifying activities that cause pain until the inflammation subsides, ice, and nonsteroidal anti-inflammatory drugs (NSAIDs) to reduce pain and inflammation.

27. A: Deposits of immune complexes trigger a generalized inflammatory response that can lead to tissue damage, such as vasculitis and ischemia, and numerous organ system abnormalities (commonly the heart and renal system). There is variety in both the presentation—acute life-threatening episodes or an indolent

manner—and how it is manifested over time in an individual (Burns & Dunn, 2012, p. 523).

28. C: Refer to an orthopedist as early as possible, ideally in the newborn nursery, because the joints are most flexible in the first hours and days of life.

29. C: In flexible MA, the forefoot can be abducted past midline.

30. A: Two techniques can be used to reduce the radial head; supination and flexion or pronation and flexion.

31. A: The Galeazzi sign can signal conditions that cause leg length discrepancies, the Barlow maneuver dislocates an unstable or dislocatable hip posteriorly, and the Ortolani maneuver reduces a posteriorly dislocated hip. All three will be positive in a dislocatable hip.

32. D: The goal of treatment in SCFE is to prevent further slippage and to stabilize the epiphysis via surgical intervention.

33. A: The X-linked dystrophies are the most common, with the most common dystrophy being Duchenne.

34. A: The female-to-male ratio increases with increasing curve magnitude. Small curves are equivalent between females and males. For curves less than 20 degrees, the risk for progression of the curve is low; these curves generally just need to be observed. However, for curves between 20 and 45 degrees, the risk for progression is high during growth, and early intervention is of paramount importance (Burns & Dunn, 2012, p. 940).

35. A: The patient with LCPD is generally afebrile, and the disorder arises from the avascular necrosis of the femoral head. The pain is referred to the knee or groin area.

36. A: DMD is a progressive disorder that affects muscles in the lower extremities, chest wall, and heart. There are no visual abnormalities or hip dislocation involved in the disorder.

37. B: Osteomyelitis is an inflammation of the bone that requires long-term antibiotic therapy (4–6 weeks). Diet, activity, and rest are supportive care as indicated.

38. A: Poor body mechanics are a common cause of sports injuries that can be lessened by proper training. Sports injuries are more commonly found in males in sports such as football, soccer, and wrestling. Not affected by socioeconomic status or preexisting conditions such as scoliosis.

39. B: Bone length occurs at the epiphyseal plates, which is also where the blood supply enters. If the blood supply is compromised growth may be jeopardized.

40. A: Growth in muscles is due to the range of motion the muscle is asked to perform as the underlying bone lengthens.

41. C: The normal growth pattern is one of slight varus (bowleg), which progresses to a neutral angle, and then slight valgus (knock-knee). Persistence of any phase beyond what is expected warrants further investigation.

42. A: Valgus up to 15 degrees is common up through the age of 8 or 9 years, but persistence beyond that may lead to problems and degenerative changes and warrants referral.

43. D: Genu varum, or bowed leg, is normal until approximately 18 months.

44. C: A fractured clavicle is not an uncommon finding following birth, especially in large babies. The spasm of the sternocleidomastoid and asymmetrical Moro reflex are classic signs of this problem.

45. B: Growing pains tend to occur during rapid growth, increasing in prevalence after 5 years of age. The pain is a muscular pain located bilaterally in the legs and thighs.

46. D: Rickets develops after several months of vitamin D deficiency and is characterized by craniotabes and enlarged anterior fontanelle with delayed closing. The enlarged costochondral junction, or rachitic rosary, is a classic sign.

47. B: Treatment of slipped capital femoral epiphysis is aimed at preventing further slippage. Since the goal is no weight bearing and avoiding flexion of the hip, no sports are recommended. Ice would not change the problem in the femoral head, and ROM and exercise are contraindicated.

48. A: Age, because younger children have more time to remodel compared with older children. Severity of pain, antalgic gait, family history, and bilateral involvement all have less impact on outcome than does age. Legg-Calvé-Perthes disease (LCPD) etiology is multifactorial and may be related to family history, environment, and or trauma.

49. D: Creatinine is formed in healthy muscle tissue from creatine at a steady rate. When muscle wasting occurs, as in muscular dystrophy, creatine excretion is dramatically increased. Deficiencies in serum calcium, phosphorus, and magnesium may result in muscle cramping and spasms but do not represent the clinical picture described.

50. B: Osgood-Schlatter disease is a benign condition resulting from overuse and is best treated with rest and supportive therapy.

51. A: Most torticollis resolves by 1 year of age. When there is no response to more conservative treatment interventions such as passive stretching and environmental stimulation, resulting in limited neck range of motion and facial asymmetry, surgery may be the recommended course of action.

52. C: Although still recommended in some sources, triple diapering is not thought to be effective because the musculoskeletal forces are greater than those exerted by diapers. Swaddling and the prone position are contraindicated and may increase the risk of dislocation. The appropriate treatment would be an evaluation by an orthopedic specialist and most likely a Pavlik harness.

53. D: After the age of 6 months, the Ortolani maneuver is less reliable due to diminished laxity in the hip. After

2 months of age, soft tissue contractures may develop, making this test unreliable.

54. A: Osteomyelitis is frequently associated with local trauma, whereas toxic synovitis is more commonly associated with a recent upper respiratory illness. The elevated WBCs, fever, and refusal to bear weight can occur in either osteomyelitis or transient (toxic) synovitis.

55. B: Observing the patella can be very helpful in differentiating internal tibial torsion from internal femoral torsion. The patella will rotate inward if the problem is above the knee. There is also general ligamentous laxity in other areas (fingers, elbows) associated with internal tibial torsion.

56. C: Metatarsus adductus is a flexural deformity of the foot related most commonly to intrauterine positioning. Flexible deformities able to be moved past the midline can be managed with stretching exercises.

57. A: This is the characteristic rash associated with systemic juvenile arthritis that occurs in 25% to 50% of children. Lyme disease rash is characteristic of erythema at the site of the tick bite with central clearing like a bull's eye. Systemic lupus erythematosus typically has a "butterfly rash" that is most often seen over the cheeks and bridge of the nose and gets worse in sunlight. Rheumatic fever often is associated with erythema marginatum, a nonpruritic, light pink macular rash that is usually on the trunk.

58. C: Little League elbow, or epicondylitis, is a result of repetitive forearm supination and pronation. Therefore, the goal is to prevent the injury by reducing the repetitive motion. Ice falsely reassures parent or coach that the injury can be prevented by applying before and after pitching.

☐ BIBLIOGRAPHY

Burns, C. E., & Dunn, A. M., et al. (2012). *Pediatric primary care* (5th ed.). St. Louis, MO: Saunders Elsevier.

Cannada, L. K. (Ed.). (2014). *Orthopaedic knowledge update* (11th ed.). Rosemont, IL: American Academy of Orthopaedic Surgeons.

Cassidy, J. T., Laxer, R., Petty, R. E., & Lindsley, C. (Eds.). (2011). *Textbook of pediatric rheumatology* (6th ed.). Philadelphia, PA: Saunders Elsevier.

Herring, J. (Ed.). (2013). *Tachdjian's pediatric orthopaedics* (5th ed.). Philadelphia, PA: Saunders Elsevier.

Kliegman, R. M., Stanton, B., St. Geme, J., & Schor, N. F. (Eds.). (2011). *Nelson's textbook of pediatrics* (19th ed.). Philadelphia, PA: W. B. Saunders.

McIlvain-Simpson, G. (2009). Juvenile rheumatoid arthritis. In P. J. Allen, J. A. Vessey, & N. Schapiro (Eds.), *Primary care of a child with a chronic condition* (5th ed.). St. Louis, MO: Mosby.

Muscular Dystrophy Association. (2014). Signs and symptoms. Retrieved from http://www.mda.org

Reuter-Rice, K., & Bollick, B. (Eds.). (2012). *Pediatric acute care*. Burlington, MA: Jones & Bartlett Learning.

Sarwark, J. F. (Ed.). (2010). *Essentials of musculoskeletal care* (4th ed.). Rosemont, IL: American Academy of Orthopaedic Surgeons.

Staheli, L. T. (Ed.). (2007). *Fundamentals of pediatric orthopedics* (4th ed.). Philadelphia, PA: Lippincott Williams & Wilkins.

Weinstein, S. L., & Flynn, J. M. (Eds.). (2013). *Lovell & Winter's pediatric orthopaedics* (7th ed.). Philadelphia, PA: Lippincott Williams & Wilkins.

Wheeless, C. R. (2014). Genu valgum in *Wheeless' textbook of orthopaedics*. Retrieved from http://www.wheeless online.com/ortho/genu_valgum

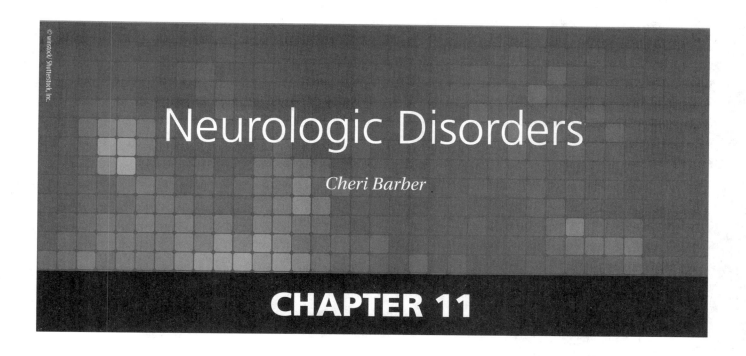

Neurologic Disorders

Cheri Barber

CHAPTER 11

❏ SEIZURE DISORDERS/EPILEPSY

- Definition
  1. Seizures—disturbances of normal nerve cell function characterized by uncontrolled, spontaneous electrical activity in the brain that may result in loss of consciousness, altered body movements, or disturbances of sensation and behavior
  2. Epilepsy—condition of recurrent seizures, associated with abnormal electrical activity in the brain
  3. Nonepileptic—mimic epileptic seizures and are a response to other events (i.e., fever, toxins, psychic stress or hypoxia)
  4. Status epilepticus—a seizure lasting for 30 minutes or a series of three seizures without any periods of consciousness between them
- Etiology/Incidence
  1. Caused by any event with potential to produce insult to the brain
  2. Multiple causes; specific etiologies remain uncertain for 50% of cases
     a. Genetic component or familial predisposition
     b. Genetic disorders—tuberous sclerosis; neurofibromatosis
     c. Hemorrhage (intracranial)
     d. Central nervous system (CNS) infection (encephalitis, meningitis)
     e. Head trauma
     f. Developmental defects of brain
     g. Biochemical factors (inborn metabolic errors, electrolyte imbalance)
     h. Intracranial tumors
     i. Toxic ingestions—e.g., alcohol

j. Poor drug compliance or altered drug metabolism because of illness
  3. Incidence varies greatly with age
     a. 1:1000 during first year of life
     b. 50% of all cases of epilepsy occur before age 25 years
  4. Variation in clinical manifestations due to location of brain involved
- Signs and Symptoms: Types of seizures
  1. Partial seizures—begin with an electrical discharge in one limited area of the brain
     a. Simple partial seizures
        (1) Characterized by seizure activity restricted to one side of body but may spread to other parts of the body
        (2) Usually last less than 2 minutes; no loss of consciousness and no postictal state
        (3) Motor—part of body or entire side (e.g., arm, leg, Jacksonian march, postural, vocalizations)
        (4) Sensory—visual, auditory, olfactory, paresthesias, visual hallucinations
        (5) Autonomic—result in changes in parts of the nervous system that automatically control bodily functions, e.g., tachycardia, pallor, sweating, flushing
        (6) Psychic—changes in how the person thinks, feels, or experiences things, e.g., memory problems, fearful, or feelings of déjà-vu
     b. Complex partial seizures—start in a limited area of the brain, typically the temporal or frontal lobes, and spread to other parts of the brain with a variety of clinical expressions
        (1) Impairment of consciousness for 30 seconds to approximately 2 minutes or longer

249

(2) Cognitive symptomatology
    (a) Abrupt alteration in mental state
    (b) Involves disruption of time relationships and memory
(3) Affective symptomatology—inexplicable feelings, e.g., fear or dread without obvious cause
(4) Somatosensory disturbances
    (a) Distortions of perception or hallucinations
    (b) May involve odd taste or smell with visual disturbances
(5) Automatisms
    (a) Occur in 50% to 75% of cases
    (b) Semi-purposeful perseverative movements
    (c) May involve walking, sucking, lip pursing, or picking at clothing

2. Generalized seizures—begin with a widespread electrical discharge of both hemispheres of the brain, usually with loss of consciousness
  a. Absence seizures (petit mal)
    (1) Onset between 4 and 8 years of age, higher incidence in girls
    (2) Brief, generalized, nonconvulsive episode with no aura and no postictal state
    (3) Characterized by interruption of activity, brief stare that begins and ends suddenly, and unresponsiveness
    (4) Usually lasts less than 10 seconds but may be as long as 20 seconds
    (5) Episode begins and ends abruptly
    (6) Child is unaware of episode and is fully alert afterward
  b. Tonic-clonic (grand mal)
    (1) Consists of motor manifestations with loss of consciousness
    (2) Prodrome stage (symptoms that occur prior to seizure—change in mood, behavior, or thinking)
    (3) Tonic phase
      (a) Sustained contraction of muscles
      (b) Occurs suddenly and without warning
      (c) Causes the person to fall to the ground
      (d) Extensor posturing and tonic contraction
      (e) Averages 10–30 seconds
    (4) Clonic phase
      (a) Bilateral and rhythmic, repetitive muscle contractions, with jerking movements
      (b) May bite tongue
      (c) Bowel or bladder incontinence may occur
      (d) Averages 30–60 seconds
    (5) Postictal phase
      (a) Period of cortical inhibition
      (b) Vomiting may occur
      (c) Confusion and lethargy
      (d) Gradual recovery of consciousness
  c. Myoclonic seizures
    (1) Brief (1 to 2 seconds), sudden muscle contractions/jerks

(2) Both sides of the body are involved but may involve only one area of body
(3) May occur as isolated events or in clusters
(4) Uncontrollable
(5) There may be no alteration in consciousness

  d. Infantile spasms (West syndrome)
    (1) Age-specific disorder with most occurring in the first 12 months of life
    (2) Sudden jerk followed by stiffening with arm extension and knees pulled up to body ("jack-knife" posture)
    (3) Approximately 60% have some brain disorder before seizures start
    (4) Often in clusters up to 150 individual spasms
    (5) Classified in two groups—infants with spasms but no basic neurologic disorder have a better prognosis, whereas those with symptomatic type have a specific etiological factor identified and an 80% to 90% risk of mental retardation
  e. Atonic
    (1) Also termed "drop" attacks
    (2) Characterized by sudden loss of muscle tone, which may result in head nodding or falling to the ground
    (3) Usually no alteration in consciousness and last <15 minutes
    (4) May require protective helmet due to drop attacks
  f. Lennox-Gastaut syndrome (rare)
    (1) Severe epileptic encephalopathy
    (2) Characterized by variety of primary, generalized seizures
    (3) Onset between 1 and 8 years of age; boys > girls
    (4) Have a preexisting brain disorder or injury
    (5) About one-third previously had infantile spasms
  g. Tonic seizures
    (1) Sudden significant increase in muscle tone lasting less than 20 seconds
    (2) Often occur during sleep, but if it happens while awake, the person will fall
    (3) Abrupt onset with rapid return to baseline
    (4) Frequently seen with Lennox-Gastaut syndrome
  h. Clonic seizures
    (1) Rhythmic jerking of arms and legs that may involve both sides of the body
    (2) Length varies
    (3) May progress to tonic-clonic seizure
    (4) Most commonly noted in arms, neck, and face but may involve other muscle groups

• Differential Diagnosis
1. Breath-holding spells—usually younger than 6 years of age
2. Sleep disorders, e.g., narcolepsy
3. Tics
4. Complicated migraine headaches
5. Syncope—more common in adolescence

6. Gastroesophageal reflux
7. Benign paroxysmal vertigo
8. Pseudoseizures
9. Vertigo

- Physical Findings
  1. Physical examination can be abnormal with underlying cerebral pathology
  2. Transient abnormal neurologic signs common during and after seizures
     a. Intention tremor
     b. Incoordination
     c. Weakness of one or more extremities
     d. Pathologic exaggeration of reflexes
     e. Confusion
  3. Warning signs of serious neurologic problems
     a. Asymmetric pupils
     b. Signs of increased intracranial pressure
     c. Focal deficits
     d. Unusual physical features, e.g., lesions seen in tuberous sclerosis that may indicate underlying genetic disorder
     e. Change in seizure pattern

- Diagnostic Tests/Findings
  1. Clinical and laboratory diagnosis
  2. Complete history
     a. Detailed description of seizure—onset, loss of consciousness, type, duration
     b. Underlying medical diagnosis
     c. Previous seizures and frequency
     d. Evidence of infection
     e. Abnormal behavior
     f. Previous static or progressive neurologic/developmental dysfunction
     g. Pica; possible ingestion of lead
     h. Trauma, including recent head injuries
     i. Birth history
     j. Current medication including anticonvulsants
     k. Family history of febrile and nonfebrile seizure
  3. Laboratory studies—to identify possible underlying etiology
     a. Complete blood count (CBC), including liver function tests—will be useful for diagnostic purposes and as a baseline for anticonvulsant therapy if necessary
     b. Serum fasting glucose, calcium, magnesium, and serum electrolyte levels
     c. Seizures and mental retardation suggestive of metabolic problem
        (1) Plasma amino acids
        (2) Blood ammonia
        (3) Blood lactate and pyruvate
        (4) Urinary organic acids
        (5) Cytogenetic analysis
     d. Other studies as determined by history/physical findings
  4. Lumbar puncture—not routine, used in patients <6 months and with older patient with obvious changes in mental status

5. Neuroimaging studies
   a. Skull radiographs—rarely indicated but helpful to rule out skull fracture
   b. Cranial CT and MRI
      (1) For detection of structural abnormalities
      (2) Indicated for:
         (a) A changing seizure pattern
         (b) Focal or lateralized abnormalities
         (c) History of trauma
         (d) Focally abnormal electroencephalogram (EEG)
         (e) Evidence of increased intracranial pressure
         (f) Known or suspected specific white or gray matter disease
         (g) First seizure in all adolescents
   c. MRI more sensitive for detection of low-grade tumors
   d. CT more sensitive to small foci or calcifications
6. Electroencephalography (EEG)—measures physiologic/electrical activity of the brain
   a. Standard in all children to diagnose and define seizure type, after first nonfebrile seizure
   b. Interpreted in context of child's age, history, and physical findings
   c. Recorded for up to 1 hour during periods of wakefulness and sleeping
   d. Normal EEG does not exclude diagnosis
   e. Video EEG (VEEG) over 1–6 days or a 24-hour ambulatory EEG often used if regular EEG is inconclusive

- Management/Treatment: Referral to neurologist for diagnosis and for initial treatment and management plan
  1. Antiepileptic drugs
     a. Principles
        (1) Utilize least number of medications
        (2) Maintain maximum level of alertness with fewest number of seizures
        (3) Emphasis is on enabling patients with seizures to lead full lifestyles consistent with their capabilities
        (4) Select drug effective for specific seizure type (see **Table 11-1**)
        (5) Use least toxic, least expensive, requiring least amount of laboratory monitoring
        (6) Begin with single drug; easier to assess side effects
        (7) Obtain baseline of child's physical status
           (a) Complete blood count (CBC)
           (b) Liver function tests (LFTs)
           (c) Blood urea nitrogen (BUN) and urinalysis
     b. Factors to consider in choice of drug
        (1) Type of seizure
        (2) Dosage
        (3) Potential side effects
        (4) Half-life
        (5) Age, sex, weight, and physical condition of child

■ **Table 11-1** Choice of Antiepileptic Drug According to Seizure Type and Epilepsy Syndrome

Type of Seizures Epileptic Syndrome	First-Choice AED	Second-Choice AED	Consider
Partial seizures with/ without generalization	Carbamazepine, phenytoin	Valproate, phenobarbitone, Lamotrigine, gabapentin, vigabatrin	Clobazam
Generalized tonic-clonic seizures	Valproate, phenytoin. carbamazepine	Phenobarbitone, primidone	Clobazam, felbamate, lamotrigine, gabapentin, Tiagabine, vigabatrine
Absence seizure	Valproate, ethosuximide	Clobazam, lamotrigine	
Juvenile myoclonic epilepsy	Valproate	Phenobarbitone	
Progressive myoclonic epilepsy	Valproate	Carbamazepine	
Lennox-Gastaut syndrome	Valproate	Clobazam, lamotrigine	Clobazam, felbamate, topiramate
Infantile spasm	ACTH or oral steroid	Vigabatrin	Benzodiazepines, felbamate, topiramate

Note: ACTH, adrenocorticotropic hormone; AED, antiepileptic drug.
Data from Singh, U. K., & Jaiswai, B. P. (2014). Pediatric oncall child health care. Retrieved from http://www.pediatriconcall.com/fordoctor/Conference_abstracts/report.aspx? reportid=457

2. Anticipatory guidance
   a. First aid measures
      (1) Protect child from injury, but do not restrain
      (2) Assess for adequate airway, breathing, and circulatory status
      (3) Do not insert items in mouth
      (4) Note time, duration, and activity
      (5) If seizure persists beyond 5 minutes, seek medical assistance, dial 911
   b. Observe for side effects of drugs
   c. Possible drug interactions
   d. Guidelines for activities/activity restrictions
      (1) Avoid activities where seizures may cause dangerous fall (e.g., high diving, rope and rock wall climbing)
      (2) Supervised swimming only
      (3) Discuss other sports participation with parents and child
   e. Importance of compliance with drug therapy
3. Intractable seizures—15% children with epilepsy
   a. Refer to epilepsy center with interdisciplinary team
   b. Alternative treatments
      (1) Ketogenic diet—very restricted, high-fat/low-carbohydrate diet
      (2) Epilepsy surgery—approximately half of children with intractable seizures are appropriate candidates for surgical procedures

☐ FEBRILE SEIZURES

- Definition: Generalized tonic or tonic-clonic seizures that occur as a consequence of an abrupt and steep rise in body temperature in young children

- Etiology/Incidence
  1. 3% to 4% of otherwise healthy children between 3 months and 5 years of age have one or more febrile seizures; peak onset between 12 and 24 months of age
  2. Exact cause unknown; hereditary influence suspected
  3. Most common nonepileptic seizure disorder and usually benign in nature
  4. Recurrence is greater with onset in the first year
  5. Cooling the child's body will not prevent a febrile seizure
- Signs and Symptoms: Two groups based on clinical features
  1. Simple febrile seizures
     a. Duration, 15 minutes
     b. No focal features
     c. If occur in series, total duration of less than 30 minutes
  2. Complex febrile seizures
     a. Duration, 15 minutes
     b. Focal features or postictal paresis present
     c. Occur in series with total duration greater than 30 minutes
- Differential Diagnosis
  1. Underlying meningitis or encephalitis
  2. Febrile shivering
  3. Breath-holding spells
  4. Underlying metabolic disorder
  5. Epilepsy
- Physical Findings
  1. Often associated with viral or bacterial illness
  2. Occur as the fever is rising
  3. Usually fever above 102°F (39°C)

- Diagnostic Tests/Findings
  1. Detailed description of seizure
  2. Complete physical assessment with careful neurologic examination
  3. Lumbar punctures not routine, but indicated for:
     a. Infants, younger than 1 year of age
     b. If the child is 12 to 18 months of age (should be considered due to elusive signs)
     c. >18 months if meningeal signs are present
  4. Skull radiographs not routine
  5. Blood laboratory studies, EEG, CT, or MRI not routine but performed if indicated by history or physical findings
- Management/Treatment
  1. Urgent treatment for unabated seizures of greater than 10 minutes
  2. Fever control for temperature >101°F to make the child feel better
     a. Sponge baths with tepid water are not recommended because they are ineffective and risk the possibility of increasing temperature through shivering
     b. Antipyretic use, e.g., acetaminophen or ibuprofen for child's comfort
  3. A comprehensive search for cause of fever and treatment of underlying illness
  4. Reassurance to parents regarding excellent prognosis
  5. Antiepileptic drugs
     a. Short-term or prolonged anticonvulsant prophylaxis not recommended
     b. On rare occasions rectal diazepam may be used when parents have significant anxiety or for prolonged seizure; the side effects of diazepam (drowsiness, lethargy, and ataxia) could mask signs of a CNS infection
     c. Parents should be taught the basic first aid measures for seizures

☐ HEADACHES

- Definition: Pain in any region of the head, may be sharp, throbbing, or dull
- Etiology/Incidence
  1. Exact etiology often unknown; pain may be extracranial and/or intracranial
     a. Possible causes
        (1) Genetic predisposition
        (2) Head trauma
        (3) Environmental factors
        (4) Illness or infection
        (5) Emotional factors
        (6) Certain foods and beverages, e.g., monosodium glutamate (MSG) and caffeine
  2. Difficult to distinguish tension headaches from migraine headaches in many children
  3. Chronic and recurrent headaches are most common neurologic complaints; 40% of children prior to 7 years of age will experience a headache and 75% by the age of 15 years
     a. Migraines—account for 50% of chronic or recurrent headaches; younger than 10 years of age males > females, and after 11 years of age females are more likely to have migraines than males
     b. Cluster headaches—less common in children younger than 20 years of age
        (1) Pain occurs in bursts, involve sharp stabbing pain on one side of the head
        (2) Painful when laying down
        (3) More frequent in males
        (4) 30–90 minutes and may reoccur several times per day
     c. Tension headaches
        (1) Affects all ages but more common in adolescence
        (2) Affects both sexes equally
        (3) Common family history with childhood onset
        (4) Diffuse, dull pain, mild-moderate intensity
        (5) Present all day with worsening in the afternoon
  4. Headache pain is produced by several factors that activate pain fibers
     a. Inflammation
     b. Stretching
     c. Torsion
     d. Contraction of innervated structures
        (1) Large intracranial arteries and veins
        (2) Dural sinuses
        (3) Periosteum of bone
        (4) Muscle/skin of scalp
        (5) Teeth and gums
- Signs and Symptoms
  1. Migraine headaches—recurrent headaches with varied frequency, intensity, and duration
     a. Diagnostic criteria—repeated episodes of headache accompanied by at least three of the following symptoms:
        (1) Recurrent abdominal pain (with or without headache), nausea, vomiting, extreme sensitivity to light or sound
        (2) Often have an aura, usually visual, but may be sensory, motor, or vertiginous
        (3) Throbbing or pounding pain (resolves after sleeping)
        (4) Pain restricted to one side of head (although may shift sides from one headache to next); bilateral before puberty
        (5) Relief of pain by brief periods of sleep
        (6) Family history of migraine in one or more immediate relatives
  2. Tension headaches—headaches occurring with most frequency and intensity during periods of increased stress
     a. Tend to involve occipital or temporal regions bilaterally and often extend to the neck, or may be diffuse

b. Nausea and vomiting may occur with chronic tension headaches, but not with episodic tension headaches

3. Intracranial headaches—may have certain distinguishing factors
   a. Severe occipital headache
   b. Exacerbated by straining, sneezing, or coughing
   c. Awaken child from sleep
   d. Exacerbated or improved markedly by position changes
   e. Associated with projectile vomiting or vomiting without nausea
   f. Associated with history of focal seizures
   g. Increase in intensity and severity if not treated

4. Sinus headache—chronic or recurrent headaches that occur in about 15% of children with chronic sinusitis
   a. Often occur same time each day, build slowly, with throbbing quality
   b. Accompanied by rhinorrhea, postnasal drip, persistent cough, recurrent ear infections, and fever
   c. Pain or pressure over frontal or maxillary sinuses

- Differential Diagnosis
1. Acute, severe headache—distinguish between intracranial and extracranial cause by thorough history and physical examination
   a. Intracranial causes
      (1) Intracranial mass
      (2) Infection—meningitis, encephalitis
      (3) Intracranial hemorrhage
      (4) Post–head injury
      (5) Postseizure
   b. Extracranial causes
      (1) Sinusitis—rare
      (2) Temporomandibular joint problem
2. Chronic headaches—stress, anxiety, or tension with resulting muscle contractions

- Physical Findings
1. Chronic migraine or tension headaches—physical examination generally normal
2. Acute headache—critical indicators of possible intracranial cause
   a. Meningismus
   b. Focal neurologic signs
   c. Papilledema
   d. Split sutures
   e. Evidence of cranial trauma (including blood in or behind ear)
   f. Depressed level of consciousness

- Diagnostic Tests/Findings
1. Unnecessary unless history/physical examination suggests intracranial etiology, e.g., infection, bleeding, tumors, sudden onset with increased severity, neurologic exam is abnormal with complaint of dizziness
   a. CT without contrast; if abnormal, then an MRI
   b. Lumbar puncture if warranted by exam
   c. EEG if seizure is suggested by history
2. Psychological evaluation may be needed with frequent tension headaches

- Management/Treatment
1. Specific treatment determined by etiology
2. Headaches with suspected intracranial etiology need evaluation by neurologist
3. Cautious use of medications for pain relief
   a. Initial treatment with simple analgesics
   b. Acetaminophen
      (1) 12–17 pounds—80 mg orally every 4 hours prn
      (2) 18–23 pounds—120 mg orally every 4 hours prn
      (3) 24–35 pounds—160 mg orally every 4 hours prn
      (4) 36–47 pounds—240 mg orally every 4 hours prn
      (5) 48–59 pounds—320 mg orally every 4 hours prn
      (6) 60–71 pounds—400 mg orally every 4 hours prn
      (7) 72–95 pounds—480 mg orally every 4 hours prn
      (8) 96+ pounds—640 mg orally every 4 hours prn
   c. If mild analgesics ineffective in children older than 11 years, may progress with caution to:
      (1) Midrin
         (a) Combination of isometheptene mucate 65 mg (constricts blood vessels); acetaminophen 325 mg, and dichloralphenazone 100 mg (mild sedative)
         (b) 1 to 2 capsules immediately; repeat 1 capsule every hour until relieved (a maximum of 3/day or 5/week)
      (2) Ergotamine tartrate—2 mg sublingual
   d. Prophylactic treatment
      (1) With headaches more than once/week and those that interfere with routine activities, e.g., school attendance
      (2) Unresponsive to symptomatic treatment
      (3) Must consider side effects
      (4) Medications used
         (a) Propranolol—0.6 to 3.0 mg/kg/day for children
         (b) Cyproheptadine hydrochloride—children >3 years 0.2–0.4 mg/kg/day
         (c) Phenobarbital—3 to 5 mg/kg/day every night (3 to 10 years)
         (d) Amitriptyline hydrochloride—1 to 1.5 mg/kg/day children
4. Stress management and relaxation techniques
5. Eliminate foods that may be triggers, e.g., chocolate, cheese, MSG, caffeine
6. Refer to specialists for further evaluation if headaches are recurrent, unresponsive (including allergist, psychiatrist, neurologist, or pain clinic)

☐ NEUROFIBROMATOSIS TYPE 1 (NF1) (VON RECKLINGHAUSEN DISEASE)

- Definition
1. A genetic disorder that causes tumors to grow around nerves (especially the eye)
2. Most common type of NF1
3. Always a progressive disorder
4. Often have learning disabilities and/or attention deficit hyperactivity disorder (ADHD)

- Etiology/Incidence
  1. Inherited autosomal dominant disorder; associated with chromosome 17, but 30% to 50% result from a spontaneous mutation of unknown cause
  2. Occurs 1:3000 to 1:4000 persons
  3. High variability and severity among individuals and within families
  4. Penetrance (likelihood that mutant gene will express itself at all if it is present) is virtually 100%
- Signs and Symptoms: Two or more of the following:
  1. Six or more light-brown spots on the skin (café au lait spots—CAL) measuring more than 5 mm in children or more than 15 mm in adolescents
  2. Freckling in armpits or groin
  3. Two or more neurofibromas—tumors around or on the peripheral nerves
  4. Two or more growths on the iris of the eye (Lisch nodules)
  5. Optic glioma
  6. Pheochromocytoma—tumor of the adrenal gland
  7. Enlargement of the liver
  8. Distinctive osseous lesions (e.g., sphenoid wing dysplasia or thinning of long bone cortex, with or without pseudoarthritis)
  9. First-degree relative (parent, sibling, child) with NF1
- Differential Diagnosis
  1. Benign condition with five or six CALs
  2. McCune-Albright syndrome
  3. Neurilemmoma
  4. Proteus syndrome
- Diagnostic Tests/Findings: Additional tests to confirm diagnosis and identify complications
  1. Slit-lamp ocular examination to identify ocular abnormalities (e.g., iris Lisch nodules and signs of optic pathway glioma)
  2. Cranial MRI—to identify gliomas
  3. Radiographs of spine, chest, skull—to identify neurofibromas and other tumors
  4. EEG—to detect epileptogenic foci
  5. Psychological evaluation of school-age child for school—to determine abilities and needs
  6. Audiogram/brain stem evoked response testing—baseline for hearing and detection of acoustic neuromas
- Management/Treatment
  1. Problems associated with NF1 most likely to require medical treatment
     a. Constipation
     b. Seizures
     c. Headaches
     d. Hyperactivity
     e. Learning disabilities
     f. Anxiety
     g. Renovascular hypertension
  2. Surgery
     a. Removing or debulking tumors
     b. Treating skeletal dysplasia
     c. Correcting scoliosis
     d. Treatment of vascular compromise

3. Frequent consultation with medical and surgical specialists, social workers, and other healthcare specialists
4. Genetic counseling
5. Referral to support group for NF1

☐ TUBEROUS SCLEROSIS (TS)

- Definition
  1. Neurocutaneous syndrome with a combination of skin abnormalities, seizures, and cognitive deficits
  2. Progressive disorder with deterioration over time, including new lesions and complications with increasing patient age
  3. Majority have ongoing debilitation from TS throughout their lives
  4. Mental retardation and seizures are most common problems
- Etiology/Incidence
  1. Autosomal dominant mutant gene, but many cases result from new mutations
  2. Previously negative family history does not exclude diagnosis
  3. Incidence—1:6000 to 1:50,000 in United States
  4. Most are diagnosed between 2 and 6 years
  5. Risk for affected person's children is 50%
- Signs and Symptoms
  1. Hypopigmented skin lesions often noted at birth
  2. Developmental delay
  3. Abnormal movements, particularly myoclonic jerking movements
  4. Abnormal heart rhythm
  5. Noncancerous tumors on the kidneys or heart
  6. Growths underneath and around the fingernails and toenails
- Differential Diagnosis: Seizures or mental retardation
- Physical Findings
  1. Establishing diagnosis of TS depends on detecting presence of two major features or one major plus two minor features
     a. Skin
        (1) Hypopigmented macules, of elliptical shape (ash-leaf spots)
        (2) Fibroadenomas—adenoma sebaceum
        (3) Distinctive brown patch on forehead
        (4) Shagreen patch (characteristic)—raised lesion in lumbosacral region
     b. Teeth—characteristic pitting of enamel
     c. Eye
        (1) Choroidal hamartomas
        (2) Hypopigmented defects of iris
     d. CNS
        (1) Periventricular tubers
        (2) Cerebral astrocytomas
        (3) Nonspecific EEG abnormalities, including hypoarrhythmia
     e. Cardiovascular
        (1) Cardiac rhabdomyomas
        (2) Aortic and major artery constrictions

f. Kidney—renal angiomyolipomas

g. Lungs—diffuse interstitial fibrosis

2. Seizures of all types, but myoclonic jerks and mental retardation most common symptoms

- Diagnostic Tests/Findings
  1. MRI scan of brain—virtually diagnostic and must be used in suspected TS
  2. Electrocardiogram
  3. Kidney ultrasound
  4. Once diagnosis is made, close follow-up surveillance is essential using appropriate clinical laboratory and radiographic techniques to monitor progression and identify new lesions

- Management/Treatment
  1. No specific medical treatment available
  2. Treat seizures and other complications (e.g., heart failure, renal failure) the same as if TS were not present
  3. Surgery on primary lesions may be indicated
  4. Genetic counseling
  5. Psychometric testing and psychoeducational techniques for cognitive needs
  6. Family and individual support and counseling
  7. Refer to tertiary care center for specialized treatment, information, and support

☐ TIC DISORDERS

- Definition
  1. Tic—repetitive, brief, involuntary, stereotypic, uncontrollable muscle movement or vocalizations
  2. Symptoms appear before 18 years of age and cannot be caused by the ingestion of substances such as stimulants or be part of another medical disease such as Huntington's disease
  3. Severity ranges, in terms of disruption and impairment, from mild and transient to more severe and permanent
  4. Types
     a. Transient tic disorder—duration less than 1 year
     b. Chronic tic disorder—duration more than 1 year, simple or complex; are either motor or vocal, but not both
     c. Tourette syndrome—most severe chronic tic disorder; symptoms include multiple motor and vocal tics, varying in nature and severity over time
        (1) Frequently have additional problems such as aggressiveness, social withdrawal, self-harming acts, and sleep disorders
        (2) Symptoms become more unpredictable during adolescence and may result in school refusal

- Etiology/Incidence
  1. Uncertain etiology; possible genetic central nervous system disturbance
  2. Believed that abnormal neurotransmitters in the brain contribute
  3. Transient tics
     a. Occur in 25% of normal children
     b. Often begin in school-age children and can be intensified by anxiety, fatigue, or excitement

4. Tourette syndrome
   a. Onset between 2 and 15 years of age with mean age 6 to 7 years
   b. Incidence—5:10,000 persons
   c. Male to female ratio 4:1

- Signs and Symptoms
  1. Characteristics of tics
     a. Variable expression—frequency, intensity, and severity
     b. Exacerbated by stress
     c. Some degree of voluntary control may be present
     d. Typically subside during sleep
  2. Simple tics
     a. Movements present that resemble nervous habits
     b. Facial "twitches," head shaking, eye blinking, shoulder shrugging, or throat clearing
  3. Tourette syndrome
     a. Simple tics
     b. Complex sequences of coordinated movements (e.g., bizarre gait, kicking, jumping, body gyrations, scratching, and seductive or obscene gestures)
     c. Involuntary vocalizations occur, ranging from simple to complex noises
     d. Expression is gender influenced
        (1) Motor and vocal manifestations more prevalent in boys
        (2) Behavioral problems, such as obsessive-compulsive disorder, more common in girls

- Differential Diagnosis
  1. Chronic tic disorder
  2. Stuttering
  3. Seizures
  4. Medication-induced tics
  5. Pervasive developmental disorder
  6. Psychiatric disorders, e.g., schizophrenia
  7. Medical conditions with associated abnormal movements, e.g., postviral encephalitis, multiple sclerosis

- Physical Findings
  1. Usually normal
  2. Some degree of voluntary ability to suppress tics is often present

- Diagnostic Tests/Findings: None
  1. Ordering of MRI scans and other blood tests typically done to rule out other diseases (such as seizure disorder)

- Management/Treatment
  1. Transient tics—support and education for child and family
  2. Chronic tics/Tourette syndrome
     a. Referral to mental health specialist
     b. May involve psychotherapy, behavior management, stress management
     c. Pharmacologic management
        (1) Consultation and/or referral—pediatric neurologist
        (2) Medications useful to suppress behavioral symptoms but interfere with daily functioning

(3) Pimozide—beginning dose of 1 mg at bedtime

  (a) Gradual increases (every 5 to 7 days) until symptoms subside

  (b) Maximum dose of 10 mg/day in children; 20 mg/day in adolescents

  (c) Side effects—sedation, lethargy, acute dystonic reactions, tardive dyskinesia

  (d) Less frequent side effects than haloperidol

(4) Haloperidol—beginning dose of 0.25 to 0.50 mg at bedtime

  (a) Gradual increases (every 4 to 5 days) until symptoms subside

  (b) Side effects similar to pimozide; tardive dyskinesia more common than with pimozide

(5) Clonidine—less effective but with fewer side effects; is sometimes used

□ HEAD INJURIES

- Definition: Any injury to the meninges, scalp, skull, or any part of the brain; classified by severity (mild, moderate, severe)
- Etiology/Incidence
  1. Injury resulting from external physical force to the cranium and internal brain structures
  2. Approximately 1 in 25 children receives medical attention each year for head injuries
  3. Twice as frequent in boys
  4. Greatest incidence in children 0–4 years and 15–19 years
  5. Very young children are especially vulnerable because of relatively larger heads with less musculoskeletal support and large-surfaced vascular scalps
  6. Age-specific etiology
     a. Infant—child abuse, falls
     b. 1 to 4 years of age—falls
     c. School age—falls, motor vehicle accidents, sports/recreation
     d. Adolescents—motor vehicle accidents, athletic injuries
- Signs and Symptoms: Important to determine specific circumstances associated with head trauma
  1. Scalp injuries—contusions and lacerations are most frequent
  2. Concussion
     a. Head injury sufficient to cause brief loss of consciousness and/or amnesia for event
     b. Presence and duration of amnesia is indicative of severity
     c. Usually brief loss of consciousness is followed in minutes by complete return to normal mental status and behavior
     d. Recovery usually complete without complications
     e. Few children experience postconcussional syndrome several hours after concussion, characterized by:
        (1) Headache
        (2) Drowsiness

        (3) Confusion or irritability
        (4) Symptoms may last for several days
  3. Diffuse axonal injury (DAI)
     a. Diffuse injury, usually resulting from violent motion, e.g., motor vehicle accidents
     b. Diagnosis of exclusion associated with:
        (1) Unconsciousness >6 hours
        (2) No other cause for symptoms, such as seizures or hematoma
     c. More serious diagnosis with less favorable prognosis than concussion
     d. Other symptoms depend on severity of injury
        (1) Abnormal movements with abnormal pupillary reaction
        (2) Difficulty regulating respirations and blood pressure
  4. Contusion
     a. Result of brain moving within the skull
     b. Bruising or tearing of cerebral structures
     c. Common locations include frontal, temporal lobes and orbital area
     d. Focal motor signs related to increased intracranial pressure (ICP) may be diagnostic
  5. Hematomas
     a. Epidural hematoma—blood clot formation between skull and dura mater of the brain
        (1) Most treatable; rare but potentially most lethal type of head injury
        (2) Classic clinical sign is delayed onset of symptoms
        (3) Initial neurologic symptoms may be minimal or absent
        (4) Secondary injury from increased ICP as hematoma enlarges, may result in neurologic symptoms
           (a) Headache
           (b) Confusion
           (c) Vomiting
           (d) One-sided weakness
           (e) Agitation
        (5) Symptoms may progress to lethargy, coma, and even death if left untreated
        (6) Prognosis is favorable if surgery is performed before secondary injury becomes irreversible, but this may not happen due to delayed presentation of symptoms
     b. Subdural hematoma—blood clot formation between the dura and arachnoid meninges of brain
        (1) Acute presentation
           (a) Symptoms appear within 48 hours of head injury
           (b) Signs of intracranial hypertension, including irritability or lethargy, vomiting, headache
        (2) Subacute
           (a) Symptoms appear between 2 and 21 days
           (b) Chronic hematoma with symptoms appearing after 21 days

(c) Signs include seizures, motor abnormalities (hypertonicity and agitation), systemic (irritability, vomiting, fever, anemia, poor weight gain)

6. Skull fracture
   a. Brain damage may not be present, or conversely, brain can be injured without skull fracture present
   b. Type, severity, symptomatology depend on area involved, age of child, and force of impact
   c. Linear
      (1) Fracture in temporoparietal region
      (2) Most common
      (3) Frequent in children younger than 2 years who fall from low heights
      (4) Outcome is usually excellent
   d. Depressed
      (1) Skull is disrupted/depressed at point of impact
      (2) Underlying structures may be bruised or lacerated
   e. Basal
      (1) Diagnosis dependent on recognition of signs, including hemorrhage in nose, nasopharynx, middle ear
      (2) Bruising over mastoid bone (Battle's sign) or around eyes (raccoon eyes sign)
      (3) Cranial nerve palsy
      (4) Cerebrospinal fluid (CSF) from ears or nose

- Differential Diagnosis
  1. Seizure disorder
  2. Child maltreatment
- Physical Findings
  1. Alterations in vital signs may indicate shock
  2. Headache, irritability, and/or crying may indicate acute pain
  3. Tense anterior fontanel in young child
  4. Alterations in level of consciousness (LOC) vary from irritability, agitation, restlessness to confusion and/or coma
  5. Skull fractures may or may not show bony displacement
  6. Unilateral swelling may present from a possible hematoma
  7. Decreased score on Glasgow Coma Scale
  8. Other signs
     a. Asymmetry of head
     b. Focal neurologic deficits
     c. Cranial nerve injuries
     d. CSF rhinorrhea or otorrhea
     e. Localized bogginess
     f. Ecchymosis
     g. Hearing impairments
  9. With cerebral edema and increasing ICP, may observe:
     a. Changes in level of consciousness
     b. Abnormal respiratory patterns
     c. Loss of protective reflexes (e.g., cough, gag, or corneal)
     d. Changes in motor function or posturing
     e. Nausea and projectile vomiting

- Diagnostic Tests/Findings
  1. Skull radiography
     a. Indicated when severity of head trauma includes:
        (1) Loss of consciousness
        (2) Presence of focal neurologic signs
     b. Only 20% of basal skull fractures can be recognized on standard skull radiographs
     c. If depressed skull fracture is suspected, obtain tangential views in addition to standard views
  2. CT scan—useful in detection of intracranial hemorrhage; investigation of localizing neurologic signs
  3. MRI—most useful in evaluation of subacute or chronic, rather than acute, injuries
- Management/Treatment
  1. For acute injury: Rapid, accurate assessment of primary injury and level of severity
  2. Most head trauma is minor, with momentary unconsciousness, then child resumes activity and does not require treatment
  3. Hospital observation may be required for:
     a. More than momentary loss of consciousness
     b. Lethargy, confusion, or irritability
     c. Severe headache
     d. Changes in speech or movements in arms and legs
     e. Significant bleeding from wound
     f. Vomiting 1 to 2 hours following injury
  4. Instructions for home observation
     a. Need to seek medical attention if child exhibits:
        (1) Increased drowsiness, prolonged sleepiness, inability to wake up
        (2) Disorientation
        (3) Confusion, trouble with blurred vision, speech, or hearing
        (4) Vomiting more than twice
        (5) Seizure
        (6) Change in swelling of scalp
        (7) Watery or bloody discharge from ear or nose
        (8) Headache that gets worse or last longer than 24 hours
        (9) Stumbling or trouble walking
  5. Anticipatory guidance and prevention
     a. Use of safety equipment for recreation and sports
     b. Never leave infant unattended on bed/furniture
     c. Evaluate play areas for risk factors
     d. Injury prevention instruction
     e. Drivers education/use of seat belts and child safety seats at all times

☐ MENINGITIS

- Definition: Inflammation of the meninges
- Etiology/Incidence of bacterial meningitis—related to age
  1. Most frequently a result of hematogenous dissemination
  2. Bacterial pathogens—related to age
     a. Newborn
        (1) *Escherichia coli*

(2) Group B streptococci

(3) *Listeria monocytogenes* (less frequent)

(4) Enterobacteriaceae

b. Etiologic agents responsible for 95% of cases that occur in children older than 2 months have been:

(1) *Haemophilus influenzae* type b (dramatic decline in incidence with *H. influenzae* immunization)

(2) *Streptococcus pneumoniae*

(3) *Neisseria meningitidis*

3. Other etiologic agents

a. Mycobacteria

b. Fungal infections

c. Viral (aseptic)—most common cause of meningitis

d. Protozoa

4. Highest risk—children 2 years of age and younger have the greatest incidence, with a peak occurring at less than 1 year of age

- Signs and Symptoms

1. Newborn

a. Often nonspecific and indistinguishable from those of septicemia

b. Most frequent signs

(1) Temperature instability

(2) Respiratory distress

(3) Irritability, lethargy

(4) Poor feeding

(5) Vomiting

c. Seizures present in 40%

2. Older infants and children

a. Nausea and vomiting

b. Irritability, confusion

c. Anorexia

d. Headache, back pain, nuchal rigidity

e. Hyperesthesia, cranial nerve palsy, ataxia

f. Photophobia

- Differential Diagnosis

1. Brain abscess

2. Spinal, epidural, or intracranial abscess

3. Bacterial endocarditis with embolism

4. Subdural empyema with or without thrombophlebitis

5. Brain tumor

- Physical Findings

1. Newborn

a. Bulging fontanel (with or without suture diastasis)

b. Increased intracranial pressure

c. Vomiting

2. Older infants and children

a. Common clinical signs associated with meningeal irritation are:

(1) Kernig's sign

(a) Flexion of the leg 90 degrees at hip

(b) Pain on extension of leg

(2) Brudzinski's sign—involuntary flexion of legs when neck is flexed

b. Headache is frequent sign of increased intracranial pressure

c. Behavior changes

d. Decreased consciousness

e. Weakness, numbness, eye movement problems, double vision

f. Seizures and/or vomiting

- Diagnostic Tests/Findings

1. Diagnosis based on examination and culture of cerebrospinal fluid

2. Lumbar puncture for CSF analysis

a. Contraindicated in following conditions:

(1) Cardiopulmonary compromise

(2) Signs of increased ICP—papilledema

(3) Infection in area overlying lumbar puncture location

b. Adverse reactions—pain, headache, bleeding

3. CSF analysis

a. Cloudy

b. Increased white blood cell count (predominantly neutrophils)

c. Increased protein >150 mg/dL

d. Decreased glucose (30% of serum glucose)

e. Gram stain

f. Culture

4. Polymerase chain reaction analysis possibly

- Management/Treatment

1. Hospitalization for bacterial meningitis—first 3 to 4 days are critical

2. Initiate antibiotic therapy once diagnosis is confirmed by clinical findings while awaiting specific CSF and blood culture results

3. Neonates

a. Fatality rate is 15% to 30% in neonates

b. Prognosis depends upon:

(1) Causative pathogen

(2) Predisposing risk factors

(3) Availability of intensive care facilities

c. Follow-up

(1) Group B *Streptococcus*

(a) 15% to 20% have sequelae—spastic quadriplegia, profound mental retardation, hemiparesis, hearing/visual deficits

(b) 11% have hydrocephalus

(c) 13% have seizure disorder

(2) Gram-negative meningitis

(a) 10% have severe sequelae of developmental delays

(b) About 25% to 35% have mild to moderate sequelae, which may not interfere with normal development

(c) Hydrocephalus develops in infants

d. Neonatal survivors without major sequelae typically develop normally

4. Older infants and children

a. Prognosis depends on several factors

(1) Patient's age at onset

(2) Duration of disease before appropriate antibiotic therapy initiated

(3) Specific microorganism involved and number of organisms

(4) Whether disorder is compromising host response to infection

b. Mortality rate 1% to 5% beyond the neonatal period

c. Up to 50% of survivors have some sequelae

(1) 10% have hearing deficits

(2) 15% have language disorder/delay

(3) 2% to 4% have vision impairment

(4) 10% to 11% have mental retardation

(5) 3% to 7% have motor problems

(6) 2% to 8% have seizures

5. Immunizations for prevention of meningitis

a. *Haemophilus influenzae* type b (Hib)

b. Pneumococcal conjugate (Prevnar13)

c. Meningococcal (Menactra or Menveo)

☐ BRAIN TUMORS

- Definition: Tumors are abnormal growth of tissue, a mass of expanding abnormal intracranial cells; brain tumors are the most common tumors in childhood
- Etiology/Incidence

1. Etiology is unknown; may be genetic predisposition, congenital factors, environmental exposures

2. The primary tumors seen in children

a. Astrocytomas

(1) Usually slow growing, noncancerous cysts

(2) Often develop between 5 and 8 years of age

b. Medulloblastoma

(1) The most common brain cancer in children

(2) Usually develops around age 5

(3) Occurs more often in boys

c. Brain stem gliomas

(1) Occur almost exclusively in children

(2) Often grow very large before symptoms develop

(3) Average age of development is 5 years

(4) Five-year survival rate is low

d. Ependymomas

(1) Are located in the ventricles

(2) Block the flow of CSF

3. In children between 4 and 11 years, infratentorial (posterior fossa; posterior third of the brain) tumors predominate (60%), including cerebellar and brain stem tumors; the others are supratentorial in the anterior two-thirds of the brain

- Signs and Symptoms

1. Infants with open sutures

a. Increased head circumference

b. Irritability

c. Head tilt

d. Loss of developmental milestones

e. Bulging fontanelle

f. No red reflex in the eye

2. Older children

a. Headache; symptoms usually increase in frequency, becoming more severe in the morning, followed by vomiting

b. 85% of children with malignant tumors have abnormal neurologic or ocular examinations within 2 to 4 months of onset of headaches

c. Gradual loss of movement or feeling in an arm or leg

d. Problems with balance, speech

e. Certain specific neurologic symptoms may occur later and suggest localization of the CNS tumor

(a) Ataxia, hemiparesis, cranial nerve palsies

(b) Somnolence

(c) Seizures

(d) Head tilt

(e) Diencephalic syndrome—failure to thrive (FTT), emaciation

(f) Diabetes insipidus

- Differential Diagnosis

1. Brain abscess

2. Intracranial hemorrhage

3. Nonneoplastic hydrocephalus

4. Arteriovenous malformations or aneurysm

5. Indolent viral infections

6. Subdural hematoma

- Physical Findings: Directly related to anatomic location, size, and to some extent the age of the child. May include:

1. Tense, bulging fontanelle at rest (in infant)

2. Cranial enlargement (present in infants and young children)

3. Papilledema once sutures are fused (edema of optic nerve)

4. Nuchal rigidity

5. Poor coordination or clumsiness

6. Poor fine motor control

7. Hypoflexia or hyperflexia

8. Positive Babinski sign

9. Spasticity/paralysis

10. Behavioral changes—may be earliest symptom in child/adolescent

- Diagnostic Tests/Findings

1. MRI—superior, sensitive neuroimaging technology

2. CT scan

a. Without contrast, can detect:

(1) Whether lesion is cystic or solid

(2) Presence of calcifications, hemorrhage, edema, and hydrocephalus

b. With contrast can detect:

(1) Small tumors

(2) Differentiation of areas of edema

3. Angiography—determines blood supply to affected structures

4. Bone scan—x-rays of the bones after a dye has been injected that is absorbed by bone tissue

5. Lumbar puncture contraindicated in presence of increased ICP

- Management/Treatment: Therapy selected depends on type and site of tumor

1. Surgery (usually treatment of choice, although some tumors cannot be removed entirely and can only be debulked)

2. Radiation therapy
3. Chemotherapy
4. Proton therapy (precise form of radiation therapy)
5. Steroids used to treat and prevent swelling in the brain
6. Follow-up
   a. EEG for seizures
   b. Visual evoked response (VER) for visual problems
   c. Brain stem auditory evoked response (BAER) for hearing problems
   d. Rehabilitation for lost motor skills and/or muscle strength
   e. Multidisciplinary approach for comprehensive health and developmental needs of child/family

❏ QUESTIONS

Select the best answer.

1. A 5-month-old boy, former 28-week-premature infant, is being evaluated in your practice because of a concern about delayed motor development. In formulating the differential diagnosis, you keep in mind that spastic cerebral palsy is characterized by:
   a. Increased deep tendon reflexes and sustained clonus
   b. Dystonic posturing
   c. Abnormal involuntary movements
   d. Nystagmus

2. A 4-year-old child with a history of myelomeningocele and a ventriculoperitoneal shunt presents to the clinic with a headache, nausea, vomiting, and lethargy. The most probable diagnosis is:
   a. Viral gastroenteritis
   b. Shunt malfunction
   c. Meningitis
   d. Shunt infection

3. An apparently healthy child, who is enrolled in Head Start, is suspected of having developmental delays based on Denver II results at two separate clinic visits. The most appropriate next step would be to:
   a. Request developmental evaluation from the Head Start program
   b. Repeat the Denver II in 6 months
   c. Refer the child for a more definitive evaluation
   d. Discuss ways in which parents can foster the child's development

4. What needs to be included when educating parents about febrile seizures?
   a. The pediatric patient is at increased risk for epilepsy than an adult is.
   b. The pediatric patient would benefit from phenytoin prophylaxis.
   c. Children may experience repeated seizures.
   d. The pediatric patient would benefit from phenobarbital prophylaxis.

5. Which of the following signs is not characteristic of generalized seizures?
   a. Unilateral motor manifestations
   b. Disturbance of consciousness
   c. Tonic stiffening of the trunk
   d. Simultaneous and symmetric cerebral hemisphere discharge

6. Which of the following is the primary diagnostic tool used in the evaluation of seizure disorder?
   a. EEG
   b. Cerebral blood flow studies
   c. CT scan
   d. MRI

7. Upon physical examination of a 4-year-old boy, you note seven café au lait spots greater than 5 mm in diameter. This finding may be indicative of:
   a. Tuberous sclerosis
   b. Sturge-Weber disease
   c. Duchenne dystrophy
   d. Neurofibromatosis

8. Michael is a 15-year-old high school student who presents for a school sports physical. He appears to be in good health but is concerned about a bad headache he had a few weeks ago. He is concerned because his mother's friend died of a brain tumor. You tell Michael that the most common type of headache with onset in adolescence is:
   a. Sinus headache
   b. Vascular headache
   c. Tension headache
   d. Migraine headache

9. An 18-year-old college freshman is seen in the student clinic with a complaint of migraine headaches. In collecting the history, you would expect him to say he experiences pain:
   a. Throughout his head without any localization
   b. Restricted to one side of his head during an episode
   c. Mostly in the occipital area
   d. Across his head from one temporal side to another

10. Which of the following history points would not alert the practitioner to the possibility of a brain tumor?
    a. Headache in the morning associated with vomiting
    b. Sleep apnea
    c. School failure and personality changes in older children
    d. None of the above

11. Which of the following signs is not scored in the Glasgow Coma Scale?
    a. Eye opening
    b. Verbal response
    c. Upper limb response
    d. Fine motor response

12. Mr. Harris calls the pediatric clinic to say that Josh, his 2-year-old son, has tripped on the sidewalk and hit his head on concrete. Which of the following symptoms reported by Mr. Harris would require that Josh be seen in the emergency room?
    a. Uncontrollable crying
    b. Loss of consciousness
    c. Scalp laceration
    d. History of febrile seizures

13. A 2-year-old child is evaluated in the emergency department for a closed head injury following a 10-foot fall from an open window. When interpreting diagnostic imaging results, you are aware that the most common and generally the least serious type of skull fracture is:
    a. Basilar fracture
    b. Compound fracture
    c. Depressed fracture
    d. Linear fracture

14. A 12-month-old child, whose parents have a history of noncompliance for routine care, presents to the clinic with fever, irritability, and nuchal rigidity. The most critical diagnostic step in the child with suspected meningitis is:
    a. The history
    b. The physical examination
    c. Evaluation of the CSF
    d. Blood culture

15. In a child with suspected meningitis, the lumbar puncture should be delayed and a CT scan obtained first in which of the following circumstances?
    a. There are signs of increased intracranial pressure.
    b. The child has tachycardia.
    c. The child has a negative Brudzinski's sign.
    d. The WBC count is greater than 10,000/mm³.

16. Absence seizures:
    a. Often begin between 1 and 2 years of age
    b. Appear as altered awareness and blank stare for a brief period
    c. More commonly occur in first-born children
    d. Usually progress to a more severe seizure disorder beyond childhood

17. The most common type of brain tumor in children is:
    a. Ependymoma
    b. Brain stem tumor
    c. Craniopharyngioma
    d. Medulloblastoma

18. In most states, a learning disability is defined on the basis of:
    a. The child's IQ as determined by a psychological evaluation
    b. A discrepancy between the child's actual and expected achievement
    c. A diagnosis of attention deficit disorder
    d. All of the above

19. Which of the following is a measure of childhood intelligence?
    a. Wechsler scales
    b. Denver II
    c. Bayley scales
    d. Vineland scales

20. In working with a child with Tourette syndrome and his family, the nurse practitioner should be aware that:
    a. Symptoms become more unpredictable during adolescence.

b. Boys are more likely than girls to exhibit behavioral problems such as obsessive-compulsive disorder.
    c. Sleep disturbance from tics increases with age.
    d. Several medications are now available to control the tics without interfering with daily functioning.

21. There are several skin features seen with tuberous sclerosis. Which of the following is most characteristic?
    a. Café au lait spots
    b. Blue or purple striae
    c. Papules in a "Christmas tree" pattern
    d. Hypopigmented macules in an "ash leaf" shape

22. A head injury in which bruising or tearing of the cerebral structures occurs is a:
    a. Contusion
    b. Concussion
    c. Hematoma
    d. Diffuse axonal injury

23. Which of the following responses during a tonic-clonic seizure is most important to teach family members of a child who has these seizures?
    a. Restrain the child
    b. Insert an airway into the mouth to prevent tongue biting
    c. Note the time, duration, and activity of the seizure
    d. Protect child from injury

24. Which of the following would not be associated with an uncomplicated concussion?
    a. Focal motor signs
    b. Brief loss of consciousness
    c. Headache
    d. Confusion or amnesia for the event

25. For children 2 to 4 years of age, the most common cause of head injury is:
    a. Motor vehicle accidents
    b. Falls
    c. Child abuse
    d. Bicycle accidents

26. An 11-year-old girl is brought in by her mother complaining of severe headaches associated with nausea and vomiting. Which of the following signs and symptoms would lead you to consider a brain tumor as part of your differential diagnosis?
    a. Throbbing pain accompanied by severe light sensitivity
    b. Bilateral throbbing pain
    c. Headache preceded by a visual aura
    d. More severe in the morning followed by vomiting

27. A neonate is being worked up for meningitis after experiencing a seizure preceded by fever, irritability, and poor feeding for 1 day. On physical examination, which of the following findings would be most consistent with a diagnosis of meningitis?
    a. Bulging fontanelle
    b. Positive Brudzinski's sign
    c. Nuchal rigidity
    d. Positive Kernig's sign

28. Which of the following statements about Tourette syndrome is true?
    a. Symptoms can improve with age.
    b. It is more common among males than among females.
    c. Mean age at onset is between 5 and 7 years.
    d. All of the above.
29. The most useful diagnostic tool for diagnosing epilepsy is:
    a. MRI
    b. EMG
    c. EEG
    d. CT scan

☐ ANSWERS AND RATIONALES

1. A: In spastic CP, a lowered reflex threshold results in increased deep tendon reflexes (DTRs) and sustained clonus. The other signs are characteristic of dyskinetic and ataxic CP.
2. B: Headache, nausea, vomiting, and lethargy are frequently associated with malfunctioning shunt systems.
3. C: If a developmental lag is suspected based on repeated performances on the Denver II (which is a screening tool), a more definitive assessment should be obtained.
4. C: Children with a diagnosis of simple febrile seizures may experience repeated febrile seizures, particularly if the first seizure occurred before 1 year of age. They are not at increased risk for epilepsy as adults, phenytoin is not efficacious as a prophylactic drug, and phenobarbital is not routinely recommended.
5. A: In generalized seizures, motor manifestations, if any, are bilateral.
6. A: In the study of seizure disorders, the electroencephalogram (EEG) has the greatest clinical applicability. The other imaging techniques are considered supplemental.
7. D: More than six café au lait spots (greater than 5 mm in diameter) in prepubertal children is an essential part of the diagnosis of neurofibromatosis.
8. C: The most common headache in adolescents is the tension, or psychogenic, headache.
9. B: After puberty, migraine headache pain is restricted to one side of the head but may switch sides from one headache episode to another.
10. B: Brain tumors can be associated with morning headaches, vomiting, and behavioral changes. Sleep apnea is associated with airway obstruction or other neuromuscular disorders.
11. D: The Glasgow Coma Scale is based on eye opening, verbal response, and best upper limb response.
12. B: Emergency care should be sought following head trauma if the child is unresponsive.
13. D: The linear fracture is the most common and has little serious clinical implication, unless it overlies a vascular channel or penetrates an air sinus.

14. C: Collection of the cerebrospinal fluid (CSF) is the most critical diagnostic step in the child with suspected meningitis, based on the history and physical examination.
15. A: If elevated intracranial pressure is suspected, a CT scan should be obtained first to avoid the complication of cerebellar or uncal herniation.
16. B: Absence seizures appear as altered awareness and blank stare, usually appear between the ages of 4 and 8 years, and the cause is predominantly genetic.
17. D: Medulloblastomas are the most common brain tumors of childhood.
18. B: In most states, a learning disability means a discrepancy between the child's actual and expected achievement.
19. A: The Wechsler scales measure intelligence, the Denver and Bayley scales measure development, and the Vineland scales measure adaptive behavior.
20. A: Changing hormones make the symptoms more unpredictable.
21. D: Hypopigmented macules in an elliptical shape are characteristic and are often described as an "ash leaf" spot.
22. A: A contusion is a head injury with bruising or tearing of the cerebral structures, whereas a hematoma is a collection of blood outside the blood vessel that occurs due to trauma of the wall of the blood vessel.
23. D: It is *most* important to protect the child from injury, never to restrain a child. Make note of the time, duration, and activity of the seizure.
24. A: Focal motor signs are more commonly seen with partial (focal) seizures and can be divided into simple and complex seizures.
25. B: Head injuries from falls are most common in children between the ages of 2 and 4 years. In older children, bicycle, vehicle, and recreational accidents are the main causes of head injuries.
26. D: Symptoms of brain tumors are headaches that are more severe in the morning followed by vomiting and sometimes with changes in personality and behavior, inability to concentrate, memory loss, and/or increased sleep.
27. A: A bulging fontanelle in an infant is indicative of meningitis (infection of the membranes covering the brain), encephalitis (swelling or inflammation of the brain caused by an infection), or hydrocephalus (a build-up of fluid).
28. D: Tourette syndrome is more common in boys than in girls and typically starts before age 18—usually between 5 and 7 years of age.
29. C: An electroencephalogram (EEG) is first line for diagnosing epilepsy by measuring the impulses in the brain; other tests such as MRI and blood tests may also be ordered.

□ BIBLIOGRAPHY

American Psychiatric Association. (2013). *Diagnostic and statistical manual of mental disorders* (5th ed.). Washington, DC: Author.

Bajaj, L., Hambidge, S., Nyquist, A. C., & Kerby, G. (2011). *Berman's pediatric decision making* (5th ed.). St. Louis, MO: Mosby.

Blair, J. L. (2009). Epilepsy and seizure disorders. In J. Allen, J. A. Vessey, & N. A. Shapiro (Eds.), *Primary care of the child with a chronic condition* (5th ed.). St. Louis, MO: Mosby.

Bourgeois, B. F., Dodson, E., Pellock, J. M., & Nordli, D. R. (2007). *Pediatric epilepsy: Diagnosis and therapy* (3rd ed.). New York, NY: Demos Medical Publishing.

Carey, W. B., Crocker, A. C., Elias, E. R., Feldman, H. M., & Coleman, W. L. (2009). *Developmental-behavioral pediatrics: Expert consult* (4th ed.). Philadelphia, PA: W. B. Saunders.

Engel, J. (2006). Report of the ILAE classification core group. *Epilepsia, 47*(9), 1558–1568.

Engorn, B., & Flerlage, J. (2014). *The Harriet Lane handbook* (20th ed.). St. Louis, MO: Elsevier Health Services.

Hockenberry, M. J. (2010). *Wong's nursing care of infants and children* (9th ed.). St. Louis, MO: Mosby.

Kliegman, R., Behman, R., Jenson, H. B., & Stanton, B. (Eds.). (2011). *Nelson textbook of pediatrics* (19th ed.). Philadelphia, PA: W. B. Saunders.

Marx, J. A. (Ed.). (2010). *Rosen's emergency medicine: Current concepts and clinical practice* (7th ed.). St. Louis, MO: Mosby.

National Institute of Neurologic Disorders and Stroke. (2011). Neurofibromatosis fact sheet. Retrieved from http://www.ninds.nih.gov/disorders/neurofibromatosis/detail_neurofibromatosis.htm

Singh, U. K., & Jaiswai, B. P. (2014). Pediatric oncall child health care. Retrieved from http://www.pediatriconcall.com/fordoctor/Conference_abstracts/report.aspx?reportid=457

Taketomo, C. K., Hodding, J. H., & Kraus, D. M. (2013). *Pediatric and neonatal dosage handbook* (20th ed.). Hudson, NY: Lexicomp.

U.S. National Library of Medicine. (2014). Childhood brain tumors. Medline Plus. Retrieved from http://www.nlm.nih.gov/medlineplus/childhoodbraintumors.html

Genitourinary/Gynecological Disorders/Adolescent Pregnancy

Marlo A. Eldridge

MaryLou C. Rosenblatt

CHAPTER 12

☐ URINARY TRACT INFECTION (UTI)

- Definition: A generic term referring to the presence of bacterial infection of the urinary tract involving the bladder (cystitis), urethra (urethritis), or kidney (pyelonephritis)
- Etiology/Incidence
  1. Multifactorial etiology, including agent virulence and host predisposing factors
     a. Agent virulence
        (1) *Escherichia coli*—pathogenic agent in 80% to 90% of all childhood UTIs
        (2) Other enteric bacteria agents— *Klebsiella, Enterobacter* sp.
        (3) *Staphylococcus saprophyticus*—common in males
        (4) Viral agents rare with exception of adenovirus
     b. Host predisposing factors
        (1) Immature kidneys associated with premature and low-birth-weight infants
        (2) Congenital urologic abnormalities, reflux, neurogenic bladder
        (3) Gender differences in anatomy of urinary tract predisposes females, e.g., short urethra and close proximity to anus
        (4) Dysfunctional voiding—urinary stasis/incomplete bladder emptying
        (5) Functional obstruction—constipation, pregnancy
        (6) Trauma/irritants—catheterization, bubble baths, sexual intercourse, sexual abuse, pinworms
  2. Incidence—most common pediatric urinary tract problem
     a. Newborns—2 per 100 live births
     b. Accounts for 4.1% to 7.5% of infant febrile episodes
     c. Infancy—increased incidence in males (2.7% of males and 0.7% of females have experienced an episode of bacteriuria by the time they reach 1 year of age)
     d. Increased incidence among females after infancy and through adolescence, affecting less than 1% of school-age boys and 1% to 3% of school-age girls
- Signs and Symptoms
  1. May be asymptomatic or with nonspecific symptoms, especially in infancy
  2. Symptom clusters by age group
     a. Newborns—irritability, poor feeding, diarrhea, fever, vomiting
     b. Infants/preschoolers—diarrhea, vomiting, fever, poor feeding, strong/foul-smelling urine
     c. School-age children/adolescents—fever, vomiting, strong/foul-smelling urine, suprapubic or urethral pain, frequency, dysuria, and incontinence
- Differential Diagnosis
  1. Acute abdomen—appendicitis, sexually transmitted diseases, ectopic pregnancy
  2. Chemical irritation—soaps, bubble baths
  3. Vulvovaginitis
  4. Dysfunctional voiding—enuresis
  5. Sexual abuse
  6. Foreign body
  7. Pelvic inflammatory disease (PID)
  8. Dysfunctional elimination syndrome (DES)—dysfunctional voiding accompanied by constipation
- Physical Findings
  1. May be normal
  2. Infancy—weight loss, poor feeding, diarrhea

3. Fever and irritability
4. Blood pressure may be elevated—reflux nephropathology
5. Abdominal examination—pain, tenderness, guarding
6. Urethral or vaginal irritation/discharge—with vulvovaginitis due to irritation or sexually transmitted disease (STD)

- Diagnostic Tests/Findings
1. Urine analysis—presence of urinary leukocyte esterase, nitrate, and blood suggestive of UTI, but it is not diagnostic
2. Urine culture mandatory for accurate diagnosis—technique for specimen collection depends on age and developmental status of child, severity of condition, and urgency of need for unequivocal results
   a. Random voids/bagged urine—minimal usefulness due to high potential for contamination from external genitalia; 93% false positives; most useful for exclusion of the diagnosis of bacteriuria, but not appropriate for culture and sensitivity. If positive, warrants second sample via appropriate means. Therefore, a bagged urine can delay diagnosis and treatment and require a second trip to the office or lab for families
   b. Clean-catch midstream—often contaminated from external genitalia, especially in young girls; more reliable from circumcised males and older girls
      (1) Appropriate for mild symptoms or follow-up
      (2) Positive with colonies of 50,000–100,000 colony forming units (CFUs)/mL of single organism
   c. Straight catheterization—used with infants/children who cannot void voluntarily; lower risk for nosocomial infection than indwelling catheters
      (1) Appropriate for moderate or severe symptoms
      (2) Positive with colonies >10,000 CFUs/mL of single or multiple organisms
   d. Suprapubic aspiration—used with infants/children unable to void voluntarily when culture is urgently needed due to severity or equivocal results from alternative techniques
      (1) Appropriate for moderate or severe symptoms
      (2) Positive with colonies >1000 CFUs/mL of single or multiple organisms
3. Blood culture—collected in infants <12 months with suspected sepsis
4. Radiologic studies—for localizing infection and to rule out urinary abnormalities as part of UTI work-up
   a. Indications for imaging studies—recommendations vary but generally include:
      (1) Symptoms of pyelonephritis regardless of age and gender
      (2) UTI in any child <3 months of age
      (3) Males with first infection and females with second infection, even if it is not pyelonephritis and the child is >3 months of age
   b. Types
      (1) Bladder and renal ultrasound—usually first step in evaluation of structural and developmental anomalies/disorders
      (2) Voiding cystourethrogram (VCUG)—detects regurgitation (reflux) of urine into ureter; delay 4 to 6 weeks after diagnosis to exclude UTI-related reflux; continue antibiotic prophylaxis until after VCUG
      (3) Intravenous pyelogram (IVP) or nuclear renal cortical scans—detect scarring and examine renal function; usually done only if VCUG is positive and there is suspicion of renal scarring
      (4) An acute DMSA (dimercaptosuccinic acid) can be done during time of infection to assess acute renal inflammation and/or uptake defects

- Management/Treatment
1. Antibiotic treatment
   a. Parenteral antibiotics—newborns, infants, or older children with vomiting or severe symptoms, systemic illness, fever, or unable to take fluids
   b. Oral antibiotic
      (1) Generally treated for 10-day regimen
      (2) Can be extended to 14-day regimen in complicated infections
      (3) Single-dose regimen remains controversial
   c. First-line drugs of choice
      (1) Trimethoprim-sulfamethoxazole (TMP/SMX)—infants >2 months of age
         (a) TMP 6 to 10 mg/kg/day 1 SMX 30 to 60 mg/kg/day bid
         (b) Recommended until sensitivities are available since most UTIs are caused by *E. coli*
      (2) Amoxicillin—30 to 50 mg/kg/day tid
      (3) Amoxicillin/clavulanate—40 mg/kg/day tid
      (4) Sulfisoxazole—150 mg/kg/day qid
      (5) Cephalexin—50 mg/kg/day tid
      (6) Nitrofurantoin—5 to 7 mg/kg/day in divided doses; ideal for treatment of bladder infections because it is highly concentrated in the urine but less effective for systemic/renal infections as it does not concentrate well in the blood
2. Follow-up urine cultures
   a. Second culture at 72 hours after initiating treatment if symptoms are not resolving
   b. Culture 1 week after completion of treatment when test of cure is indicated
   c. Close monitoring of periodic urine cultures with recurrent infections and/or unexplained fevers
3. Prophylactic antibiotics—very controversial due to 2011 American Academy of Pediatrics (AAP) guidelines. Guidelines conclude that prophylactic antibiotics (abx) are not indicated for infants 2–24 months without reflux or with reflux Grades I–IV because they did not prevent recurrent febrile UTIs in six studies. This is a guideline, and the AAP states that this is not

an exclusive treatment recommendation; decisions should also be made on a case-by-case basis and on the basis of clinical judgment. If prophylaxis is chosen for vesicoureteral reflux (VUR): trimethoprim-sulfamethoxazole, one-half daily dose, usually at bedtime, until reflux resolves spontaneously or via endoscopic/surgical intervention and is proven with a negative VCUG. Alternately, nitrofurantoin/macrodantin 1–2 mg/kg/day given in a single daily dose.

4. VCUG
   a. Most VUR grades I to III resolve as child grows if there is no underlying dysfunctional voiding or dysfunctional elimination syndrome
   b. VCUG to assess status of reflux every 12 to 18 months in children older than 24 months
5. Education/prevention
   a. Increased fluid intake
   b. Frequent voiding with complete emptying of bladder
   c. Good perineal hygiene with front-to-back wiping
   d. Avoid bubble baths and other urethral irritants

❏ ENURESIS

- Definition: Involuntary urination after child has reached age when bladder control is usually attained; may occur during daytime (diurnal) or at night, especially while sleeping (nocturnal); usually resolves by 5 to 7 years of age and is considered outside the norm if occurring after the 7th birthday
  1. Primary enuresis—child has never attained control
  2. Secondary enuresis—recurrence of incontinence following a period of at least 6 months of dryness
- Etiology/Incidence
  1. Many causes suggested
     a. Primary—small bladder capacity; toilet-training problems; delayed maturation of voiding inhibitory reflex; sleep problems ("deep sleeper"); lack of inhibition of antidiuretic hormone (ADH); ingestion of increased amounts of fluid; dysfunctional voiding (inattention/too busy to void)
     b. Secondary
        (1) Diseases—UTI, diabetes, genitourinary (GU) abnormalities
        (2) Medications—e.g., theophylline, diuretics
        (3) Family disruptions, stress
  2. Primary enuresis most common form in children—75% to 80%
  3. Older than 12 years—50% have secondary enuresis
  4. Familial predisposition
     a. One parent—44% increased risk
     b. Both parents—77% increased risk
- Signs and Symptoms
  1. Bedwetting or daytime urine leakage
  2. Odor of urine on clothing and/or bedding
  3. May have withdrawal/isolation from peers, diminished self-esteem

- Differential Diagnosis
  1. UTI
  2. GU anomalies—ectopic ureter
  3. Mechanical obstruction
  4. Dysfunctional voiding
  5. Dysfunctional elimination syndrome—constipation
- Physical Findings: Genitalia
  1. Hypospadias, epispadias
  2. Labial fusion
  3. Dribbling of urine during examination
- Diagnostic Tests/Findings
  1. Urinalysis/urine culture—to rule out UTI or hypercalciuria
  2. Renal ultrasound/vesicoureterogram—with abnormal urine studies; GU anomaly on examination
- Management/Treatment
  1. Primary nocturnal
     a. Limit fluid intake after dinner
     b. Double voiding before bedtime
     c. Avoid punishment/criticism
     d. Usually self-limited; spontaneous resolution of 10% per year after 5 years of age
  2. Motivational therapy
     a. May be unsuccessful as exclusive treatment
     b. Verbal praise for dryness
     c. Reward system
     d. Dryness calendar
  3. Conditioning therapy—enuresis alarm
     a. Triggered by urine
     b. Children awakened by alarm
     c. Alarm sensitizes child to sensation of full bladder
     d. Restrictions
        (1) Expensive ($50–$150)—not covered by all insurance plans
        (2) Treatment takes 2 to 3 months, often up to 6 months for greater success rate; relapse rate is high following discontinuation
        (3) May awaken other family members
        (4) Child's age, motivation, cooperation, family support important success factors
     e. Pharmacologic treatment
        (1) Desmopressin acetate
           (a) Synthetic analog of antidiuretic hormone/vasopressin
           (b) Dose—oral tablet (0.2 mg to 0.6 mg, 1 hour before bedtime)
           (c) Rapid response—1 to 2 weeks once initiated
           (d) Increase or decrease according to response—dose is not weight based
           (e) Relapse 90% once discontinued if ADH production has not increased with child's maturation
           (f) Side effects—headache, congestion, nasal irritation, epistaxis

(2) Imipramine (use is controversial due to the potentially serious, dose-related adverse effects, including depression, seizures, cardiac arrhythmias. An electrocardiogram [ECG] is recommended before beginning therapy)

    (a) Tricyclic antidepressant; unclear mechanism of action; may depress bladder contractions

    (b) Used in children older than 6 years

    (c) Dose—0.9 to 1.5 mg/kg/day, 1 to 2 hours before bedtime (dose not to exceed 25–50 mg per day)

    (d) Results seen within a few weeks

    (e) Treat 3 to 6 months, then taper

    (f) Relapse after treatment—75% to 90%

    (g) Side effects—cardiotoxicity, arrhythmias, sedation, dry mouth

4. Secondary enuresis

  a. Evaluation of underlying etiology—disease process, medication, aggressive/interdisciplinary treatment of dysfunctional voiding/DES

  b. Therapeutic intervention for individual/family stress

❐ CRYPTORCHIDISM (UNDESCENDED TESTES)

- Definition: Absence of one or both testes in scrotal sac due to failure of normal descent from abdomen during fetal development
- Etiology/Incidence
  1. Normal fetal descent of testes
     a. Hormonal mediation of normal testicular descent
        (1) Abdominal descent to inguinal ring—12 to 14 weeks gestation
        (2) Inguinal descent into scrotum—28 to 36 weeks
     b. Increased incidence among premature infants secondary to gestational development
  2. Failure of normal descent associated with hormonal imbalance, chromosomal abnormalities, structural disorders
  3. May be unilateral (usually right-sided) or bilateral
  4. Incidence
     a. Common (20% to 30%) among premature male births with birth weight <1500 g
     b. Lower incidence (3% to 5%) among full-term male infants
     c. Incidence decreases to approximately 1% by 1 year due to spontaneous descent in approximately 75% of full-term and up to 95% of preterm cases
- Signs and Symptoms
  1. May be asymptomatic
  2. Family history of undescended testes
  3. Testes may be palpable or nonpalpable
- Differential Diagnosis
  1. Retractile testes
  2. Ectopic testes

3. Anorchia
4. Chromosomal disorders
- Physical Findings
  1. Palpable testes—may be retractile or ectopic
  2. Nonpalpable testes—may be abdominal or absent
  3. Presence or absence of testes should always be documented
- Diagnostic Tests/Findings
  1. Unilateral—usually none
  2. Bilateral nonpalpable testes
     a. Karyotyping for chromosomal abnormalities
     b. Follicle-stimulating and luteinizing hormones may suggest anorchia
     c. Imaging studies occasionally utilized
- Management/Treatment
  1. Routine assessment at each well-child visit during first year of life; most spontaneous descents occur by 6 months
  2. Refer to urologist if undescended by 1 year
     a. Hormonal therapy—human chorionic gonadotropin (hCG); gonadotropin-releasing hormone (GnRH) currently used in Europe, but not yet approved for use in United States (response rates = hCG 19%, GnRH 21%, compared to 4% in placebo)
     b. Surgical intervention—orchiopexy usually recommended when child is between 12 and 18 months
  3. Family education and support regarding potential complications
     a. Infertility—greater risk in bilateral cryptorchidism
     b. Testicular malignancy—up to 40 times increased risk
     c. Hernia

❐ HYDROCELE

- Definition: Painless scrotal swelling due to collection of peritoneal fluid within the tunica vaginalis surrounding the scrotum
  1. Noncommunicating type—tunica vaginalis is closed, limiting fluid collection to scrotum; size of hydrocele is constant
  2. Communicating type—tunica vaginalis remains open, allowing fluid to flow between peritoneum and hydrocele sac; often associated with hernia
- Etiology/Incidence
  1. Incomplete closure of processus vaginalis, which usually isolates tunica vaginalis from peritoneum
  2. Most common cause of painless scrotal swelling; uncertain incidence
- Signs and Symptoms
  1. Swelling in scrotum—alternating or fixed
     a. Usually asymptomatic
     b. May become painful if full or tense, secondary to coughing or straining
     c. Variable size with child's state; larger when active/distressed, decreases with rest
     d. Smaller on awakening—enlarges as day progresses

- Differential Diagnosis
  1. Cryptorchidism
  2. Retractile testes
  3. Hernia
  4. Inguinal lymphadenopathy
  5. Patent processus vaginalis
- Physical Findings
  1. Scrotal swelling or asymmetry—tense appearance; scrotal skin normal, nontender
  2. Fluctuance
  3. Translucent with transillumination
- Diagnostic Tests/Findings: Abdominal ultrasound to differentiate hydrocele from hernia
- Management/Treatment
  1. Noncommunicating
     a. Most resolve spontaneously without intervention
     b. Refer for evaluation
        (1) Persists beyond 1 year
        (2) Significant increase in size
        (3) Causes discomfort
  2. Communicating
     a. Occasional spontaneous resolution
     b. Frequently develops into hernia requiring surgical intervention
     c. Refer for surgical evaluation if persists beyond 1 year

HYPOSPADIAS

- Definition: Congenital defect with urethral meatus on ventral surface of penis
- Etiology/Incidence
  1. Urethral folds along midline fail to fuse
  2. Common disorder—1 in 250 male births
  3. Occurs more frequently in Caucasians
  4. Both genetic and environmental factors have been implicated; a positive family history increases risk to 1 in 100 to 1 in 80 births
  5. Increasing incidence in Western cultures over the past 15 years
- Signs and Symptoms: Deflected urinary stream
- Differential Diagnosis: Ambiguous genitalia; female masculinization
- Physical Findings
  1. Ectopic opening of the urethral meatus
     a. Anterior—glans, corona, anterior shaft
     b. Midshaft
     c. Posterior—scrotal, penoscrotal junction, posterior shaft
  2. Inguinal hernia, undescended testes, incomplete foreskin
  3. Chordee—ventral curvature of penis due to fibrous band of tissue
- Diagnostic Tests/Findings
  1. Radiography if meatus in perineum (severe)
  2. Karyotype for chromosomal analysis

- Management/Treatment
  1. Avoid circumcision—foreskin used for repair
  2. Refer to pediatric urology for evaluation and planning
  3. Mild cases—primarily cosmetic surgery
  4. Increasing severity—functional, psychological, and cosmetic surgery
     a. Repair early—6 to 18 months
     b. Family preparation for procedure and expected results

PHIMOSIS AND PARAPHIMOSIS

- Definition
  1. Phimosis—narrow, nonretractile foreskin of childhood; not fully retractable to expose glans
     a. Newborns normally have adhesions, glans to foreskin
     b. May not be fully retractable until 10 years of age or older
  2. Paraphimosis—inability to replace foreskin over glans after retraction
- Etiology/Incidence
  1. Primary phimosis physiologically normal
  2. Secondary phimosis due to a scarring process such as balantis xerotica obliterans
  3. Phimosis may be due to congenital narrowing/tightness
  4. Phimosis may be due to inflammation/infection under foreskin
  5. Paraphimosis may be due to forcible retraction of foreskin for "cleaning" purposes
- Signs and Symptoms
  1. May be asymptomatic
  2. Painful urination
  3. Weak urine stream
  4. Pain/tenderness with paraphimosis
  5. Ballooning of foreskin when urinating; may be normal if voiding uncompromised
- Differential Diagnosis
  1. Balanitis (inflammation of glans penis)
  2. Balanoposthitis (inflammation of glans penis and prepuce)
- Physical Findings
  1. Phimosis—unretractable foreskin
  2. Paraphimosis—edema/discoloration of foreskin and glans
- Diagnostic Tests/Findings—none indicated
- Management/Treatment
  1. Maintain good hygiene
  2. Gentle stretch of foreskin during bath—advise family against forceful retraction; scarring and balanitis may occur
  3. Paraphimosis—goal is reduction of swelling to reduce foreskin; may be accomplished with ice, application of granulated sugar to the penis, or wrapping distal penis in saline-soaked gauze and applying pressure

for 5 to 10 minutes; will occasionally inject hyaluronidase beneath the band to release it; rarely a surgical emergency

4. Surgery—circumcision in phimosis with urinary obstruction

MEATAL STENOSIS

- Definition: Narrowing of distal end of urethra
- Etiology/Incidence
  1. Postcircumcision—11%
     a. Mechanical irritation by diaper
     b. Ischemia from frenular artery damage during procedure
     c. Inflammation secondary to dermatitis
  2. Almost never seen in uncircumcised males
- Signs and Symptoms
  1. Penile pain/discomfort with urination
  2. Narrow, dorsally diverted urine stream
  3. High-velocity urine stream
  4. Occasional bleeding following void
- Differential Diagnosis
  1. Hypospadias
  2. Chordee
- Physical Findings
  1. Inflammation of glans
  2. Slit-like or narrowed meatus—best to observe urination; appearance alone may be misleading
- Diagnostic Tests/Findings: None
- Management/Treatment
  1. Air exposure
  2. Warm soaks/baths
  3. Frequent diaper changes
  4. Meatotomy may be necessary in some cases
  5. Prevention
     a. Care exercised at circumcision to avoid damage to frenular artery
     b. Cover glans following procedure—petrolatum gauze commonly used
     c. Observe for early sign of irritation/inflammation

TESTICULAR TORSION

- Definition: Torsion of the spermatic cord; can result in gangrene of testes (emergency)
- Etiology/Incidence
  1. Abnormal fixation of testis to scrotum—permits testis to twist/rotate; impedes lymphatic and blood flow
  2. Not unusual to awaken with pain, but can also develop after scrotal trauma or increased activity
  3. Most common in adolescent males
- Signs and Symptoms
  1. Acute, painful swelling of scrotum
  2. Nausea, anorexia, vomiting
  3. Minimal fever, if any
  4. Lack of urinary symptoms is the norm

- Differential Diagnosis
  1. Trauma
  2. Orchitis
  3. Acute epididymitis
  4. Hydrocele
- Physical Findings
  1. Enlarged, highly tender testis
  2. Scrotum on involved side edematous, warm, erythematous
  3. Anxious patient, resistant to movement
  4. Lifting testis does not relieve pain (Prehn's sign)
  5. Solid mass may be visualized with transillumination
- Diagnostic Tests/Findings
  1. Complete blood count (CBC)—may see slight increase in white blood count
  2. Doppler ultrasound—reveals diminished blood flow
  3. Urinalysis (U/A)—often normal, but leukocytosis may develop rapidly
- Management/Treatment: Immediate referral for surgery
  1. Emergently performed within first 6 hours—preservation of fertility great concern; prevention of atrophy and abscess
  2. Untreated torsion can lead to testicular loss

LABIAL ADHESIONS (LABIAL FUSION, SYNECHIA VULVAE, LABIAL AGGLUTINATION)

- Definition: Generally benign fusion of labial minora
- Etiology/Incidence
  1. Thought to result from tissue irritation/inflammation and hypoestrogenization of labia minora
  2. Potential sources of irritation—trauma, superficial infection, poor hygiene (damp skin), sexual abuse
  3. Incidence—rarely present at birth (newborns are spared due to maternal estrogen); usually occurs after 2 months of age
     a. Estimated incidence is 2% of all girls in first year
     b. Highest incidence between 3 months and 6 years of age, but may occur any time up to menarche
- Signs and Symptoms
  1. Generally asymptomatic
  2. Parental concern regarding potential anatomic abnormality
  3. Difficulty voiding, general discomfort
  4. Enuresis—primarily diurnal
     a. Pooling of urine behind adhesion after voiding may occur depending upon degree of meatal obstruction
     b. Results in dribbling of urine throughout the day
- Differential Diagnosis
  1. Intersex anomalies
  2. Imperforate hymen
  3. Genital scarring
- Physical Findings: Thin, flat membrane of variable length found midline extending from clitoris to posterior fourchette when labia majora are gently separated

1. Complete fusion—entire vestibule covered; may see pinpoint opening
2. Partial fusion—much of genital structures visible
- Diagnostic Tests: None indicated
- Management/Treatment
1. In most cases, parental reassurance and observation for resolution without intervention
2. Previous practice of mechanical lysis no longer recommended due to high frequency of re-fusion
3. Observation for UTI symptoms and recurrent UTIs
4. Topical application of conjugated estrogen cream; applied sparingly twice a day for 2 to 3 weeks results in separation within 8 weeks in 90% of cases
   a. Overuse may stimulate signs of precocious puberty, such as breast buds, which resolve when cream is discontinued. Careful not to tear tissue.
   b. Transient hyperpigmentation of labia may occur during treatment
   c. Following separation
      (1) Maintain good hygiene
      (2) Topical applications of bland creams or petroleum jelly
   d. Inspection of vulva on routine well-child visits to monitor baseline anatomy, hygiene, and sexual development and to detect problems

❒ VULVOVAGINITIS

- Definition: Perineal inflammation and/or infection of the vulva (vulvitis) or vagina (vaginitis); often associated with vaginal discharge, vaginal odor, vaginal itching/irritation
- Etiology/Incidence
1. Sources of vulvovaginitis may be noninfectious or infectious
2. Noninfectious vulvovaginitis
   a. Chemical irritation—bubble bath, powder, detergents, soaps, over-the-counter (OTC) douches
   b. Mechanical irritation—tight clothing, nylon underwear
   c. Foreign body irritation—toilet tissue, retained tampon
   d. Trauma/sexual abuse
   e. Masturbation
   f. Allergy to latex condoms
3. Infectious vulvovaginitis
   a. Nonspecific—bacterial overgrowth due to poor hygiene
   b. Specific
      (1) Bacterial—Group A beta-hemolytic *Streptococcus*, pneumococcus, enterococcus, *Shigella flexneri*, *Gardnerella vaginalis*, *Mycoplasma hominis*, *Neisseria gonorrhoeae*, *Chlamydia trachomatis*
      (2) Viral—herpes simplex virus (HSV), human papillomavirus (HPV)

      (3) Parasitic—*Enterobius vermicularis* (pinworms); *Trichomonas vaginalis*
      (4) Mycotic/fungal—candidiasis (common following antibiotic use)
4. Uncertain incidence; 25% to 75% are noninfectious/nonspecific inflammation with normal flora
- Signs and Symptoms
1. Vaginal discharge
2. Genital discomfort/itching
3. Dysuria/burning
4. Erythema/edema of vulva or vagina
5. Vaginal odor
- Differential Diagnosis
1. Physiologic leukorrhea—thin, clear, or white discharge
2. UTI
3. Dermatologic disorders—psoriasis, seborrheic dermatitis, atopic dermatitis
- Physical Findings
1. May have no physical findings
2. Discharge
   a. White to yellow—chemical, mechanical, *Chlamydia trachomatis*
   b. Pale yellow to gray green—trichomoniasis
   c. White, thick, cheesy—candidiasis ("yeast")
   d. Thin, white, frothy—bacterial vaginosis
   e. Brown, bloody, foul odor—foreign body
3. Genital erythema
4. Lesions
5. Perianal soiling
6. Examination techniques—sensitive, gentle
   a. Prepubertal female
      (1) Pelvic examination usually deferred; visual inspection only
      (2) Exploratory procedure under anesthesia may be needed for vaginal bleeding and should be referred
   b. Pubescent female
      (1) Visual inspection of external genitalia, pelvic examination if symptoms of abdominal pain
      (2) Vaginal swab for gonorrhea (GC), *Chlamydia*, *Trichomonas*
      (3) Wet mount and potassium hydroxide (KOH) testing may be performed with vaginal pool secretions
- Diagnostic Tests/Findings
1. Urinalysis for presence of white blood cells (WBCs), trichomonads
2. Tape test for pinworms
3. Saline preparation for wet mount
   a. Clue cells—bacterial vaginosis
   b. Presence of WBCs—may indicate vaginitis or cervicitis
   c. Trichomonads
4. Potassium hydroxide (KOH) 10% preparation
   a. Hyphae—candidiasis
   b. "Whiff test"—positive (fishy odor of bacterial vaginosis)

5. pH testing of vaginal secretions
   a. pH of <4.5—normal or candidiasis
   b. pH of >4.5—bacterial vaginosis, *Trichomonas*
- Management/Treatment (see section on sexually transmitted diseases for specific management)
  1. Foundation of treating childhood vulvovaginitis is improvement of local perineal hygiene
  2. Nonspecific vaginitis often resolves without intervention
  3. Discontinue genital irritants—bubble bath, harsh bath soap and laundry detergents
  4. Cotton or cotton-lined underwear—avoid tight-fitting clothing (tights, pants, undergarments)
  5. Bacterial vaginosis
     a. Metronidazole—1 g/day orally in two divided doses for 7 days (adolescents/adults) and 15 mg/kg per day (children <45 kg) with maximum dose of 1 g/day; OR metronidazole gel, 0.75%, 5 g (1 applicator) intravaginally daily for 5 days (adolescents) or 15 mg/kg per day
     b. Clindamycin cream 2%, 5 g (1 applicator) intravaginally at night for 7 days
     c. Alternative treatments are less effective
     d. Pregnant women should be treated for bacterial vaginitis
  6. Parasitic
     a. Pinworms—mebendazole, pyrantel pamoate, or albendazole in single dose repeated in 2 weeks. Treat household members and wash linens, bedding, clothing
     b. *Trichomonas* vaginalis—metronidazole 15 mg/kg per day orally in three divided doses for 7 days (<45 kg) with maximum of 1 g/day; OR 2 g orally in single dose or 1 g/day in two divided doses for 7 days (>45 kg); partner must be treated
  7. Fungal—candidiasis
     a. Oral agent—fluconazole 150 mg single dose
     b. Various topical agents include clotrimazole, miconazole, butoconazole nitrate, terconazole, which are more effective than nystatin
  8. Foreign body
     a. Prepubertal—attempt irrigation; warm saline via small feeding tube
     b. Postpubertal
        (1) Pelvic examination to locate object
        (2) Moistened cotton-tip applicator or forceps for removal
     c. Unsuccessful irrigation/pelvic or anxious child—refer for examination under general anesthesia
  9. Positive cultures suspicious for sexual abuse or sexual activity—see section on sexually transmitted diseases
  10. Physiologic leukorrhea
      a. Educate about normal pubertal changes
      b. Some benefit from "mini-pads" in underwear to absorb moisture/prevent wetness from staining clothing
      c. Avoid use of douches and creams
  11. Nonlatex condoms for suspected latex allergy

❑ DYSMENORRHEA

- Definition: Pain during menstrual cycle; usually first 1 to 2 days; cramping discomfort felt mid-to-lower abdomen
  1. Primary dysmenorrhea—no pelvic abnormality, common in adolescents, usually develops 6 to 12 months after menarche, ovulation is necessary component
  2. Secondary dysmenorrhea—underlying pelvic pathology
     a. Congenital anomalies (septate uterus)
     b. Cervical stenosis or strictures
     c. Cysts, tumors of ovary or uterus
     d. Endometriosis
     e. Pelvic inflammatory disease
- Etiology/Incidence (Primary Dysmenorrhea)
  1. Increased production of uterine prostaglandins; uterine contractions, ischemia
  2. Ovulation is required for development of primary dysmenorrhea
  3. Most common gynecological complaint
  4. 20% to 90% of adolescent women report dysmenorrhea
     a. Significant limitation for 10% to 15% of females
     b. School absenteeism—14% of those reporting dysmenorrhea frequently missed school
- Signs and Symptoms
  1. Pain usually starts with flow or several hours later, or may precede flow by several hours to 2 days
  2. Crampy/spasmodic pain, primarily lower abdominal area; may radiate to inner thighs, lower back
  3. Systemic symptoms
     a. Nausea/vomiting/diarrhea
     b. Lightheadedness/dizziness
     c. Fatigue or general malaise
- Differential Diagnosis
  1. Reproductive system malformations
  2. Endometriosis
  3. Pelvic inflammatory disease (PID)
  4. Psychogenic problems
- Physical Findings: May be none; defer pelvic examination only if adolescent is not sexually active
  1. Bimanual and rectovaginal exams indicated
  2. Cervical motion tenderness with PID
- Diagnostic Tests/Findings
  1. Suspicion of PID—see section on sexually transmitted diseases
  2. Pelvic ultrasound for palpable masses or concern of GU abnormalities
- Management/Treatment
  1. Primary dysmenorrhea—mild
     a. Heat to abdomen
     b. Exercise
     c. Acetaminophen
     d. Ibuprofen—400 mg orally immediately at onset of pain, then every 6–8 hours for 1 to 3 days; take with food, milk, antacid to avoid GI distress. Titrate to max dose 800 mg TID
     e. Well-balanced diet
     f. Acknowledgment of symptoms; the pain is real

2. Primary dysmenorrhea—moderate to severe; unresponsive to treatment for mild disorder
   a. Nonsteroidal anti-inflammatory drugs (NSAIDs)
      (1) Inhibit prostaglandin synthesis
      (2) Naproxen sodium—500 mg orally at onset, then 250 mg every 6 to 8 hours
      (3) Mefenamic acid—500 mg orally at onset, then 250 mg every 6 to 8 hours
      (4) Assess efficacy of NSAIDs after three to four cycles before using another medication
      (5) NSAIDs contraindicated in clotting disorders, renal or peptic ulcer disease, pre-op patients, NSAID or aspirin allergy, aspirin-induced asthma
3. Severe dysmenorrhea—unresponsive to NSAIDs alone
   a. Low-dose combination oral contraceptives (OCPs); effective in 90% of cases with severe pain
   b. Minimum three to four cycles for symptom improvement
   c. Continuous symptoms after 4 months
      (1) OCPs can be used in conjunction with NSAIDs
      (2) Consider gynecological referral
4. Secondary dysmenorrhea
   a. Begin PID treatment immediately, if indicated
   b. Gynecological referral if persistent dysmenorrhea after PID treatment or if pelvic pathology exists

☐ PREMENSTRUAL SYNDROME

- Definition: Cluster of symptoms, physical, cognitive, and behavioral, that occur in second half of menstrual cycle (last week of luteal phase); usually resolve with onset of menses; symptoms exist over several cycles and cause disruption of normal activities.
- Etiology/Incidence
  1. Numerous mechanisms postulated
     a. Vitamin deficiencies, inconsistent evidence
     b. Fluid retention
     c. Steroid hormone fluctuation
     d. Alteration in serotoninergic neuronal mechanisms
     e. Inappropriate prostaglandin activity
  2. Studies note 14% to 61% adolescent women reporting at least one symptom
- Signs and Symptoms
  1. Onset of symptoms usually within 1 week of menses
     a. Breast tenderness
     b. Headache, muscle aches
     c. Weight gain, bloating
     d. Mood swings, lethargy, anxiety, irritability, depression
     e. Fatigue
     f. Appetite changes
     g. Lower back pain
     h. Loss of concentration
     i. Acne
     j. Constipation
     k. Hot flashes, chills

- Differential Diagnosis
  1. Pregnancy
  2. Primary/secondary dysmenorrhea
  3. Premenstrual dysphoric disorder (PMDD), *Diagnostic and Statistical Manual of Mental Disorders*, 4th Edition (*DSM-IV*) diagnosis for severe form of premenstrual syndrome (PMS); requires mental health referral
- Physical Findings: Pelvic examination normal
- Diagnostic Tests/Findings: None indicated
- Management/Treatment
  1. Diet/nutrition
     a. Frequent small meals
     b. Increase intake—complex carbohydrates, protein, fresh fruits, vegetables, foods rich in pyridoxine (vitamin B_6)
     c. Vitamin/mineral supplement—vitamin B_6, magnesium
     d. Limit intake—refined sugar, salt, red meat, alcohol, coffee, tea, chocolate
  2. Lifestyle
     a. Regular exercise (especially aerobic)
     b. Stress management
     c. Address psychosocial issues
     d. Chart symptoms for two to three cycles to clarify/treat symptoms
     e. Avoid alcohol
     f. Sleep 9 hours per day
  3. Pharmacological management
     a. Diuretics
     b. NSAIDs
     c. Selective serotonin reuptake inhibitors (SSRIs), e.g., fluoxetine, sertraline, paroxetine—for adult women with diagnosis of PMDD
     d. Oral contraceptive pills may reduce symptoms for some women; some women feel worse; a 24/4 formulation may improve symptoms more than a 21/7 formulation; OCPs may improve physical symptoms more than mental/emotional symptoms; close follow-up indicated

☐ GENITOURINARY TRAUMA

- Definition: Injury to the genitourinary tract; refers to accidental injury (for nonaccidental trauma, refer to section on sexual abuse)
- Etiology/Incidence
  1. Blunt insult generally from athletic activities, motor vehicle accidents, falls
  2. No specific incidence—commonly seen; over 50% associated with trauma to intraperitoneal organs
- Signs and Symptoms
  1. Frank urethral bleeding
  2. Hematuria
  3. Bluish-red mass in perineal area
- Differential Diagnosis
  1. Hemorrhagic cystitis
  2. Vaginitis
  3. Sexual abuse

- Physical Findings
  1. Hematomas—urethral/scrotal/perineal
  2. Periurethral lacerations
- Diagnostic Tests/Findings: Referral necessary if extensive injury suspected; radiographic evaluation of urinary tract is the cornerstone of treatment; usually done once referral to specialist has been made
- Management/Treatment
  1. Urethral/vulvar trauma
     a. Mild bruising, superficial lacerations (symptomatic relief)—ice pack, sitz baths, analgesics
     b. Blunt or penetrating trauma—surgical intervention
  2. Testicular trauma—surgical referral
  3. Suspected renal injury—referral
  4. Penetrating injury—immediate surgical exploration

☐ GLOMERULONEPHRITIS (GN)

- Definition: Disease characterized by diffuse inflammatory changes in the glomeruli; immune-mediated response
  1. Primary acute form—poststreptococcal glomerulonephritis; most common form in children; true incidence unknown
  2. Primary chronic form
     a. Primarily seen with IgA nephropathy
     b. Other types—membranoproliferative glomerulonephritis (MPGN), mesangial proliferative glomerulonephritis
  3. Secondary forms—associated with other disorders, e.g., systemic lupus erythematosus, anaphylactoid purpura, vascular problems
- Etiology/Incidence
  1. Multifactorial etiology—not completely understood
  2. Combination of factors induce injury
     a. Immune complex deposits in glomerular basement membrane
     b. Coagulation factors—fibrin deposits
     c. Exogenous nephrotoxins
        (1) Penicillamine, trimethadione, captopril, probenecid
        (2) Heavy metals—gold, mercury
  3. Uncertain incidence
- Signs and Symptoms
  1. Acute disease
     a. Hematuria
     b. Decreased urine output
     c. Edema
     d. Dark urine—acute poststreptococcal glomerulonephritis (APSGN)
  2. Chronic disease
     a. Fatigue
     b. Failure to thrive
- Differential Diagnosis
  1. Benign hematuria
  2. Hereditary nephropathy
  3. Systemic lupus erythematosus

  4. Anaphylactoid purpura
  5. IgA nephropathy—most common GN leading to chronic renal failure worldwide
  6. Henoch-Schönlein purpura (HSP)
- Physical Findings
  1. May be asymptomatic or severely ill depending upon extent of renal involvement
  2. Gross hematuria
  3. Edema—facial (especially periorbital) in the morning
  4. Hypertension—with or without renal insufficiency
  5. Costovertebral angle (CVA) tenderness
- Diagnostic Tests/Findings
  1. Urinalysis
     a. Casts—red blood cells (RBCs), leukocytes, and/or casts indicate glomerular inflammation
     b. Hematuria
     c. Protein—correlates with degree of hematuria
     d. pH—low
     e. Specific gravity—increased
  2. Titers—serum ASO, AHT, anti-DNase B
  3. Cultures—throat, skin; may be negative by the time signs of nephritis appear
  4. Chest radiograph—assess pulmonary edema
  5. Serum complement
     a. Returns to normal in APSGN
     b. Chronic elevation in MPGN
- Management/Treatment
  1. All treatment is supportive
     a. Hypertension/relieve edema
        (1) Fluid restriction
        (2) Diuretics
        (3) Vasodilators
     b. Antibiotic (penicillin) if throat or skin infection persists

☐ HYDRONEPHROSIS

- Definition: Unilateral or bilateral dilation of kidney(s)
- Etiology/Incidence
  1. Caused by anatomic block of urine flow from kidney
  2. Obstruction in 1 per 1000 births—slight male prevalence
  3. Ureteropelvic junction (UPJ)—most common site of obstruction
- Signs and Symptoms
  1. Nausea
  2. Abdominal or flank pain
  3. Decreased urine output
- Differential Diagnosis
  1. Prune belly syndrome
  2. UPJ obstruction
  3. Ectopic ureterocele
  4. Urethral/ureterovesical obstructions
  5. Vesicoureteral reflux
  6. Posterior urethral valves
- Physical Findings
  1. Pain—abdominal/flank

2. Failure to thrive
3. May be asymptomatic in older children
- Diagnostic Tests/Findings
  1. May be detected during prenatal ultrasound
  2. IVP—late emptying of renal pelvis
  3. Renal scan—reveals impact of obstruction on total renal function
- Management/Treatment
  1. Surgery to relieve obstruction
  2. Obstruction will lead to destruction of renal parenchyma; early exploration and repair advocated
  3. Must follow up long term for continued assessment of renal function

□ RENAL TUBULAR ACIDOSIS (RTA)

- Definition: Defect in normal urine acidification with resulting persistent metabolic acidosis; primary RTA includes two types
  1. Type 1 (distal tube)—defect in distal tube secretion of hydrogen ions
  2. Type 2 (proximal tube)—defect in reabsorption of bicarbonate
- Etiology/Incidence
  1. Cellular basis of defect is unknown; distal RTA may have genetic transmission as autosomal dominant disorder
  2. Incidence of primary RTA is unknown
- Signs and Symptoms
  1. Growth failure
  2. Gastrointestinal complaints
  3. Muscle weakness
- Differential Diagnosis
  1. Diarrhea
  2. Diabetes mellitus
  3. Renal failure
  4. Lactic acidosis
- Physical Findings: Growth failure
- Diagnostic Tests/Findings
  1. Urine pH—first morning specimen; pH less than 5.5 supports diagnosis of proximal RTA; 5.8 or greater indicates distal RTA
  2. Serum electrolytes—serum bicarbonate less than 16 mEq; hyperkalemia
  3. Various low-molecular-weight proteins are used as markers
- Management/Treatment: Goals: Achieve optimal growth and bone mineralization and prevent nephrocalcinosis and progression to renal failure
  1. Correction of acidosis; balance serum bicarbonate to normal level
     a. Intravenous therapy for infants with severe hyperkalemia/acidosis
     b. Oral therapy for most children
  2. Alkali administration as sodium bicarbonate or sodium citrate
     a. Potassium supplement if needed
     b. Sodium bicarbonate tablets—325 mg and 650 mg

3. Mineralocorticoid deficiency corrected; diuretics reduce serum potassium
4. Carnitine supplements if needed
5. Risk of nephrocalcinosis, renal failure—continuous alkali therapy and long-term clinical monitoring
6. Normal growth resumes with corrected acidosis

□ SEXUALLY TRANSMITTED INFECTIONS

Gonorrhea

- Definition: Acute infectious process primarily involving genital tract, anorectum, throat, and ophthalmic epithelium
- Etiology/Incidence
  1. *Neisseria gonorrhoeae*—Gram-negative diplococcus
  2. Reportable disease in all states; estimated 321,849 new cases in 2011 in the United States, per the Centers for Disease Control and Prevention (CDC)
  3. Women younger than 25 years of age are at the highest risk for gonorrhea infection
  4. Other risk factors include previous gonorrhea infection, other sexually transmitted infections, new or multiple sex partners, inconsistent condom use, commercial sex work, and drug use
  5. Associated with sexual abuse in children beyond newborn period and nonsexually active adolescents
  6. Persons at risk for extragenital infection should be screened at extragenital sites
- Signs and Symptoms
  1. Varies by site and gender; asymptomatic in 10% to 40% males and 50% to 80% females
  2. Vaginal or penile creamy discharge
  3. Perineal discomfort
  4. Menstrual irregularities
  5. Frequent, urgent, painful urination
  6. Rectal pain/itching
  7. Sore throat
  8. Fever, malaise, chills
- Differential Diagnosis
  1. *Chlamydia trachomatis* infection (may be concurrent)
  2. Genital mycoplasmas (may be concurrent)
  3. Bacterial vaginosis (may be concurrent)
  4. Trichomoniasis (may be concurrent)
  5. Complications include pelvic inflammatory disease, epididymitis, disseminated infection
- Physical Findings: Exam may be normal or include the following:
  1. External genitalia
     a. Erythema, edema
     b. Thick, purulent, greenish-yellow discharge (penile or vaginal)
  2. Female—pelvic examination
     a. Cervical erythema, friability, exudate
     b. Vaginal wall discharge/erythema
     c. Cervical/adnexal tenderness

3. Male
   a. Thick, creamy penile discharge
   b. Enlarged, tender prostate
   c. Scrotal or groin pain (unilateral)
   d. Tender swelling above testis
4. Disseminated gonococcal infection (DGI): bacteremic spread of *N. gonorrhoeae*
   a. Typically present with one or both of two syndromes: polyarthralgias, tenosynovitis, dermatitis triad, and purulent arthritis
   b. Acute stage of tenosynovitis illness includes fever, chills, general malaise, fever, which diminish as illness progresses. Those with purulent arthritis (usually knees, wrists, ankles) present without systemic symptoms
   c. Diagnosis based on history, physical, and laboratory studies
   d. Risk factors include recent menstruation, pregnancy, or immediate postpartum; congenital or acquired complement deficiencies; systemic lupus erythematosus (SLE)
   e. Treatment includes IV antibiotics. Purulent arthritis requires joint drainage
   f. Nucleic acid amplification test (NAAT) testing for genital sites, pharynx, rectal, synovial fluid, skin lesions
- Diagnostic Tests/Findings
  1. Nucleic acid amplification tests (NAATs)
     a. Best sensitivity and specificity of any other test to detect gonorrhea (CDC)
     b. Preferred sites are vaginal swab for women and first-part void for men
     c. Culture is needed in cases of child sexual assault of boys and rectal and pharyngeal infection in prepubescent girls
     d. Culture is needed in cases of treatment failure to assess susceptibility and to monitor drug resistance
  2. Screening recommendations include annual for sexually active persons; more frequent screening for pregnant women and those at risk due to new, anonymous, and/or multiple partners, and those in communities with high burden of disease
  3. No useful serologic test available to distinguish current from past infection
  4. Evaluate for possible concurrent syphilis, hepatitis B, HIV, and *Chlamydia trachomatis*
- Management/Treatment (see AAP *Red Book* for most current treatment guidelines)
  1. Uncomplicated infections
     a. Children <8 years weighing <45 kg
        (1) Ceftriaxone sodium, 125 mg, IM in single dose (drug of choice)
        (2) Concomitant treatment for possible *Chlamydia trachomatis*; azithromycin, 20 mg/kg (maximum 1 g) orally in single dose; OR erythromycin, 50 mg/kg per day (maximum 2 g/day) orally in four doses for 14 days

     b. Children/adolescents weighing >45 kg and older than 8 years
        (1) Ceftriaxone, 125 mg, IM in single dose (drug of choice); OR cefixime 400 mg oral, single dose
        (2) Fluoroquinolones not recommended due to growing resistance
        (3) Concomitant treatment for possible *Chlamydia trachomatis*—azithromycin, 1 g orally in single dose OR doxycycline, 100 mg orally bid for 7 days
  2. Complicated (disseminated) infections
     a. Children <8 years weighing <45 kg
        (1) Ceftriaxone, 50 mg/kg/day (maximum 1 g/day) in single dose (IV or IM) for 7 days
        (2) Concomitant treatment for possible *Chlamydia trachomatis* with azithromycin or erythromycin
     b. Children/adolescents >8 years weighing >45 kg
        (1) Ceftriaxone, 1 g (IV or IM) in single dose for 7 days OR cefotaxime, 1 g (IV) every 8 hours for 7 days
        (2) IV administration may change to oral antimicrobial agent such as ciprofloxacin (500 mg bid for 7 days) after 1 to 2 days of initial improvement
        (3) Concomitant treatment for *Chlamydia trachomatis* with azithromycin, 1 g orally in single dose OR doxycycline, 100 mg, orally bid for 7 days
  3. Prophylaxis after sexual victimization
     a. Antimicrobial prophylaxis no longer recommended for abused prepubertal victims
     b. Prophylaxis for postpubertal females seen within 72 hours of sexual victimization
        (1) Ceftriaxone, 125 mg IM in single dose
        (2) Concomitant treatment for possible *Chlamydia trachomatis* with:
            (a) Azithromycin, 20 mg/kg (maximum of 1 g) orally in single dose for patients weighing <45 kg
            (b) Azithromycin, 1 g orally in single dose for patients >45 kg
  4. Prevention strategies
     a. Risk reduction education
     b. Condom use
     c. Routine screening for sexually active adolescents

Chlamydia

- Definition: Most common reported sexually transmitted infection in United States, with primary sites of infection being genital tract, cornea, and respiratory system
- Etiology/Incidence
  1. *Chlamydia trachomatis*; obligate intracellular bacteria; at least 18 variants
  2. Reportable disease in most states; 1,412,791 new cases in the United States in 2011, per CDC

3. Prevalence is consistently highest among adolescent females
4. Complications include endometritis, salpingitis, perihepatitis, acute/chronic pelvic inflammatory disease (may result in ectopic pregnancy, infertility) for females; epididymitis, Reiter syndrome for males
5. Congenital chlamydia
   a. Perinatal transmission from infected mothers to infants estimated from 40% to 70%
   b. Manifestation primarily as conjunctivitis or pneumonia
6. Screening is recommended for all women younger than 25 years, pregnant women, men who have sex with men (MSM) who have anal receptive intercourse and young men in high-prevalence areas
- Signs and Symptoms: Genital tract infection
   1. Often asymptomatic for months to years
   2. Abdominal/pelvic pain
   3. Dysuria/burning
- Differential Diagnosis
   1. Gonorrhea
   2. Genital mycoplasmas
   3. Trichomoniasis
   4. Bacterial vaginosis
   5. Pelvic inflammatory disease
- Physical Findings: Genital tract infection
   1. May be normal
   2. Erythema of external genitalia
   3. Vaginal/penile discharge—yellowish, watery
   4. Tenderness on bimanual examination
- Diagnostic Tests/Findings
   1. NAATs—most sensitive screening tests for genital chlamydia infection
      a. Specimens can be vaginal or urine for asymptomatic women, urine for males, and cervical for symptomatic women
      b. CDC recommends NAATs for rectal and pharyngeal sites due to increased sensitivity and ease of use. However, Food and Drug Administration (FDA) has not cleared for use due to issues with cross reactivity and false positives. Laboratories must have performance specifications when using these tests to meet CLIA (Clinical Laboratory Improvement Amendment) regulatory requirements
      c. NAATs can also detect gonorrhea
   2. Tissue culture
      a. Culture specimen must contain epithelial cells to be accurate
      b. Necessary for suspected child abuse. Culture sent for boys and for extragenital infections in girls
      c. Processing takes 2–3 days
- Management/Treatment—see AAP *Red Book* for additional treatment guidelines
   1. Antibiotic treatment for uncomplicated genital tract infection
      a. Adolescents—doxycycline, 100 mg two times daily for 7 days OR azithromycin 1 g in single dose

   b. Alternate therapies—erythromycin base 500 mg po four times daily for 7 days, erythromycin ethylsuccinate 800 mg po four times daily for 7 days, levofloxacin 500 mg daily for 7 days, ofloxacin 300 mg two times daily for 7 days
   c. Pregnancy
      (1) Doxycycline is contraindicated in pregnancy
      (2) Treatment regimen in pregnancy
         (a) Azithromycin 1000 mg po × 1
         (b) Erythromycin base, 500 mg four times daily for 7 days; may be given in half doses for 14 days if not tolerated well
         (c) Amoxicillin 500 mg po three times daily for 7 days
   d. Children (6 months to 12 years)—erythromycin, 50 mg/kg/day four times daily for 7 days OR azithromycin 20 mg/kg in single dose (not to exceed 1 gram)
   e. Infants <6 months of age
      (1) Erythromycin, base or ethylsuccinate, 50 mg/kg/day four times daily for 14 days
      (2) Second course may be required
      (3) Association between oral erythromycin and infantile hypertrophic pyloric stenosis (IHPS) has been reported in infants <2 weeks of age; requires informing parents of potential risks and need for careful follow-up
   f. Identify, examine, test, and treat any sexual contacts
   2. Evaluate for other STDs, e.g., gonorrhea, syphilis, and treat as necessary
   3. No need for retest following treatment with doxycycline, azithromycin, unless symptoms persist or if possibility of reinfection
   4. Retest may be recommended at 3 or more weeks following treatment with erythromycin or amoxicillin
   5. Partners must be treated to avoid recurrence

Acquired Syphilis

- Definition: A contagious systemic infectious disease characterized by three progressive clinical stages
   1. Primary stage—painless chancres on skin or mucous membranes at site of exposure that may go unnoticed
   2. Secondary stage—between 1 and 2 months after inoculation, characterized by skin rash, cutaneous lesions, lymphadenopathy
   3. Latent stage—no lesions: early latent is less than 1 year, and late latent is more than 1 year in duration
   4. Tertiary stage—multisystem involvement that may occur from years after primary infection, including aortitis or gummatous changes of skin, bone, or viscera
   5. Neurosyphilis may occur at any stage of infection, particularly in HIV patients
   6. Congenital syphilis: Transplacental transmission from infected mother to fetus

- Etiology/Incidence
  1. Infectious agent—*Treponema pallidum*, a thin, motile spirochete
  2. Transmission—sexual contact, transplacental, direct contact with infected tissue
  3. Reportable communicable disease in all states; 46,042 new cases in the United States in 2011
  4. CDC (2014c) reports cases increased from all-time low of 2.1 cases per 100,000 in 2000 to 5.3 cases per 100,000 in 2011
     a. Men who have sex with men had the largest increase in cases. May be due in part to multiple or anonymous partners
     b. Importance of taking complete sexual history, finding and treating contacts
     c. HIV screening in all positive cases as MSM have increased rates of co-infection, thought to be due to genital sores, making it easier for HIV transmission
- Signs and Symptoms
  1. Primary stage—one or more painless lesions, usually on genitalia but may be on lips, tongue, or extremities. Chancres are very infectious and resolve in 1–6 weeks. Painless regional lymphadenopathy
  2. Secondary stage—fever, malaise, sore throat, skin rash, hair loss. Up to 25% of untreated persons relapse with secondary symptoms in 1 year
  3. Latent stage—no lesions. May occur between primary and secondary stages, between secondary and relapse of secondary symptoms, and after secondary stage
     a. Early latent—less than 1 year in duration
     b. Late latent—more than 1 year in duration. May be difficult to determine
  4. Tertiary stage—symptoms recur years after initial untreated infections; rarely seen among adolescents. Cardiac or gummatous lesions
  5. Neurosyphilis—may be asymptomatic and may occur at any stage; neurologic signs include fever, headache, photophobia, meningismus, cranial nerve palsies; less frequently confusion, delirium, and seizures
  6. Congenital syphilis—most infectious when untreated mother has primary or secondary syphilis. May result in stillbirth, infants with neurologic impairment and bone deformities
- Differential Diagnosis
  1. Primary syphilis
     a. Genital herpes
     b. Chancroid, granuloma inguinale, lymphogranuloma venereum
     c. Traumatic lesion, excoriation
     d. Behçet's lesion
  2. Secondary syphilis
     a. Pityriasis rosea
     b. Psoriasis
     c. Condylomata acuminata
     d. Drug-sensitivity reactions
     e. Infectious mononucleosis
     f. Lupus erythematosus
- Physical Findings
  1. Primary stage
     a. Chancre—one or more painless ulcers
     b. Most common on genitalia but seen at other sites of inoculation
  2. Secondary stage
     a. Generalized polymorphic maculopapular rash—classic if palms and soles included
     b. Round to oval, reddish-brown, "copper-colored" lesions
     c. Lymphadenopathy, arthralgia, fever, malaise, sore throat, headaches, splenomegaly
     d. Hypertrophic papular lesions of vulva/anus—condylomata lata
  3. Latency period—no lesions
  4. Tertiary phase
     a. 15 or more years after chancre
     b. Aortitis, gummous changes of bone, skin, or viscera
  5. Neurosyphilis, infection of the central nervous system
     a. May occur at any stage
     b. HIV-positive persons at higher risk
- Diagnostic Tests/Findings
  1. Dark-field microscopic tests or direct fluorescent antibody (DFA) tests—presence of spirochetes from scrapings or washings of primary lesions; inexpensive, definitive diagnosis
  2. Serologic tests—presumptive diagnosis
     a. Nontreponemal tests—rapid plasma reagin (RPR), Venereal Disease Research Laboratory (VDRL), toluidine red unheated serum test (TRUST), unheated serum reagin (USR)
        (1) Measure nonspecific antigens
        (2) False-positive rate of 1% to 2%
        (3) False negatives with recently acquired infections prior to seroconversion or latent syphilis of long duration
        (4) Serial testing, using the same test, used to monitor response to treatment
        (5) Takes time to return to nonreactive after treatment
     b. Treponemal tests—fluorescent treponemal antibody absorption (FTA-ABS) and *Treponema pallidum* particle agglutination (TP-PA)
        (1) Detect specific treponemal antigens
        (2) Greater specificity than nontreponemal methods
        (3) Usually reactive for life
        (4) More expensive and time-consuming
        (5) Useful to distinguish/confirm positive vs. false-positive nontreponemal results
        (6) May show false-positive results in presence of Lyme disease, acute infections, autoimmune disorders, and narcotic addiction
     c. High probability of infection in sexually active person with reactive nontreponemal and treponemal tests

    d. VDRL/RPR screening in early pregnancy and at delivery for all women to prevent/identify transplacental transmission
- Management/Treatment: See AAP *Red Book* for additional treatment guidelines
  1. Primary, secondary, and early latent syphilis (less than 1 year in duration) without neurologic symptoms
     a. Children—penicillin G benzathine, 50,000 U/kg IM up to adult dose of 2.4 million units in single dose
     b. Adults—penicillin G benzathine, 2.4 million units, IM in single dose
        (1) If allergic to penicillin and NOT pregnant—doxycycline, 100 mg orally twice daily for 14 days OR
        (2) Tetracycline, 500 mg orally four times daily for 14 days
  2. Late latent (more than 1 year in duration) and tertiary syphilis
     a. Children—penicillin G benzathine, 50,000 U/kg, IM up to adult dose of 2.4 million units, as three single doses administered at 1-week intervals
     b. Adults—penicillin G benzathine 7.2 million units total administered as three doses of 2.4 million units IM per dose at 1-week intervals
        (1) If allergic to penicillin and NOT pregnant—doxycycline, 100 mg orally twice daily for 4 weeks OR
        (2) Tetracycline, 500 mg orally four times daily for 4 weeks
  3. Neurosyphilis
     a. Children—aqueous crystalline penicillin G, 200,000 to 300,000 U/kg per day given every 4 to 6 hours for 10 to 14 days, not to exceed adult dose
     b. Adults—aqueous crystalline penicillin G, 18 million to 24 million units per day in doses of 3 million to 4 million units, IV every 4 hours for 10 to 14 days OR penicillin G procaine, 2.4 million units, IM once daily PLUS probencid, 500 mg, four times per day orally, both for 10 to 14 days
     c. See *Red Book* for penicillin allergic regimens
  4. Evaluation of patient and all recent sexual contacts for syphilis and other sexually transmitted infections (STIs)
  5. Prevention and control
     a. Patient education/discussion of sexuality, contraception, and STIs as part of adolescent well-child visits
     b. Counseling regarding safe sexual practices, including abstinence and proper use of condoms
     c. Treatment of sexual contacts
     d. Report each case to local health authorities for contact investigation
     e. All women should be screened early in pregnancy and at delivery
     f. Follow-up of treated cases: Primary and secondary—6 and 12 months; latent—6, 12, and 24 months; co-infections with HIV—primary and secondary, 3, 6, 9, 12, and 24 months, and latent, 6, 12, 18, and 24 months
     g. Jarisch-Herxheimer reaction is a sepsis-like reaction to an antibiotic when endotoxins are released from the death of harmful organisms. This requires medical evaluation and treatment

Genital Herpes Simplex Virus (HSV)

- Definition: Most common HSV infection among adolescents characterized by clusters of painful lesions of the genital tract, perineum, mouth, lips, or pharynx
- Etiology/Incidence
  1. Agent (herpes simplex viruses)—large DNA viruses of two major types
     a. Type 2 (HSV-2)—primary source of genital herpes, usually, but not always, affecting skin below the waist
     b. Type 1 (HSV-1)—less common source of genital herpes, usually, but not always, sites include face and skin above the waist
  2. Primary transmission through sexual contact and/or direct contact with open lesions; may be transmitted by autoinoculation of HSV-1 to genital area
  3. Transplacental transmission results in congenital herpes
  4. Genital herpes is rare in prepubertal children except in cases of child abuse
  5. Estimated prevalence of 1 in 16 Americans aged 14–49 years
  6. Symptoms can be severe and persistent in immunosuppressed persons
  7. Recent HSV infection is a risk factor for acquisition of HIV
- Signs and Symptoms
  1. Painful genital lesions
  2. Burning with urination
  3. Tender, swollen lymph nodes
  4. Fever, malaise
- Differential Diagnosis
  1. Chancre of early syphilis
  2. Chancroid
  3. Lymphogranuloma venereum, granuloma inguinale
  4. Behçet's lesion
  5. Excoriation
  6. Allergic reaction
- Physical Findings
  1. Vesicular/ulcerated lesions—genital tract, perineum, mouth, lips, pharynx
  2. Genital, perianal erythema, and/or edema
  3. Cervical friability, discharge
  4. Lymphadenopathy
  5. Primary HSV rare complications include aseptic meningitis, encephalitis, proctitis in MSM and extragenital lesions

- Diagnostic Tests/Findings
  1. Tissue culture
     a. Sensitivity varies by stage of disease—highest with vesicular lesions; lowest with recurrent infections and crusted lesions
     b. Results available within 1 to 5 days
  2. Newer diagnostic techniques
     a. PCR-DNA probe test of choice for cerebrospinal fluid (CSF) specimens—technique with good sensitivity and specificity; results available within 1 to 3 days
     b. Direct fluorescent antibody/enzyme immunoassay—more rapid results than cultures, but less sensitive results
     c. Polymerase chain reaction (PCR)—very sensitive; useful to detect shedding in clinical trials
  3. Serologic testing—may show rise in HSV antibodies; of limited value
     a. May be used to confirm initial diagnosis
     b. Often shows no rise in titers with recurrences
- Management/Treatment: See AAP *Red Book* for additional treatment guidelines
  1. Primary episode of genital infection
     a. Acyclovir, 200 mg orally, five times/day for 7 to 10 days or 400 mg three times per day for 7 to 10 days
     b. Initiation of treatment within 6 days of onset of lesions may reduce duration and severity of symptoms
     c. Valacyclovir 1 g po twice daily for 7–10 days and famciclovir 250 mg orally three times daily for 7–10 days provide alternatives for adult (pediatric formulations not yet available) treatment with advantage of less frequent dosing
  2. Recurrent episodes—alternative doses/frequency. Start as soon as lesions appear
     a. Acyclovir, 200 mg orally, five times per day for 5 days or 800 mg po twice daily for 5 days or 800 mg orally three times daily for 2 days. Famciclovir 1000 mg twice daily for 1 day or 500 mg po followed by 250 mg po twice daily for 2 days. Valacyclovir 500 mg po twice daily for 3 days or 1000 mg po daily for 5 days
     b. Acyclovir less effective in treatment of recurrent vs. primary episodes
  3. Topical acyclovir no longer recommended; limited benefit
  4. Suppressive therapy—with frequent recurrences of more than six per year
     a. Acyclovir 400 mg, two times per day, famciclovir 250 mg twice daily, or valacyclovir 500 mg daily, 1000 mg daily if more than 10 recurrences per year
     b. Discontinue after 1 year to reassess recurrences
  5. Sitz baths may provide relief
  6. Education—recurrences, viral shedding, abstinence when lesions are present, use of condoms during sexual activities

Genital Warts (Condylomata Acuminata)

- Definition: Most common symptomatic viral reproductive tract infection in United States; characterized by epithelial warts/tumors of mucous membranes and skin
- Etiology/Incidence
  1. Causative agent—human papillomavirus (HPV), a small DNA virus with more than 100 subtypes; types 6 and 11 usually cause genital warts; types 16, 18, 31, 33, 35 cause vaginal, anal, and cervical dysplasia
  2. Primary mode of transmission is sexual contact; sexual abuse must be considered when present in prepubertal child
  3. Genital HPV infection may be as high as 40% among sexually active female adolescents
  4. Most infections are transient and clear spontaneously
- Signs and Symptoms
  1. Firm bumps in anogenital area
  2. Occasional local symptoms—burning, pain, itching, bleeding
  3. Often asymptomatic
- Differential Diagnosis
  1. Chancre of secondary syphilis
  2. Molluscum contagiosum
- Physical Findings
  1. Firm, flesh-colored anogenital lesions resembling cauliflower in configuration
  2. Range in size from few millimeters to centimeters
  3. Males—warts on shaft of penis, meatus, scrotum, and perianal areas
  4. Females—warts usually seen on labia and perianal areas
  5. Anal genital warts—primarily from anal-receptive intercourse but may be due to proximity in genital region
- Diagnostic Tests/Findings
  1. Diagnosis usually based on clinical inspection; no culture is available
  2. Colposcopy to detect cervical lesions—application of 3% to 5% acetic acid (vinegar) causes lesion to blanch; not definitive
  3. Pelvic examination—Pap smear for cytological analysis may be diagnostic
  4. Biopsy of lesion for histologic examination—may be diagnostic
  5. DNA probe—may detect asymptomatic HPV infection
- Management/Treatment
  1. No definitive treatment yet available to eradicate HPV; palliative treatment focusing on removal of lesions, symptom relief, and close follow-up for recurrences and sequelae. Unclear if treatment decreases infectivity
  2. Spontaneous resolution within 3 months in 25% cases; recurrences are common
  3. External visible lesions
     a. Self-treatment

(1) Podophyllum resin solution or gel 0.5% (contraindicated in pregnancy and not yet tested for safety/efficacy in children)

    (a) Topical application bid for 3 days; need not be washed off

    (b) First application should be done in office to ensure proper technique

    (c) Treatment may be repeated up to four cycles with 4-day rest period between cycles

    (d) Not approved in pregnancy

(2) Imiquimod 5% cream

    (a) Three times per week for 6 to 10 hours, then wash off

    (b) Maximum is 16 weeks

(3) Sinecatechin 15% ointment

    (a) Apply three times per day up to 16 weeks

    (b) May cause pruritus, ulcer, pain, burning

    (c) Not recommended in pregnancy, HSV infection, HIV infection

  b. Clinician applied

    (1) Podophyllin, 10% to 25% in compound tincture of benzoin (contraindicated in pregnancy)

      (a) Weekly treatment up to total of six applications

      (b) Must be washed off in 1 to 4 hours

    (2) Trichloracetic acid (TCA 80% to 90%)

      (a) Topical application followed by careful drying and application of talc or baking soda

      (b) Weekly treatments up to total of six applications

      (c) Causes more local discomfort than podophyllin

    (3) Liquid nitrogen or cryotherapy—performed by a trained provider

    (4) Laser surgery, cryosurgery, excision, electrodessication—reserved for extensive, severe, and/or resistant cases

4. Gynecologic referral necessary for cervical warts
5. Monitoring of Pap smears for cervical cancer

  a. First Pap smear at 21 years old. Do not get HPV testing until age 30 years

  b. Repeat every 3 years if normal

  c. For ASCUS (atypical squamous cells of undetermined significance) or LSIL (low-grade squamous intraepithelial lesions)—repeat in 12 months

  d. For ASCUS, cannot rule out high-grade SIL—refer to GYN colposcopy

  e. For high-grade SIL (squamous intraepithelial lesions), CIN1 (cervical intraepithelial neoplasia 1), CIN 2—refer to GYN colposcopy

  f. Obtain Pap smear for suspicious cervical exam

6. Screening serology for syphilis; evaluate for any other concomitant STDs and treat accordingly
7. Education regarding safer sexual practices
8. Prevention—HPV vaccine (for types 6, 11, 16, 18) for males and females aged 9–26 years. Typically administered at age 11, three injections given over 6 months on a schedule of 0, 1–2 months, and 6 months

Trichomoniasis

- Definition: Common sexually transmitted infection of the genital tract
- Etiology/Incidence
  1. Causative agent—*Trichomonas vaginalis*, a flagellated protozoan
  2. Transmitted primarily through sexual contact; presence in prepubertal child should alert practitioner to possible sexual abuse
  3. Often associated with other STDs, e.g., gonorrhea, chlamydia
  4. Unknown incidence since it is not reportable
  5. Increases risk of getting or spreading STDs
  6. Known co-infection with other STDs and bacterial vaginosis
  7. Strong evidence that trichomoniasis in HIV-infected individuals increases the risk of transmission of HIV to uninfected partners as well as acquisition of HIV in *Trichomonas*-infected women
- Signs and Symptoms
  1. Females—asymptomatic in 25% to 50% of all cases
     a. Vaginal discharge
     b. Vulvovaginal irritation and itching
     c. Vaginal odor
     d. Dysuria, urinary frequency, abdominal pain, dyspareunia
     e. Risk of preterm birth and low-birth-weight infants of infected mothers.
  2. Males—usually asymptomatic
     a. Mild dysuria
     b. Itching
- Differential Diagnosis
  1. Candidiasis
  2. Chemical vaginitis
  3. Bacterial vaginosis
  4. UTI
  5. Poor hygiene
  6. Gonorrhea
- Physical Findings
  1. Vaginal discharge—frothy, light yellow to gray-green, musty odor with a pH >4.5
  2. Pelvic examination—evidence of vaginitis, cervicitis, punctate hemorrhage known as "strawberry cervix," erythema, edema, and pruritus of external genitalia may be present
  3. Males generally asymptomatic
- Diagnostic Tests/Findings
  1. Wet mount of vaginal secretions or spun urine sediment—presence of motile trichomonads
  2. Trichomonads may also be seen on Pap smears and urinalysis
  3. Culture

4. NAATs, DNA hybrid probes, positive rapid antigen tests, PCR analysis
- Management/Treatment: See AAP *Red Book* for additional treatment guidelines
  1. Metronidazole—treatment of choice
     a. Prepubertal—15 mg/kg/day orally three times daily for 7 days (maximum 2 g for 7 days) or 40 mg/kg (maximum 2 g) orally in single dose
     b. Adolescent—2 g orally in single dose or 375 mg two times per day for 7 days
     c. Avoid alcohol during treatment and for 24 hours after treatment
     d. During pregnancy—2 g single dose of metronidazole or 7-day regimen
  2. Tinidazole 2.0 g po × 1. No alcohol consumption for 72 hours
  3. No sexual activity during treatment
  4. Partners should receive concurrent therapy
  5. Evaluate for presence of other STIs—treat accordingly
  6. HIV-infected women may need the 7-day course of metronidazole
  7. Encourage condom use for STD prevention

Bacterial Vaginosis (BV)

- Definition: Clinical syndrome characterized by vaginal symptoms, primarily in sexually active adolescents/adults
- Etiology/Incidence
  1. Not an actual infection but classified as a sexually transmitted disease
  2. Results from replacement of normal vaginal flora (*Lactobacillus*) with high concentrations of anaerobes—*Gardnerella vaginalis*, *Mycoplasma hominis*
  3. Transmission may be sexual or nonsexual
  4. Incidence unknown
- Signs and Symptoms
  1. Profuse vaginal discharge with "fishy" odor
  2. May be asymptomatic
- Differential Diagnosis
  1. Foreign body
  2. Gonorrhea/chlamydia/trichomoniasis
  3. Vulvovaginitis—group A streptococci, *Shigella* organisms
  4. Candidiasis
  5. Physiologic leukorrhea
- Physical Findings
  1. Vaginal/cervical discharge—thin, white-gray, malodorous; adherent to vaginal wall
  2. Itching, swelling, redness of external genitalia
- Diagnostic Tests/Findings
  1. Vaginal secretions
     a. pH greater than 4.5
     b. KOH 10% mixed with vaginal discharge—releases amine, "fishy odor" (whiff test)
     c. Saline wet mount—clue cells: Epithelial cell covered in bacteria, obliterating the nucleus

2. Culture available—rarely helpful, expensive
- Management/Treatment—see AAP *Red Book* for additional treatment guidelines
  1. Metronidazole
     a. 500 mg, orally, twice daily for 7 days OR
     b. 2 g orally, single dose with 2nd dose in 48 hours
  2. Alternative treatment
     a. Clindamycin cream 2%, one full applicator (5 g) intravaginally at bedtime for 7 days
     b. Metronidazole gel 0.75%, one full applicator (5 g) intravaginally twice daily for 5 days
     c. Clindamycin, 300 mg, orally, twice daily for 7 days
  3. Education
     a. Avoid douching
     b. Common recurrence
     c. Treatment of male partner not recommended, does not decrease female recurrence
     d. Increased risk for PID
     e. Pregnancy risk for chorioamnionitis and premature delivery

❑ CONTRACEPTION

- Abstinence—most effective method
  1. Half of all adolescents select this option
  2. Should be discussed as viable option regardless of prior history
- Male Condoms—most effective barrier method.
  1. Mechanism—mechanical barrier preventing semen from entering vagina; types of male condoms—over 100 brands currently on the market
     a. Latex—recommended. Helps to prevent pregnancy and STDs
     b. Polyurethane (latex-free) if latex sensitive. Helps prevent pregnancy and STDs
     c. Natural skin (lambskin)—not recommended (inadequate STD and HIV protection)
  2. Failure rates
     a. Theoretical—3%
     b. Actual—18%, primarily due to nonuse/misuse
     c. Combined with spermicide—no more effective than lubricated condoms in protecting against STIs and HIV
  3. Risks/precautions
     a. Breakage rate is approximately 1% to 2%
     b. Only water-based lubricants should be used—latex breaks down in contact with petroleum-based products
     c. Latex breakdown over time and when exposed to heat
- Female Condoms
  1. Worn by the woman
  2. Available over the counter.
  3. Packaged with a lubricant.
  4. Can be inserted up to 8 hours before intercourse.
  5. Failure rates: Typical use 21%

- Vaginal Spermicides—topical creams, jellies, foams, suppositories, and films to prevent pregnancy; used alone or in combination with condoms
  1. Active spermicidal agent—nonoxynol-9 or octoxynol-9
  2. Failure rate is approximately 6%
  3. Risks/precautions (CDC, 2010)
     a. Not effective in preventing cervical gonorrhea, *Chlamydia*, or HIV
     b. Frequent use may disrupt genital epithelium, may be associated with an increased risk of HIV transmission
     c. Increased risk for UTIs in women using diaphragm/spermicide
     d. Should not be used as a lubricant or microbicide for anal intercourse due to rectal cell damage
- Diaphragm—female barrier contraceptive method
  1. Thin latex dome with flexible ring with spermicide applied, for vaginal insertion prior to intercourse; positioned with posterior rim on posterior fornix and anterior rim behind pubic bone. A cervical cap is a smaller, thimble size cup that is fitted to cover the cervix
  2. Requires pelvic examination for proper fitting for appropriate size
  3. Failure rate among adolescents—10% to 25%
  4. Risks/precautions
     a. Requires technical skill/comfort with body for correct placement
     b. Must be kept in place for 6 hours postintercourse
     c. Spermicidal agent must be used for subsequent intercourse
     d. Side effects—UTI, vaginitis
- Combined Hormonal Contraceptives—oral contraceptives (OCs), transdermal contraceptive patch, vaginal contraceptive ring
  1. Mechanisms
     a. Prevents ovulation
     b. Increases viscosity of cervical mucus, inhibiting sperm penetration
     c. Alters endometrium to resist implantation
  2. Health benefits
     a. Decreased risk of endometrial and ovarian cancer
     b. Improved androgen insensitivity
     c. Decreased risk of hospitalization for GC-PID
     d. Suppresses endometriosis
     e. Decreases iron-deficiency anemia
     f. Improves dysmenorrhea
  3. Oral contraceptive pills; estrogen-progestin combinations
     a. Estrogens—ethinyl estradiol and mestranol
        (1) Ethinyl estradiol—1.2 to 1.4 times stronger than mestranol
        (2) Ethinyl estradiol effective at doses as low as 20 μg
        (3) Usually select lowest effective estrogen dose (20 to 35 μg)
     b. Basic progestins—norethindrone, norethindrone acetate, norethynodrel, ethynodiol diacetate, norgestrel
     c. Newer progestins—norgestimate, desogestrel, gestodene
     d. Monophasic, biphasic, or triphasic combinations—deliver constant or progressively increasing progestin during cycle
  4. Transdermal contraceptive patch
     a. Ethinylestradiol/norelgestromin
     b. Wear one patch for 1 week, repeat with a new patch weekly for 2 more weeks
     c. Patch must be correctly applied to dry skin and site rotated
     d. Failure rate may be higher in women who weigh more than 198 pounds
  5. Vaginal contraceptive ring
     a. Ethinylestradiol/etonorgestrel
     b. Inserted ring must remain in place for 3 weeks
     c. User must learn how to place and check for ring
  6. Failure rates—0.5% (theoretical) to 9% with typical use
  7. Risks/precautions
     a. Drug interactions
        (1) Drugs that may reduce OCP effectiveness—antibiotics, antifungals, anticonvulsants, antacids
        (2) Drugs that enhance OC effectiveness—ascorbic acid, co-trimoxazole
     b. Major side effects—thrombosis
     c. Minor side effects—vaginal spotting, nausea, bloating, irritability
     d. Does not protect against HIV and other STIs
     e. Absolute contraindications for use
        (1) History of clotting disorder
        (2) Impaired liver function
        (3) Abnormal vaginal bleeding (undiagnosed)
        (4) Pregnancy
        (5) Estrogen-dependent carcinoma
     f. Relative contraindications for use
        (1) Severe hypertension
        (2) Migraines
        (3) Chronic diseases, e.g., diabetes, heart disease, sickle cell
        (4) Rheumatologic disorders
- Long-Acting Progestins—injectable and implantable to inhibit ovulation
  1. Depo-medroxyprogesterone acetate (injectable)
     a. Dosage and administration—150 mg/mL intramuscular injection every 3 months during first 5 days of normal period to ensure nonpregnant status. Quick start method can be used without waiting for menses; requires negative pregnancy test and plan to repeat pregnancy test 2 weeks after injection. EC can be given if there was intercourse in the prior 5 days. Education regarding small risk of pregnancy

b. Failure rate—0.25%
c. Precautions/risks
  (1) If more than 13 weeks between injections, pregnancy test as precaution
  (2) Should not be given to pregnant, postpartum, lactating adolescent mothers
  (3) Contraindicated: Active thrombophlebitis, undiagnosed vaginal bleeding, breast malignancy, significant liver disease
  (4) Side effects: Spotting, weight gain, bloating, headaches, mood changes
  (5) Risk of decreased bone density. May reduce bone mass and may not be completely irreversible
  (6) Assess for adequate calcium and vitamin D intake
  (7) Manufacturer recommends not to be used long term (more than 2 years) unless other methods are considered inadequate

2. Nexplanon (Etonogestrel 68 mg), long-acting reversible contraception (LARC)
  a. One rod implanted in subcutaneous tissue of upper, inner arm
  b. Effective for 3 years
  c. Vaginal bleeding and spotting are not predictable
  d. Does not protect against STIs
  e. Radiopaque
  f. Typical use failure rate 0.05%

• IUD—a long-acting reversible contraceptive
1. Safe, effective, long-term contraception. Placed by a clinician
2. Copper T 380A increases uterine and tubal fluids that impair sperm function; lasts up to 10 years. Typical use failure rate 0.8%
3. LNG-IUS (Mirena) releases levonorgestrel 20 mcg per day, which thickens cervical mucus, inhibits sperm, suppresses endometrium. Lasts up to 5 years. Typical use failure rate 0.2%
4. Reduces risk of ectopic pregnancy
5. LNG-IUS decreases blood loss
6. Fertility rebounds when discontinued
7. Does not protect against STIs

• Emergency Contraception (EC)—use of oral contraceptive within 72 hours of unprotected intercourse
1. Evaluate for pregnancy risk
2. EC will not terminate existing pregnancy
3. Plan B is progesterone only (levonorgestrel), 2 tabs. Plan B One-Step is one pill, approved for OTC purchase by any age. Generic products may apply to the FDA in 2016 for OTC status
4. Schedule of doses from 20 OCPs brands, given in two doses 12 hours apart; may cause nausea, vomiting (see Hatcher et al., *Contraceptive Technology*, 18th edition, p. 280)
5. Meclizine HCI 25 to 50 mg may be given before first dose of OCP method to reduce nausea
6. Provide counseling to prevent future need for EC

7. Perform pregnancy test if no menses after 3 weeks
8. Failure rate 1.6%
9. Since Plan B One-Step is OTC, individual insurances may or may not cover with prescription benefit

• Contraceptive Methods Less Suitable for Adolescents
1. Coitus interruptus—failure rate >27%
2. Natural family planning—high failure rate
3. Cervical cap—difficulties with proper placement; risk of infection
4. Progestin-only mini-pill—failure rates up to 13% among mature adults, increased risk of ectopic pregnancy when method fails

☐ ISSUES OF PREGNANCY AND BIRTH FOR THE ADOLESCENT

• Pregnancy: Diagnosis and Counseling
1. Risk factors
  a. Early onset of sexual activity; inadequate concept of fertility and contraception
  b. Low socioeconomic level
  c. Poor academic achievement
  d. Low self-image; few options for future
  e. Early pregnancy in mother or sister
  f. Substance abuse
  g. Physical/sexual abuse
  h. Barriers to contraceptive use, including misinformation, lack of health care, poor communication with partner
  i. Exposure to irresponsible media portrayal of sex
2. Incidence
  a. United States has the highest rates of adolescent pregnancy and births among developed nations; estimates of 614,000 each year
  b. Rates have shown a decline from 1990 (116.9:1000) to 2010 (57.4:1000) among 15- to 19-year-olds, with largest decline among African American teens
  c. Birth rate among 15- to 19-year-old females—34.4:1000 (2010)
  d. Subsequent pregnancy common—12% to 44% pregnant again within 1 year, 20% to 37% within 2 years
  e. Teen mothers are more likely to drop out of school than teens without babies
3. Signs and Symptoms
  a. First trimester
    (1) Irregular menses/amenorrhea
    (2) GI—nausea, vomiting
    (3) Urinary frequency
    (4) Breast tenderness/tingling
    (5) Other—headache, vertigo, abdominal cramps
  b. Second trimester
    (1) Increased/darkening skin pigmentation
    (2) Fetal movement—"quickening" 16 to 20 weeks
    (3) Contractions—Braxton-Hicks 16 to 27 weeks
  c. Third trimester—increased contractions

4. Physical Findings
  a. First trimester
    (1) Breast—fullness/tenderness, nipple tingling/discharge/darkening areola
    (2) Abdomen—uterine fundus at symphysis pubis at 12 weeks
    (3) Pelvic examination
      (a) Softening of uterine isthmus (Hegar sign) 6 to 8 weeks
      (b) Bluish hue to cervix/vaginal epithelium (Chadwick sign) 6 to 8 weeks
      (c) Cervical softening (Goodell sign) 6 to 8 weeks
      (d) Increased leukorrhea
    (4) Weight gain—2 pounds (1 kg)
    (5) Fetal heart tones (FHTs)—by Doppler at 10 to 12 weeks
  b. Second trimester
    (1) Stretch marks "striae" on abdomen and breasts
    (2) Fundus midway between symphysis pubis and umbilicus by 14 to 15 weeks, at umbilicus 20 to 22 weeks
    (3) Fetal heart tones by fetoscope at 20 weeks
    (4) Weight gain—11 pounds (5 kg)
  c. Third trimester
    (1) Colostrum from breasts 28 to 40 weeks
    (2) Fundus between umbilicus and xiphoid, 28 weeks; at xiphoid, 38 weeks
    (3) Weight gain—11 pounds (5 kg)
    (4) Bloody show—impending labor
    (5) Ruptured membranes
  d. Labor
    (1) Stage 1—effacement and dilatation of cervix
    (2) Stage 2—delivery of fetus
    (3) Stage 3—separation and delivery of placenta
5. Differential Diagnosis
  a. Ectopic pregnancy
  b. Incomplete spontaneous abortion
  c. Molar pregnancy
  d. UTI
6. Diagnostic Tests/Findings
  a. Urine for human chorionic gonadotropin (hCG)—positive 7 to 10 days after conception
  b. Blood test for pregnancy—more expensive, takes longer to get results, positive 7 to 10 days after conception; hCG can be quantified if needed.
  c. Cervical cultures—gonorrhea/chlamydia screen
  d. Wet mount—saline, KOH
  e. Papanicolaou smears
  f. Serology—syphilis, hepatitis B surface antigen, blood type/Rh factor, glucose, CBC with indices, rubella, human immunodeficiency virus
  g. Blood pressure (BP) checks
  h. Urinalysis and culture (if indicated)
  i. Pelvic ultrasound (if indicated)
7. Counseling/Education
  a. Impact on future plans, finances, family structure
  b. Identity and age of father—anticipated involvement

  c. Options
    (1) Continue pregnancy and maintain custody
    (2) Continue pregnancy and place child for adoption
    (3) Termination of pregnancy
  d. Prenatal care—examinations, adequate diet, prenatal vitamins (includes folic acid). Iron and calcium as needed
  e. Avoidance of medications/drugs/alcohol/x-rays/smoking
- Prenatal Diagnosis—identify potential inherited/acquired defects
  1. Variety of causes—genetic factors (25%); environmental (15%); combination of both genetic and environmental (30%); unaccountable (30%)
  2. Incidence—3% to 5% infants in United States
  3. Risk factors—maternal
    a. Disease—diabetes, thyroid, immune deficiency or compromise
    b. Age—young, especially younger than 16 years; older than 35 years
    c. Previous child with Down syndrome, anencephaly, meningomyelocele
  4. Screening tools
    a. Family pedigree—graphic record, family medical history
    b. Alpha-fetoprotein
      (1) Screens for neural tube defects, trisomy 21, trisomy 18
      (2) Serum levels less accurate than amniotic fluid analysis but can be done earlier in pregnancy for initial screen
      (3) High levels may be due to inaccurate pregnancy dates or to multiple pregnancy
    c. Amniocentesis—collection of amniotic fluid, 15 to 16 weeks gestation; karyotype/chromosomal analysis; inborn errors of metabolism; confirmatory test with abnormal serum alpha-fetoprotein
    d. Chorionic villus sampling—tissue (villus) sample from fetal placenta at 9 to 11 weeks gestation; chromosomal abnormality; usually reserved for women older than 35 years
    e. Metabolic disease, hemoglobinopathies from DNA analysis
- Genetic Counseling—communication process regarding risk/problems surrounding certain disorders
  1. Often initiated following birth of affected child
  2. Both parents included—family history, medical/psychological consequences for child/family, possibility of future children affected, options
  3. Utilizes results from prenatal diagnostic tools/tests
- Pregnancy Termination
  1. Spontaneous termination—miscarriage
    a. Miscarriage/spontaneous abortion of pregnancy prior to fetal viability
    b. May be complete or incomplete
    c. Occurs in 20% of all pregnancies, including adolescents

d. Often associated with genetic abnormality in fetus

2. Elective termination—induced abortion

a. Induced or elective abortion—35% of adolescent pregnancies

b. Procedural options—dependent on trimester of termination

c. First trimester abortion options—rule out STI prior to procedure

  (1) Manual syringe evacuation/early suction curettage—4 to 6 weeks of pregnancy

    (a) Cannula positioned into uterus with aspiration or suction of conceptus (menstrual extraction)

    (b) Low risk of genital injury or complications

  (2) Suction curettage/vacuum aspiration—up to 12 to 14 weeks of pregnancy

    (a) Cervical dilation 61 hours prior to procedure using *Laminaria* (hydrophilic seaweed sticks)

    (b) Cannula position into uterus with suction followed by curettage

    (c) Considered safest in first trimester

  (3) Medical abortion—induces abortion when administered in early pregnancy (49 days or less)

    (a) Acts as antiprogesterone

    (b) Initial dose of mifepristone 600 mg followed with 400 mcg of misoprostol (a prostaglandin) 2 days later

    (c) Risks include pain, excessive bleeding

d. Second trimester

  (1) Dilatation and evacuation curettage (D&E)—20 to 24 weeks of pregnancy

    (a) Cervical dilation prior to procedure with osmotic dilators

    (b) Conceptus removed via curettage, aspiration, or ring forceps under general anesthesia; risk of cervical trauma

    (c) Antibiotics recommended postprocedure

  (2) Prostaglandin suppository technique—16 to 24 weeks of pregnancy; rarely used

    (a) Cervical dilation with osmotic dilators followed by vaginal suppositories of prostaglandin E; has largely replaced more controversial intra-amniotic instillation techniques

    (b) 20-mg prostaglandin suppositories used every 3 to 4 hours, induces labor and subsequent abortion within 4 to 60 hours

    (c) Complications include significant flu-like symptoms and possible delivery of live fetus

e. Referral and follow-up

  (1) Referral to obstetrician/gynecologist or family planning clinic once decision to terminate pregnancy is made

  (2) Continue supportive care and counseling options on follow-up

- Birthing Methods: May have greater risk of cesarean delivery due to immature pelvic skeletal development; cephalopelvic disproportion

- Prematurity/Low Birth Weight

1. Maternal risk factors—maternal age less than 16 years; poor prenatal care/poor nutrition

2. Prevention aimed at prenatal management

a. Good nutrition; avoid dieting—daily calories 2500 to 2700 kcal/day

b. Supplements—vitamins (include folic acid), iron (anemia possible), calcium

3. Early/consistent prenatal care

a. Avoid all medications unless specifically approved by healthcare provider

b. Potential for multisystem complications—infant

  (1) Respiratory—respiratory distress syndrome, bronchopulmonary dysplasia, apnea

  (2) Cardiovascular—patent ductus arteriosus, bradycardia, malformations

  (3) Hematologic—hyperbilirubinemia, subcutaneous hemorrhage

  (4) Gastrointestinal—poor motility

  (5) Metabolic/endocrine—hypocalcemia, hypoglycemia or hyperglycemia, hypothermia

  (6) Central nervous system—intraventricular hemorrhage, hypotonia

  (7) Renal abnormalities

  (8) Infections

- Home Monitoring/Follow-Up Care

1. Frequent contact with mother/infant—early discharge follow-up recommended within 48 hours

a. Infant feeding patterns

b. Adaptation of mother to sleep changes

c. Social support—father of baby, mother's family

2. Follow-up (well-child visits)

a. Adolescent problems—repeated pregnancy, STI

b. Optimal health of mother/infant

c. Future plans—completion of high school, college/technical training, career

- Maternal Substance Abuse

1. Risk of substance abuse among adolescents—requires assessment

2. Drug/alcohol use

a. Counsel at initial prenatal visit

b. Reinforce impact of all substances on developing fetus—tobacco, alcohol, marijuana, inhalants, cocaine, heroin, designer and other medicines and drugs

- Screening for potentially abusive partner

1. Increased risk of battering by partner when pregnant

a. Assess relationship between girl and partner

b. Some states require mandatory reporting of victims of domestic violence

2. Risk factors for child abuse

a. Parental factors

  (1) Young and/or immature adolescent parents

  (2) Minimal education

(3) Financial stress
(4) Lack of social support
(5) Unplanned or unwanted pregnancy
(6) Unrealistic expectations of parenting
b. Infant factors
(1) Prematurity
(2) Perception as "different/bad"; difficult temperament
(3) Congenital defect/malformation

- Perinatal complications of neonate
1. Low birth weight and prematurity—see earlier section
2. Infant mortality, linked with low birth weight and prematurity
3. Cognitive/social development—possible low self-esteem, less responsive/expressive, decreased ability to trust others
4. Sudden infant death syndrome (SIDS)

☐ QUESTIONS

Select the best answer.
Questions 1 and 2 refer to the following scenario.
A 10-year-old boy comes to your clinic for evaluation of a suspected urinary tract infection (UTI).

1. Which of the following signs would lead you to include diagnoses other than UTI in the differential?
   a. Urinary frequency
   b. Penile discharge
   c. Suprapubic or urethral pain
   d. Incontinence
2. The culture indicates sensitivity to trimethoprim/sulfamethoxazole. The boy is treated with this antibiotic for 10 days. The most appropriate follow-up in this case would include:
   a. Obtaining a urinalysis in 2 weeks
   b. Instructing the parents that the child should return to the clinic if symptoms persist
   c. Teaching parents home monitoring with nitrite sticks
   d. Referring the child for a renal ultrasound
3. The most important laboratory test to be performed when a UTI is suspected in a school-age child is a:
   a. CBC with differential
   b. Urine dipstick
   c. Clean catch urine for U/A and C/S
   d. Voiding cystourethrogram (VCUG)
4. Jay is a 9-year-old boy who has had no significant health problems by history, but his mother is very concerned because he is "wetting himself." As you begin your history and physical examination, you keep in mind that the most common type of enuresis in school-age children is:
   a. Primary nocturnal enuresis
   b. Occasional daytime enuresis
   c. Secondary nocturnal enuresis
   d. Primary diurnal enuresis

5. Which of the following statements is not true with regard to primary nocturnal enuresis?
   a. There is often a positive family history of enuresis.
   b. It appears to be related to maturational delay.
   c. Some nighttime wetters stop wetting without any form of treatment.
   d. The incidence is higher in girls than in boys.
6. Which of the following is not true about the use of imipramine for the treatment of enuresis?
   a. It is not generally recommended for this nonfatal disorder due to the potentially lethal side effects.
   b. The lasting cure rate is approximately 17%.
   c. Imipramine should only be given to children who have had a baseline EEG.
   d. The most appropriate imipramine treatment group is adolescent boys with both ADHD and persistent nocturnal enuresis.
7. While examining a 4-month-old boy, you are unable to palpate one of the testes. The next most appropriate step is to:
   a. Reassure the parents that this is a normal finding
   b. Refer the child to an endocrinologist
   c. Reexamine the baby in 2 months
   d. Refer the child to a urologist
8. Which of the following is not true with regard to hypospadias?
   a. The meatus is formed along the dorsum of the penis.
   b. It is one of the most common penile abnormalities.
   c. Circumcision should be deferred.
   d. A referral for an endocrine evaluation may be indicated.
9. Upon examination of a 2-month-old boy, you notice a swelling in the right inguinal canal. Your differential diagnosis would not include:
   a. Diastasis recti
   b. Hydrocele of the spermatic cord
   c. Inguinal hernia
   d. Lymphadenopathy

Questions 10 and 11 refer to the following scenario.
A 12-year-old girl presents to your clinic with symptoms of vaginitis, including odor, dysuria, frequency, and discomfort.

10. Which of the following causes of vaginitis is most likely due to sexual transmission?
    a. *Candida*
    b. *Chlamydia*
    c. Pinworms
    d. *Gardnerella*
11. Upon further history, physical examination, and laboratory screening, the girl is diagnosed with *Candida albicans* vaginitis. Appropriate treatment would include:
    a. Avoiding bubble baths
    b. Topical acyclovir
    c. Ceftriaxone
    d. Clotrimazole

12. A labial adhesion extending from the posterior four-chette to the clitoris is noted during the routine assessment of a 4-year-old girl. There is no history of difficulty voiding, dysuria, or discomfort. The most appropriate initial management is to:
    a. Recommend mechanical lysis using petrolatum ointment
    b. Prescribe a topical application of estrogen cream
    c. Refer to a GU specialist
    d. Reassure parents that no specific treatment is needed at this time
13. Patients with acute nephrotic syndrome may present with all but which of the following signs?
    a. Edema
    b. Hypertension
    c. Dark amber-colored urine
    d. History of weight loss
14. It is important to look for evidence of a preceding streptococcal infection when ruling out acute nephritis. This is best done by:
    a. Throat culture
    b. Skin examination
    c. ASO titer
    d. ESR
15. An adolescent boy presents to the clinic with a painless mass in the left side of his scrotum. The most likely diagnosis is:
    a. Epididymitis
    b. Testicular torsion
    c. Incarcerated hernia
    d. Hydrocele
16. A foul-smelling vaginal discharge that emits a fishy odor when combined with 10% potassium hydroxide is most likely due to:
    a. *Gardnerella vaginalis*
    b. *Candida albicans*
    c. *Chlamydia trachomatis*
    d. *N. gonorrhoeae*
17. A 17-year-old sexually active girl with chancres in the genital area is noted to have a positive Venereal Disease Research Laboratories (VDRL) test. The next step should be to:
    a. Treat with ceftriaxone
    b. Perform a specific treponemal antibody test
    c. Culture for *C. trachomatis*
    d. Discuss safer sex practices
18. The most common bacterial cause of a sexually transmitted infection (STI) is:
    a. *Neisseria gonorrhoeae*
    b. *Trichomonas vaginalis*
    c. *Chlamydia trachomatis*
    d. Herpes simplex
19. Which of the following is an absolute contraindication for use of combined hormonal contraceptives in adolescent women?
    a. History of thromboembolism
    b. Diabetes

c. Smokes five cigarettes per day
d. Sickle cell disease

20. A 15-year-old girl, who had menarche at 13 years of age, complains of monthly menstrual pain on the first day of her periods for 1 year. She has never been sexually active. Which of the following is not a characteristic of dysmenorrhea?
    a. Increased production of uterine prostaglandins
    b. Pain usually starts within hours of menstrual flow or may precede flow by up to 2 days
    c. Anovulatory cycles
    d. Crampy, spasmodic pain in the lower abdominal area, which might radiate to inner thighs
21. Which of the following is a risk factor for adolescent pregnancy?
    a. Good grades in school
    b. Asks for contraceptive at the school health clinic
    c. Plans to study nursing in college
    d. Unsure if monogamous partner uses condoms
22. Cara is a 16-year-old adolescent who has been sexually active with a male partner for 6 months. They have used condoms consistently. Cara is interested in a hormonal method as well. Your advice includes all of the following except which one?
    a. Combined oral contraceptives prevent ovulation.
    b. Transdermal contraceptive patches must be correctly applied and the site rotated.
    c. The vaginal contraceptive ring must be changed weekly.
    d. Long-acting progestins might cause weight gain.
23. Dan is a healthy 17-year-old student. He is thinking about having sex but asks for more information about condoms. You give him all of the following advice except which one?
    a. Male condoms are the most effective barrier method.
    b. Latex condoms are the most recommended and are heat tolerant.
    c. Condoms have a theoretical failure rate of 3%.
    d. It is only safe to use water-based lubricant with latex condoms.
24. Which of the following is true about LARCs (long-acting reversible contraception)?
    a. Nexplanon is radiopaque.
    b. Mirena IUD can stay in place for 3 years.
    c. Vaginal bleeding is predictable.
    d. Adolescents should avoid using IUDs.
25. The following are true about *Trichomonas* except which statement?
    a. *Trichomonas* infection increases the risk of spreading other STIs.
    b. Males are often asymptomatic.
    c. Once trichomoniasis is cured the person is considered immune to reinfection.
    d. Latex condoms help reduce the risk of getting *Trichomonas*.

26. According to the 2011 American Academy of Pediatric guidelines for UTI management in children 2–24 months, a 6-month-old baby girl diagnosed with her first UTI should be treated with an appropriate antimicrobial agent. Which additional intervention should be ordered for this child?
    a. A test of cure
    b. A voiding cystourethrography (VCUG)
    c. An ultrasound of the kidneys and bladder
    d. Prophylactic antibiotics

27. Urinary tract infections (UTIs) are the most common pediatric urinary tract problems seen in primary care. Which of the following statements is not true regarding UTIs?
    a. Symptoms are often nonspecific, especially in infancy.
    b. Urine culture is required for definitive diagnosis.
    c. Trimethoprim-sulfamethoxazole is the drug of choice for most children.
    d. Radiologic studies are rarely indicated with first infection.

28. A 2-year-old girl presents with symptoms of painful urination, frequency, and occasional incontinence over the past week. When seen in your office, she has a temperature of 101.6°F. Which of the following would be your approach in establishing a definitive diagnosis?
    a. Clean-catch midstream collection of specimen for urine analysis
    b. Clean-catch midstream collection of specimen for urine culture
    c. Straight catheterization collection of specimen for urine culture
    d. Voiding cystourethrogram (VCUG)

29. The most likely organism to cause a UTI in the pediatric population is:
    a. *Staphylococcus saprophyticus*
    b. *Klebsiella*
    c. *Chlamydia*
    d. *E. coli*

30. One of the most commonly suggested reasons for primary enuresis is:
    a. Certain medications, such as theophylline
    b. Genitourinary abnormalities
    c. Family disruptions and stress
    d. Delayed maturation of voiding inhibitory reflex and arousal response

31. Suzanne, a 7-year-old, comes to you for a physical examination prior to participation in soccer. Suzanne's mother is concerned that the child "still has accidents at night." You determine that Suzanne has primary nocturnal enuresis and your first recommendation to her mother is to:
    a. Avoid use of criticism or punishment
    b. Use a sticker/star chart
    c. Treat with medication
    d. Purchase an enuresis alarm

32. The incidence of cryptorchidism at 1 year of age is about 1%. The best explanation for this is:
    a. Examination of the scrotum begins at this age.
    b. A child can usually stand, making palpation of the testes easier.
    c. Spontaneous resolution often occurs in first 6 months.
    d. Surgical repair can now be done in neonatal period.

33. In counseling parents when their child is diagnosed with mild hypospadias, suggest that the following may be part of the management:
    a. Circumcision
    b. Radiography
    c. Consult with pediatric urology
    d. Surgical correction at 2 years of age

34. On physical examination of a 2-year-old uncircumcised male, you note that the foreskin is retracted and discolored. There is swelling of the glans. The most likely diagnosis is:
    a. Phimosis
    b. Balanitis
    c. UTI
    d. Paraphimosis

35. Meatal stenosis, narrowing of the distal urethra, is seen following:
    a. Orchiopexy
    b. Circumcision
    c. Epididymitis
    d. Hypospadias repair

36. During a track meet, a 14-year-old male pole-vaulter falls to the ground screaming in pain. He complains of intense, searing pain in his right scrotum. He vomits twice while waiting for the ambulance. He most likely has:
    a. Orchitis
    b. Hydrocele
    c. Acute epididymitis
    d. Testicular torsion

37. Treatment for testicular torsion is primarily:
    a. Scrotal elevation
    b. Ice
    c. Immediate surgical referral
    d. Bed rest

38. Labial adhesions are a relatively common finding among infants and young girls. Which of the following statements about this condition is true?
    a. Adhesions are usually present at birth but may be missed on examination.
    b. Highest incidence is from birth to 3 years.
    c. Simple lysis of adhesions is often recommended.
    d. Most cases resolve without intervention.

39. Which of the following statements is true regarding the use of topical application of conjugated estrogen cream with labial adhesions?
    a. It is highly successful in resolving most adhesions within 2 months.
    b. It is no longer recommended because it may stimulate precocious puberty.

c. Topical applications of bland creams or petroleum jelly are equally effective.

d. Mechanical lysis is preferred treatment today.

40. In cases of accidental genitourinary trauma, which of the following is not commonly seen?

   a. Extensive tears of the vaginal wall
   b. Hematuria
   c. Hematoma of the urethra, scrotum, lower abdomen
   d. Periurethral lacerations

41. The most common form of glomerulonephritis in children is:

   a. Mesangial proliferative
   b. Poststreptococcal
   c. Membranoproliferative
   d. Mesangiostreptococcal

42. Which of the following signs/symptoms is not associated with acute forms of glomerulonephritis?

   a. Edema
   b. Hematuria
   c. Increased urine output
   d. Dark urine

43. Which of the following is true of renal tubular acidosis type 1?

   a. Genetically transmitted as autosomal recessive disorder
   b. Distal tube defect affecting secretion of hydrogen ions
   c. Distal tube defect affecting bicarbonate reabsorption
   d. Most children remain short in stature despite early treatment

44. Meatal stenosis can be identified by all of the following with the exception of:

   a. Crying with urination
   b. Inflammation of glans penis
   c. Slit-like meatus
   d. Wide urinary stream

45. Most patients with uncomplicated UTI can be treated on an outpatient basis. The first antibiotic you would consider using is:

   a. Amoxicillin
   b. Trimethoprim-sulfamethoxazole
   c. Cephalexin
   d. Amoxicillin/clavulanate

46. Cryptorchidism is more prevalent in:

   a. Term infants
   b. Premature infants
   c. Babies at 1 year of age
   d. Toddlers

47. A 3-year-old boy is in the process of toilet training. The parents come to see you because when the child urinates, all of the urine goes on the floor. You suspect hypospadias because:

   a. It is a rare disorder and would indicate a more serious problem.
   b. Normally, the urine stream is directed from the meatal opening at the tip of the penis, in a straight path.

c. The child is circumcised.

d. Fusion of the urethral folds has occurred.

48. Which of the following is not used in the management of the child with phimosis?

   a. Ice packs
   b. Gentle stretching when bathing
   c. Circumcision in cases of urinary obstruction
   d. Good hygiene

49. Treatment of a child with glomerulonephritis would not include:

   a. Vasoconstrictors for hypotension
   b. Antibiotics for persistent infection
   c. Increased fluids to maintain hydration
   d. Avoidance of diuretics

❒ ANSWERS AND RATIONALES

1. B: Classic signs of a UTI include enuresis, frequency, dysuria, urgency, fever, and pain. Discharge may indicate balanitis or a sexually transmitted disease.

2. D: Older boys with a first infection should be examined for urinary tract abnormalities. The other laboratory tests do not assess for urinary tract anomalies.

3. C: The gold standard for the diagnosis of a UTI is quantitative urinary culture via clean-catch urine sample. The urinalysis is also useful in supporting the diagnosis.

4. D: The recurrence risk for a child to be affected by enuresis is 40% if one parent and 70% if both parents had been enuretic as children.

5. D: Primary nocturnal enuresis is seen in boys almost three times as often as in girls.

6. C: While imipramine therapy is helpful in approximately 50% of children, care should be taken to stay within the recommended 25–50 mg po qHS. Baseline electroencephalogram (EEG) is not necessary.

7. D: Testes rarely descend after the first 6 months.

8. A: The incidence of hypospadias has increased over the past 15 years in Western culture. The meatus of the penis forms ventrally.

9. A: Diastasis recti is a midline fascial attenuation extending from the umbilicus to the xiphoid process.

10. B: Papillomas, *Trichomonas*, herpes simplex, gonococcal, and chlamydial disease carry a high suspicion for sexual transmission. *Candida* typically occurs after a course of antibiotics, *Gardnerella* is indigenous vaginal flora, and pinworms is a parasitic disease.

11. D: In *Candida albicans*, local application of clotrimazole, miconazole, and ticonazole appear to be equally effective.

12. D: The majority of labial adhesions resolve spontaneously during hormonal changes at puberty. In general, labial adhesions do not warrant treatment.

13. D: Patients with nephritic syndrome can present with periorbital edema, hyper- or hypotension and associated tachycardia, as well as weight gain due to fluid overload.

14. C: The antistreptolysin O (ASO) titer is elevated in 80% of patients with a preceding streptococcal infection, and although ASO titers peak 2–4 weeks after an acute episode, antibody titers can remain elevated for up to 6 months.

15. D: Typically, a hydrocele manifests as a painless scrotal swelling of variable size and an inguinal hernia as intermittent inguinal swelling.

16. A: Bacterial vaginosis, often caused by an overgrowth of *Gardnerella vaginosis*, is suspected on the basis of a malodorous vaginal discharge and positive "whiff" test when the discharge is mixed with potassium hydroxide.

17. B: If the VDRL test is positive, a specific treponemal test such as FTA-ABs should be done to confirm the diagnosis. Treatment is with benzathine penicillin G.

18. C: *Chlamydia* is the most common bacterial cause of STD, with over 4 million cases annually.

19. A: Estrogen-containing combined hormonal contraceptives increase hepatic production of extrinsic clotting factors and increase the relative risk for thromboembolic events in women with a history of deep vein thrombosis (DVT) or pulmonary embolism (PE).

20. C: Primary dysmenorrhea usually begins within 1 to 3 years of menarche and is associated with the establishment of ovulatory cycles.

21. D: Poor communication with one's partner is a definite risk factor for adolescent pregnancy.

22. C: The vaginal contraceptive ring is worn for 3 weeks, removed, and then a new ring is inserted 1 week later.

23. B: Heat can cause latex condoms to break down.

24. A: Nexplanon is radiopaque, which can be useful if it is difficult to remove the implant.

25. C: Treating trichomoniasis does not confer immunity to reinfection. In fact, 1 in 5 people are reinfected within 3 months.

26. C: Data from six recent studies do not support the use of antimicrobial prophylaxis in infants with grades I–IV vesicoureteral reflux. Therefore, VCUG is not recommended routinely after first UTI. Ultrasonography of the kidneys and bladder should be performed to detect abnormalities.

27. D: Initial febrile UTI should be followed up with ultrasonography of kidneys and bladder.

28. C: In a non-toilet-trained child, the most accurate method for nonemergent urine collection is a sterile straight catheterization for urine culture.

29. D: *E. coli* accounts for 80–90% of all UTIs.

30. D: Many children who experience primary nocturnal enuresis have not yet developed a normal arousal response.

31. D: Use of criticism or punishment for a child with voiding difficulties can be detrimental to their self-esteem and is not productive in achieving the desired outcome.

32. C: Typically, in cryptorchidism, the testes will descend in the first 3–6 months of life. Rarely will they descend after the first 6 months.

33. C: Circumcision is not recommended because the foreskin may be needed for repair at a later time. Consult with a pediatric urologist is recommended for optimization of surgical intervention, timing, and outcomes.

34. D: Paraphimosis occurs when the narrow tip of the prepuce is withdrawn behind the glans and constricts the penile shaft, leading to edema of the distal penis, preventing repositioning of the prepuce over the glans.

35. B: For some boys following circumcision the then exposed meatus will rub against the diaper and result in meatal stenosis. Meatal stenosis can also be seen at an older age for a variety of other reasons.

36. D: Testicular torsion typically presents as acute onset, intense pain. Patients often, but not always experience vomiting during the intense pain period.

37. C: Surgical intervention for testicular torsion must occur within 6 hours of the onset to prevent testicular loss.

38. D: Asymptomatic labial adhesions typically resolve with the onset of puberty and the accompanying hormones. Intervention is needed only if symptomatic.

39. A: In cases where labial adhesions are symptomatic or causing other urologic issues, conjugated estrogen cream applied bid is quite successful in resolving adhesions in 2 weeks to 2 months.

40. A: It is rare to see extensive tears of the vaginal wall with genitourinary trauma. Other causes of tearing should be explored.

41. B: Postinfectious glomerulonephritis (PIGN) is the most common cause of acute nephritis in the pediatric population.

42. C: Patients with glomerulonephritis are typically fluid overloaded and have decreased urine output due to varying degrees of renal dysfunction.

43. C: Bicarbonate reabsorption is sometimes dramatically affected in renal tubular acidosis type 1.

44. D: Meatal stenosis results in a narrowed, often pressurized urinary stream that is often deviated right or left depending on the location of the area of stenosis.

45. B: TMP/SMX is the first-line drug of choice for uncomplicated UTIs.

46. B: Cryptorchidism is seen in 3% of term and 30% of preterm infants.

47. B: A downward stream of urine originating from the underside of the glans is always suspicious for hypospadias.

48. A: Proper hygiene, gentle stretching of the foreskin, and circumcision in cases of urinary obstruction are the main management strategies for phimosis.

49. B: Antibiotics are not indicated for the treatment of postinfectious glomerulonephritis.

☐ BIBLIOGRAPHY

American Academy of Pediatrics. (2011). Urinary tract infection: Clinical practice guideline for the diagnosis and management of the initial UTI in febrile infants and children 2–24 months. *Pediatrics, 128*(3), 595–610. Doi 10.1542/peds.2011-1330

American Academy of Pediatrics. (2012). *Red book: 2012 report of the committee on infectious diseases* (29th ed.). Elk Grove Village, IL: Author.

Bakwin, H. (1973). The genetics of enuresis. *Clinics in developmental Medicine, 48/49*, 73–77.

Behrman, R. E., Kliegman, R. M., & Jenson, H. B. (Eds.). (2007). *Nelson textbook of pediatrics* (18th ed.). Philadelphia, PA: W. B. Saunders.

Berkowitz, C. D. (Ed.). (2008). *Pediatrics: A primary care approach* (3rd ed.). Philadelphia, PA: W. B. Saunders.

Bower, W. F., Moore, R. B., Sheperd, R. D., & Adams, A. (1996). The epidemiology of childhood enuresis in Australia. *British Journal of Urology, 78*, 602–606.

Burns, C. E., Dunn, A. M., Brady, M. A., Starr, N. B., & Blosser, C. (Eds.). (2008). *Pediatric primary care* (4th ed.). St. Louis, MO: Elsevier Saunders.

Center for Young Women's Health. (2014, July). Pregnancy: How to have a healthy pregnancy. Retrieved from http://youngwomenshealth.org/2013/07/16/healthy-pregnancy/

Centers for Disease Control and Prevention. (2010). 2010 STD Treatment Guidelines. Retrieved from http://www.cdc.gov/std/treatment/2010/clinical.htm

Centers for Disease Control and Prevention. (2010). Genital warts. Retrieved from http://www.cdc.gov/std/treatment/2010/genital-warts.htm

Centers for Disease Control and Prevention. (2014a). Contraception. Retrieved from http://www.cdc.gov/reproductivehealth/unintendedpregnancy/contraception.htm

Centers for Disease Control and Prevention. (2014b). Recommendations for the Laboratory-Based Detection of *Chlamydia trachomatis* and *Neisseria gonorrhoeae*—2014. Retrieved from http://www.cdc.gov/std/laboratory/2014LabRec/default.htm

Centers for Disease Control and Prevention. (2014c). Syphilis—CDC fact sheet. Retrieved from http://www.cdc.gov/std/syphilis/STDFact-Syphilis-detailed.htm

Centers for Disease Control and Prevention. (2015). Trichomonas—CDC fact sheet. Retrieved from http://www.cdc.gov/std/trichomonas/STDFact-Trichomoniasis.htm

Chand, D. H., & Valentini, R. P. (Eds.). (2011). *Clinicians manual of pediatric nephrology*. Singapore: World Scientific.

Emans, S. J., Laufer, M. R., & Goldstein, D. P. (Eds.). (2011). *Pediatric and adolescent gynecology* (6th ed.). Philadelphia, PA: Lippincott-Raven.

Forsythe, W. I., & Redmond, A. (1974). Enuresis and spontaneous cure rate: Study of 1129 enuretics. *Archives of Disease in Children, 49*, 259–263.

Gearhart, J. P., Rink, R. C., & Mouriquand, P. (Eds.). (2010). *Pediatric urology* (2nd ed.). Philadelphia, PA: Elsevier Saunders.

Goldenberg, D, & Sexton, D. (2014). Disseminated gonococcal infection. Retrieved from http://www.uptodate.com/contents/disseminated-gonococcal-infection?source=search_r

Hatcher, R. A., Trussell, J., Stewart, F., Cates, W., Jr., Stewart, G. K., Guest, F., & Kowal, D. (2007). *Contraceptive technology* (19th ed.). New York, NY: Ardent Media.

Kim, S., Lee, J. W., Park, J., Na, K. Y., Joo, K. W., Ahn, C., . . . Han, J. S. (2004). The urine- blood PCO gradient as a diagnostic index of H(+)-ATPase defect distal renal tubular acidosis. *Kidney International, 66*, 761–767.

Kliegman, R. M., Behrman, R. E., Jenson, H. B., & Stanton, B. M. D. (Eds.). (2007). *Nelson textbook of pediatrics* (18th ed.). Philadelphia, PA: W. B. Saunders.

Kost, K., & Henshaw, S. (2014). *U.S. teenage pregnancies, births and abortions, 2010: National and state trends by age, race and ethnicity*. Guttmacher Institute. Retrieved from https://www.guttmacher.org/pubs/USTPtrends10.pdf

Martin, I. G. (1971). Imipramine pamoate in the treatment of childhood enuresis. *American Journal of Diseases of Children, 122*, 42–47.

Neinstein, L. S. (2008). *Adolescent health care: A practical guide* (5th ed.). Philadelphia, PA: Wolters Kluwer/Lippincott Williams & Wilkins.

Schwartz, G. J., & Al-Awati, Q. (2005). Role of hensin in mediating the adaptation of the cortical collecting duct to metabolic acidosis. *Current Opinion in Nephrology and Hypertension, 14*(4), 383–388.

Yin Sinhoe, J. D., Wong, S., & Yeung, C. K. (2005). Voiding disorders. In D. F. Geary & F. Schaefer (Eds.), *Comprehensive pediatric nephrology* (pp. 587–606). Philadelphia, PA: Mosby.

Zieman, M. (2015). Overview of contraception. UpToDate. Retrieved from http://www.uptodate.com/contents/overview-of-contraception

Zitelli, B., McIntire, S. C., & Nowalk, A. J. (2012) *Atlas of pediatric physical diagnosis* (6th ed.). Philadelphia, PA: Elsevier.

Author's Note

The older references in this chapter are from the Gearhart, Rink, and Mouriquand textbook, which is a premier textbook in pediatric urology. Experts in this field still consider these to be seminal references on the subjects of imipramine and nocturnal enuresis, and they are still widely cited in the world of pediatric urology.

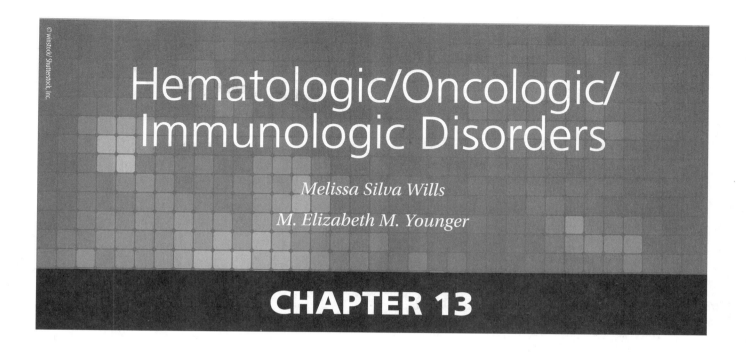

Hematologic/Oncologic/Immunologic Disorders

Melissa Silva Wills

M. Elizabeth M. Younger

CHAPTER 13

❒ ABO INCOMPATIBILITY

- Definition: Incompatibility between the ABO blood group of the fetus and mother (mother is blood type O and baby is A, B, or AB)
- Etiology/Incidence
  1. Occurs in approximately 20% of pregnancies
  2. Approximately 33% of the infants in these pregnancies are Coombs test positive
  3. Approximately 20% of these infants develop significant hyperbilirubinemia and may also develop anemia in the first several weeks of life
- Signs and Symptoms
  1. Mild cases—asymptomatic
  2. Severe cases—yellow discoloration of skin, sclerae, and gums or inside of mouth
- Differential Diagnosis
  1. Physiologic jaundice—most common
  2. Infection
  3. Hyperbilirubinemia of prematurity
  4. Metabolic disorder
- Physical Findings
  1. Jaundice usually occurring within first 24 hours of life; may be present or appear up to a week later
  2. May have hepatosplenomegaly
- Diagnostic Tests/Findings
  1. Blood type—mother usually O; baby A, B, or AB
  2. Coombs test (direct antiglobulin test, or DAT)—positive in approximately 13% of cases
  3. Hemoglobin—moderately low; hemolysis occasionally occurs up to 2 to 3 months
  4. Elevated indirect bilirubin level
  5. Presence of antibodies in infant and maternal serum

- Management/Treatment
  1. Monitor indirect bilirubin levels
  2. Phototherapy if indicated based on bilirubin, gestational, and postdelivery age of neonate
  3. If anemia is severe, may require exchange transfusion

❒ RH INCOMPATIBILITY

- Definition: Incompatibility between the Rh blood group of the mother and fetus (mother is Rh negative and baby is Rh positive)
- Etiology/Incidence: Relatively uncommon; 5% occurrence in first susceptible newborn; becomes more severe with each pregnancy if untreated
- Signs and Symptoms
  1. Causes hemolysis, resulting in anemia and hyperbilirubinemia
  2. In severe cases causes fetal death secondary to fetalis
- Differential Diagnosis
  1. Physiologic jaundice—most common
  2. Anemia secondary to another etiology
  3. Infection
  4. Hyperbilirubinemia of prematurity
  5. Metabolic disorder
- Physical Findings
  1. Jaundice
  2. Hepatosplenomegaly; varies with severity
- Diagnostic Tests/Findings
  1. Blood type—mother Rh negative, baby Rh positive
  2. Direct Coombs test—positive
  3. Hemoglobin—below normal, may be very low; hemolysis often continues up to 3 months
  4. Serum indirect bilirubin—markedly elevated

- Management/Treatment
  1. Mother
     a. Rh isoimmunization screen at first prenatal visit
     b. If mother Rh negative, test father; if father is Rh positive, then the pregnancy is at risk
     c. Risk for problems increases with each pregnancy as antibody levels rise
     d. Administration of Rh immune globulin after any invasive procedure during pregnancy and after the termination of each pregnancy (including any miscarriage and/or abortion)
  2. Infant
     a. Antenatal treatment—once diagnosis has been established, transfusion of fetus with Rh-negative blood
     b. Postpartum treatment
        (1) Phototherapy, with exchange transfusion if indicated by bilirubin level
        (2) Transfusion of packed red blood cells if indicated by hemoglobin level
        (3) Multiple studies have reported on efficacy of administration of gamma globulin, but there is no recommendation for this treatment at this time

☐ NEONATAL HYPERBILIRUBINEMIA

- Definition: An increased amount of bilirubin in the blood; if untreated and bilirubin levels continue to rise, can cause encephalopathy (kernicterus)
- Etiology/Incidence
  1. Unconjugated (indirect) types—may be caused by overproduction of bilirubin, impaired conjugation, transport or uptake of bilirubin
     a. Physiologic hyperbilirubinemia
        (1) Indirect bilirubin 5 to 7 mg/dL
        (2) Usually peaks within 3 to 5 days of life
        (3) Usually resolves within 10 days
        (4) Occurs in approximately 50% of full-term infants
        (5) Higher incidence among preterm infants and low-birth-weight (LBW) infants
        (6) Occurs in approximately 13% of breastfed infants within the 1st week of life (breastfeeding jaundice)
     b. Breastmilk jaundice
        (1) Occurs in approximately 2% of breastfed infants
        (2) Develops after the 7th day of life with maximum bilirubin concentrations of 10 to 30 mg/dL reached during the 2nd to 3rd week of life
        (3) Levels fall rapidly with discontinuation of breastfeeding for 1 to 2 days, after which breastfeeding can resume
     c. Prolonged (nonphysiologic) neonatal hyperbilirubinemia—associated with breastfeeding, maternal diabetes, induced labor, prematurity, Asian ethnicity, and male gender
        (1) Common in infancy
        (2) Less common in older children, but can be associated with hemoglobinopathies and some metabolic syndromes

  2. Conjugated (direct) types—caused by range of pathologic conditions (rare in newborns), including biliary obstruction, infection, drugs (aspirin, acetaminophen), and other metabolic disorders
     a. Direct bilirubin >1.5 to 2 mg/dL
     b. Jaundice in 1st day of life
     c. Total bilirubin >12.9 mg/dL (full-term), >15 mg/dL (preterm)
     d. Persistence >1 week (full term), >2 weeks (preterm)
- Signs and Symptoms: Yellow discoloration of skin, whites of eyes, gums, and oral mucosa
- Differential Diagnosis
  1. Transient neonatal hyperbilirubinemia
     a. Physiologic
     b. Breastfeeding associated
     c. Breastmilk jaundice
  2. Infection
  3. Hepatic disease
  4. Intestinal obstruction
- Physical Findings
  1. Clinical jaundice varies based on bilirubin level—5 mg/dL appears first on head, progresses down chest/abdomen as bilirubin increases; usually at least 15 mg/dL when noted on distal extremities
  2. Hepatosplenomegaly
  3. Edema
- Diagnostic Tests/Findings
  1. Evaluate for pathologic causes for jaundice—sepsis, polycythemia
  2. Coombs test (DAT)
     a. Blood group incompatibilities—DAT usually positive
     b. Membrane disorders, red cell enzyme disorders, bacterial or viral sepsis, drug toxin—DAT usually negative
  3. Bilirubin
     a. Indirect hyperbilirubinemia—unconjugated bilirubin increased
     b. Direct hyperbilirubinemia—conjugated bilirubin increased
     c. Reticulocyte count—may be increased with both indirect or direct
- Management/Treatment: Based on etiology, age of child, and bilirubin level
  1. Indirect (unconjugated) hyperbilirubinemia
     a. Hydration and feeding
     b. Phototherapy
     c. Exchange transfusion
  2. Direct (conjugated) hyperbilirubinemia—treat underlying disease or refer as appropriate

☐ HEMOGLOBINOPATHIES

- Definition: Production of abnormal hemoglobin as a result of inherited genetic mutation in globin genes
- Etiology/Incidence: Incidence associated with specific ethnic groups
  1. Beta (β) thalassemia
     a. β-chain synthesis decreased in β-thalassemia intermedia; absent in β-thalassemia major (Cooley's anemia)

b. Increased but ineffective erythropoiesis

c. Shortened red cell life span

2. Alpha (α) thalassemia

a. Deletion of one or more of the α-globin genes

b. Increased but ineffective erythropoiesis

c. Shortened red cell life span

3. Hemoglobin C and E

a. Amino acid substitution of lysine for glutamic acid

b. Hemoglobin C—carrier state in 2% of African Americans

c. Hemoglobin E—prevalent in populations from Southeast Asia

4. Ethnic groups—individuals of African, Asian, and Mediterranean descent are at highest risk

- Signs and Symptoms

1. β-thalassemia major and intermedia

a. Pale skin or mucous membranes

b. Weakness

c. Characteristic facies (frontal bossing, exposure of frontal teeth, prominence of malar eminences)

2. β-thalassemia minor (trait), α-thalassemia trait, hemoglobin C, hemoglobin E—usually asymptomatic

- Differential Diagnosis

1. Iron-deficiency anemia

2. Lead poisoning

3. Chronic infection

4. Sideroblastic anemia

5. Malignancy

- Physical Findings

1. β-thalassemia major and intermedia

a. Splenomegaly, occasional hepatosplenomegaly

b. Jaundice, usually mild

c. Abnormal facies secondary to extramedullary hematopoiesis—prominence of malar eminences, frontal bossing, depression of bridge of nose, exposure of upper incisors

d. Growth retardation

2. β-thalassemia minor, α-thalassemia trait, and hemoglobin C trait—physical examination normal

3. Hemoglobin C and E—splenomegaly

- Diagnostic Tests/Findings

1. β thalassemia

a. Complete blood count (CBC) with red cell indices

(1) Hemoglobin—decreased

(2) Hypochromia, microcytosis, low mean corpuscular volume (MCV), anisocytosis, target cells

(3) Reticulocyte count—increased

b. Hemoglobin electrophoresis

(1) β⁺ thalassemia

(a) Hemoglobin A (Hgb A)—present

(b) Hgb A_2—increased

(c) Hgb F—normal or slightly increased

(2) β⁰ thalassemia

(a) Hgb A—absent

(b) Hgb A_2—increased

(c) Hgb F—normal or slightly increased

2. β thalassemia (minor or trait)—usually discovered on routine examination or in family investigation

a. CBC with red cell indices

(1) Hemoglobin—slightly decreased (9 to 11 g/dL)

(2) Hypochromic, microcytic cells, target cells, anisocytosis, basophilic stippling, low MCV, low mean corpuscular hemoglobin (MCH), normal red cell distribution width (RDW)

b. Hemoglobin electrophoresis

(1) Hgb A_2—increased

(2) Hgb F—may be mildly elevated

3. α-thalassemia trait

a. CBC with red cell indices

(1) Hemoglobin—may be slightly decreased

(2) Microcytosis, hypochromia

b. Hemoglobin electrophoresis—Hgb Barts on newborn screen; disappears by 1 to 3 months of age (2-gene deletion approximately 2%, 3-gene deletion ~2% to 6%)

4. Hemoglobin C and hemoglobin E

a. CBC with red cell indices

(1) Hemoglobin—may be decreased

(2) Hemoglobin C—target cells, spherocytes, increased reticulocytes

(3) Hemoglobin E—target cells, microcytosis

b. Hemoglobin electrophoresis

(1) Hemoglobin C (Hgb C)—present

(2) Hemoglobin E (Hgb E)—present

- Management/Treatment

1. β-thalassemia major

a. Refer to hematologist

b. Chronic transfusion protocol—to maintain hemoglobin, support growth, and prevent extramedullary hematopoiesis

c. Chelation therapy (deferoxamine) once serum ferritin is greater than 2000 ng/mL; to remove excessive intracellular iron

d. Prophylactic penicillin initiated by 2 months of age, until at least 5 years of age; recommendations for prophylaxis after the age of 5 are equivocal

e. Splenectomy—may reduce transfusion requirements

(1) Postsplenectomy care: All immunizations, including pneumococcal, meningococcal, and annual influenza immunizations as recommended by the Centers for Disease Control and Prevention (CDC); prophylactic penicillin or amoxicillin daily; because of the increased risk for infection with an encapsulated bacteria, any fever greater than 101.5°F (38.5°C) requires immediate evaluation with a physical exam, CBC, and blood culture and administration of a broad-spectrum antibiotic (ceftriaxone)

2. β-thalassemia intermedia

a. Observe hemoglobin

b. Splenectomy may help

3. β-thalassemia minor, a-thalassemia trait, hemoglobin C and E

a. No therapy

b. Genetic counseling

❑ IRON-DEFICIENCY ANEMIA

- Definition: A microcytic, hypochromic anemia caused by inadequate supply of iron, associated with low reticulocyte count and elevated red cell distribution width
- Etiology/Incidence
  1. Causative factors
     a. Deficient dietary intake
     b. Increased demand—growth (low birth weight, prematurity, adolescence, pregnancy), cyanotic congenital heart disease
     c. Blood loss—GI tract is most common site
     d. Malabsorption—rare except for after a bowel resection
  2. Incidence
     a. Most common nutritional deficiency in children
     b. Most common between 8 and 18 months of age and in adolescence, not during early infancy because infants are born with sufficient iron stores to prevent anemia for first 4 to 5 months of life
     c. Higher incidence in lower socioeconomic groups
- Signs and Symptoms: Vary with severity of anemia
  1. Mild anemia—usually asymptomatic
  2. More severe anemia
     a. Fatigue
     b. Irritability
     c. Delayed motor development
     d. Decreased attentiveness, shorter attention span, poor school performance
     e. Eating nonnutrient substances such as ice, plaster, clay, paint, fabric (pica)
- Differential Diagnosis
  1. Hemoglobinopathies
  2. Lead poisoning
  3. Anemia of chronic disease or inflammation
  4. Malignancy
- Physical Findings: Vary with severity of anemia
  1. Mild—normal physical examination
  2. More severe—pallor, tachycardia, systolic murmur, hepatomegaly, congestive heart failure (CHF)
- Diagnostic Tests/Findings
  1. Hemoglobin—falls 2 standard deviations below the mean for age and gender
  2. Peripheral blood smear—hypochromic, microcytic red cells, confirmed by red blood cell (RBC) indices, MCV decreased by two standard deviations below the age-appropriate mean
  3. Wide red cell distribution width (RDW), >17
  4. Serum ferritin—decreased (this is the first value to fall)
  5. Serum iron and iron-binding capacity
     a. Decreased total serum iron
     b. Increased iron-binding capacity (TIBC)
     c. Decreased iron saturation (16% or less)
  6. Free erythrocyte protoporphyrin (FEP)—elevated
- Management/Treatment: According to American Academy of Pediatrics guidelines, children should routinely be screened between the ages of 9 and 12 months, and additionally for child at risk, between 1 and 5 years of life
  1. Nutritional counseling—prevention
     a. Maintain breastfeeding for at least 6 months if possible; supplemental iron drops or iron-fortified cereal by 4 to 5 months of age
     b. If not breastfed, use iron-fortified infant formula until 1 year of age
     c. Use iron-fortified cereals from 6 to 12 months of age
     d. No cow's milk before 1 year of age, then limit to 18 to 24 oz/day
     e. Prescribe 2 to 3 mg/kg/day elemental iron in 1 to 2 doses/day for prophylaxis in low-birth-weight infants
  2. Oral iron medication
     a. Prescribe as elemental iron—3 to 6 mg/kg/day in 1 to 3 doses until hemoglobin normal, then 2 to 3 mg/kg/day for 4 months to replace iron stores. It is best absorbed on an empty stomach
     b. Failure to respond—consider the following reasons in this order:
        (1) Failure or inconsistent administration of medication
        (2) Inadequate iron dose
        (3) Persistent or unrecognized blood loss
        (4) Incorrect diagnosis
        (5) Impaired GI absorption
  3. Parenteral iron dextran—consider for use in cases of noncompliance, severe bowel disease, genuine intolerance, chronic hemorrhage, chronic diarrhea
  4. Packed red cell transfusion—is seldom necessary but may be considered in children who are debilitated or chronically ill and are symptomatic (especially with cardiac dysfunction) or when hemoglobin level is 4 g/dL or less

❑ SICKLE CELL DISEASE

- Definition: A collection of autosomal recessive, recessive genetic disorders characterized by the hemoglobin S variant of the beta-globin gene
- Etiology/Incidence
  1. Hemoglobin S results from a single base pair substitution of valine for glutamic acid at the sixth position of the beta (β) globin gene; this results in distorting of the red blood cells into classic crescent or sickle shapes when deoxygenated; this leads to hemolysis and intermittent episodes of vascular occlusion that can cause tissue ischemia and acute and chronic organ dysfunction
  2. Sickle cell disease occurs in individuals of African, Mediterranean, Indian, and Middle Eastern descent; incidence and clinical severity of sickle cell disease and trait in U.S. African American population is listed in **Table 13-1**

■ **Table 13-1**   Differential Diagnosis and Incidence of Sickle Cell Disease and Sickle Cell Trait in U.S. African Americans

Syndrome (Genotype)	Incidence	Clinical Severity	Hgb (g/dL)[a]	MCV (fl)[a]	Reticulocytes (%)[a]	Newborn Screening[b]	Electrophoresis (%)
Sickle cell anemia (SS)	1:400	Usually marked	6.5–9.5	>80	5–20	FS	S 80–90 F 2–20 A_2 <3.6
Sickle hemoglobin C (SC)	1:1000	Mild to moderate	9.5–13.5	75–95	5–10	FSC	S 45–55 C 45–55
Sickle beta plus ($S\beta^1$) thalassemia	1:4000	Mild to moderate	8.5–12.5	<75	5–10	FSA or FS[c]	S 65–90 A 5–30 F 2–20 A_2 >3.6
Sickle beta zero ($S\beta^0$) thalassemia	1:10,000	Marked to moderate	6.5–9.5	>80	5–20	FS	S 80–92 F 2–10 A_2 > 3.6
Sickle cell trait (AS)	1:10	Asymptomatic	Normal	Normal	Normal	FAS	S 35–45% A 55–65%

[a] Hematologic values are approximate; results apply to older children

[b] Hemoglobins reported in order of quantity (e.g., FSA = F > S > A); F, fetal hemoglobin; S, sickle hemoglobin; C, hemoglobin C; A, hemoglobin A.

[c] Quantity of Hb A at birth; sometimes insufficient to quantitate

Data from American Academy of Pediatrics. (2002). Health super- vision for children with sickle cell disease. Pediatrics, 109(3), 526–535; National Institutes of Health. (2002). Management of sickle cell disease (4th ed.) (NIH Publication No. 20– 2117) Washington, DC: U.S. Government Printing Office.

- Signs and Symptoms: Vary with associated problems (see **Table 13-2**)
  1. Infection (peak incidence between 1 and 3 years of age)
     a. Fever
     b. Malaise
     c. Anorexia
     d. Poor feeding
  2. Acute painful events—"pain crisis," "vaso-occlusive crisis"
     a. Pain—most often in bones, but can occur in any part of body (chest, stomach, hands or feet, back, etc.); in children <2 years of age usually in hands or feet (dactylitis)
     b. Swelling—sometimes seen at site of pain
     c. Low-grade fever—sometimes occurs
  3. Splenic sequestration
     a. Weakness
     b. Irritability
     c. Unusual sleepiness
     d. Paleness
     e. Large spleen
     f. Fast heart rate
     g. Pain in the left side of the abdomen—does not always occur
  4. Aplastic crisis (is associated with parvovirus B19)
     a. Pale
     b. Malaise
     c. Headache
     d. Fever
     e. Mild upper respiratory infection symptoms

■ **Table 13-2**   Associated Problems of Sickle Cell Disease

Hemolysis
Chronic anemia
Jaundice
Aplastic crisis[a]
Cholelithiasis
Delayed growth and sexual maturity
Vaso-occlusion
Recurrent acute pain (e.g., dactylitis, musculoskeletal, abdominal)
Functional asplenia (bacterial infections[a])
Splenic sequestration[a]
Acute chest syndrome[a]
Stroke[a]
Hyposthenuria and enuresis
Papillary necrosis of kidneys
Chronic nephropathy
Priapism
Avascular necrosis of humeral heads, femoral heads
Proliferative retinopathy
Leg ulcers

[a] Potential cause of mortality.

Data from American Academy of Pediatrics. (2002). Health super- vision for children with sickle cell disease. Pediatrics, 109(3), 526–535; National Institutes of Health. (2002). Management of sickle cell disease (4th ed.) (NIH Publication No. 20– 2117) Washington, DC: U.S. Government Printing Office.

- Differential Diagnosis
  1. Infection
     a. Septicemia
     b. Meningitis
     c. Pneumonia
     d. Osteomyelitis
     e. Viral illness
  2. Acute painful events
     a. Bone pain
        (1) Bone infarct
        (2) Osteomyelitis
        (3) Rheumatoid arthritis
        (4) Leukemia
     b. Abdominal pain
        (1) Cholelithiasis—right upper quadrant
        (2) Splenic infarct—left upper quadrant
        (3) Functional abdominal pain
        (4) Gas pain
  3. Splenic sequestration—chronic splenomegaly
  4. Aplastic crisis—other viral illnesses
- Physical Findings: Presence variable
  1. Jaundice
  2. Cardiac murmur
  3. Splenomegaly
  4. Pallor
- Diagnostic Tests/Findings (see Table 13-1)
  1. Prenatal diagnosis—can be done by analysis of DNA obtained through chorionic villus sampling (9 to 11 weeks of gestation) or amniocentesis (11 to 17 weeks of gestation)
  2. Usual diagnostic hemoglobin electrophoresis and hematologic results in infants and adults with sickle cell disease are presented in Table 13-1
  3. "Sickle prep" (metabisulfite solution)—should not be used as diagnostic test because it does not distinguish among sickle cell anemia, other forms of sickle cell disease, and sickle cell trait or common interacting hemoglobinopathies such as Hgb C or thalassemia
  4. Splenic sequestration
     a. Hemoglobin—below baseline (steady state)
     b. Platelets—decreased
  5. Aplastic crisis
     a. Hemoglobin—below steady state
     b. Reticulocyte count— >1.0%
- Management/Treatment
  1. Maintenance care—should be directed toward prevention of complications and crisis precipitating factors, and include:
     a. Administer all immunizations as recommended by American Academy of Pediatrics, including pneumococcal, meningococcal, and annual influenza vaccines
     b. In addition to routine conjugate pneumococcal (PCV 13) vaccine received at 2, 4, 6, and 12 or 15 months, should also receive polysaccharide pneumococcal vaccine (PPV) every 5–10 years as recommended by current guidelines

     c. Prophylactic penicillin—initiate by 2 months of age and continue until at least 5 years of age
     d. Family education regarding increased risk of infection due to functional asplenia and the need to seek medical attention promptly for evaluation of febrile illnesses
     e. Because of the increased risk for infection with encapsulated bacteria, any fever greater than 101.5°F (38.5°C) requires immediate evaluation with a physical exam, CBC and blood culture, and a dose of broad-spectrum antibiotics (ceftriaxone). (A second dose of ceftriaxone may be necessary if the preliminary blood culture is not back.)
     f. For children with frequent complications, daily hydroxyurea has been reported to decrease hemolysis and painful crises
  2. Acute painful events
     a. Prevention
        (1) Education regarding factors that may precipitate painful events, i.e., dehydration, hypoxia, fever, exposure to extreme temperatures
        (2) Education regarding how to manage mild to moderate pain and how to recognize signs of serious problems
     b. Home-based management
        (1) Analgesia as prescribed
        (2) Nonpharmacologic treatment such as hydration, heat, localized massage
     c. Emergency department (ED) management
        (1) Parenteral fluids
        (2) Analgesics
     d. Inpatient management—if pain not reduced by ED management
        (1) Hydration
        (2) Parenteral analgesics, and concomitant NSAID
  3. Acute exacerbations of anemia (such as aplastic crisis)
     a. Packed red blood cell transfusions may be indicated
     b. Exchange transfusions may be indicated for severe vaso-occlusive associated problems (e.g., organ failure, stroke)
  4. Management of other problems associated with sickle cell disease—consultation with or referral to a pediatric hematologist
  5. Frequent reinforcement of education regarding fever and pain management
  6. Anticipatory guidance regarding physiologic and psychological effects of chronic illness and sickle cell disease specifically, including delayed growth, enuresis, school attendance, physical endurance
  7. Genetic counseling
  8. School problems/learning disabilities: Some children have attention or learning problems believed to be related to stroke, severe anemia, or silent cerebral infarction. Problems may include memory issues, difficulties

with focusing or sustaining attention, organization, and/or processing issues. Developmental or neurocognitive assessments and intervention may be necessary

☐ LEAD POISONING (PLUMBISM)

- Definition: A chronic disease caused by the accumulation of toxic amounts of lead in the body; the CDC defines lead poisoning as a whole blood lead level (BLL) >5 µg/dL; however, no safe blood level of lead has been identified
- Etiology/Incidence
  1. Ingestion or inhalation of lead or lead compounds; transplacental transmission may also occur
  2. Sources of lead exposure
     a. Lead-based paint in older homes built prior to 1978, especially housing built before 1950
     b. Lead-contaminated soil and dust from automobile emissions (decreasing with use of lead-free gasoline)
     c. Lead-contaminated drinking water (lead or lead-soldered pipes)
     d. Certain lead-containing folk remedies, cosmetics, and other imported items
     e. Lead-based paint on imported items, including toys
  3. Highest prevalence among poor, inner-city children living in older, deteriorating housing
  4. Children between 1 and 3 years of age are at greatest risk
  5. Lead toxicity may contribute to neurobehavioral, as well as cognitive, morbidities of childhood
- Signs and Symptoms: Vary with degree of exposure
  1. Low-level exposure may be asymptomatic
  2. Mild acute lead poisoning—resembles gastroenteritis, e.g., anorexia, nausea, vomiting, constipation or diarrhea, and abdominal pain; other possible symptoms are sleep disturbances, metallic taste in mouth, limb pain, and headaches
  3. Severe lead poisoning—lethargy, difficulty walking, tingling, cognitive impairment, personality changes
  4. Approximately 90% of children with lead poisoning will have pica
- Differential Diagnosis
  1. Iron-deficiency anemia
  2. α or β thalassemia
  3. Metabolic disorders
  4. Developmental or cognitive delay secondary to other causes
- Physical Findings
  1. May see bluish discoloration of gingival border (Burtonian blue lines)
  2. Bradycardia
  3. Neuropathy
  4. Papilledema
  5. Ataxia

- Diagnostic Tests/Findings
  1. CDC revised guidelines (2012) recommend universal screening for Medicaid children and those deemed at risk, such as those who live in homes built before 1978
  2. Whole blood lead level test (BLL) by categories of risk
     a. Lead level <5 µg/dL—not considered blood poisoning
     b. Lead level >5 µg/dL—elevated BLL that is associated with lead-exposure hazards
     c. Lead level of 10 to 19 µg/dL—venipuncture confirmation within 1 week–1 month
     d. Lead level of 20 to 44 µg/dL—venipuncture confirmation within 1 week to 1 month
     e. Lead level of 45 to 69 µg/dL—diagnostic venous blood testing within 24 to 48 hours
     f. Lead level of >70 µg/dL—medical emergency, retest immediately
- Management/Treatment
  1. Follow-up BLL monitoring—frequency determined based on whether low or high risk and BLL obtained
     a. Lead level <5 µg/dL—if high risk, retest in 6 months; if low risk, no further testing needed
     b. Lead level of 5 to 14 µg/dL—at risk for lead poisoning, early follow-up within 3 months; if follow-up level is 15 to 19 µg /dL or higher 3 months apart, retest every 1 to 2 months until results <15 µg/dL for at least 6 months, then every 6 to 9 months
     c. Lead level of 15 to 19 µg/dL—at risk for lead poisoning, early follow-up within 2 months; if follow-up level is >15, retest every 1 to 2 months until results <15 /dL for at least 6 months, then every 3 months until child is 36 months old; include educational and nutritional counseling
     d. Lead level of 20 to 44 µg/dL—early follow-up in 1 to 2 months for BLLs 20 to 24 µg/dL; 2 weeks to 1 month for BLLs 25 to 44 µg/dL, retest every 1 to 2 months until results <15 µg/dL for at least 6 months, then every 3 months until child is 36 months old
     e. Lead level of 45 to 69 µg/dL—early follow-up as soon as possible; retest every month until results <15 µg/dL for at least 6 months, then every 3 months until child is 36 months old
     f. Lead level of >70 µg/dL—early follow-up as soon as possible, retest every month until results <15 µg/dL for at least 6 months, then every 3 months until child is 36 months old
  2. For blood lead level >20 µg/dL, refer for further medical evaluation, interventions, and follow-up
     a. Test for iron deficiency
     b. Environmental assessment and removal of known sources of lead in environment
     c. Medical evaluation for symptoms and possible pharmacologic management
        (1) Lead level of 20 to 44 µg/dL may require pharmacologic management

(2) Lead level of >45 µg/dL will require chelation therapy with Succimer

(3) Parenteral chelation with dimercaprol and calcium edentate is used for cases of lead encephalopathy

3. Primary prevention
   a. Outreach education regarding nutrition and avoidance of exposure
   b. Assessment of potential risk with specific environmental and health questions during routine well-child visits

□ GLUCOSE-6-PHOSPHATE DEHYDROGENASE (G-6-PD) DEFICIENCY

- Definition: X-linked or autosomal recessive genetic disorder in which activity of red cell enzyme G-6-PD is decreased or absent, causing hemolytic anemia
- Etiology/Incidence
  1. Lack of G-6-PD decreases the ability to deal with oxidative stress and results in hemolysis; episodes of hemolysis may be induced by the following:
     a. Drugs such as aspirin, sulfonamides, antimalarials, nitrofurans
     b. Fava beans, ingestion or exposure to pollen from the bean's flower (occurs in Mediterranean- and Canton-type deficiencies)
     c. Infection (in more susceptible individuals)
  2. Many genetic variants described with altered enzyme levels, which determine the severity of disorder
     a. A type—enzyme activity decreases with age of cell; hemolyzes only old RBCs; occurs in 11% African American males, 2% African American females
     b. Mediterranean type—associated with severe deficiency of enzyme
     c. Canton type—severe disease in Asians
  3. Most common among individuals of African, Mediterranean, or Asian descent
- Signs and Symptoms: Symptoms develop 24 to 48 hours after ingestion of substance having oxidant properties
  1. Weakness
  2. Pale appearance
  3. Severe case
     a. Blood in the urine
     b. Yellow discoloration of skin, whites of eyes, and gums or inside of mouth
- Differential Diagnosis
  1. Other causes of hemolytic anemia
  2. Hemoglobinopathies
- Physical Findings
  1. Hyperbilirubinemia in infants—usually associated with Mediterranean and Canton individuals
  2. Older children are asymptomatic between episodes of hemolysis
- Diagnostic Tests/Findings
  1. G-6-PD fluorescence-based screen (may give false negative)

2. Red blood cell indices during or just after hemolytic episode
   a. Heinz bodies present
   b. Fragmented cells and blister cells
3. Reticulocytosis
4. Hemoglobin—usually normal between episodes of hemolysis; may be decreased in Mediterranean or Canton types
5. Acute self-limiting hemolytic anemia with hemoglobinuria (type A variant)
6. Acute life-endangering hemolysis often leads to acute renal failure (all other variants)

- Management/Treatment
  1. Generally mild symptoms require minimal intervention
  2. Identification and avoidance of foods and drugs that cause hemolysis
  3. Transfusion for severe hemolysis
  4. Genetic counseling; routine screening not generally recommended

□ BLEEDING DISORDERS

Hemophilia

- Definition: Bleeding disorder caused by congenital deficiency or absence of clotting factor VIII or IX
- Etiology/Incidence
  1. Hemophilia A (factor VIII deficiency, classical hemophilia)
     a. Third most common X-linked disorder, but 20% to 30% are caused by spontaneous mutation
     b. Approximately 1:5000 male births
     c. 10% to 30% of patients develop antibodies against the functional activity of factor VIII
     d. Factor VIII deficiency is four times more common than factor IX deficiency
  2. Hemophilia B (factor IX deficiency, Christmas disease)—X-linked disorder, with 20% to 30% spontaneous mutation
- Signs and Symptoms: Vary based on severity of factor deficiency
  1. Easy bruising at injection sites
  2. Prolonged bleeding following circumcision—not all severe hemophiliacs bleed postcircumcision
  3. Excessive bruising after child begins walking
  4. Mucosal bleeding
  5. Prolonged bleeding in any part of the body
  6. May have pain at the site of the bleed
  7. Hemarthrosis (bleeding into joint spaces)
- Differential Diagnosis
  1. Thrombocytopenia
  2. Von Willebrand disease
  3. Vitamin K deficiency
  4. Disseminated intravascular coagulation (DIC)
  5. Child abuse
- Physical Findings: Signs of bleeding, including ecchymosis, swelling and pain in joints, and prolonged bleeding from lacerations or injections

- Diagnostic Tests/Findings
  1. Prenatal diagnosis—can be done by fetal blood sampling (periumbilical blood sampling [PUBS]) (18 to 20 weeks gestation) through fetoscopy or by analysis of DNA obtained through chorionic villus sampling (9 to 11 weeks gestation) or amniocentesis (11 to 17 weeks gestation)
  2. Diagnostic test—direct assay of plasma factor activity level for hemophilia A and B—see **Table 13-3**
  3. Screening tests
     a. Activated partial thromboplastin time (APTT)—prolonged
     b. Prothrombin time (PT)—normal
     c. Bleeding time (not indicated)—normal
- Management/Treatment
  1. Collaborative interdisciplinary approach facilitated by regional hemophilia treatment center
  2. Factor replacement therapy
     a. Hemophilia A—factor VIII concentrate intravenously
     b. Hemophilia B—factor IX concentrate intravenously
     c. Approximately 10% to 15% of patients develop anti-factor antibodies (inhibitors) and may require other therapy (immune tolerance)
  3. Prophylaxis
     a. Primary prophylaxis—regular infusions of factor VIII or IX given to prevent joint hemorrhage and bleeding episodes
     b. Secondary prophylaxis—started after a joint has developed hemarthrosis; used to prevent further bleeding into the joint
  4. Desmopressin intranasally or intravenously—for mild FVIII deficiency
  5. Antifibrinolytic therapy—for oral mucosal bleeds
  6. Physical therapy—for musculoskeletal bleeds
  7. Surgery—synovectomy, arthroscopic or with use of isotopes
  8. Anticipatory guidance regarding developmental issues such as discipline, child care, and schooling
  9. Genetic counseling

■ **Table 13-3** Relationship of Factor Levels to Severity of Clinical Manifestations of Hemophilia A and B

Type	% Factor VIII/IX	Type of Hemorrhage
Severe	<1	Spontaneous hemarthrosis and deep-tissue hemorrhages
Moderate	1–5	Gross bleeding following moderate trauma; some hemarthrosis; rare spontaneous hemorrhage
Mild	6–25	Severe hemorrhage only following moderate to severe trauma or surgery

Von Willebrand Disease (VWD)

- Definition: An inherited hemorrhagic disorder characterized by defective primary hemostasis and due to a quantitative or qualitative abnormality in Von Willebrand factor (VWF)
- Etiology/Incidence
  1. The most common congenital bleeding disorder
  2. Six variant types
     a. Type 1—mild to moderate decrease in VWF
     b. Type 2A—decreased platelet-dependent VWF
     c. Type 2M—affinity to platelet binding
     d. Type 2B—rare form
     e. Type 2N—an abnormal VWF molecule that does not bind with factor VIII
     f. Type 3—severe bleeding disorder with deficits in primary and secondary hemostasis
  3. Affects at least 1% of the population, but only 10% are symptomatic
- Signs and Symptoms: Great variation in frequency, severity, and bleeding manifestations
  1. Nosebleeds
  2. Bleeding gums
  3. Heavy menstrual bleeding
  4. Prolonged oozing from cuts
  5. Increased bleeding after trauma or surgery
- Differential Diagnosis
  1. Thrombocytopenia
  2. Hemophilia
  3. Vitamin K deficiency
  4. Disseminated intravascular coagulation
- Physical Findings
  1. Easy bruising
  2. Multiple sites of bruising
  3. Oozing or bleeding at trauma or surgical site
- Diagnostic Tests/Findings
  1. Variation in findings by specific type of VWD as well as within same patient over time
  2. Bleeding time—usually prolonged
  3. Von Willebrand factor—usually decreased or absent
  4. Von Willebrand factor antigen—usually decreased or absent
  5. Blood group—VWF factor decreased in type O
- Management/Treatment
  1. Desmopressin acetate—used to treat bleeding complications or as preoperative preparation for Type 1; contraindicated in the treatment of Type 2B
  2. Alternative treatment if desmopressin not indicated or effective—treatment with factor concentrates with intact Von Willebrand factor should be considered
  3. Antifibrinolytic agents—particularly effective in areas where fibrinolysis appears to contribute to bleeding, i.e., in mucous membranes (nose, mouth, throat, and menorrhagia), trauma, and dental procedures and surgery

Immune Thrombocytopenia (ITP; Idiopathic Thrombocytopenic Purpura)

- Definition: Immune-mediated disorder characterized by production of antiplatelet antibodies
  1. Primary ITP—isolated thrombocytopenia (platelet count of 100,000/mm³ in the absence of other causes)
  2. Chronic ITP—disease lasting for more than 12 months; approximately 10% of children with ITP
  3. Persistent ITP—disease that continues between 3 and 12 months from diagnosis
  4. Secondary ITP—all forms of immune-mediated thrombocytopenia except primary ITP
- Etiology/Incidence
  1. Autoimmune disorder, sometimes related to sensitization by viral infection
  2. 4 to 5.3 cases/100,000 children
  3. Most prevalent during early- to mid-childhood and in older adults, although it affects all ages
  4. Chronic ITP—more common in children >7 years of age; more prevalent in females (3:1 ratio)
- Signs and Symptoms
  1. Bruising
  2. Nosebleeds
  3. Bleeding of gums and lips
  4. Petechiae
  5. Menorrhagia
  6. Child appears well, except for signs of bleeding
- Differential Diagnosis
  1. Thrombocytopenia of other causes
     a. Bone marrow infiltration
     b. Septicemia
     c. Aplastic anemia
  2. Disseminated intravascular coagulation
  3. Hemolytic uremic syndrome
  4. Acute leukemia
  5. Evan's syndrome (thrombocytopenia and hemolytic anemia)
  6. In young children
     a. Congenital amegakaryocytic thrombocytopenia-absent radius syndrome
     b. Wiskott-Aldrich syndrome (only in males)
  7. In older children, especially those with chronic symptoms
     a. Systemic lupus erythematosus
     b. HIV infection
     c. Lymphoma
- Physical Findings
  1. Petechiae, purpura, and ecchymoses
  2. Hemorrhages in mucous membranes
  3. Pallor usually not present (unless there has been significant bleeding)
  4. Splenomegaly
- Diagnostic Tests/Findings
  1. CBC—generally the only required test
  2. Hemoglobin—normal or slightly reduced with prior bleeding; can drop with bruising only

3. Platelet count
   a. <20,000/mm³ (diagnostic for acute ITP); often <10,000/mm³
   b. <100,000/mm³ for <12 months (diagnostic for chronic ITP)
4. White blood cell (WBC) count—normal; if active infection, may have increased neutrophils, lymphocytes, or atypical mononuclear cells
5. Bleeding time test (unnecessary)—always abnormal if platelets <50,000 mm³
6. Blood group and Rh analysis should be performed if treatment with anti-D immunoglobin is considered
- Management/Treatment: Controversial
  1. Acute ITP
     a. Treatment usually not indicated if platelet count >50,000/mm³
     b. Treatment usually considered if platelet count <20,000/mm³, especially with extensive cutaneous (and especially mucosal) bleeding or if protective environment cannot be ensured
     c. Acute bleeds, especially intracranial or gastrointestinal, may require therapy
     d. Pharmacologic management: Inhibit autoantibody-mediated platelet clearance
        (1) High-dose corticosteroids (prednisone 2 to 5 mg/kg/day orally for 1 to 3 weeks) with slow wean
        (2) Intravenous gamma globulin (IVIG)—1 g/kg/day for 1 to 3 days is the treatment of choice for acute bleeds; platelets may also be given but are short-lived
        (3) Anti-D immunoglobulin—50 mcg/kg
  2. Chronic ITP
     a. Referral to a hematologist
     b. Pharmacologic management—when thrombocytopenia worsens during viral illness or prior to elective surgery, prednisone or IVIG can be administered
     c. Prolonged use of high-dose steroids should be avoided, but low-dose maintenance steroids may be necessary for a prolonged period of time
     d. Antacids, H₂ blockers, or proton pump inhibitors need to be taken with steroids
     e. Monoclonal antibody therapy (e.g., rituximab) may be effective in refractory ITP
     f. Splenectomy—treatment of choice when disease is severe or symptomatic
     g. Postsplenectomy care
        (1) All immunizations, including meningococcal, pneumococcal polysaccharide, and annual influenza vaccines, should be given as per CDC recommendations
        (2) Prophylactic penicillin or amoxicillin daily
        (3) Because of the increased risk for infection with an encapsulated bacteria, any fever greater than 101°F requires immediate evaluation with a physical exam, CBC, blood culture, and a dose of ceftriaxone

3. Patient/family education
   a. Avoid all competitive contact sports that could result in head trauma or ruptured spleen
   b. Avoid aspirin and aspirin-containing medications and nonsteroidal anti-inflammatory drugs (NSAIDs)
   c. Monitor for signs of occult bleeds
   d. Seek medical care if signs of bleeding are noted

☐ CANCERS

Leukemias

- Definition: A malignant neoplasm of bone marrow characterized by proliferation of immature white cells
- Etiology/Incidence
  1. Etiology is usually unknown
  2. Accounts for 25% to 30% of all childhood cancers
  3. Acute leukemia constitutes 97% of all childhood leukemias and includes most common types
     a. Acute lymphoblastic leukemia (ALL)—75%; survival rate is 60% to 85%
     b. Acute myeloid leukemia (AML)—20%; survival rate is 40% to 60%
  4. Chronic myelogenous leukemia (CML) constitutes 3% of childhood leukemia
  5. 1 per 25,000 of population up to 14 years of age
  6. Peak incidence between 2 and 5 years of age
- Signs and Symptoms
  1. Fatigue, headache
  2. Bruising
  3. Fever
  4. Nosebleeds
  5. Bone pain, limp
- Differential Diagnosis
  1. Chronic infections such as Epstein-Barr virus (EBV) or cytomegalovirus (CMV)
  2. ITP
  3. Transient erythroblastopenia of childhood
  4. Aplastic anemia
  5. Juvenile rheumatoid arthritis
- Physical Findings
  1. Pallor
  2. Purpura, ecchymosis
  3. Organomegaly (liver/spleen)
  4. Lymphadenopathy
  5. Testiculomegaly
  6. Cranial nerve palsy
- Diagnostic Tests/Findings
  1. CBC—presence of blast cells on peripheral blood smear highly suggestive; requires confirmatory bone marrow examination
  2. Bone marrow aspiration/biopsy (required for diagnosis)—bone marrow replaced by >25% blasts, usually 80% to 100%
- Management/Treatment
  1. Combination chemotherapy (protocol length 1 to 3½ years)

2. Central nervous system (CNS) prophylaxis
   a. Radiation therapy (for high-risk patients)
   b. Combined intrathecal chemotherapy
3. Patient/family education regarding side effects of therapy, anticipatory guidance on coping
4. For relapse on therapy, bone marrow transplant is recommended; relapse after therapy is completed, a second course of chemotherapy may provide cure; for AML, bone marrow transplant is treatment of choice; if no suitable donors available, standard chemotherapy is utilized
5. Primary care considerations—immunizations held while on therapy and resume 6 to 12 months after therapy completed (institution-specific policy); sibling immunizations not affected; fever on therapy requires CBC/blood cultures and hospitalization for neutropenia with fever or if patient has central line
6. Long-term follow-up for delayed effects of chemotherapy and/or radiation

Neuroblastoma

- Definition: A neoplasm of the primitive cells from the sympathetic nervous system
- Etiology/Incidence
  1. Etiology—possible genetic factors; familial predisposition
  2. Most common malignancy in infancy, accounts for 8–10% of all childhood malignancies
  3. Metastases at onset in 70% to 75% of cases
  4. 10 per 1 million live births annually
  5. Survival rate for patients:
     a. Low risk—95%
     b. Intermediate risk—greater than 90%
     c. High risk—35%
- Signs and Symptoms: Dependent on primary site, presence of metastases
  1. Listlessness
  2. Poor feeding
  3. Pale
  4. Weight loss
  5. Abdominal pain
  6. Weakness
  7. Irritability
- Differential Diagnosis
  1. Trauma
  2. Lymphadenopathy
  3. Leukemia
  4. Lymphoma
  5. Wilms' tumor
- Physical Findings: Related to site of primary tumor
  1. Lymph node enlargement
  2. Hepatomegaly
  3. Abdominal or flank mass
  4. Proptosis and periorbital ecchymoses (raccoon eyes)
  5. Scalp or skin nodules (often bluish coloration)

- Diagnostic Tests/Findings
  1. CT or MRI scan to determine site and location of any suspected masses
  2. Tissue biopsy to confirm diagnosis
  3. Bone marrow aspiration and biopsy to evaluate for infiltrating tumor
  4. Serum or urine catecholamine levels—may be increased and followed for tumor response/recurrence
- Management/Treatment: Based on stage and site of tumor
  1. Treatment of emergent symptoms
  2. Surgery
     a. Staging excision of tumor
     b. Evaluation of treatment (early stage/low-risk disease may have observation only)
  3. Radiation therapy (for resistant/relapse disease)
  4. Combination chemotherapy
  5. Bone marrow transplant for high-risk disease
  6. Immune-mediated therapy—a monoclonal antibody that targets the neuroblastoma antigen GD2
  7. Patient/family education regarding side effects of therapy
  8. Anticipatory guidance on developmental issues such as sleep, toileting, discipline, and child care
  9. Primary care considerations—immunizations held while on therapy and resume 6 to 12 months after therapy completed (institution-specific policy); sibling immunizations not affected; fever on therapy requires CBC/blood cultures and hospitalization for neutropenia with fever or if patient has central line
  10. Long-term follow-up for delayed effects of chemotherapy and/or radiation

Retinoblastoma

- Definition: Congenital malignant intraocular tumor
- Etiology/Incidence
  1. Abnormal fetal neural crest cell maturation
     a. Hereditary—germinal mutation (40%); siblings and subsequent offspring at risk
     b. Acquired—somatic mutations
  2. Most common intraocular childhood tumor
     a. 1:10,000 live births
     b. Accounts for 2.5–4% of all childhood cancers; 15% childhood cancer mortality
  3. Majority diagnosed before 5 years—are bilateral; usually diagnosed in first year
  4. Prognosis varies with age and tumor staging
     a. Overall survival rate >90%
     b. High incidence of secondary malignancies with hereditary form may limit survival into 3rd or 4th decade of life
- Signs and Symptoms
  1. Squinting
  2. Eyes turning inward or outward
  3. Painful red eye

- Differential Diagnosis
  1. Cataract
  2. Retinal detachment
  3. Persistent hyperplastic primary vitreous
  4. Coloboma
  5. Retinopathy of prematurity
- Physical Findings
  1. Leukocoria—yellow-white pupillary reflex (most common presentation)
  2. Strabismus
  3. Hyphema may be present
- Diagnostic Tests/Findings
  1. Fundoscopic examination under anesthesia or sedation—findings may include:
     a. Creamy-pink mass
     b. White avascular tumor mass
  2. CT of the orbits to evaluate extent of tumor and to determine optic nerve or bony structure involvement
  3. MRI to assess for optic nerve invasion
  4. Ultrasound to detect calcification and the proximity of the tumor
- Management/Treatment: Determined by stage and extent of disease
  1. Surgery
     a. Resection
     b. Enucleation
  2. Radiation therapy
  3. Photocoagulation (laser therapy)
  4. Cryotherapy
  5. Chemotherapy—advanced or recurrent disease
  6. Patient/family education regarding side effects of therapy
  7. Anticipatory guidance on developmental issues such as sleep, toileting, discipline, and child care; refer family to genetic specialist
  8. Long-term follow-up for recurrence or delayed effects of chemotherapy or radiation

Lymphomas

- Definition: Malignant disorders characterized by proliferation of cells, usually restricted to lymphoid cells but may be found in bone marrow; includes Hodgkin's (HL) and non-Hodgkin's (NHL) lymphomas
- Etiology/Incidence
  1. Etiology unknown—possible etiologic factors
     a. Genetic predisposition
     b. Environmental exposures
     c. Epstein-Barr virus
     d. Immunologic disorders
  2. Third most common childhood cancer—10%
     a. HL—1:100,000 children
        (1) Peak age—bimodal age incidence curve
           (a) 15 to 35 years
           (b) >50 years
        (2) Survival—related to patient age and gender, disease subtype, and extent of involvement

(a) Overall survival is 85% to 95%

(b) Children younger than 10 years have a 10-year disease-free survival of 92%

(c) Adolescents have a 10-year disease-free survival of 86%

b. NHL—15:100,000 children between 5 and 10 years

(1) Peak age—5 to 15 years

(2) Survival—85% to 95% in localized disease and 70% to 90% in advanced stage disease

- Signs and Symptoms
  1. Hodgkin's
     a. Painless, firm swelling of lymph nodes
     b. Fatigue (B symptom)
     c. Decreased appetite and unintentional weight loss (>10% weight loss; B symptom)
     d. Unexplained fever (B symptom)
     e. Drenching night sweats (B symptom)
  2. Non-Hodgkin's
     a. Asymptomatic if not disseminated
     b. Difficulty swallowing, breathing, or cough
     c. Swelling in neck, face, upper extremities
     d. Lymphadenopathy
     e. Abdominal pain
- Differential Diagnosis
  1. Other malignancy
  2. Lymphadenopathy associated with infection
- Physical Findings
  1. Hodgkin's
     a. Affected nodes—often fixed, firm, nontender, discrete; cervical and supraclavicular areas most common
     b. Splenomegaly
  2. Non-Hodgkin's
     a. Similar to Hodgkin's
     b. May vary depending on degree of involvement
     c. Distended neck veins and respiratory distress due to superior vena cava syndrome
- Diagnostic Tests/Findings
  1. Hodgkin's
     a. Chest radiograph—to explore possibility of mediastinal involvement and examine airway patency
     b. PET scan to evaluate disease involvement
     c. Biopsy—tumor giant cells (Reed-Sternberg cells)
     d. CBC with red cell indices
        (1) Hemoglobin—decreased
        (2) Normocytic and normochromic or microcytic and hypochromic
     e. Serum ferritin—increased
     f. Erythrocyte sedimentation rate (ESR)—increased
  2. Non-Hodgkin's—tissue diagnosis necessary before treatment is started, findings vary based on specific histologic type
     a. Isolated peripheral nodes—excisional or fine-needle biopsy
     b. Mediastinal mass—thoracotomy or mediastinoscopy, parasternal fine-needle biopsy, or thoracentesis (if associated pleural effusion)

c. Abdominal mass—open biopsy usually necessary

d. Lactic dehydrogenase (LDH)—increased due to rapid cell turnover

- Management/Treatment: Plan developed based on stage of involvement
  1. Multiagent chemotherapy
  2. Radiation
  3. Patient/family education regarding side effects of therapy
  4. Primary care considerations—immunizations held while on therapy and resume 6 to 12 months after therapy completed (institution-specific policy); sibling immunizations not affected; fever on therapy requires CBC/blood cultures and hospitalization for neutropenia with fever or if patient has central line
  5. Long-term follow-up for delayed effects of chemotherapy or radiation

Wilms' Tumor (Nephroblastoma)

- Definition: A primary malignant renal tumor
- Etiology/Incidence
  1. Etiology unknown; predisposing factors
     a. Genetic factors
        (1) Associated with aniridia, Beckwith-Wiedemann syndrome
        (2) Familial predisposition
     b. Environmental factors—chronic chemical exposure (hydrocarbons, lead)
  2. 6% of all cancer in children; 9:1 million Caucasian children/year
  3. Equal frequency in males and females
  4. 78% diagnosed between 1 and 5 years of age; peak incidence 3 to 4 years of age
  5. Survival rate—70% to 90%
- Signs and Symptoms
  1. May be asymptomatic
  2. Abdominal mass—usually nonpainful
  3. Occasionally abdominal pain
  4. Malaise, fever, loss of appetite
  5. Vomiting
  6. Blood in urine
- Differential Diagnosis
  1. Hydronephrosis
  2. Polycystic kidney disease
  3. Neuroblastoma
  4. Rhabdomyosarcoma
  5. Lymphoma
- Physical Findings
  1. Abdominal mass—usually asymptomatic
  2. Hypertension
  3. Associated congenital anomalies—aniridia, hemihypertrophy, genitourinary anomalies
- Diagnostic Tests/Findings
  1. CBC and urine analysis for anemia, hematuria
  2. CT of abdomen to evaluate:
     a. Presence and function of opposite kidney

b. Evidence of bilateral involvement
c. Evidence of involvement of blood vessels of tumor
d. Lymph node involvement
e. Liver involvement
3. Abdominal and pelvic ultrasound—may indicate that the tumor is intrarenal
4. Chest radiograph, CT of chest to evaluate for metastasis to lung

- Management/Treatment: Plan developed based on stage of involvement
  1. Surgical excision
     a. If unilateral—complete nephrectomy
     b. If bilateral—nephrectomy of more involved site, excision biopsy/partial nephrectomy of smaller lesion in remaining kidney; or no surgery with radiation
  2. Multiagent chemotherapy
  3. Radiation therapy
  4. Patient/family education regarding side effects of therapy
  5. Primary care considerations—immunizations held while on therapy and resume 6 to 12 months after therapy completed (institution-specific policy); sibling immunizations not affected; fever on therapy requires CBC/blood cultures and hospitalization for neutropenia with fever or if patient has central line
  6. Long-term follow-up for disease recurrence and delayed effects of chemotherapy and radiation

Osteosarcoma

- Definition: A solid tumor of the bone in which malignant spindle cell stroma produce osteoid; most common form of bone cancer in children
- Etiology/Incidence
  1. Etiology unknown
  2. Associated factors
     a. Genetic factors and family predisposition
        (1) Increased risk with hereditary retinoblastoma
        (2) Increased risk with chromosome 13 abnormalities
     b. Environmental factors—increased risk associated with previously irradiated bone
     c. Increased risk with taller children (may appear during growth spurt)
  3. Incidence—approximately 400 children and adults younger than 20 years of age
     a. Peak incidence during adolescent growth spurt between 15 and 19 years of age
     b. Male incidence slightly higher than female incidence
- Signs and Symptoms
  1. Local pain
  2. Local swelling
  3. Mass at end of long bone
  4. Decreased range of motion
- Differential Diagnosis
  1. Growing pains
  2. Trauma

3. Osteomyelitis
4. Tendonitis
5. Septic arthritis
6. Leukemia (due to bone pain)
- Physical Findings
  1. Pain over involved site
  2. Palpable mass
  3. Swelling
  4. Decreased range of motion of affected extremity
- Diagnostic Tests/Findings
  1. Radiograph of affected bone
  2. MRI of affected bone
  3. Biopsy of area
  4. CT of the chest and bone scan or PET scan to evaluate for metastatic disease
- Management/Treatment
  1. Multiagent chemotherapy
  2. Surgery—amputation/limb-sparing surgery
  3. Patient and family education regarding side effects of therapy, anticipatory guidance on coping
  4. Primary care considerations—immunizations held while on therapy and resume 6 to 12 months after therapy completed (institution-specific policy); sibling immunizations not affected; fever on therapy requires CBC/blood cultures and hospitalization for neutropenia with fever or if patient has central line
  5. Long-term follow-up for delayed effects of chemotherapy

☐ IMMUNE DEFICIENCIES

- Definition: Primary or secondary disorders of immune function classified according to the arm of the immune system affected:
  1. Humoral (B cell) immunodeficiencies
  2. Cellular (T cell) immunodeficiencies
  3. Combined B and T cell immunodeficiencies
  4. Complement deficiencies
  5. Phagocyte disorders

Severe Combined Immunodeficiency (SCID)

- Definition: Absence of T- and B-cell function leading to susceptibility to infection from virtually any pathogen
- Etiology/Incidence: Approximately 45% are X-linked; occurs in 1:100,000 live births
- Signs and Symptoms:
  1. Failure to thrive
  2. Diarrheal illness (may develop rotavirus after vaccination)
  3. Morbilliform rash
  4. Opportunistic infections
  5. Infections from any pathogen
- Differential Diagnosis: Other immune deficiency
- Physical Findings: Specific to manner of presentation

- Diagnostic Findings
  1. Lymphopenia
  2. T-cell cytopenia
  3. Absence of lymphocyte function on proliferation assays
- Management/Treatment
  1. Bone marrow transplant is the standard of care
  2. Enzyme replacement *if* the cause is adenosine deaminase deficiency
  3. SCID undiagnosed or untreated is universally fatal within the first year of life
  4. Profound lymphopenia in an infant is *always* SCID until proven otherwise

Common Variable Immunodeficiency (CVID)

- Definition: Hypogammaglobulinemia and impaired antibody responses to antigenic stimuli
- Etiology/Incidence: Genetic defect or predisposition
- Signs and Symptoms (specific to manner of presentation): Recurrent or severe bacterial infections of respiratory tract (sinusitis, otitis, pneumonia) or skin (cellulitis, abscesses); initial presentation may be autoimmune disease (e.g., inflammatory bowel disease, cytopenia) or lymphoreticular cancer
- Differential Diagnosis: Other immune deficiencies
- Physical Findings: Specific to manner of presentation
  1. Sinusitis—fever, periorbital edema, tenderness on percussion over sinuses, mucosal thickening or opacification on sinus CT, purulent drainage from sinuses
  2. Otitis—hyperemic, opaque, bulging tympanic membrane with poor mobility
  3. Pneumonia—retractions, flaring nares, diminished breath sounds, crackles on affected side
  4. Cellulitis or abscess—erythema, swelling, purulent drainage
- Diagnostic Tests/Findings: Serum immunoglobulin
  1. IgG—decreased
  2. IgA—may be decreased
  3. IgM—may be decreased
- Management/Treatment: Immunoglobulin replacement therapy given intravenously every 3–4 weeks or subcutaneously given daily up to every 2 weeks. Replaces IgG, *not* IgA or IgM

Transient Hypogammaglobulinemia of Infancy

- Definition: Maturational delay in humoral immune development
- Etiology/Incidence
  1. Etiology: maturational delay
  2. Incidence is unknown; it is suspected many children are undiagnosed
- Signs and Symptoms
  1. Recurrent infections

  2. Infections with unusual pathogens
  3. Infections recalcitrant to appropriate antibiotic therapy
- Differential Diagnosis: Other immune deficiencies
- Physical Findings: Specific to manner of presentation
- Diagnostic Tests/Findings—hypogammaglobulinemia and nonprotective antibody levels in response to vaccination
- Management/Treatment
  1. Serial monitoring of immunoglobulin levels (should trend upward)
  2. Revaccination may be necessary
  3. Hold live viral vaccines until immunocompetence is demonstrated
  4. Prophylactic antibiotics may be considered
  5. Immunoglobulin replacement is rarely necessary

X-Linked Agammaglobulinemia (Bruton's Tyrosine Kinase, or BTK)/ Agammaglobulinemia

- Definition: Panhypogammaglobulinema caused by absence of B cells secondary to the lack of Bruton's tyrosine kinase, the enzyme that enables B-cell precursors to become mature B cells
- Etiology/Incidence
  1. X-linked disorder (85%); 15% is autosomal recessive
  2. Affected infants usually asymptomatic for 3 to 6 months due to passive transmission of maternal antibodies, then show frequent infections and failure to thrive
  3. Incidence 1–9/1,000,000
- Signs and Symptoms (specific to manner of presentation): Recurrent or severe infections
- Differential Diagnosis: Other immune deficiencies
- Physical Findings: Specific to manner of presentation
  1. Signs and symptoms of infection (fever, elevated WBC count, etc.)
  2. Absence of or very small tonsils (B-cell organ)
- Diagnostic Tests/Findings
  1. Serum immunoglobulins
     a. IgG—undetectable or decreased
     b. IgA—undetectable or decreased
     c. IgM—undetectable or decreased
  2. Blood T and B lymphocytes—B cells absent or decreased and T cells normal
  3. Absence of protective levels of antibody to vaccine antigens
- Management/Treatment
  1. Immunoglobulin replacement therapy (either intravenous or subcutaneous)
  2. Prophylactic antibiotics are rarely necessary
  3. Appropriate antibiotic therapy for infections; infections should be treated aggressively and the causative pathogen should be identified if possible
  4. *Live viral vaccines are contraindicated*; routine vaccination is not necessary once immunoglobulin replacement therapy has been initiated

Thymic Hypoplasia (DiGeorge Syndrome), 22q11 Deletion Syndrome

- Definition: Autosomal dominant disorder characterized by syndrome features (phenotype is extremely variable, even in the same family):
  1. Congenital heart disease (particularly midline defects, e.g., atrial septal defect [ASD]/ventricular septal defect [VSD], truncus arteriosus, tetralogy of Fallot)
  2. Abnormal facies
  3. Thymic aplasia or hypoplasia (T-cell immunodeficiency)
  4. Cleft lip or palate
  5. Hypocalcemia
  6. Adolescent onset schizophrenia
- Etiology/Incidence
  1. Dysmorphogenesis occurs during embryogenesis, resulting in hypoplasia of the thymus and parathyroid glands
  2. Occurs in males and females equally
  3. Presentation usually results from cardiac failure or, after 24 to 48 hours of age, from hypocalcemia
  4. Sometimes diagnosed during cardiac surgery when no thymus is found in mediastinum
  5. May have increased susceptibility to viral, fungal, and bacterial infections dependent on the degree of immunodeficiency present
- Signs and Symptoms: Specific to manner of presentation
- Differential Diagnosis: Other immune deficiencies
- Physical Findings
  1. Characteristic features—hypertelorism; shortened lip frenulum; low-set, notched pinnae; and nasal cleft
  2. Other physical findings—specific to manner of presentation
- Diagnostic Tests/Findings
  1. Routine chest radiograph may reveal absent thymus
  2. Labs
     a. Lymphopenia
     b. Decreased T cells
     c. Hypocalcemia
- Management/Treatment
  1. Prophylactic antibiotics are rarely necessary
  2. Antibiotic therapy for infections
  3. Thymus transplant if patient is athymic
  4. Bone marrow transplant if patient is athymic
  5. May require immunoglobulin replacement therapy if there is an associated humoral deficiency present

Wiskott-Aldrich Syndrome (WAS)

- Definition: X-linked disorder characterized by small, dysfunctional platelets, eczema, and abnormal B- and T-cell function
- Etiology/Incidence
  1. X-linked recessive inheritance; carrier detection is possible
  2. Caused by a mutation in the WAS gene, resulting in decreased expression of WASp protein
  3. Incidence—approximately 4:1 million male births
- Signs and Symptoms
  1. Neonatal—bloody diarrhea, prolonged bleeding from circumcision
  2. Later—eczema and frequent infections
  3. Patients have increased risk for autoimmune disease (specifically cytopenias) and lymphoreticular malignancies
- Differential Diagnosis: Usually made during neonatal period due to thrombocytopenia
  1. Other causes of bleeding
- Physical Findings: Specific to manner of presentation
- Diagnostic Tests/Findings
  1. Small platelet size (decreased MPV) is pathognomonic
  2. Thrombocytopenia
  3. May have lymphopenia, decreased T-cell numbers
  4. May have hypogammaglobulinemia or impaired antibody responses
- Management/Treatment
  1. Aggressive treatment of eczema to prevent suprainfection
  2. Platelet transfusions for acute bleeding
  3. Immunoglobulin replacement therapy if humoral defect present
  4. Appropriate, aggressive antibiotic therapy for infections
  5. Splenectomy—for treatment of thrombocytopenia
     a. Conjugate or polysaccharide pneumococcal vaccines as recommended by the American Academy of Pediatrics; should be given at least 2 weeks or longer prior to surgery, if possible, to increase the likelihood of eliciting a protective antibody response
     b. Prophylactic penicillin 250 mg bid for at least 1 to 2 years postsplenectomy
     c. Increased risk for bacterial infections postsplenectomy—for fever (T >101.5°F) immediate referral for blood culture and empiric parenteral antibiotics against encapsulated organisms
  6. Bone marrow transplant if human leukocyte antigens (HLA)-matched donor is available

Chronic Granulomatous Disease (CGD)

- Definition: Neutrophil oxidative burst dysfunction: phagocytes go to sites of infection but are unable to produce hydrogen peroxide and other chemicals needed to kill pathogen
- Etiology/Incidence: 70% are X-linked, 30% are autosomal recessive caused by four other mutations
- Signs and Symptoms: Infections of any organ (skin, bones, liver, lungs, lymph nodes) caused by catalase-producing organisms. Frequent pathogens include *Staphylococcus aureus*, *Serratia marcescens*, *Burkholderia*, and *Aspergillis*
- Differential Diagnosis:
  1. Infection without underlying immunodeficiency
  2. Infection in setting of a humoral immunodeficiency

- Physical Findings: consistent with underlying infection (fever, pain, inflammation, elevated neutrophil count with or without a PMN predominance), lymphadenopathy
- Diagnostic Tests/Findings: Nitroblue tetrazolium test or dihydrorhodamine test; both demonstrate failure of oxidative burst
- Treatment/Management
  1. Interferon gamma subcutaneously three times/week
  2. Staph prophylaxis with twice daily trimethoprim/sulfamethoxazole
  3. Fungal prophylaxis with daily itraconazole
  4. Aggressive treatment of infections; pathogen should be identified if possible; may need prolonged treatment courses to eradicate pathogen
  5. Affected children should not be allowed to play where there is the possibility of mold contamination (areas of new construction, landscaping with mulch, swimming in fresh water)

❑ QUESTIONS

Select the best answer.

1. Baseline management of all neonates with ABO incompatibility includes:
   a. Phototherapy
   b. Serial monitoring of bilirubin and hemoglobin levels
   c. Exchange transfusion
   d. Simple transfusion of packed red blood cells

2. Which of the following is not associated with Rh incompatibility?
   a. Mother Rh negative, baby Rh positive
   b. Mother Rh positive, baby Rh negative
   c. More severe in subsequent sensitized pregnancies
   d. Hemolysis may occur up to 6 weeks or more

3. Clinical jaundice of the distal extremities would be noted at a bilirubin level of:
   a. <5 mg/dL
   b. 5 mg/dL
   c. 10 mg/dL
   d. >15 mg/dL

4. β-chain synthesis is absent in:
   a. β-thalassemia minor
   b. β-thalassemia intermedia
   c. β-thalassemia major
   d. α-thalassemia trait

5. Which of the following is most often associated with hemoglobin C?
   a. Growth retardation
   b. Hepatosplenomegaly
   c. Usually asymptomatic
   d. Frontal bossing

6. Diagnostic findings inconsistent with β thalassemia would be
   a. Hemoglobin—normal
   b. Reticulocytes—increased
   c. Hgb A_2 > 3.6
   d. Hypochromia, microcytosis

7. Asplenic children are at increased risk for which of the following?
   a. Bacterial infections
   b. Fungal infections
   c. Viral infections
   d. Parasites

8. Which of the following is not considered preventive management for iron-deficiency anemia?
   a. Iron-fortified cereal from 6 to 12 months of age
   b. Iron-fortified formula until 6 months of age
   c. No cow's milk until 1 year of age
   d. If breastfeeding, supplemental iron drops or iron-fortified cereal by 4 to 5 months of age

9. The expected clinical severity of hemoglobin sickle C disease (Hgb SC) is:
   a. Asymptomatic
   b. Marked to moderate
   c. Mild to moderate
   d. Severe

10. The expected hemoglobin range for sickle cell anemia is:
    a. 6.5–9.5 g/dL
    b. 13.5–16.5 g/dL
    c. 8.5–12.5 g/dL
    d. 9.5–13.5 g/dL

11. Prophylactic penicillin should be initiated in children with sickle cell anemia by:
    a. 3 years of age
    b. 12 months of age
    c. 2 to 3 months of age
    d. 9 months of age

12. Which of the following blood lead levels is not considered lead poisoning?
    a. <5 μg/dL
    b. 10–14 μg/dL
    c. >15 μg/dL
    d. >25 μg/dL

13. Which of the following is not a precipitating factor for hemolysis in G-6-PD deficiency?
    a. Drugs
    b. Exposure to extreme temperatures
    c. Ingestion of fava beans
    d. Infection

14. What type of hemorrhage would be expected with severe factor VIII deficiency?
    a. Severe hemorrhage following moderate to severe trauma
    b. Gross bleeding following mild to moderate trauma
    c. Gynecologic hemorrhage
    d. Spontaneous hemarthrosis

15. A newly circumcised infant is still bleeding an hour after the circumcision. Your differential diagnosis would include all except:
    a. Hemophilia
    b. Sickle cell anemia
    c. Von Willebrand disease
    d. Wiskott-Aldrich syndrome

16. Which of the following medications should be avoided in a child with ITP?
    a. Decongestants
    b. Aspirin
    c. Acetaminophen
    d. Sulfa drugs

17. A 5-year-old is brought to the clinic. Her mother reports that she has been lethargic and has been running a low-grade fever for about 2 weeks. Physical examination reveals no significant findings other than pallor and lymphadenopathy. A complete blood count reveals decreased hematocrit, neutropenia, and thrombocytopenia. The practitioner's next action should be to:
    a. Prescribe a broad-spectrum antibiotic and ferrous sulfate
    b. Instruct parents on the appropriate use of acetaminophen to treat the child's fever
    c. Reassure parents that their daughter's signs and symptoms are indicative of a viral infection
    d. Refer child to a pediatric hematologist/oncologist for further evaluation

18. A 1-day-old child is evaluated in the newborn nursery for a fever. A CBC reveals a WBC count of 18 K/mm³ with a differential of 82% PMNs, 4% lymphs, 9% monos, 3% eo's, and 2% bands. Which of the following would be highest on your list of differential diagnoses?
    a. Necrotizing enterocolitis (NEC)
    b. Maternally transmitted bacterial infection (e.g., group B Strep)
    c. Severe combined immunodeficiency (SCID)
    d. TORCH infection

19. Which of the following tests is required to diagnose leukemia?
    a. CBC with differential
    b. Bone marrow aspiration/biopsy
    c. Chest radiograph
    d. Biopsy of an enlarged lymph node

20. Which of the following is not included as part of the initial therapy for ALL?
    a. Chemotherapy
    b. Radiation therapy
    c. Bone marrow transplant
    d. Intrathecal chemotherapy

21. Which malignancy is associated with genitourinary anomalies?
    a. Acute lymphocytic leukemia
    b. Chronic myelogenous leukemia
    c. Osteosarcoma
    d. Wilms' tumor

22. Which of the following statements is true about immunizations during treatment of childhood cancer?
    a. Children continue to receive immunizations as usual.
    b. Immunizations are not given during active chemotherapy.

c. Only live vaccines are held during active chemotherapy.
d. No family member should be immunized while the child is receiving chemotherapy.

23. The peak incidence of osteosarcoma is:
    a. 4–7 years of age
    b. 8–11 years of age
    c. 12–14 years of age
    d. 15–19 years of age

24. Which of the following types of infection is not associated with humoral immunodeficiencies such as common variable immunodeficiencies?
    a. Sinusitis
    b. Pneumonia
    c. Urinary tract infection
    d. Cellulitis

25. Which of the following diagnostic findings is consistent with X-linked agammaglobulinemia?
    a. IgG—normal
    b. B cells—decreased
    c. T cells—decreased
    d. IgA—normal

26. Which of the following characteristics is not a feature of DiGeorge syndrome?
    a. Hypertelorism
    b. Cleft palate
    c. Cardiac defects
    d. Frontal bossing

27. The diagnostic finding that is pathognomonic for Wiskott-Aldrich syndrome is:
    a. Absent B cells
    b. Small platelets (low mean platelet volume)
    c. CD4 cytopenia
    d. Decreased hemoglobin

28. Management of a patient with a splenectomy does not include:
    a. Pneumococcal vaccines at least 2 weeks prior to surgery
    b. Prophylactic penicillin
    c. Blood culture and parenteral antibiotics for febrile illnesses
    d. Treating fever with antipyretics only and observing for resolution

☐ ANSWERS AND RATIONALES

1. B: Only 20% of infants with ABO incompatibility require acute intervention; these interventions are based on the degree of hyperbilirubinemia or anemia present.

2. B: Incompatibility issues occur only if the infant is Rh positive and the mother is negative.

3. D: Jaundice proceeds in a progressive fashion, starting on the head, down to the chest and abdomen, and appears on the extremities only when the bilirubin is >15 mg/dL.

4. C: β-chain synthesis is absent only in β-thalassemia major; it is decreased or impaired in the other thalassemic conditions.

5. C: Hemoglobin C is considered a minor hemoglobinopathy that is usually picked up as an incidental finding on hemoglobin electrophoresis.

6. A: Hemoglobin is generally decreased in patients with β thalassemia.

7. A: Bacterial infections, particularly those with encapsulated organisms, can be life-threatening in asplenic children.

8. B: If not breastfeeding, iron-fortified formula is recommended until 12 months of age.

9. C: Sickle cell C is generally considered to be a milder form of the disease.

10. A: Higher hemoglobins are associated with sickle cell C or sickle thal; those with sickle cell trait have normal hemoglobins.

11. C: Penicillin prophylaxis is critical because of the risk of potential life-threatening infection with encapsulated bacteria.

12. A: The CDC defines lead poisoning as lead levels greater than 10 µg/mL.

13. B: Extreme temperatures (either heat or cold) are not factors in precipitating episodes of hemolysis in children with G-6-PD.

14. D: Spontaneous hemorrhage or hemarthrosis can occur in patients with untreated severe factor VIII deficiency disease.

15. B: Sickle cell anemia does not usually cause acute bleeding problems; thrombocytopenia and clotting problems are associated with the other conditions.

16. B: Aspirin can cause bleeding problems in people without thrombocytopenia; aspirin and nonsteroidal anti-inflammatory drugs (NSAIDs) should be avoided in people with low platelet counts.

17. D: An abnormality of more than one formed element of the blood (red blood cells, white blood cells, or platelets) may indicate aplastic anemia (bone marrow dysfunction) or cancer and should be evaluated by a specialist.

18. C: Although all the conditions are possible, this child's profound lymphopenia gives him a diagnosis of severe combined immunodeficiency (SCID); immediate lymphocyte subset evaluation should be undertaken. He should be treated as though he has SCID until it is proven that he does not.

19. B: The diagnosis of leukemia is made by a bone marrow examination that shows a homogeneous infiltration of leukemic blasts replacing normal marrow elements.

20. C: Chemotherapy (oral, IV, and intrathecal) is typically the first line of treatment, with radiation sometimes added. Bone marrow transplantation is rarely used as initial treatment for leukemia because most patients are cured with chemotherapy alone. It is considered for initial treatment in patients with very high risk acute lymphoblastic leukemia (ALL).

21. D: Wilms' tumor is also known as nephroblastoma and is a cancer of the kidneys.

22. B: Cancer chemotherapy suppresses immune response. Therefore, immunizations should be withheld during chemotherapy because they are likely to be ineffective. Non-live-virus immunizations may be resumed 6 months after therapy is completed. Live virus immunizations may be resumed 12 months after therapy is completed.

23. D: Osteosarcoma incidence peaks during the growth spurt of adolescence, between 15 and 19 years of age, with males slightly more likely to be affected than girls.

24. C: Urinary tract infections (UTIs) are not generally problematic for these patients; the most frequent infections are sinopulmonary infections as well as cellulitis and abscesses.

25. B: B-cell precursors in children with X-linked agammaglobulinemia (XLA) cannot grow into mature B cells; decreased or absent levels of IgG, IgA, and IgM are present. Cellular immunity (T cells) is not affected.

26. D: Dysmorphia associated with DiGeorge syndrome includes hypertelorism, low-set ears, and not frontal bossing. Congenital heart disease and cleft lip and palate are associated syndromic features.

27. B: Patients with Wiskott-Aldrich syndrome (WAS) have small, dysfunctional platelets; they are not always profoundly thrombocytopenic. B-cell and T-cell numbers vary.

28. D: Asplenic patients are at risk for the development of potentially life-threatening illness secondary to infection with encapsulated organisms. They need vaccine and antibiotic prophylaxis, and any febrile illness needs to be immediately evaluated with a physical exam, complete blood count, and blood culture. Additionally, a dose of ceftriaxone should be given if the patient appears toxic.

☐ BIBLIOGRAPHY

Abdelaziz, Y. E., Harb, A. H., Hisham, M. N., Bruder, S., Oh, W., & Whitley, R. (Eds.). (2014). *Textbook of clinical pediatrics* (2nd ed.). New York, NY: Springer Berlin Heidelberg.

American Academy of Pediatrics. (2012). *Red book online*. Retrieved from http://aapredbook.aappublications.org/

American Academy of Pediatrics Subcommittee on Hyperbilirubinemia. (2004). Management of hyperbilirubinemia in the newborn infant 35 or more weeks of gestation. *Pediatrics*, *114*(1), 297–316.

Baggott, C. R., Kelly, K. P., Fochtman, D., & Foley, G. V. (Eds.). (2011). *Nursing care of the child and adolescents with cancer* (4th ed.). Glenview, IL: Association of Pediatric Hematology/Oncology Nurses.

Behrman, R. E., Kliegman, R. M., & Jensen, H. B. (Eds.). (2007). *Nelson textbook of pediatrics* (18th ed.). Philadelphia, PA: W. B. Saunders.

Burns, C. E., Dunn, A. M., Brady, M. A., & Starr, N. B. (2012). *Pediatric primary care* (5th ed.). Philadelphia, PA: Elsevier Saunders.

Centers for Disease Control and Prevention. (2012). *Low level lead exposure harms children: A renewed call for primary prevention report of the Advisory Committee on Childhood Lead Poisoning Prevention.* Atlanta, GA: Author.

Centers for Disease Control and Prevention. (2014). *Managing elevated blood lead levels among young children: Recommendations from the Advisory Committee on Childhood Lead Poisoning Prevention.* Atlanta, GA: Author.

Centers for Disease Control and Prevention. (2014). Newborn screening. Retrieved from http://www.cdc.gov/newbornscreening

Fioredda, F., Cavillo, M., Banov, L., Plebani, A., Timitilli, A., & Castagnola, E. (2009). Immunizations after the elective end of antineoplastic chemotherapy in children. *Pediatric Blood Cancer, 52*(2), 165–168.

Hay, W. W., Levin, M. J., Deterding, R., & Abzug, M. (Eds.). (2014). *Current pediatric diagnosis and treatment* (19th ed.). Stamford, CT: McGraw-Hill/Appleton & Lange.

Imbach, I., Kuhne, T., & Arceci, R. (Eds.). (2006). *Pediatric oncology: A comprehensive guide.* Heidelberg, Germany: Springer.

Jackson, P. L., & Vessey, J. A. (Eds.). (2009). *Primary care of the child with a chronic condition* (5th ed.). St. Louis, MO: Mosby

Kavanagh, P. L., Sprinz, P. G., Vinci, S. R., Bauchner, H., & Wang, C. J. (2011). Management of children with sickle cell disease: A comprehensive review of the literature. *Pediatrics, 128*(6), e1553–e1571.

Kumar, R., & Carcao, M. (2013). Inherited abnormalities of coagulation: Hemophilia, Von Willebrand disease, and beyond. *Pediatric Clinics of North America, 69*(6), 1419–1441.

Lanzkowsky, P. (2010). *Manual of pediatric hematology and oncology* (5th ed.). New York, NY: Churchill Livingstone.

Nathan, P., Patel, S., Dilley, K., Goldsby, R., Harvey, J., Jacobsen, C., & Armstrong, F. (2007). Guidelines for identification of, advocacy for, and intervention in neurocognitive problems in survivors of childhood cancer: A report from the Children's Oncology Group. *Archives of Pediatrics & Adolescent Medicine, 161*(8), 798–806.

Neunert, C., Lim, W., Crowther, M., Cohen, A., Solberg, L., Jr., & Crowther, M. S. (2011). American Society of Hematology 2011 evidence-based practice guideline for immune thrombocytopenia. *Blood, 117*(16), 4190–4207.

Newman, T. B., Kuzniewicz, M. W., Liljestrand, P., Wi, S., McCulloch, C., & Escobar, G. J. (2009). Numbers needed to treat with phototherapy according to American Academy of Pediatrics guidelines. *Pediatrics, 123*(5), 1352–1359.

Pizzo, P. A., & Poplack, D. G. (Eds.). (2011). *Principles and practice of pediatric oncology* (6th ed.). Philadelphia, PA: Lippincott.

Quinn, C. T. (2013). Sickle cell disease in childhood: From newborn screening through transition to adult medical care. *Pediatric Clinics of North America, 60*(6), 1363–1381.

Sullivan, K. E., & Stiehm, E. R. (2014). *Stiehm's immune deficiencies.* London, England: Elsevier.

Tepoele, E., Tissing, W., Kamps, W., & de Bont, E. (2009). Risk assessment in fever and neutropenia in children with cancer: What did we learn? *Critical Reviews in Oncology/Hematology, 72*(1), 45–55.

World Health Organization. (2010). *Childhood lead poisoning.* Geneva, Switzerland: WHO Document Production Services.

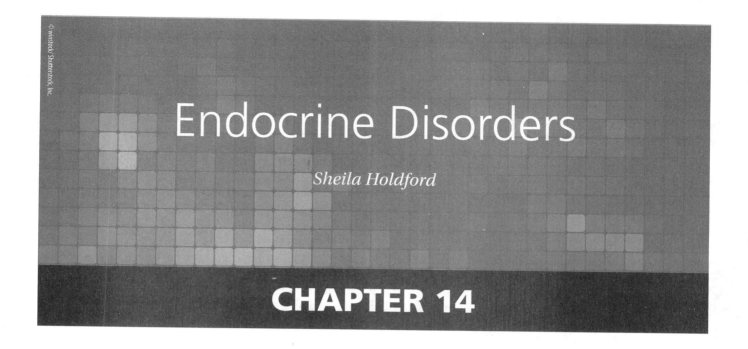

© winstock/Shutterstock, Inc.

Endocrine Disorders

Sheila Holdford

CHAPTER 14

☐ THYROID DISORDERS

Hypothyroidism

- Definition
  1. Congenital vs. acquired (based on timing of disorder)
     a. Congenital can cause severe mental retardation unless treated early; newborn screening can identify hypothyroid infants by 3 weeks of age, allowing early treatment to avoid the effects of severe neurologic devastation
     b. Acquired may have onset within first year of life, usually onset occurs in childhood or adolescence
  2. Primary, secondary, tertiary (based on site of disorder)
     a. Primary disease or disorder of thyroid gland (thyroid gland failure)
     b. Secondary disease or disorder of the pituitary gland that compromises thyroid gland function
     c. Tertiary disease or disorder of the hypothalamus compromises thyroid gland function
- Etiology/Incidence (most common acquired endocrinopathy)
  1. Congenital hypothyroidism
     a. Absence (athyreosis) or underdevelopment (dysgenesis) of ectopic gland most common
     b. Inherent dysfunction in transport or assimilation of iodine, or in synthesis or metabolism of thyroid hormone (e.g., thyroid enzyme defects, familial dyshormonogenesis)
     c. Maternal disease adversely affecting fetal thyroid development and function (prenatal exposure to iodine-containing or goitrogenic drugs and agents, e.g., propylthiouracil [PTU], methimazole, iodines;

maternal exposure to radioactive iodine; placental crossing of maternal antibodies to fetal thyroid gland)
     d. Iodine deficiency causing endemic goiter and cretinism
     e. Hypothalamic or pituitary disorder (e.g., pituitary agenesis, anencephaly)
     f. Affects 1 infant in every 4000 live births, female-to-male ratio 2:1
     g. Higher incidence in Hispanic and Native American infants
     h. Higher incidence in areas with endemic iodine deficiency
     i. Higher incidence in women, affecting 2% of women and 0.2% of men
  2. Acquired hypothyroidism
     a. Chronic lymphocytic thyroiditis (Hashimoto's, autoimmune) most common cause beyond perinatal period; often with positive family history; two types: goitrous (more common) and atrophic
     b. Late manifestation of congenital absence, underdevelopment (dysgenesis), or atrophy of thyroid gland
     c. Late manifestation of congenital defects in synthesizing or metabolizing thyroid hormone
     d. Ablation of thyroid through medical procedures (e.g., surgery, irradiation, radioactive iodine)
     e. Exposure to iodine-containing drugs and agents; drug-induced (e.g., antithyroid drugs, excessive iodide, lithium, cobalt); exposure to naturally occurring goitrogens in foods, water pollutants
     f. Disease of hypothalamus or pituitary (e.g., pituitary tumors, trauma), rare; child will show other signs of hypothalamic or pituitary disease

313

g. Endemic goiter from nutritional iodide deficiency—most common thyroid disease worldwide

3. Hypothyroidism, depending on cause, may be a permanent or transient disorder

4. Severity, compensated or uncompensated hypothyroidism reflects the ability to maintain normal T_4

- Signs and Symptoms
  1. Affects multiple systems; many nonspecific, insidious signs and symptoms; severity depends on age of onset and degree of thyroid deficiency; symptoms vary for infants vs. children
  2. May be familial history of thyroid and pituitary diseases; may have maternal prenatal history of thyroid disease or ingestion of antithyroid medications or foods
  3. May be associated with other autoimmune disease or syndromes (e.g., Down, Turner's, type 1 diabetes)
  4. Neonates/infants
     a. Infants may have no obvious symptoms during 1st month of life
     b. History of lethargy, poor feeding, prolonged physiologic hyperbilirubinemia elevated bilirubin (>10 mg/dL at 3 days of age)
     c. May be postmature; increased birth weight (>4000 g)
  5. Older infants, children, adolescents
     a. History of poor growth, intolerance to cold, poor appetite, constipation
     b. Mental and physical sluggishness, developmental delay
- Differential Diagnosis
  1. Differentiate primary hypothyroidism due to intrinsic thyroid gland defects from secondary thyroid deficiency caused by pituitary or hypothalamic disorders
  2. Congenital thyroxine-binding globulin (TBG) deficiency is a normal variant of thyroid physiology; TBG deficiency is defined as low T_4 with normal thyroid-stimulating hormone (TSH) and free T_4; both TBG is low and T_3 uptake is elevated
  3. "Euthyroid sick syndrome" seen in small or sick newborns or in children with acute or chronic severe illnesses, surgery, trauma, or malnutrition; commonly have low T_3; normal, low, or free T_4; and normal TSH
- Physical Findings
  1. Affects multiple systems; severity of findings depends on age of onset and degree of thyroid deficiency; no findings are entirely sensitive or specific
  2. Neonates/infants
     a. Prolonged jaundice; poor feeding
     b. Growth deceleration
     c. Hypothermia, skin mottling
     d. Large fontanels, especially posterior; wide sutures, hirsute forehead, coarse facial features, dull expression, facial edema, nasal discharge, macroglossia
     e. Normal, slightly enlarged or goitrous thyroid gland; if thyroid ectopic, may see mass at base of tongue or in midline of neck

f. Hoarse cry

g. Axillary, prominent supraclavicular fat pads

h. Respiratory distress in term infant

i. Bradycardia (<100 beats/min)

j. Distended or protuberant abdomen, umbilical hernia, constipation

k. Lumbar lordosis, hypotonia

3. Infants, children, and adolescents
   a. Low energy level, increased weight for height, myxedema with hypothyroidism of long duration
   b. Linear growth retardation or growth deceleration; delayed bone maturation, dentition, tooth eruption
   c. Decreased concentration, memory impaired, developmental delay, poor motor coordination, dull appearance
   d. Delayed puberty, occasionally precocious puberty or pseudoprecocity; menstrual disorders
   e. Skin cool, dry, pale, gray, mottled, thickened, increased pigmentation, carotenemia
   f. Hair dry, brittle; lateral thinning of eyebrows
   g. Possible enlarged thyroid gland (goiter); may feel cobblestone-like
   h. Galactorrhea, constipation
   i. Myopathy, muscular hypertrophy, poor muscle tone; prolonged relaxation phase of deep tendon reflexes (DTRs)
   j. Delayed bone age
   k. If advanced hypothyroidism and myxedema, may be "chubby" and have periorbital edema

- Diagnostic Tests/Findings
  1. Newborn screening for congenital hypothyroidism is routine in all 50 states
     a. Abnormal newborn screen—repeat thyroid screen for confirmatory diagnosis with thyroid-stimulating hormone (TSH) and thyroxine (T_4)
     b. Elevated serum TSH and low T_4 diagnostic of transient or permanent primary hypothyroidism
     c. Positive TSH receptor-blocking antibodies (TRBAb)—diagnostic for transient congenital hypothyroidism (maternal antibodies)
     d. Additional thyroid function tests—serum thyroxine-binding globulin (TBG); triodothyronine resin uptake (T_3RU)
  2. Acquired hypothyroidism secondary to pituitary or hypothalamic disorders
     a. Low free (unbound) thyroxine (free T_4), usually normal TSH, and low thyroxine-binding globulin
     b. Abnormal pituitary function tests
  3. Euthyroid sick syndrome (nonthyroidal illness syndrome) secondary to coexisting acute or chronic illness; low T_4 level with normal TBG; low T_3; normal TSH; free T_4 and reverse T_3 levels high, normal, or elevated
  4. Autoimmune (Hashimoto's) thyroiditis (with goiter present)—elevated serum thyroid peroxidase or thyroglobulin antibody titers; autoantibodies are present in 95% of cases; begin treatment therapy when TSH rises above normal and T_4/free T_4 is low or normal

5. Repeat thyroid function tests if clinical suspicion of hypothyroidism, history of thyroid disease in pregnancy, positive history of thyroid dyshormonogenesis

6. May have abnormal thyroid scan, ultrasound, imaging, or bone age results

- Management/Treatment
  1. Consultation or referral to pediatric endocrinologist for suspected or confirmed hypothyroidism
  2. For congenital hypothyroidism, rapid and adequate thyroid hormone replacement critical to avoid irreparable neurologic impairment and mental retardation; treat within first month of life for best prognosis for optimal intellectual development
  3. Drug of choice daily oral levothyroxine (L-thyroxine); after treatment initiated for hypothyroidism in infancy, monitor T_4 and TSH levels monthly during first 3 months of age, every 2 to 3 months for the remainder of the 1st year, every 3 to 4 months during 2nd and 3rd years, and every 4 to 12 months thereafter until growth complete; more frequent checks if compliance issues, changes in physical symptoms (especially poor growth), or abnormal values; monitor additionally as needed whenever dose adjusted
  4. Recommended dosages of levothyroxine (T_4) vary by age; with higher doses for infants and lower doses over time to 2–3 mcg/kg/day for children >12 years of age
  5. In older children and adolescents, increase thyroid dose gradually to full replacement dose to avoid undesirable side effects and clinical symptoms of thyrotoxicosis (e.g., headaches, abrupt personality changes)
  6. Once older children and adolescents in euthyroid state, monitor adequacy of levothyroxine therapy with regular, periodic T_4 and TSH levels
  7. Levothyroxine is administered as a single oral dose on an empty stomach approximately 30–60 minutes before breakfast for maximum absorption. Oral tablets can be crushed and mixed with a small amount of water for infants and young children. It should not be mixed with infant formula or breast milk, and iron may interfere with absorption
  8. Educate parents and child about disease, treatment regimen, and routine monitoring; with thyroid replacement, child will be more lively, less docile, may lose water weight, hair of normal texture will replace dry hair, may have transient stomachaches or headaches
  9. Genetic counseling may be indicated if familial etiology
  10. Trial off of medication may be indicated at age 3 years, if possibility child had transient congenital hypothyroidism, once the brain is more mature and there is less risk of neurologic sequelae

Hyperthyroidism

- Definition: Excessive production and secretion of thyroid hormone (TH) by thyroid gland (thyrotoxicosis)

resulting in increased basal metabolism, goiter, autonomic nervous system disorders, and problems with water and electrolyte metabolism

1. Caused by excess production of thyroid hormone (e.g., Graves' disease or autoimmune hyperthyroidism, pituitary tumor) or excess release of thyroid hormone (e.g., subacute thyroiditis, Hashimoto's toxic thyroiditis, iodine-induced hyperthyroidism), or hot nodules

2. Most common cause is autoimmune response (Graves')—body produces thyroid-stimulating immunoglobulins (TSIs), which stimulate TSH receptors in thyroid gland, causing overproduction of TH and thyroid hypertrophy; has genetic predisposition

3. If mother is thyrotoxic prenatally or has history of Graves' disease, infants may have transient congenital hyperthyroidism (neonatal Graves' disease) since thyroid-stimulating immunoglobulins cross placenta to fetus; rare

- Incidence
  1. Graves' disease is rare: 0.8 per 100,000 children per year and six times more common in girls, usually in second decade and commonly associated in children with other autoimmune disorders
- Signs and Symptoms
  1. May have family history of thyroid disorder (e.g., Graves' disease) or maternal history of antithyroid drug ingestion for treatment of Graves' disease during pregnancy
  2. Neonates/infants
     a. Very rare in neonate; signs and symptoms usually present shortly after birth or may present days or weeks later; not common, but can have severe consequences if untreated; diagnosis rarely made in newborn period
     b. Prematurity, low birthweight, poor weight gain, poor feeding
     c. Restlessness, irritability, tachycardia
     d. Can be neonatal Graves' disease, due to transplacental passage of stimulatory maternal antibodies, or autosomal dominant hyperthyroidism requiring antithyroid treatment prior to thyroidectomy
  3. Child/adolescent
     a. Weight loss, although increased appetite; may have accelerated growth and advanced bone age with long-term illness
     b. Nervousness, irritability, decreased attention span, behavior problems, decline in school performance, emotional lability, restlessness, fatigue, weakness, heat intolerance, increased perspiration
     c. Sleeplessness or sleep restlessness, insomnia, nightmares
     d. Visual disturbances, e.g., increased lacrimation, diplopia, photophobia, blurring
     e. Palpitations
     f. Frequent urination and loose stooling, may have enuresis
     g. Amenorrhea

- Differential Diagnosis
  1. Neonates—systemic illness, sepsis, and narcotic withdrawal
  2. Children and adolescents
     a. Nodular thyroid disease
     b. Thyroid cancer
     c. Euthyroid goiter
     d. Chronic disease, e.g., pituitary disease, severe anemia, leukemia
     e. Thyroiditis
     f. Accidental or deliberate excessive thyroid hormone or iodine ingestion
     g. Chorea
     h. Psychiatric illness, e.g., anxiety disorder, anorexia
- Physical Findings
  1. Neonates and infants
     a. May be small for gestational age
     b. Lid retraction, proptosis, periorbital edema
     c. Face may be flushed
     d. Enlarged thyroid (goiter)
     e. Tachycardia without underlying heart disease
     f. Increased gastrointestinal motility
     g. Severely affected neonates may have jaundice, microcephaly, frontal bossing, craniosynostosis, ophthalmopathy, exophthalmia, thrombocytopenia, cardiac problems, hepatosplenomegaly, and other signs of severe illness
  2. Children and adolescents
     a. Increased energy (with periods of lethargy), decreased sleep, decreased school performance and concentration, personality changes: irritability and emotional lability
     b. Eye findings, e.g., proptosis, exophthalmos, upper lid lag with downward gaze, lid retraction, stare appearance, periorbital and conjunctival edema
     c. Variable-size enlarged, tender or nontender, spongy or firm thyroid with palpable border; may have thyroid bruit or thrill
     d. Tachycardia, systolic hypertension, increased pulse pressure, palpitations
     e. Proximal muscle weakness, diminished fine motor control, tremor, short DTR relaxation phase
     f. Advanced skeletal maturation radiographically
     g. Warm, moist, smooth, diaphoretic skin; face may be flushed; heat intolerance; increased bowel movements
- Diagnostic Tests/Findings
  1. If signs or symptoms of thyrotoxicosis or enlarged thyroid, do confirmatory laboratory thyroid function tests
  2. Thyroiditis indicated by elevated T_4, free T_4, T_3 resin uptake (T_3RU) with TSH suppression and low serum cholesterol
  3. Circulating thyroid-stimulating immunoglobulin and other thyroid antibody tests, including thyrotropin receptor antibody (TRAb) titers, are elevated and in most cases thyroid peroxidase (TPO) antibodies are also positive
  4. Although rare in childhood, a child developing acute onset of hyperthermia, severe tachycardia, and restlessness needs evaluation for thyroid crisis or storm, a rare and potentially life-threatening emergency
  5. Graves' disease—elevated T_4 and low TSH; advanced bone age
  6. Radioactive iodine uptake scan shows increased uptake if excess TH production; if increased release of TH only, will have decreased radioactive iodine uptake
  7. High plasma T_4 does not necessarily indicate hyperthyroidism as there is a physiologic transient peak of plasma T_4 on day 2 of life; diagnosis of true hyperthyroidism requires low or undetectable TSH with high T_4 or T_3 or both
- Management/Treatment
  1. Consultation or referral to pediatric endocrinologist for suspected or confirmed hyperthyroidism
  2. Treatment dictated by identified etiology for hyperthyroidism and degree of thyrotoxicity; attempt medical management as primary initial therapy
  3. Prompt diagnosis and treatment especially important in neonates as condition may be life threatening
  4. Treatment goal is prompt return to euthyroidism with use of:
     a. Antithyroid drugs to inhibit thyroxine (T_4) synthesis and conversion of T_3 to T_4, e.g., such as methimazole. In 2010, the Food and Drug Administration (FDA) added a "black box warning" for the use of propylthiouracil (PTU) because of the risk of severe liver disease. The use of PTU should be reserved for children who cannot tolerate methimazole
     b. Beta-adrenergic receptor blockers to control nervousness and cardiovascular symptoms, e.g., propranolol, atenolol (*not* in asthmatics)
     c. Side effects of antithyroid medications include rashes, urticaria, arthralgias, and decreased white blood cell count; all children on treatment require a complete blood count (CBC) for fever or sore throat
     d. Ablative therapy with radioiodine permanently suppresses thyroid function; hypothyroidism is induced without side effects of medication
     e. Thyroid surgery no longer considered primary form of treatment except in restricted physical activity if hyperthyroidism severe or in preparation for surgery
  5. Educate parent and child about disease, duration of treatment, side effects of medications or complications if surgery required, adherence to treatment regimen, and, if Graves' disease, need for lifelong monitoring; advise of complications, e.g., thyrotoxicosis
  6. Genetic counseling may be indicated if familial etiology

Thyroiditis

- Definition: Inflammation of thyroid gland caused by autoimmune response to the thyroid gland (chronic lymphocytic thyroiditis [Hashimoto's]); infectious agents (acute suppurative and subacute or nonsuppurative); or from exposure to radiation or trauma; occasionally idiopathic

- Etiology/Incidence
  1. Acute suppurative thyroiditis with bacterial etiology—e.g., group A streptococci, pneumococci, *Staphylococcus aureus*, and anaerobes; rare
  2. Subacute nonsuppurative thyroiditis caused by viruses—e.g., mumps, influenza, echovirus, coxsackie, Epstein-Barr, adenovirus; rare in United States
  3. Chronic lymphocytic thyroiditis (chronic autoimmune or Hashimoto's thyroiditis)—noninfectious autoimmune inflammatory disease of thyroid most common cause of goiter and hypothyroidism in childhood; highest incidence in children 8 to 15 years; more common in females than in males (4:1); increasing incidence may be associated with rising incidence of type 1 diabetes and improved diagnostic techniques and an active search among family members of known patients
- Signs and Symptoms
  1. With infectious thyroiditis, may have recent history of or concurrent upper respiratory illness
  2. With chronic autoimmune thyroiditis, may have family history of autoimmune thyroid disease
  3. Onset in acute thyroiditis rapid; insidious onset in subacute and chronic lymphocytic thyroiditis
  4. Fever, malaise; may feel quite ill with acute suppurative or subacute thyroiditis, particularly with former
  5. With acute and subacute thyroiditis, pain and tenderness of thyroid with radiation to other areas of neck, ear, chest; with acute suppurative thyroiditis, severe pain with neck extension; no tenderness with chronic lymphocytic thyroiditis
  6. Complaints of unilateral or bilateral swelling of the thyroid, complaints of fullness in anterior neck; sensation of tracheal compression
  7. May have sore throat, hoarseness, dysphagia
  8. May have nervousness, irritability, other symptoms of mild hyperthyroidism
- Differential Diagnosis
  1. Infectious toxic thyroiditis must be distinguished from chronic lymphocytic autoimmune thyroiditis; simple goiters due to inborn errors of T_4 synthesis; and chronic autoimmune thyroiditis (Hashimoto's) associated with adolescence in girls; and thyroglossal duct abscesses
  2. Goiters induced by drugs—(e.g., from iodine, lithium, para-amino salicylic acid, thionamides [methimazole], white turnip plants); by transplacental exposure to TH by breastfeeding of newborns when mothers are on antithyroid therapy
  3. Cancerous or cystic thyroid nodules
     a. Benign causes include multinodular goiter, cysts, follicular adenomas, or thyroiditis
     b. Malignant causes include papillary, follicular, Hurthle cell, medullary, or anaplastic carcinomas or metastatic lesions

- Physical Findings
  1. Findings variable depending on etiology—i.e., infectious vs. autoimmune
  2. May be toxic-appearing if infectious etiology, but not necessarily thyrotoxic
  3. In infectious thyroiditis—thyroid gland unilaterally or bilaterally enlarged, tender, firm
  4. In chronic lymphocytic thyroiditis, usually symmetric, nontender, firm, freely movable, diffusely enlarged "pebbly" goiter
- Diagnostic Tests/Findings
  1. Laboratory findings variable depending on etiology
  2. In acute suppurative thyroiditis—usually no consistently associated endocrine disturbances, moderate to marked shift to left in differential, elevated sedimentation rate
  3. Subacute nonsuppurative thyroiditis—radioiodine uptake usually reduced; serum TH levels normal or elevated
  4. In chronic lymphocytic thyroiditis—usually normal T_4, free T_4, T_3 RU, but may be elevated or depressed; thyroid autoantibodies usually present, abnormal thyroid scan, surgical or needle biopsy diagnostic but rarely indicated
- Management/Treatment
  1. Physician consultation or referral to pediatric endocrinologist for suspected or confirmed thyroiditis
  2. Specific antibiotic therapy required for acute suppurative thyroiditis and may be needed for subacute nonsuppurative thyroiditis since latter is difficult to distinguish from former; acetylsalicylic acid or other anti-inflammatory drugs
  3. Treatment for autoimmune chronic lymphocytic thyroiditis controversial; levothyroxine may be used to decrease goiter, but efficacy in preventing progression of hypothyroidism in long term is not supported
  4. Adolescents with autoimmune chronic lymphocytic thyroiditis need lifelong monitoring since development of hypothyroidism is possible, subacute thyroiditis self-limiting
  5. All children with type 1 diabetes should be annually screened for thyroid dysfunction; increased risk of thyroid microsomal antibody
  6. Genetic counseling may be indicated for familial etiology

☐ PITUITARY DISORDER: DIABETES INSIPIDUS (DI)

- Definition: Excretion of large amounts of dilute urine due to insufficient function of antidiuretic hormone (ADH), arginine vasopressin, disorder in ADH receptors in kidney, primary renal disease, or, rarely in children, primary polydipsia; compromised ability to concentrate urine
- Etiology/Incidence
  1. Central (hypothalamic, neurogenic, vasopressin-sensitive) DI caused by hypofunction of hypothalamus/

posterior pituitary or increased vasopressin metabolism, resulting in ADH deficiency
  a. Genetic, familial autosomal dominant trait, rare
  b. Congenital, e.g., anatomic defects in brain
  c. Acquired secondary to accidental or surgical trauma, infection, cerebral anoxia, neoplasm, or infectious disease; trauma following removal of hypothalamic area tumors major cause
  d. Secondary to autoimmune or infiltrative disease, e.g., histiocytosis, lymphocytic hypophysitis
  e. Idiopathic
  f. Others: Brain death, increased vasopressin metabolism, drugs, e.g., ethanol
 2. Nephrogenic (vasopressin-resistant) DI caused by reduced renal responsiveness to ADH (not central nervous system mediated)
  a. Familial—X-linked inherited disorder of ADH receptor sites in kidney in males primarily; females rarely affected, less common etiology but more severe
  b. Acquired
   (1) Renal failure, e.g., obstructive uropathy, polycystic kidney disease
   (2) Electrolyte disorders (hypercalcemia, hypokalemia)
   (3) Nephrotoxic drugs, e.g., lithium, demeclocycline, amphotericin, methicillin, and rifampin
   (4) Other illness, e.g., sickle cell
- Signs and Symptoms
 1. Symptoms vary depending on etiology, age, anterior pituitary function, and preservation of normal thirst, diet
 2. Central (neurogenic) DI
  a. May have family history of congenital ADH deficiency
  b. Generally rapid onset; disease may be masked as failure to thrive
  c. History of poor weight gain, deficient growth if long duration
  d. Unexplained fever, irritability
  e. Intense thirst, polydipsia, desire for cold drinks, preference for cold water; irritable when fluid withheld; unable to sleep through night without water intake
  f. Vomiting, constipation; unexplained fever in infants
  g. Tendency to avoid diets high in protein and salt
  h. Polyuria, nocturia, enuresis in previously toilet-trained child; clear urine; unable to concentrate urine after fluid restriction
  i. May have symptoms of intracranial tumor (headaches, strabismus, double vision, vomiting, precocious puberty)
  j. May follow intracranial surgical procedures or trauma; central nervous system (CNS) disease; rarely idiopathic
 3. Nephrogenic DI
  a. Genetic or acquired causes—may have family history of congenital nephrogenic DI or maternal

history of polyhydramnios; infants may do well on breastfeeding until weaning (breastmilk has low renal solute load), infection, or introduction of solids, then may fail to thrive; often present with fever, vomiting, dehydration
  b. Female carriers of trait have varying severity of disease
  c. Poor weight gain, deficient growth if long duration; may be malnourished
  d. Increased thirst, polydipsia, history of large water intake, poor food intake because of preference for water over milk or solids
  e. Dehydration, absence of tears, perspiration; if dehydration severe, may have seizures
  f. Irritability; may have poor attention span, poor school performance
  g. Vomiting, polyuria, nocturia
- Differential Diagnosis
 1. Distinguish DI caused by suppression of vasopressin secretion (congenital vs. acquired central DI) from DI caused by reduced renal responsiveness to arginine vasopressin (congenital vs. acquired nephrogenic DI)
 2. Psychogenic polydipsia (compulsive water drinking) and other causes of polyuria (e.g., drug-induced polydipsia [e.g., thioridazine, tricyclics]; hypokalemia; hypercalcemia [including hypervitaminosis D]; primary and secondary renal disease; diabetes mellitus)
- Physical Findings
 1. Central (neurogenic) DI
  a. Variable levels of dehydration; if disease unrecognized, infants may have high fever, vomiting, seizures, circulatory collapse
  b. Poor weight gain, deficient growth if long duration, may be malnourished
  c. Irritability, may have poor attention span
  d. May have symptoms of brain tumor (e.g., strabismus, nystagmus)
 2. Nephrogenic DI
  a. Variable levels of dehydration; dry skin, no tears, no perspiration; if severe, infants may have high fever, convulsions, circulatory collapse
  b. Failure to thrive, malnourished; if long duration, may have growth retardation, delayed sexual maturation, CNS damage
  c. Fever, irritability
  d. Large or distended bladder except immediately after voiding; nonobstructive hydronephrosis, hydroureter
- Diagnostic Tests/Findings
 1. History of pathological polydipsia and polyuria (>2 L/m^2/day) in children
 2. Urine specific gravity (<1.005; osmolality <280 mOsm/kg)
 3. Inability to concentrate urine after fluid restriction
 4. Hyperosmolality of plasma
 5. Water deprivation test—to establish diagnosis of DI and differentiate central vs. nephrogenic DI

a. Serum osmolality >300 mOsm/kg and urine osmolality <600 mOsm/kg diagnostic of DI

6. Vasopressin challenge with desmopressin acetate (DDAVP) performed immediately after water deprivation test to determine if DI is central or nephrogenic
   a. Central DI—decreased urine volume and increased urine osmolality
   b. Nephrogenic DI—no further changes in urine volume or osmolality

7. With MRI, absence or diminished "bright spot" in posterior pituitary; diminished blood flow to posterior pituitary; classic finding for a mass of the optic chiasm—bitemporal hemianopsia

8. Low serum ADH concentration in central DI; high serum ADH level in nephrogenic DI

- Management/Treatment
  1. Immediate physician consultation or referral to pediatric endocrinologist for suspected or confirmed DI
  2. Careful adequate rehydration to avoid seizures, intellectual impairment due to CNS damage from hypernatremia and dehydration, particularly in infants who may not be able to make known their need for water or to obtain water necessary to quench thirst; early recognition and management needed to avoid sequelae of stunted growth and cognitive impairment
  3. Treat treatable underlying causes of nephrogenic DI, e.g., hypokalemia, drug-induced obstructive uropathy
  4. Treatment of choice for diabetes insipidus—intranasal DDAVP; in infants, sometimes given extra free water rather than DDAVP for normal hydration and prevention of unwanted hyponatremia; with nephrogenic DI, may need diuretics, e.g., thiazides, prostaglandin synthesis inhibitors, e.g., indomethacin
  5. Breastfeeding preferable; adequate calories for growth; with nephrogenic DI, water allowed as demanded, sodium intake restricted; teach regarding avoidance of severe dehydration
  6. Genetic counseling may be indicated for familial etiology
  7. Treat other identified causes, e.g., germinomas, histiocytosis, craniopharyngiomas

☐ GROWTH DISTURBANCES

Short Stature

- Definition
  1. Variation from average pattern of growth; associated with normal variants of growth and pathologic conditions
  2. Growth adequacy determined by consideration of both growth rate and absolute height; severe form of short stature defined as height <3 standard deviations below the mean
  3. Centers for Disease Control and Prevention (CDC) growth chart should be used to evaluate growth of children; see http://www.cdc.gov/growthcharts

- Etiology/Incidence
  1. Multiple etiologies—genetic, constitutional, physiologic, environmental, psychosocial
     a. Normal growth variations (most common)
        (1) Familial or genetic normal variant of average growth pattern that is familial, racial, or genetic; child "constitutionally small" and remains small as adult
        (2) Constitutional delay of growth with delayed growth pattern resulting in delayed physical maturity but normal final adult height
     b. Non-endocrine causes of short stature
        (1) Syndromes of short stature
            (a) Turner syndrome and its variants
            (b) Noonan syndrome (pseudo-Turner syndrome)
            (c) Prader-Willi syndrome
            (d) Laurence-Moon and Bardet-Biedl syndromes
        (2) Chronic disease
            (a) Cardiac disorders—left to right shunt, congestive heart failure (CHF)
            (b) Pulmonary disorders—cystic fibrosis, asthma
            (c) GI disorders—malabsorption, celiac disease, disorders of swallowing
            (d) Hepatic disorders
            (e) Hematologic disorders—sickle cell disorder, thalassemia
            (f) Renal disorders—renal tubular acidosis, chronic uremia
            (g) CNS disorders
            (h) Malnutrition—decreased availability of nutrients, fad or voluntary dieting anorexia nervosa, anorexia of cancer chemotherapy
        (3) Genetic short stature
        (4) Intrauterine growth delay and small for gestational age (SGA)
     c. Endocrine causes of short stature
        (1) Growth hormone (GH) deficiency and variants
            (a) Congenital GH deficiency—with midline defects, with other pituitary hormone deficiencies, isolated GH deficiency, pituitary agenesis
            (b) Acquired GH deficiency—hypothalamic pituitary tumors, histiocytosis X, CNS infections, head injuries, GH deficiencies following cranial irradiation, central nervous system vascular accidents, empty sella syndrome
            (c) Abnormalities of GH action—GH insensitivity (Laron dwarfism), primary IGF-1 deficiency, pygmies, insulin-like growth factor (IGF) receptor defect
            (d) Psychosocial dwarfism
            (e) Hypothyroidism
            (f) Glucocorticoid excess (Cushing syndrome)—endogenous, exogenous

    (g) Pseudohypoparathyroidism

    (h) Disorders of vitamin D metabolism

    (i) Diabetes mellitus, poorly controlled

    (j) Diabetes insipidus, poorly controlled

- Signs and Symptoms
  1. Normal growth variations
     a. Familial short stature—usually small at birth (<3%) but consistent with family pattern
     b. Constitutional growth delay—usually normal size at birth with declining height and weight to <5% between 1 and 3 years of age; delayed pubescence; family history of similar growth pattern in parents or other family members and will reach height that is normal for their genetic potential
  2. Pathologic growth variations
     a. History of poor nutritional intake, malabsorption syndromes
     b. Symptoms of GH deficiency—failure to grow, headaches, delayed dental development, visual field defects, polyuria, polydipsia, delayed sexual maturation, CNS abnormalities, history of trauma, infection, radiation to CNS
     c. Signs and symptoms of other endocrine disorders—fever, lethargy, irritability, developmental delay, dull appearance, failure to thrive (FTT), increased weight for height, polyuria, polydipsia, constipation, delayed sexual maturation, CNS symptoms, CNS surgery
     d. Intrauterine growth retardation (IUGR) and low birth weight (LBW); normal BW or normal growth pattern with subsequent onset of decelerated or delayed growth; history of premature aging
     e. Symptoms of other systemic or chronic illness—FTT, congenital defects, including intrinsic diseases of bone
     f. Dysmorphism at birth, chromosomal abnormalities, syndromes, congenital skeletal defects or anomalies, e.g., abnormal upper-to-lower-body ratio, abnormal or disproportionate features
     g. Signs and symptoms of neglect, emotional maltreatment; abnormalities in psychosocial development; parents may be overwhelmed or disorganized and not intentionally neglectful or abusive
     h. Chronic drug intake, e.g., glucocorticoids, high doses of estrogens, androgens
- Differential Diagnosis: Distinguish normal variants of familial short stature and constitutional growth delay from pathologic causes
- Physical Findings
  1. Familial or constitutional short stature—height, weight, occipital-frontal circumference (OFC) growth curve patterns generally consistent, symmetric
     a. Familial—growth chart showing BW <3% but consistent with family pattern; follows growth curve; normal physical examination; radiographic bone age consistent with chronological age
     b. Constitutional delay—growth chart showing normal size at birth with declining height and weight throughout 1 to 3 years to <5%; normal physical examination; bone maturation 2 to 3 years behind chronological age
  2. Pathologic short stature
     a. GH deficiency—BW may be normal, birth length 50% that of normal child; height and weight growth deficits; infantile fat distribution; youthful facial features; midfacial hypoplasia; visual field defects; small hands and feet; newborn may have microphallus (stretched penile length of <2.5 cm vs. normal mean length of 4 cm); may have CNS findings
     b. Primordial short stature
        (1) IUGR—BW and birth length below normal for gestational age, OFC normal or <3rd percentile; subsequent growth parallel to or <3rd percentile
        (2) Primordial dwarfism with premature aging—child appears older than age
        (3) Short stature with and without dysmorphism—height, weight <3rd percentile, may have normal physical examination other than small size or may have various abnormal physical findings, e.g., microcephaly
     c. Short stature associated with chromosomal abnormalities—may have dysmorphism or stigmata of specific congenital or familial disorders, e.g., Turner syndrome (webbed neck, small jaw, prominent ears, epicanthal folds, low posterior hairline, broad chest, cardiac defects) or Down syndrome
     d. Short stature associated with bone or cartilage development disorders, e.g., skeletal dysplasia, short extremities with normal-size head and trunk, frontal bossing, abnormal upper-to-lower-body ratio, abnormal or disproportionate features, rickets, leg bowing
     e. Short stature associated with symptoms of endogenous cortisol excess, e.g., Cushing disease with moon facies, hirsutism, "buffalo hump," striae, hypertension, fatigue, voice deepening, obesity, amenorrhea
     f. Chronic drug intake, e.g., glucocorticoid excess with hypertension, plethora, moon facies, purple striae, interscapular fat pad, truncal obesity, muscle wasting
     g. Abnormalities in psychosocial development; parental neglect
- Diagnostic Tests/Findings
  1. Abnormalities in previous sequential, consistent recordings of height, weight, and OFC plotted on age-standardized growth charts
  2. In familial short stature and constitutional delay, height may be <3rd percentile but growth rate normal; careful family history of familial growth patterns may elucidate familial vs. constitutional delay as etiology of short stature

3. In growth failure, slower than normal growth rate results in flattened growth curve or decrease in growth parameter percentiles
4. May have abnormal complete and segmental growth measurements and upper-to-lower-body ratio measurements
5. Laboratory tests to confirm diagnosis based on clinical findings and to rule out systemic disease or hormonal deficiency; findings depend on etiology
   a. Abnormal CBC—chronic anemia, infection, leukemia
   b. Elevated sedimentation rate—collagen vascular disease, cancer, chronic infection
   c. Abnormal biochemical profiles—adrenal insufficiency, renal disease
   d. Abnormal stool examination—inflammatory bowel disease, severe parasitism
   e. Abnormal thyroid function studies—hypothyroidism
   f. Low serum human growth hormone (hGH), insulin-like growth factor 1 (IGF-1), IGF-binding protein—growth hormone deficiency (GHD)
   g. Abnormal urinalysis—renal disease
6. Delayed maturity on radiographic bone age indicates constitutional delay (generally 2 to 3 years behind chronological age), GH deficiency, hypothyroidism, severe systemic illness; normal bone age found in familial short stature
7. Nutritional evaluation may show inadequate calories
8. Abnormal home/social evaluation may suggest psychosocial etiology
9. Abnormalities on skull radiograph, CT, MRI of cranium if intracranial lesion
10. Karyotype analysis in short girls with pubertal delay may indicate Turner syndrome
- Management/Treatment
  1. Physician consultation or referral to appropriate pediatric specialists for children with other than familial or constitutional growth delay
  2. If familial or constitutional growth delay, only periodic monitoring of growth pattern needed; reassurance
  3. If marked psychosocial problems arise in boys because of pubertal delay, short-term testosterone may initiate sexual development
  4. Optimize treatment for other endocrine or systemic or chronic illnesses to minimize compromised growth; adequate calories for growth
  5. GH therapy is FDA approved for children with known GH deficiency, SGA, or IUGR without "catch-up," chronic renal failure (CRF), Turner syndrome, and Noonan syndrome

Excessive Growth

- Definition: Variation from average pattern of growth in linear height with height >2 SD above the mean; excess height for age
- Etiology/Incidence
  1. Normal variation in growth—constitutional tall structure (familial, genetic) most common, familial tendency to mature early
  2. Pathologic variations in growth
     a. Endocrine disorders
        (1) Infant of diabetic mother (IDM)
        (2) GH excess—usually due to pituitary adenoma; pituitary gigantism
        (3) Precocious puberty—androgen or estrogen excess prior to puberty from CNS disorder; adrenal or gonadal disorder, e.g., excess of androgens, estrogens, or both; or idiopathic cause leads to accelerated linear growth, early bone and sexual maturation, and adult short stature; more common in females than in males; males have more pathologic etiologies, e.g., CNS disease; females have more idiopathic precocious puberty
     b. Genetic causes
        (1) Marfan syndrome—autosomal dominant, connective tissue disorder
        (2) Chromosomal abnormalities (e.g., Klinefelter syndrome in males with two X chromosomes with usual normal adult stature), XYY, XXYY
        (3) Fragile X syndrome
     c. Other
        (1) Idiopathic or exogenous obesity—early puberty with accelerated growth; usually adult height not beyond expected genetic potential
        (2) Homocystinuria—inherited inborn error of metabolism
        (3) Cerebral gigantism (Sotos syndrome)—possible hypothalamic dysfunction; adult stature normal to excessive
        (4) Beckwith-Wiedemann syndrome
        (5) McCune-Albright syndrome
- Signs and Symptoms
  1. Concern about tall stature or excessive growth primarily with adolescent girls/parents
  2. Symptoms accompanying tall stature variable depending on underlying etiology
  3. Familial or constitutional tall stature—length normal at birth, tall stature evident by 3 to 4 years; growth rate slows after 4 or 5 years with curve, then parallel to normal curve
  4. IDM—history of maternal diabetes, large for gestational age (LGA)
  5. Beckwith-Wiedemann—LGA, rapid growth in childhood; concern about height; symptoms of hypoglycemia
  6. GH excess—symptoms vary depending on age when excess GH secretion occurs; concern about height, other symptoms of GH excess (e.g., headache, excessive perspiration, visual impairment, coarsening of facial features, enlargement of nose, ears, jaw, increases in hands and feet, galactorrhea, menstrual irregularity, polyuria, polydipsia, joint pain)

7. Precocious puberty—concern about height, increase in growth rate, and early development of pubic hair common presenting signs
   a. True precocity of familial or idiopathic origin—causes early secondary sex characteristics with testicular enlargement and spermatogenesis in boys, menarche and mature ova in girls
   b. Incomplete or pseudoprecocity—adrenal or gonadal tumor or dysfunction causes early secondary sex characteristics but no testicular enlargement, no ovulation
   c. CNS disorders/tumors—more common in males, may have seizure
8. Marfan syndrome—concern about height, vision, and cardiac problems
9. Klinefelter syndrome—concern about height, school, and behavior problems, lowered verbal IQ, vision problems, delayed adolescent development, testes before puberty normal or small
10. Obesity—normal height, weight at birth
11. Homocystinuria—concern about height, mental retardation, vision problems, CNS symptoms, back pain
12. Cerebral gigantism (Sotos)—concern about height; normal height at birth, rapid growth 1st year of life (>97% height at 1 year) to 3 to 4 years, feeding problems, developmental delay

- Differential Diagnosis: Normal variants of constitutional tall structure need to be distinguished from pathologic causes; distinguish pseudoprecocity from true sexual precocity; cause of testicular enlargement may be testicular tumor; ovarian tumor may cause early menarche
- Physical Findings
1. Constitutional tall stature—variant of normal; 2 to 4 SD above average height for age; normal body proportions; normal physical examination and appropriate pubertal development and timing
2. Endocrine disorders
   a. IDM—LGA at birth; >90% for height and weight
   b. GH excess—tall; soft tissue growth; prominent mandible; supraorbital ridge; large nose; space between teeth; hypertension; heart failure; large hands and feet, thickened bones, overgrowth of joints of extremities; visceral enlargement; osteoporosis, kyphosis, may have signs of CNS symptoms
   c. Precocious puberty—tall stature; in males, secondary sexual development before age 9 years; in females, breast development before 8.0 years, sexual pubic hair before 9.0 years, or menses before 9.5 years
3. Genetic disorders
   a. Marfan syndrome—tall stature, dolicocephaly (disproportionately long and narrow head), abnormal body proportions, thin extremities, increased arm and leg length, lowered upper/lower segment ratio, increased arm span, arachnodactyly (long, slender fingers), myopia and other visual abnormalities, external ear abnormalities, pectus excavatum, heart murmur, scoliosis or kyphosis, laxity and hyperextension of joints, hypotonicity
   b. Klinefelter syndrome—tall stature, underweight for height and age, mental retardation, long legs, low upper/lower body segment ratio, gynecomastia, normal penile size and pubic hair but small and firm testes with decreased sensitivity to pressure, cryptorchidism, hypospadias
4. Other causes of tall stature
   a. Obesity—accelerated height and weight, generally normal examination otherwise
   b. Homocystinuria—tall stature, myopia and other ocular problems, CNS symptoms, possible convulsions, mental retardation, osteoporosis, vertebral collapse
   c. Cerebral gigantism (Sotos syndrome)—large BW and height, dysmorphic features, abnormal body proportions with increased arm span, mental retardation, macrocephaly, wide-set eyes, prominent forehead, hypertelorism with other ocular abnormalities, high-arched palate, pointed chin, CNS findings, poor motor coordination
   d. Beckwith-Wiedemann syndrome—large BW and height, oomphalocele, umbilical hernia, accelerated growth in childhood, macroglossia, high-arched palate, midface hypoplasia, hemihypertrophy

- Diagnostic Tests/Findings
1. Previous sequential, consistent recordings of height, weight, and OFC plotted on age-standardized growth charts show height >2 SD above mean for age
2. Careful family history of tall growth patterns may elucidate familial etiology of tall stature; growth rate normal, growth curve parallels normal curve in familial tall stature
3. Laboratory tests to confirm diagnosis based on clinical findings and to rule out endocrine disease
   a. GH excess—low adrenocorticotropic hormone (ACTH), follicle-stimulating hormone (FSH), luteinizing hormone (LH); high or normal GH; abnormal glucose tolerance test (GTT)
   b. Cerebral gigantism—normal GH secretion
   c. Klinefelter—high pituitary gonadotropin, LH, FSH; azoospermia
   d. True precocious puberty—elevated basal LH, FSH concentrations; pubertal LH response to gonadotropin-releasing hormone (GnRH)
   e. Beckwith-Wiedemann—low blood glucose (hyperinsulinemia)
4. Radiographic bone age not advanced in constitutional tall stature; advanced in cerebral gigantism, obesity, precocious puberty
5. Abnormal echocardiogram with Marfan; may have abdominal mass on ultrasound with precocious puberty

6. Abnormalities on skull radiograph, CT, or MRI of cranium with intracranial lesion
7. Karyotype analysis may indicate chromosomal abnormalities, syndromes
- Management/Treatment
  1. Consultation or referral to appropriate pediatric specialists for children with other than constitutional tall stature
  2. Pharmacologic management controversial; if marked concern about calculated predicted adult height, endocrinologist may accelerate epiphyseal closure with gonadal steroids; if precocious puberty, may slow growth with GnRH agonist
  3. Homocystinuria—restrict dietary methionine, supplement dietary cystine
  4. GH excess from CNS tumor or adrenal or gonadal tumor—surgery as indicated
  5. Management of endocrine disease associated with tall stature
  6. Beckwith-Wiedemann—treat excess insulin production

☐ ADRENAL GLAND DISORDERS

Adrenocortical Insufficiency

- Definition: Inadequate production and secretion of adrenal hormones caused by failure of adrenals to secrete glucocorticoids, mineralocorticoids, and adrenal androgen (primary adrenal insufficiency, Addison's) or deficient secretion of ACTH from pituitary (secondary adrenal insufficiency)
- Etiology/Incidence
  1. Primary adrenal insufficiency
     a. Congenital adrenal hyperplasia (CAH)—hereditary
     b. Chronic adrenal insufficiency (hypo-adrenocorticism, Addison's disease) with destruction of adrenals from infection or hereditary autoimmune disease or adrenal calcification
     c. Congenital absence or underdevelopment of adrenals; newborn adrenal hemorrhage (with complicated or traumatic delivery)
     d. Malignancy (adrenal tumor)
  2. Secondary adrenal insufficiency
     a. Hypopituitarism—deficient secretion of one or more pituitary hormones due to congenital brain malformations, head trauma, histiocytosis, infection, tumors, radiation
     b. Cessation of glucocorticoid therapy after prolonged large-dose administration of glucocorticoids (e.g., asthma, nephrosis, leukemia)
     c. Other—postsurgical, infants of steroid-treated mothers, respiratory distress syndrome, anencephaly, pituitary defects
- Signs and Symptoms
  1. Acute adrenal insufficiency (adrenal crisis)
     a. Known or unknown diagnosis of Addison's—"crisis" may be first presentation of illness
     b. Recent or concurrent infection or febrile illness; surgery; exposure to excessive heat in susceptible individuals
     c. History of abrupt withdrawal of large-dose steroid therapy
     d. Hypotension, shock, muscle weakness, weight loss, confusion, fever, fatigue, nausea, vomiting, diarrhea, dehydration, abdominal pain, anorexia, salt craving despite anorexia, symptomatic hypoglycemia
  2. Chronic adrenal insufficiency—weakness, fatigue, anorexia, hypotension, hyperpigmentation, poor weight gain, weight loss, lethargy, exercise intolerance, headache, nausea, vomiting which may be forceful or projectile, diarrhea, dehydration, salt craving, increased pigmentation, hypotension
- Differential Diagnosis
  1. Differentiate acute adrenal insufficiency from severe acute infections, diabetic coma, CNS disturbances, acute poisoning; in newborn, distinguish from respiratory distress, intracranial hemorrhage, sepsis
  2. Differentiate chronic adrenal insufficiency from anorexia nervosa, muscular disorders (e.g., myasthenia gravis), nephritis, chronic infection (e.g., tuberculosis); consider chronic form of disease if patient has recurrent spontaneous hypoglycemia
- Physical Findings
  1. Acute adrenal insufficiency (adrenal crisis)—moribund, fever followed by hypothermia, cachexia, acutely dehydrated, vomiting, hypotension, confusion, coma, weakness, abdominal pain, nausea, increased skin pigmentation
  2. Chronic adrenal insufficiency (Addison's)—lethargy, dehydration, poor weight gain, weight loss, vomiting, hypotension, small heart size on radiograph; bronze skin pigmentation, especially of areola, mucous membranes, hand creases, axilla and groin, extensor surfaces of joints, and along surgical scars
- Diagnostic Tests/Findings
  1. Laboratory studies—decreased serum sodium and bicarbonate, $PaCO_2$, blood pH, and blood volume; hyperkalemia and increased blood urea nitrogen (BUN); urinary sodium and sodium-to-potassium ratio elevated relative to degree of hyponatremia; eosinophilia; moderate neutropenia
  2. Confirmatory tests to assess functional capacity of adrenal cortex
     a. ACTH stimulation test—involves a baseline, fasting cortisol, an injection of a synthetic hormone that should trigger an adrenal response, a second cortisol level which should double from baseline; a low level indicates adrenal insufficiency
     b. Increased baseline serum ACTH in primary adrenal failure; and measurement of TSH, FSH, LH, and prolactin
     c. Decreased urinary free cortisol and 17-hydroxycorticosteroid excretion

d. Insulin tolerance test—considered the "gold standard," causing significant symptomatic hypoglycemia to activate the hypothalamic-pituitary axis to increase ACTH stimulation; not always used in children because of the risks of hypoglycemia and hypokalemia; adrenal insufficiency is suspected with a cortisol concentration of <18 mcg/dL

e. Corticotropin-releasing hormone (CRH) test—abnormal

- Management/Treatment
  1. Immediate treatment of life-threatening acute adrenal crisis
  2. Referral to endocrinologist for suspected or confirmed adrenal insufficiency
  3. Pharmacologic—after initial stabilization, chronic corticosteroid replacement with glucocorticoids (e.g., hydrocortisone), mineralocorticoid (e.g., fluorocortisone), and/or sodium chloride (table salt); increased dosages will be needed during severe illness, trauma, stress, or surgery
  4. Monitor for steroid excess, particularly for decreasing height and weight; monitor for insufficient glucocorticoid treatment (headache, weight loss, nausea, hypotension); monitor blood glucose, ACTH, sodium, and potassium
  5. Avoid abrupt withdrawal of corticosteroids to avoid adrenal crisis
  6. Education regarding risk of acute episodes; medical alert identification tag; consider emergency hydrocortisone injection kit for use in accident or severe stress

Adrenocortical Hyperfunction

- Definition: Excessive production and secretion by the adrenal gland of cortisol, adrenocortical androgens, estrogen, and/or aldosterone
- Etiology/Incidence
  1. Hypercortisolism (Cushing syndrome)—excess cortisol (ACTH) secretion by adrenals
     a. Adrenal tumors (Cushing syndrome)—relatively rare but occurs in all ages
     b. Pituitary adenomas (Cushing disease)
     c. Chronic exposure to glucocorticoids to treat inflammation and for immunosuppression (iatrogenic hypercortisolism)
     d. Ectopic ACTH-secreting tumors—nonpituitary tumors stimulate the adrenal cortex, causing excess ACTH secretion; rare; usually seen in children <12 years
  2. Adrenogenital syndrome—virilizing adrenal tumor causes elevated adrenal androgen secretion
  3. Feminizing adrenal tumors—causes elevated adrenal estrogen secretion
  4. Hyperaldosteronism
     a. Secondary—physiologic attempts to maintain homeostasis with serum electrolytes and fluid volume due to renal compromise or physiologic response to severe illness
     b. Primary—due to adrenal tumor or hyperplasia
- Signs and Symptoms
  1. Ubiquitous effects of adrenal hormones lead to multiple and varied signs and symptoms
  2. Hypercortisolism (Cushing syndrome)—slowed growth and development, obesity, emotional lability (depression and euphoria), delayed pubertal onset, easy bruising, increased appetite, back pain
  3. Adrenogenital syndrome—increase in linear growth rate and muscle development, acne, premature pubarche, development of secondary sex characteristics in boys, enlarged and erectile clitoris in females, menstrual irregularities in older girls
  4. Feminizing adrenal tumors—rapidly increasing height, development of secondary sex characteristics in girls with possible breakthrough vaginal bleeding; gynecomastia in males
  5. Hyperaldosteronism—in infants, FTT, vomiting, weakness; may have history of recent diarrhea, increased sweating, heat exposure; history of renal or liver disease (e.g., cirrhosis, nephritis, renal ischemia); in primary hyperaldosteronism, muscle weakness, unusual periodic paralysis; paresthesias, tetany; polyuria; polydipsia
- Differential Diagnosis
  1. Hypercortisolism should be distinguished from exogenous obesity; virilizing adrenal tumors from virilizing gonadal tumors; and feminizing adrenal tumors from premature thelarche and idiopathic sexual precocity
  2. Hyperaldosteronism due to physiologic response to maintain homeostasis in severe illness vs. pathology (e.g., renal disease, adrenal tumor) should be determined
- Physical Findings
  1. Ubiquitous effects of adrenal hormones lead to multiple and varied clinical findings
  2. Hyperadrenocorticism—poor growth rate may precede obesity or other symptoms; relatively short stature; obesity; purple striae; truncal obesity; "buffalo type" adiposity of face, neck, and trunk; fat pad in interscapular area; plethoric or moon facies; delayed onset of secondary sex characteristics; muscle weakness; may have virilism; may have hemihypertrophy; delayed skeletal maturation; osteoporosis, especially of spine
  3. Adrenogenital syndrome—increase in linear growth rate; hirsutism; acne; deepening voice; increased muscle mass; masculinization of prepubertal children (boys with pubic, axillary, and sometimes facial hair with adult-size penis, frequent erections, prepubertal or slightly enlarged testes) (girls with pubic and axillary hair with enlarged and erectile clitoris); advanced bone age
  4. Feminizing adrenal tumor—increase in linear growth rate; gynecomastia in males; prepubertal testes, pubic

hair; breast development in females, may have pubic hair; advanced bone age

5. Primary hyperaldosteronism—in infants, FTT; weakness; dehydration; tetany; hypertensive or normotensive; nocturnal enuresis; muscle weakness, unusual periodic paralysis

- Diagnostic Tests/Findings
1. Various confirmatory tests are used to determine specific etiology of adrenal hyperfunction
2. Plasma cortisol concentrations elevated; may be loss of normal diurnal variation in cortisol secretion
3. Low serum chloride and potassium levels; may have elevated sodium, pH, CO_2
4. Serum ACTH slightly elevated with adrenal hyperplasia (Cushing disease), decreased with adrenal tumor, and very elevated with ACTH-producing pituitary or ectopic (extrapituitary) tumors
5. Low eosinophil counts; leukocyte counts with polymorphonuclear leukocytosis with lymphopenia, possibly elevated red blood cells (RBCs)
6. Elevated urinary free cortisol and urinary 17-hydroxycorticosteroid excretion; abnormal urinary 17-ketosteroid excretion; may have glycosuria
7. Abnormal patterns of dexamethasone suppression and abnormal CRH stimulation tests
8. Adrenogenital syndrome, androgen secretion not suppressed by dexamethasone administration; advanced bone age
9. Feminizing adrenal tumor—elevated adrenal steroids in urine; elevated urinary and plasma estrogen levels; advanced bone age
10. Hyperaldosteronism, hypokalemia, high aldosterone; may have low or elevated plasma renin level; may have increased chloride, potassium, and prostaglandin excretion in urine
11. CT and MRI to assess for adrenal tumors; pituitary imaging to assess for pituitary tumor
- Management/Treatment
1. Referral to pediatric endocrinologist for management of suspected or confirmed adrenocortical hyperfunction
2. Surgery indicated for adrenal tumors, pituitary adenomas, and ectopic ACTH-producing tumors
3. ACTH pre- and postoperatively to stimulate nontumerous contralateral adrenal cortex
4. Discontinue excessive glucocorticoid therapy if adrenocorticol hyperfunction

Hypoglycemia

- Definition: Hypoglycemia is a symptom rather than a diagnosis and indicates an abnormally low blood glucose level. When a child presents with hypoglycemia, the practitioner needs to distinguish the cause and treat the underlying condition. A definition is challenging because there is little correlation between glucose concentration, the onset of clinical symptoms, the

duration of hypoglycemia, and long-term neurocognitive sequelae. In neonates a blood glucose value of <45 mg/dL and in older infants, children, and teens of <60–70 mg/dL are reasonable targets for hypoglycemia

- Etiology/Incidence
1. Hyperinsulinism
   a. Transient—low blood glucose levels that persist beyond 24 hours of life; caused by various disorders and occurs in <0.5% of infants. These infants have low glycogen and fat reserves and delayed maturity of enzymes needed for gluconeogenesis and fatty acid oxidation; generally, they cannot tolerate a 4-hour fast. Treatment is frequent feedings to maintain glucose levels >60 mg/dL. Hypoglycemia generally resolves with steady weight gain; also seen in infants of diabetic mothers (IDM) with poor glycemic control during pregnancy, which leads to chronic intrauterine exposure to elevated maternal blood sugar. This causes increased fat deposition in the infant (AGA). Treatment is needed for 2–3 days with a combination of oral feedings and intravenous glucose infusions to maintain blood glucose between 70 and 90 mg/dL
   b. Congenital—include defects in fatty acid metabolism, insulinomas, or carbohydrate-deficient glycoprotein syndromes
   c. Hormonal deficiency—cortisol, growth hormone, ACTH, glucagon, epinephrine
   d. Defects in hepatic glycogen-release/storage—including G6PD
   e. Defects in gluconeogenesis
   f. Defects of fatty acid oxidation and carnatine metabolism
   g. Defects of ketone body synthesis/utilization
   h. Metabolic conditions—including organic acidemias, maple-syrup urine disease (MSUD), galactosemia, fructosemia
   i. Drug-induced—including sulfonylureas, insulin, beta blockers, salicylates, alcohol; consider Munchausen or Munchausen by proxy
   j. Miscellaneous causes—including infections, such as sepsis/malaria or congenital heart disease, or idiopathic ketotic hypoglycemia
- Signs and Symptoms and Physical Findings: The physical symptoms of hypoglycemia may be very nonspecific; and any nonspecific symptom may indicate hypoglycemia
1. Neonatal hypoglycemia
   a. Poor feeding, irritability, lethargy, stupor, apnea, cyanotic spells, hypothermia, hypotonia, limpness, seizures, coma
   b. Infant may demonstrate:
      (1) Cachexic or macrosomic infant
      (2) Irritability, lethargy, weak cry
      (3) Hypothermia, cyanosis, diaphoresis, pallor
      (4) Uncoordinated eye movements, eye-rolling
      (5) Apnea, irregular breathing, tachycardia
      (6) Twitching, jitteriness, convulsions, semiconsciousness, or coma

2. Childhood hypoglycemia: Symptoms are caused by deprivation of glucose in the brain; classified
    a. Autonomic symptoms (activation of the fight-flight response), including diaphoresis, palpitations, shaking, and/or hunger
    b. Neuroglycopenic—including confusion, drowsiness, odd behavior, speech difficulty, coordination problems, and/or nonspecific malaise, hunger, or headache
    c. This author uses two familiar children's stories to help parents of children with diabetes to remember the nonspecific symptoms of hypoglycemia:
        (1) "Goldilocks and the Three Bears": Your child looks like he or she has just seen these characters to explain the autonomic symptoms, including diaphoresis, elevated heart rate, and blood pressure
        (2) Your child turns into one of Snow White's Seven Dwarfs or their extended cousins—explains the neuroglycopenic symptoms, including "Sleepy," "Dopey," "Grumpy," or "Clingy"
- Differential Diagnosis: Distinguish among various possible etiologies of hypoglycemia (e.g., functional ketotic vs. inherited metabolic and endocrine disease) because of underlying implications for management
- Management/Treatment
    1. Consultation with or referral to endocrinology provider for delineation of etiology and management
    2. Treat hypoglycemic episodes promptly and adequately to prevent neurocognitive injury; especially important for infants and younger children
    3. Hypoglycemic reactions in children with diabetes—follow the "Rule of 15"
        a. Provide 15–20 g of a quick-acting source of glucose (3–4 glucose tablets, 4 oz fruit juice, 6 oz regular (sugar-containing) soda; administration of a glucose source with added fat/protein (chocolate candy bar) may delay the response to glucose; check the blood glucose level if not done initially
        b. Wait 15 minutes (while conserving energy by sitting or playing quietly)
        c. Recheck blood glucose level; repeat as necessary if blood glucose levels are <70 mg/dL
        d. Use good judgment if the episode of hypoglycemia is immediately preceding a meal; encourage the patient to eat quick-acting carbohydrates first; "treat the child and not the blood glucose level" because the blood glucose measures a "point in time" and it may not reflect how quickly the blood glucose level is changing
        e. For severe hypoglycemia, including change in consciousness, coma, or stupor making oral intake unsafe, use injectable glucagon (prescription)
    4. Surgery for pancreatic adenoma, partial pancreatomy if insulin secretion suppression unsuccessful
    5. Children with functional (fasting, ketotic) hypoglycemia—treat with liberal carbohydrate diet with bedtime snacks, moderate restriction on ketogenic foods; avoid prolonged fasting, especially if child is ill; parents may need to check urinary ketones

Diabetes Mellitus (DM)

- Definition: Chronic illness that requires a complex, multidisciplinary team, including patient and the family, to maintain glycemic control as close to normal. There are a number of disorders of insulin production or insulin action that result in hyperglycemia
- Etiology/Incidence
    1. Classification of Diabetes: There are four clinical categories of diabetes, two of which are discussed in this chapter
        o Type 1 diabetes (T1DM): Due to destruction of beta cells of pancreas, leading to absolute insulin deficiency; uncommon in infancy and toddlerhood, increases until adolescence, and then drops sharply; peaks occur between 5 and 7 years and at time of puberty; boys and girls equally affected; more frequently diagnosed in winter, especially with adolescents; environmental factors may increase or decrease expression of diabetes in susceptible individuals; multifactorial, associated with genetic predisposition and environmental factors, including viruses (e.g., mumps, coxsackie, congenital rubella), environmental toxins, nutrition, and physical and emotional stress. Previously called "juvenile onset" because a majority of persons are diagnosed before the age of 18 years
        o Type 2 (T2DM): Due to insulin resistance (in muscle, fat, and liver) as well as progressive beta-cell failure; the metabolic decline may evolve over months or years; previously called "adult-onset"; however, there is an increased incidence of T2DM in children and teens, most with a BMI >85th percentile
        o Other specific types of diabetes due to other causes—associated with administration of drugs or chemicals (steroids in renal disease, rheumatoid arthritis, asthma, leukemia, or chemotherapeutic agents), genetic defects in beta-cell function and/or insulin action, exocrine diseases, such as cystic fibrosis (treatments are similar to those for type 1), or rare genetic defects, such as maturity onset diabetes of youth (MODY), which affects 1–2% of persons diagnosed with diabetes and may be treated with sulfonylureas
        o Gestational diabetes (GDM): Diabetes diagnosed during pregnancy—beyond the scope of this chapter
- Signs and Symptoms
    1. May present along a continuum from very mild symptoms to diabetic ketoacidosis, a life-threatening

medical emergency; most T1DM patients experience a rapid progression of symptoms and are likely to get medical attention

2. Symptoms of type 1 diabetes mellitus
   a. Polyuria, polydipsia, polyphagia (primary complaints)
   b. Weight loss or failure to gain weight; variable decrease in linear growth
   c. Behavioral changes, headache, emotional lability, fatigue, recent "flulike" illness
   d. Abdominal pain, nausea, vomiting, constipation, nocturia, enuresis
   e. History of recent illness/stress, missed insulin if known diabetes

3. Symptoms of type 2 diabetes mellitus
   a. Many of the above symptoms but generally less severe than in type 1 diabetes mellitus
   b. Mild to moderate polyuria and polydipsia
   c. Weight loss
   d. History of high caloric intake and sedentary lifestyle
   e. Positive family history of type 2 diabetes mellitus or maternal gestational diabetes

- Differential Diagnosis
  1. Diabetes insipidus
  2. Nondiabetes causes of polyuria, e.g., psychogenic polydipsia, CNS injury, tumors
  3. Other causes of fatigue, weight loss, behavioral change, e.g., Hashimoto's hypothyroidism, systemic illness

- Physical Findings
  1. Type 1 diabetes mellitus
     a. May appear ill or toxic—depending on blood glucose level and degree of metabolic acidosis
     b. Hyperglycemia—as high glucose is filtered through the kidneys, osmotic balance causes excess urination
     c. Fatigue, weakness—results of decreased glucose utilization and subtle electrolyte abnormalities
     d. Weight loss, dehydration—loss of water, muscle, and fat mass contributes to acute or subacute weight loss
     e. Polydipsia—as more water is excreted, body requires more water, thirst mechanism is intact, thirst increases
     f. Visual disturbances—intraocular osmotic shift related to hyperglycemia
     g. Long-term complications—joint contractures, diabetic retinopathy, compromised renal function

  2. Type 1 diabetes with diabetic ketoacidosis
     a. Marked dehydration, irritability, lethargy, drowsiness, stupor, coma
     b. Tachycardia, cardiac arrhythmias, Kussmaul breathing (long, deep, labored breathing)
     c. Dry mucous membranes, cherry-red lips, hypotension, rapid and thready pulse, hyperventilation, low temperature, "fruity" acetone breath
     d. Vomiting, abdominal spasm, tenderness

  3. Type 2 diabetes mellitus
     a. Marked obesity
     b. Acanthosis nigricans
     c. Vaginal candidiasis in females

- Diagnostic Tests/Findings
  1. Glycosuria; urinary or blood ketones
  2. Elevated blood glucose—random blood glucose level ≥200 mg/dL or fasting blood glucose levels ≥126 mg/dL sufficient to make diagnosis of diabetes. Point-of-care blood glucose testing should be repeated with a venous sample
  3. Elevated plasma glucose—repeated findings of fasting plasma glucose level ≥126 mg/dL or plasma glucose level ≥200 mg/dL when taken either randomly (with symptoms of diabetes)
  4. Oral glucose tolerance test—75 g glucose load (2 g/kg for children younger than age 10 years); blood glucose levels are measured at baseline, 1 hour, and 2 hours
  5. Elevated glycosylated hemoglobin A1c >6.5% performed in a laboratory using a method that is certified by the National Glycohemoglobin Standardization Program (NGSP) or traceable to the Diabetes Control and Complications Trial (DCCT)
  6. Measurement of diabetes islet cell antibodies—present in >85% of patients with T1DM insulin antibody and confirms T1DM, including
     a. Insulin antibody
     b. Glutamate decarboxylase (GAD)
     c. Islet antigens (IA-2)
  7. For patients with T2DM, measurement of C-peptide level indicates endogenous insulin secretion
  8. In diabetic ketoacidosis (DKA), pH <7.30, bicarbonate <15 mmol/L—occurs in three clinical settings:
     a. New-onset T1 diabetes
     b. Insulin omission in a patient with established T1 diabetes
     c. Acute severe illness in a patient with established T1DM with inadequate insulin dosing related to metabolic needs
  9. In type 2 diabetes in children—criteria: overweight, BMI >85th percentile for age and sex; weight for height >85th percentile, *plus* any two of the following risk factors:
     a. Family history of type 2 diabetes in first- or second-degree relative
     b. Race/ethnicity: Native American, African American, Latino, Asian American, or Pacific Islander
     c. Signs/symptoms of insulin resistance (e.g., acanthrosis nigricans, hypertension, dyslipidemia, polycystic ovary syndrome [PCOS] or small for gestational age)
     d. Maternal history of diabetes or GDM

- Management/Treatment
  1. Immediate hospitalization for severe diabetic ketoacidosis
  2. The goals of treatment are to use insulin, diet, and exercise to minimize episodes of hypo- and

hyperglycemia and to promote normal growth and development

3. Consultation with physician or referral to pediatric endocrinology team for diagnostic evaluation, initial care, and ongoing management, including pediatric endocrinologists, nurse practitioners, nurses, dietician, and social worker

4. After initial stabilization, for children with type 2 diabetes, slow gradual weight loss, exercise regimen, and diabetes education

5. Patients with type 1 diabetes *must* continue insulin

6. Education is a critical component of diabetes care. The American Association of Diabetes Educators (AADE) describes AADE-7, seven healthcare behaviors necessary for educating patients and families with diabetes:
   a. Healthy eating
   b. Being active
   c. Monitoring
   d. Taking medication
   e. Problem solving
   f. Decreasing risks
   g. Healthy coping

Healthy Eating

1. Importance of consistent eating patterns
   a. Balance of protein, carbohydrates, and fats to promote normal growth and development
   b. Flexible meal plans (and insulin doses) can accommodate the child's appetite, lessen food conflicts while respecting family cultural traditions
   c. Carbohydrate counting—adding the total grams for a meal/snack and dosing insulin based on an insulin-to-carbohydrate ratio (such as 1 unit per 20 g of carbohydrates) allow for tighter glycemic control and insulin dose adjustment using rapid-acting analogs. The child with diabetes can also partake of meals/snacks with high-carbohydrate offerings (such as cake at a birthday party)

2. For patients with T2DM, weight loss of 5–7% of body weight can improve glycemic goals and decrease the risk of long-term complications

Being Active

1. Exercise—physical exercise and resistance training increase insulin sensitivity and improve blood glucose levels, strengthen the heart, and increase high-density lipoprotein (HDL) cholesterol levels, promote better sleep, improve mood with the release of endorphins, and promote overall fitness

2. Blood glucose may drop in the first 30–60 minutes of exercise—a 15-g to 20-g carbohydrate snack (without corresponding insulin dose) may prevent "postexercise hypoglycemia"

3. Some patients may experience (and some exercises may cause) a sharp rise in the blood glucose level in the first 45–60 minutes of exercise, and then a drop to hypoglycemia range 90 minutes after exercise initiation; due to a catecholamine response; insulin doses and snacks will need to be individually adjusted

4. Late hypoglycemia may appear 6–12 hours after prolonged physical activity due to muscle glycogen depletion—extra snacks and a basal insulin adjustment may be needed

Monitoring

1. Blood glucose goals vary with age (and developmental stage) of child (American Diabetes Association, 2014) (See **Table 14-1**)

2. Blood glucose management and home blood glucose targets
   a. Minimum of four blood glucose checks per day—before meals and at bedtime
   b. Additional tests may be recommended 2 hours after meals, before/during/after exercise, between 2 and 3 a.m., and whenever there is a concern of hypo- or hyperglycemia
   c. May be as many as 8–10 tests per day; patients will need prescriptions for the meter, blood glucose test strips, lancets, and a lancet device
   d. In setting blood glucose goals, the long-term health benefits of a lower A1c need to be balanced against the risk of hypoglycemia and the individual/family burden of an intensive regimen of diabetes care

Taking Medication

1. The most "physiologic" insulin regimen includes a combination of a rapid-acting analog with 1–2 doses of a long-acting analog, which may be as many as 5–8 injections daily; use of an insulin pump with a rapid-acting analog is an option (see **Table 14-2**)

2. Discuss with parents additional topics such as use of insulin pumps; successful insulin pump therapy requires parental motivation, ability to understand pump technology, frequent blood glucose monitoring, and willingness to work closely with the diabetes multidisciplinary team

3. Insulin can be taken with vial and syringe (each 10-mL vial contains ~950 units of "usable" insulin)

■ **Table 14-1**   Blood Glucose and A1c Goals for Children with T1DM

Age in Years	Before Meals	Bedtime/Overnight	A1c
0–6 years	100–180 mg/dL	110–200 mg/dL	<8.5%
6–12 years	90–180 mg/dL	100–180 mg/dL	<8.0%
13–19 years	90–130 mg/dL	90–150 mg/dL	<7.5%

■ Table 14-2

Insulin preparation	Onset of action	Peak	Duration of action
Lispro (Humalog)	<15 minutes	1–2 hours	3–6 hours
Aspart (Novolog)	<15 minutes	1–2 hours	3–6 hours
Glulisine (Apidra)	<15 minutes	1–2 hours	3–6 hours
Regular (Novolin R, Humulin R)	30–60 minutes	2–4 hours	6–10 hours
Humulin R Regular U-500	30–60 minutes	2–4 hours	Up to 24 hours
NPH (Novolin N, Humulin N, ReliOn)	2–4 hours	4–8 hours	10–18 hours
Glargine (Lantus)	1–2 hours	Usually no peak	Up to 24 hours
Detemir (Levemir)	1–2 hours	Usually no peak**	Up to 24 hours**
Premixed Insulins*			
Novolin 70/30, Humulin 70/30	30–60 minutes	2–10 hours	10–18 hours
Humalog 75/25, Novolog 70/30, Humalog 50/50	10–30 minutes	1–6 hours	10–24 hours

Data from D-life website, reviewed by James Bennett 1/12; accessed on-line 8/14, AADE Reference: The Art and Science of Diabetes Education.

*Information derived from a combination of manufacturer's prescribing information and clinical studies. Individual response to insulin preparations may vary.

**Peak and length of action may depend on size of dose and length of time since initiation of therapy

***Premixed insulins are more variable in peak and duration of action. For instance, even though the literature states that the effects may last for up to 24 hours, many people find that they will need to take a dose every 10–12 hours.

and single-use syringes or with the use of insulin pens (each 3-mL pen contains 300 units of insulin) and requires a prescription for single-use pens and needles (available in 4-mm, 5-mm, 6-mm, and 8-mm lengths)

4. For patient with T2DM, insulin is usually needed to stabilize blood glucose levels and reverse "glucose toxicity"; oral hypoglycemic agents can be given as a single agent or added with insulin; metformin is the only antidiabetic agent approved by the FDA for pediatric patients 10 years of age or older

Problem Solving

1. Definition, recognition, treatment, and prevention of hypo- and hyperglycemia
   a. Follow "the rule of 15"—see section on hypoglycemia earlier in this chapter
   b. Total daily insulin dose may need to be adjusted (+/– 10–50%) for exercise, decreased appetite, illness, or concurrent steroid use
   c. Severe hypoglycemia—generally defined as needing the assistance of another person due to confusion/change in consciousness; rates of severe hypoglycemia are higher in children <6 years old due to the lack of ability to recognize and/or articulate the symptoms
   d. Symptoms of severe hypoglycemia include disorientation, unconsciousness, seizures, and convulsions
   e. Hypoglycemic unawareness—refers to the lack of awareness of low blood glucose generally caused by an abnormal response to counterregulatory hormones and may account for prolonged and unpredictable hypoglycemia
2. Review the method to check for blood or urinary ketones if the blood glucose level remains elevated ≥250 mg/dL or *any* vomiting illness—prompt

treatment of DKA with insulin and extra fluids may prevent further morbidity

3. Glucagon is a prescription emergency kit with a lyophilized powder and sterile diluent that is mixed and injected IM or SC to treat acute hypoglycemic episodes. Dose for children <20 kg = 0.5 mg, and for children >20 kg through adult = 1 mg. Once reconstituted, Glucagon must be used immediately; if using an insulin syringe to deliver, 1 mg = 100 units
4. Information about obtaining medical identification bracelets
5. Communication with extended family and school personnel about child's management plan, school diabetes health plans (504 plans—sample plans available at http://www.childrenwithdiabetes.org)

Decreasing Risks

1. Hemoglobin A1c done quarterly to assess overall blood glucose levels and to help in ascertaining compliance with treatment regimen; gives reliable measurement of long-term glycemic control during preceding 3 months
   a. In adults, HbA1c values below or around 7% have been shown to reduce microvascular and neuropathic complications
   b. Goals should be individualized and based on reasonable benefit–risk assessment and should be less strict in children with frequent hypoglycemia or hypoglycemic unawareness
2. Sexually active adolescents need instruction regarding pregnancy; oral contraceptives are acceptable if blood pressure is normal
3. Annual blood tests to screen for diabetes complications and comorbidities, including:
   a. T_4 and TSH and thyroid antibodies for autoimmune thyroid disease

b. Total serum IgA and tissue transglutaminase antibodies (tTG-IgA) to screen for celiac disease—positive tests need diagnostic intestinal biopsy

c. Urine for microalbuminuria to screen for kidney disease

d. Fasting lipids to screen for hypercholesterolemia

4. Annual dilated eye examination to screen for diabetic retinopathy—patients with T2DM should have an eye exam shortly after diagnosis; while patients with T1DM should have regular dilated eye exams beginning 5 years after diagnosis

5. Children and adolescents with diabetes should receive immunizations as scheduled as well as annual flu vaccines (the CDC does *not* recommend the live-attenuated vaccine for patients with diabetes) and a single dose of pneumococcal vaccine

Healthy Coping

1. Recognize phases of diabetes:
   a. Development of clinical symptomatology
   b. Clinical remission or "honeymoon" period of variable duration due to improved beta-cell function after initial therapy started; lower insulin requirements
   c. Relapse with progressive increase in insulin requirement for glycemic control

2. The Juvenile Diabetes Research Foundation (JDRF) is a leading organization funding T1 diabetes research whose goal is "to remove the impact on T1s until there is a world without type 1"
   a. Online diabetes support team—match families with a local mentor
   b. T1DM toolkits—*School Advisory Toolkit for Families*
   c. Bag of Hope—free resource for newly diagnosed families filled with child- and adult-friendly books, a Rufus bear (bear with diabetes), as well as *A First Book for Understanding Diabetes,* reference books, and a DVD

3. Encourage parents to obtain user-friendly resources for helping them to better understand the disease and its management

4. Diabetes camps—search for diabetes camps by state name

☐ DISORDERS OF PUBERTAL DEVELOPMENT

- Definition: Abnormal development or delay in initiation of secondary sexual characteristics
- Etiology/Incidence: Abnormalities in pubertal development associated with CNS or gonadal disorder or dysfunction; includes temporary and permanent delays of pubertal onset or true (complete) or pseudoprecocious (incomplete) puberty

1. Intersex—ambiguous genitalia or inappropriate for gonadal sex due to endocrinopathy

2. Normal pubertal development—in females, Tanner II breast development occurs 8.0 to 10.4 years (white girls); 6.6 to 9.5 years (black girls); and 6.8 to 9.8 years (Hispanic girls); in males, Tanner II pubic hair median age 12.0 years (white boys); 11.2 (black boys); and 12.3 years (Hispanic boys)

3. Precocious puberty—secondary sexual characteristics before 9 years in males; in females, onset of breast development before 8 years, sexual pubic hair before 9.0 years, or menses before the age of 9.5 years; however, breast and pubic hair development in females may occur normally for some younger girls, see above
   a. True (complete) precocious puberty is mediated by pituitary gonadotropin secretion involving all secondary sex characteristics
      (1) Gonadotropin-releasing hormone-dependent (central)
         (a) Idiopathic (sporadic or familial)
         (b) CNS abnormalities
         (c) Tumors (e.g., LH-secreting adenoma, astrocytoma, craniopharyngioma)
      (2) Gonadotropin-releasing hormone-independent (peripheral)
         (a) Genetic (i.e., congenital adrenal hyperplasia [CAH] in males, McCune-Albright syndrome)
         (b) Tumors (e.g., adrenal, ovarian, or testicular)
         (c) Limited (e.g., chronic primary hypothyroidism, ovarian cysts)
   b. Pseudoprecocious (incomplete) puberty involves one type of secondary sexual characteristic (e.g., premature thelarche [breast development] or pubarche [pubic hair development]) mediated by excessive estrogen/androgen stimulation for age from ovaries/testes, adrenal cortex, or exogenous sources

4. Hypogonadism—causes lack of secondary sexual characteristics (sexual infantilism)
   a. In boys, lack of secondary sexual characteristics after 17 years suggests abnormal testicular maturation; may be due to testicular failure or dysfunction (primary failure due to anorchia, castration, Klinefelter syndrome, mumps, radiation, trauma, tumor, endocrinopathies, etc.) or to pituitary/hypothalamic dysfunction (panhypopituitarism, empty sella syndrome, gonadotropin deficiency, LH and FSH deficiencies, endocrinopathies, etc.)
   b. In girls, may have lack of onset of secondary sex characteristics and amenorrhea due to primary ovarian failure (due to gonadal dysgenesis, enzyme defects, infection, surgery, radiation, chemotherapy, etc.) or to secondary ovarian failure (hypothalamic disorder or dysfunction, CNS irradiation, eating disorders, excessive exercise, chronic illness, etc.)

- Signs and Symptoms
1. If intersex, history of confusion of sex assignment at birth
2. May have normal growth and development through childhood; at puberty, may have abnormal sexual

development; females may have virilization, primary amenorrhea; males may have incomplete virilization
3. May have history of underlying disease, dysfunction, or systemic illness causing delay in/or premature pubertal onset; history of exposure to radiation, drugs, etc.
4. May have history of early development of one or all secondary sex characteristics, tall stature, symptoms of endocrine disease (e.g., hypothyroidism, congenital adrenal hyperplasia), intracranial disease (e.g., visual disturbances), abdominal disease (e.g., adrenal or gonadal tumor) or dysfunction (see growth disturbances, this chapter)
5. May have delayed development of secondary sex characteristics and symptoms of metabolic or endocrine disturbances (e.g., constipation), intracranial disease (e.g., failure to grow, seizure), syndrome stigmata (e.g., developmental delays), abdominal disease (abdominal enlargement) or dysfunction (see growth disturbances and adrenal gland disorders, this chapter)
- Differential Diagnosis
1. Ambiguous genitalia or suspected intersex—distinguish true hermaphroditism (both ovarian and testicular tissue present), female pseudohermaphroditism (female genotype, only ovaries), and male pseudohermaphroditism (male genotype, only testes)
2. Structural abnormalities of genital tract and associated intracranial, endocrine, abdominal, or pelvic disease
3. Precocious puberty—distinguish between true (complete) precocious puberty mediated by pituitary gonadotropin secretion involving all secondary sex characteristics vs. pseudoprecocious (incomplete) puberty involving one type of secondary sexual characteristics
4. Premature sexual development—distinguish normal variants of premature thelarche (isolated premature breast development) and pubarche (early pubic hair development) in girls from pathologic causes; distinguish normal variants of premature adrenarche in boys (adrenal maturation with pubic hair and body odor) from pathologic causes
- Physical Findings
1. May have normal or abnormal physical examination depending on underlying etiology of pubertal disorder (e.g., normal examination in constitutional delay, findings of chronic or systemic illness, or midfacial defects in pathologic pubertal delay, tall stature in Klinefelter syndrome)
2. May have normal or abnormal genitalia depending on underlying etiology of pubertal disorder and timing (e.g., genitalia may be ambiguous in congenital adrenal hyperplasia); may have cryptorchidism in sexual infantilism or in pituitary insufficiency; may have abdominal mass or testicular mass in gonadal tumor; may have microphallus in human GH deficiency; may have small testes in testicular failure; may have abnormal pelvic examination, etc.

3. With precocious puberty, may have tall stature, premature secondary sex characteristics
4. With contrasexual pubertal development may have gynecomastia in males due to hypogonadism from Klinefelter syndrome; excessive virilization of prepubertal girls with pubic hair, oily skin, acne, clitoromegaly, hirsutism
5. With delayed pubertal development for age (constitutional delay of puberty), may have normal examination except for delayed growth and development (short stature but low-normal growth rate) during childhood; delayed bone age; relatively short legs for height or greater upper-to-lower-body ratio; descended normal testes that are prepubertal in size, consistency
6. With delayed or interrupted pubertal development may have findings consistent with endocrine disorder (e.g., anosmia, the lack of ability to smell; micropenis in gonadotropin abnormalities; hirsutism and dry hair and skin in hypothyroidism)
- Diagnostic Tests/Findings
1. Tanner staging of breasts, genitals, pubic hair development
2. Laboratory findings variable depending on etiology of pubertal disorder; tests may include plasma or serum LH, FSH, GH, electrolytes, thyroid tests, blood and urinary pH, urine specific gravity, sedimentation rates, BUN, creatinine
3. Tests of hormonal function as needed (e.g., GnRH to differentiate hypogonadotropic hypogonadism and constitutionally delayed puberty)
4. CT, MRI, or ultrasound as needed to rule in or rule out central CNS, adrenal, renal, gonadal, or thyroid disease; bone age
5. Other laboratory tests as needed—karyotype if ambiguous genitalia or Klinefelter syndrome suspected
- Management/Treatment
1. Physician consultation or referral to pediatric endocrinologist for suspected pathologic cause of pubertal delay or abnormal development
2. Treatment dictated by identified etiology for pathologic cause of pubertal delay or abnormality in pubertal development (e.g., hormonal therapy may be immediate, as with congenital adrenal hyperplasia, or at puberty with testosterone for testicular failure)
3. Management of underlying endocrine disorders and diseases and systemic illness (e.g., hypothyroidism, poorly controlled diabetes, anorexia, inflammatory bowel disease)

☐ GYNECOMASTIA

- Definition: Visible or palpable glandular enlargement of the male breast occurring commonly in healthy adolescent males (pubertal gynecomastia); occasionally indicative of underlying disease (pathologic gynecomastia); seen frequently in newborns (neonatal gynecomastia)

- Etiology/Incidence
  1. Neonatal gynecomastia—due to cross-placental transfer of maternal hormones; usually resolves by 2 to 3 weeks, may be longer in breastfed infants
  2. Pubertal gynecomastia—influence of too little androgen and/or too much estrogen on mammary tissue; transient, may occur in 40% to 66% of normal boys during puberty; onset between 10 and 12 years, peak occurrence 13 and 14 years, usually self-limiting; resolves by 16 to 17 years of age
  3. Pathologic gynecomastia—secondary to drug side effects (e.g., cimetidine, digitalis, phenothiazine, treatment with hCG, testosterone, or estrogen), underlying disease or syndromes (e.g., Klinefelter), injury to the nervous system, chest wall, or testes; or may be idiopathic
- Signs and Symptoms—breast development in other than pubertal females
- Differential Diagnosis
  1. Transient pubertal gynecomastia from obesity (lipomastia) and pathologic causes; tumor (lipoma, neurofibroma, cancer)
  2. Breast infection
  3. Fat necrosis due to injury
  4. Drugs (estrogens, anabolic steroids, marijuana)
  5. Klinefelter gonadal dysfunction
- Physical Findings
  1. Neonatal; usually bilateral, often asymmetric breast tissue enlargement; resolves within 1 to 2 weeks
  2. Pubertal (physiologic) gynecomastia—breast tissue enlargement glandular, movable, disk-shaped, below areola, nonadherent to skin or underlying tissue; typically breasts unequal in size and <3 cm in diameter; breasts may be tender, nipples irritated due to rubbing on clothing; if tissue >4 to 5 cm in diameter and breasts dome-shaped, macrogynecomastia present; Tanner stages II to IV pubertal development with testes >3 cm length
  3. Pathologic gynecomastia—malnourishment, lymphadenopathy, delayed sexual maturity with undermasculinization, signs of chronic disease (e.g., goiter, liver or renal disease, endocrinopathies, cancer, colitis, cystic fibrosis, AIDS); breast tissue >3 cm in diameter, asymmetric, hard, fixed, indurated, not directly beneath areola; may have absent, underdeveloped, or asymmetric testes
- Diagnostic Tests/Findings
  1. Endocrinology studies as indicated
  2. Imaging techniques as appropriate—ultrasonography of testes to identify impalpable testicular tumor; CT, MRI of abdomen to identify adrenal tumors
  3. Karyotyping if Klinefelter suspected
- Management/Treatment
  1. Neonatal—parent education and reassurance about etiology, transience, and normalcy of condition
  2. Pubertal (physiologic) gynecomastia <4 cm—explanation, reassurance, and observation; regression usually spontaneous, within a few months, rarely beyond 2 years

  3. Physiologic macrogynecomastia (>4 cm mass)—medical or surgical treatment usually required as regression is rare, especially if gynecomastia present for >4 years; pharmacologic therapy (e.g., tamoxifen, danazol, testosterone) sometimes used
  4. Gynecomastia usually very upsetting to adolescent but often not discussed because of embarrassment; reassure about transience and spontaneous regression

☐ MENSTRUAL DISORDERS: AMENORRHEA

- Definition
  1. Primary amenorrhea—failure of onset of menarche in females who are 16 years and have normal pubertal growth and development; 14 years with absence of normal pubertal growth and development; or in girls who have not begun menstruation 2 years after completed sexual maturation
  2. Secondary amenorrhea—absence of menstruation for >3 cycles or at least 6 months after menstruation established
- Etiology/Incidence
  1. Primary amenorrhea
     a. Constitutional/familial (common)
     b. Obstructions of menstrual flow (e.g., fusion or stenosis of labia, imperforate hymen)
     c. Estrogen deficiency
        (1) Primary ovarian insufficiency—organic or functional ovarian failure (e.g., anatomic anomalies, pelvic irradiation, enzyme defects, autoimmune disease, infection)
        (2) Secondary ovarian insufficiency—organic or functional ovarian failure from hypothalamic/pituitary disorders (e.g., decreased gonadotropin secretion, effects of chronic diseases such as DM, CF, anorexia; excessive exercise; endocrine disease)
     d. Androgen excess (e.g., polycystic ovaries, adrenal androgen excess [Cushing])
     e. Ovarian tumors
  2. Secondary amenorrhea; many causes same as primary amenorrhea
     a. Pregnancy (most common)
     b. Hypothalamic, pituitary, and adrenal disorders or tumors; chromosomal abnormalities (e.g., Turner syndrome); endocrinopathies; chronic illness, especially those causing severe weight loss or malnutrition; conditions affecting gonadal function
     c. Pharmacologic agents (discontinuance of birth control pills, use of tranquilizers)
     d. Significant emotional stress or strenuous exercise programs, especially with runners, ballet dancers, and gymnasts; major weight loss
     e. Uterine dysfunction after abortion, infection, C-section
     f. Hysterectomy

- Signs and Symptoms
  1. Primary amenorrhea—no history of menses in adolescence; may have symptoms of marked psychosocial stress, adrenal dysfunction or gonadal disease, pituitary or hypothalamic disease, chronic illness, including eating disorders, chromosomal abnormalities, pregnancy; may have cyclic abdominal pain without menstruation in pseudoamenorrhea
  2. Secondary amenorrhea—sudden or gradual cessation of menses; symptoms vary depending on underlying etiology; also caused by excessive exercise; athletes have high rates of amenorrhea as well as eating disorders
- Differential Diagnosis
  1. Determine whether underlying etiology due to chronic illness, CNS disease, anorexia nervosa, inflammatory bowel disease, diabetes, pituitary adenoma, or thyroid dysfunction
  2. Distinguish primary amenorrhea due to constitutional or familial etiology from pregnancy
  3. Distinguish secondary amenorrhea due to pregnancy (most common cause), underlying disease or disorder
  4. Determine amenorrhea vs. "pseudoamenorrhea" (menstruation occurs but obstruction prevents release of menstrual blood)
- Physical Findings
  1. May have normal physical examination or signs of chronic, systemic illness or syndromes (e.g., underweight, CNS tumor or dysfunction, endocrinopathies, autoimmune disease, anorexia, malnourishment, unusually tall or short stature); may show signs of pregnancy
  2. May have lack of development of secondary characteristics or normal sexual development
  3. Pelvic examination may show pregnancy, reproductive system abnormalities (e.g., cervical atresia, imperforate hymen)
- Diagnostic Tests/Findings
  1. Pregnancy test
  2. Careful family history to rule out constitutional/familial delay, then consultation with physician and/or referral to specialists as needed
- Management/Treatment
  1. Constitutional/familial primary amenorrhea—education, reassurance, monitoring
  2. Amenorrhea associated with other etiologies requires further evaluation, physician consultation, or referral to appropriate specialist (e.g., reproductive endocrinologist, surgeon, pediatric neurologist, obstetrician, psychologist)
  3. Treatment directed at management or correction of underlying cause of abnormal menstrual processes (e.g., surgery if imperforate hymen, adrenal tumors)
  4. Sensitivity to significant concern of delayed development by child and family very important
  5. Parent and child education regarding amenorrhea and adherence to any treatment regimen
  6. Genetic counseling may be indicated if genetic etiology

❏ OBESITY

- Definition: A multifactorial disorder of energy balance characterized by increased adipose tissue. The CDC does not use the term *obese* for children and teens (ages 2–20 years)
  1. "At risk for overweight"—children with body mass index (BMI = kg/m^2) between the 85th and 95th percentile for age
  2. "Overweight"—children with a BMI >95th percentile for age
  3. Age- and gender-specific BMI growth charts can be found on the CDC website at http://www.cdc.gov
  4. For adults:
     a. "Overweight" is defined as a BMI >25 kg/m^2
     b. "Obese" is defined as a BMI >30 kg/m^2
- Etiology/Incidence
  1. In the past 30 years, the incidence of obesity in children has more than doubled and has quadrupled in the adolescent population
  2. In 2012, more than one-third of American children were overweight or obese
  3. Obesity remains the number one public global health problem, representing a complex multifactorial disease with behavioral, environmental, and genetic factors
- Signs and Symptoms
  1. Cardiovascular disease, including hypertension and dyslipidemia
  2. Increased risk of impaired glucose tolerance (IGT), insulin resistance, and type 2 diabetes
  3. Respiratory disease, including asthma and obstructive sleep apnea (OSA)
  4. Gastrointestinal disease, including gastroesophageal reflux disease (GERD), gallstones, nonalcoholic fatty liver disease (NAFLD), and cholelithiasis
  5. Joint problems and musculoskeletal discomfort, including slipped capital femoral epiphysis (SCFE), Blount disease, Legg-Calvé-Perthes disease, flatfoot, and osteoarthritis
  6. Reproductive—menstrual irregularities, polycystic ovarian syndrome (PCOS), and increased androgenic symptoms, including acne, hirsutism, acanthosis nigricans, and infertility
  7. Psychosocial problems, including low self-esteem, and increased risk for being bullied
  8. Other—pseudotumor cerebri
- History
  1. Age of onset—review of growth charts and family photos, early onset (<5 years of age suggests a genetic cause)
  2. Duration of obesity—a short history suggests an endocrine or central cause
  3. CNS history—previous infection, trauma, hemorrhage, radiation therapy, or seizures suggest pituitary disease; whereas morning headaches, vomiting, and visual disturbance may indicate a hypothalamic tumor

4. History of dry skin, constipation, intolerance to cold, or fatigue may indicate hypothyroidism

5. Hyperphagia—specifically waking at night to eat and/or demanding food shortly after a meal suggests a genetic cause of obesity

6. Developmental delay—review developmental milestones, educational and behavioral history—may indicate a structural and/or genetic cause

7. Visual or hearing impairment—may suggest genetic cause

8. Onset and progression of pubertal development—can be early or delayed in children and teens; primary hypogonadotropic hypogonadism or hypogenitalism can be associated with genetic causes

9. Family history—maternal diabetes status, birthweight, parental height and weight

10. Previous medications use—including glucocorticoids, sulfonylureas, monoamine oxidase inhibitors (MAOIs), oral contraceptives, and/or atypical antipsychotics

- Physical Findings to assess underlying causes and/or comorbidities
  1. Vital signs—assess blood pressure (BP) using the correct cuff size; hypertension is defined as BP reading greater than the 95th percentile for age, gender, and height on three separate occasions
  2. Skin—acanthosis nigricans (sign of insulin resistance), acne, striae, and/or hirsutism (PCOS), any irritation or inflammation (consequence of obesity)
  3. HEENT (head, eyes, ears, nose, and throat)—fundoscopic examination to rule out papilledema (pseudotumor cerebri), tonsillar hypertrophy (OSA), palpate thyroid (goiter/hypothyroidism)
  4. Chest—assess for wheezing (asthma, exercise intolerance)
  5. Abdomen—tenderness (GERD, gallbladder disease, and hepatomegaly [NAFLD])
  6. Extremities—abnormal gait, limited hip range of motion (SCFE), bowing of tibia (Blount disease), small hands and feet, polydactyly (Prader-Willi syndrome or Bardet-Biedl syndrome), arches and bottom of feet (flatfoot)
  7. Reproductive—Tanner stage (premature puberty age <7 years in white girls, age <6 years in black girls; age <9 years in boys); apparent micropenis (may be normal-size penis under abdominal fat pads); undescended testis/micropenis (Prader-Willi syndrome)
- Diagnostic Tests/Findings
  1. Labs—liver function tests, fasting lipid panel, fasting glucose and insulin level
  2. Other diagnostic tests as determined by the result of the H&P—including 2-hour oral glucose test, hemoglobin A1c, sleep study, radiology studies of knees/hips
  3. Severe obesity in toddler may require genetic testing and leptin levels
  4. Measurements—growth velocity, body mass index, body fat measurement

5. 3-day dietary history (2 weekdays and 1 weekend day, ideally) to determine modifiable risk factors, overall dietary quality and quantity (portion sizes, balance of protein/fat/carbohydrate), meal frequency and snacking, quantity of sugar-sweetened beverages, intake of fast food and packaged foods, dietary intake of fruits and vegetables and calcium and fiber, consumption of breakfast, meals and snacks consumed while watching TV

6. Assess daily "screen time," including phone, texting, computer, hand-held games, and tablets; quality and quantity of activity at school (physical education) and outside of school (sports teams), and presence of "distractions" in the child's room—TV, technology—lack of regular bedtime routine

- Management/Treatment
  1. Lifestyle modification—weight maintenance is recommended for most children
     a. Dietary intervention—elimination of sugar-containing beverages and change to low-glycemic-load diet, increase fruit and vegetable consumption to 5 servings per day, encourage breakfast eating, turn off technology during meals
     b. Physical activity intervention—minimum 30 minutes of vigorous exercise 5 days per week; decrease sedentary behaviors (TV, hand-held games) and increase physical education and after-school programs
     c. School intervention—model health promotion ideals and encourage in-school vigorous activity; the White House and other organizations are promoting and encouraging healthier school lunches
     d. Family intervention—usually child is not the only obese member of the family; promote parenting skills that include healthy dietary choices and avoiding food as a reward
  2. Pharmacotherapy
     a. A number of medications for adults are FDA approved for treatment of obesity; only orlistat has been approved for treatment of obesity in adolescents age 12 or older
     b. Orlistat works by decreasing fat absorption from the gut by ~30%; unabsorbed fat is excreted in the feces, causing a side effect of transient diarrhea, abdominal discomfort, and flatulence
  3. Surgery
     a. Bariatric surgery—induces weight loss, improves medical comorbid conditions, improves quality of life, and extends survival; has increased from 13,000 operations in 1998 to ~121,000 operations in 2004
     b. Patients younger than age 18 years comprise about 0.1% to 1% of bariatric surgery patients
     c. Types of procedures—have resolved some medical comorbidities; complications include nutrient deficiency, wound infection, postoperative bleeding, intestinal obstruction, pulmonary embolism
        (1) Laproscopic adjustable gastric banding (LAGB)
        (2) Roux-en-Y gastric bypass (RYGB)

(3) Vertical banded gastroplasty (VPG)

(4) Biliopancreatic diversion with duodenal switch (BPD/DS)

(5) Laproscopic sleeve gastrectomy (LSG)

4. Prevention is critical in limiting the epidemic

☐ QUESTIONS

Select the best answer.

1. You receive the results of newborn screening and find that the TSH done at day 2 is 82 mIU/L. What is your best option?
   a. Have the child come to the clinic next week for a reevaluation.
   b. Rescreen the child in 1 month
   c. Begin thyroid supplementation immediately.
   d. Reassure the family that these are normal results.

2. You are evaluating a 13-year-old girl for Graves' disease. Which of the following signs would not support this diagnosis?
   a. An enlarged thyroid
   b. Exophthalmos
   c. A positive family history
   d. An elevated TSH level

3. The routine screening of a newborn in your practice indicates that the baby has congenital hypothyroidism and is in need of a referral to a pediatric endocrinologist. The treatment of choice for congenital or acquired hypothyroidism is:
   a. Levothyroxine
   b. Methimazole
   c. Potassium iodide
   d. Radiation therapy

4. A child in your clinic is being evaluated for short stature. Pertinent findings include delayed bone age, delayed onset of puberty, and a stature that is normal for the child's bone age. In addition, the mother states that the child's father grew taller in college and wonders if this will happen with their son. The most likely cause of these findings is:
   a. Familial short stature
   b. Chromosomal abnormality
   c. Constitutional delay of growth and puberty
   d. Endocrine abnormality

5. Which chromosomal abnormality is associated with short stature in girls?
   a. Down syndrome
   b. Turner syndrome
   c. Klinefelter syndrome
   d. Prader-Willi syndrome

6. Achondroplasia refers to a growth delay that is:
   a. Due to malabsorption
   b. Associated with Noonan syndrome
   c. Associated with endocrine disorders
   d. Manifested by disproportionately short stature

7. You are following a 4-year-old girl in your practice with a history of breast development that appeared 12 months ago and that appears to be progressing. She is growing rapidly. The PNP considers ordering a bone age because she knows that most cases of premature thelarche in girls are:
   a. A result of enzymatic defects
   b. Due to systemic CNS disease
   c. Idiopathic
   d. A result of hypothyroidism

8. The mother of an 11-year-old boy is concerned that her son is developing secondary sexual characteristics too early. Your counseling for this family is based on the knowledge that puberty is considered precocious in boys if secondary sexual characteristics appear prior to age:
   a. 12 years
   b. 11 years
   c. 10 years
   d. 9 years

9. Treatment of true (central) precocious puberty is best achieved with:
   a. Synthetic follicle-stimulating hormone
   b. Gonadotropin-releasing hormone
   c. Dexamethasone
   d. Thyroid hormone

10. The pathophysiology of type 1 diabetes is:
    a. Autoimmune destruction of the pancreatic beta cells
    b. Primary insulin receptor resistance
    c. Increased hepatic glucose production
    d. Reduced glucose uptake by target tissue

11. An 11-year-old girl presents at a well-child visit with symptoms of polyuria and polydipsi. Which of the following diagnoses must be ruled out?
    a. Diabetes mellitus
    b. Hyperthyroidism
    c. Adrenocortical insufficiency
    d. Nephrotic syndrome

12. For children with diabetes, in addition to home monitoring of blood glucose and urine ketone levels, glycosylated hemoglobin (A1c) should be measured:
    a. Once a week
    b. Once a month
    c. Once every 3 months
    d. Once every 6 months

13. Mrs. W. has brought her 1-year-old baby to the clinic for a well-baby examination. She is pregnant with her second child and is concerned about possible risks to the fetus because she has gestational class A_1 diabetes (diet controlled). For which of the following conditions is the fetus not at risk?
    a. Congenital anomalies
    b. Hypoglycemia
    c. Birth trauma
    d. Congenital hearing loss

14. Infants with IUGR are prone to hypoglycemia primarily because they:
    a. Have a decreased metabolic rate
    b. Have little glucose stores in the form of glycogen and fat

c. Become acidotic

d. Are prone to sepsis

15. During the first well-baby visit of Joshua, 2 weeks old, his mother says that she is concerned because his penis looks different from his 3-year-old brother's penis. During the physical exam, you notice that the baby's scrotum is hyperpigmented. You know that the most common cause of ambiguous genitalia is:

a. Idiopathic

b. A chromosomal defect

c. Congenital adrenal hyperplasia (CAH)

d. An embryologic disorder

16. Which of the following signs or symptoms is not associated with congenital adrenal hyperplasia?

a. Hypernatremia

b. Progressive weight loss

c. Dehydration

d. Hyperkalemia

17. For families of children with congenital adrenal hyperplasia, it is critical to educate them about:

a. The self-limiting aspect of the disorder

b. The need for genetic counseling

c. Dietary restrictions

d. The need for strict replacement therapy

18. The mother of a 14-year-old girl indicates that she is concerned because the girl has not yet started to menstruate. The history is noncontributory and the physical examination is normal. Breast development and pubic hair have been present for 12 months. The most appropriate initial step would be to:

a. Do a pregnancy test

b. Obtain a buccal smear for chromosomal analysis

c. Reassure, educate the family, and follow up

d. Draw LH and FSH levels

19. Primary dysmenorrhea is due to:

a. Elevated prostaglandin level

b. Pelvic inflammatory disease (PID)

c. Endometriosis

d. Fibroids

20. The differential diagnosis of dysfunctional uterine bleeding (DUB) includes all but which of the following?

a. Pregnancy-related disorders

b. Anemia

c. Foreign body

d. Endometriosis

21. An 11-month-old African American boy has just started walking and is found to have severely bowed legs. In the history, you learn that he is exclusively breastfed with very little other food intake. You must consider:

a. Trauma

b. Developmental variation

c. Chromosomal abnormality

d. Rickets

22. Secondary hypothyroidism results from:

a. Excess release of thyroid hormone beyond the newborn period

b. Intrauterine exposure to thyrotoxic drugs

c. Disease or disorder of the thyroid gland itself

d. Disease or disorder of the hypothalamus or pituitary gland compromising thyroid function

23. Congenital hypothyroidism has a higher incidence in which of the following populations?

a. African Americans

b. Hispanic and Native Americans

c. Asian Americans

d. Euro-Americans

24. Which of the following is not a sign or symptom of congenital hypothyroidism?

a. Hoarse cry

b. Frequent stooling

c. Coarse features

d. Lethargy

25. The most common cause of hyperthyroidism in children and adolescents is:

a. Graves' (autoimmune) disease

b. Thyroid cancer

c. Thyroid nodules

d. Pituitary tumor

26. Which of the following is not found in an adolescent with untreated Graves' disease?

a. Behavioral problems

b. Sleep disturbances

c. Tendency to gain weight easily

d. Tachycardia

27. In which one of the following children would you most suspect hyperthyroidism?

a. A 16-year-old male who complains about restlessness

b. A 14-year-old adolescent female who is heat intolerant and has amenorrhea

c. A male preteen with behavior problems

d. A 6-year-old female who complains of tiredness

28. The most common thyroiditis is:

a. Subacute thyroiditis caused by a viral infection of the gland

b. Acute suppurative thyroiditis caused by bacterial infection

c. Caused by exposure to radiation or trauma

d. Hashimoto's or chronic autoimmune thyroiditis

29. Nephrogenic, or vasopressin-resistant, diabetes insipidus:

a. Is caused by anatomic defects in the brain causing hypofunction of the pituitary or hypothalamus

b. Results from damage to the hypothalamus or pituitary from surgical trauma or infection

c. Is caused by reduced renal responsiveness to antidiuretic hormone (ADH)

d. Has oliguria as a primary presenting symptom

30. An infant with polydipsia, polyuria, irritability, and failure to thrive should be evaluated for:

a. Diabetes insipidus

b. Homocystinuria

c. Growth hormone deficiency

d. Hyperglycemia

31. Which one of the following is not characteristic of constitutional growth delay?
    a. There is generally no history of a similar growth pattern in other family members.
    b. The child usually remains constitutionally small as an adult.
    c. Final adult stature tends to be normal.
    d. Weight and height at birth are generally in the normal range.

32. A newborn infant with birth length <50th percentile and micropenis should be suspected of having:
    a. Growth hormone deficiency
    b. Congenital hypothyroidism
    c. Primordial short stature
    d. Down syndrome

33. An adolescent male who fails to develop secondary sex characteristics at puberty and who has small, underdeveloped testes should be suspected of having:
    a. Adrenal hyperplasia
    b. Klinefelter syndrome
    c. Marfan syndrome
    d. Cerebral gigantism (Sotos syndrome)

34. Individuals with chronic adrenal insufficiency often have:
    a. Frequent otitis media
    b. High energy levels
    c. Love for physical activity
    d. A craving for salt

35. In the newborn period, infants of diabetic mothers (IDMs) are particularly at risk for:
    a. Small size for gestational age
    b. Intrauterine growth retardation (IUGR)
    c. Disorders in bone development
    d. Hypoglycemia

36. Which statement is true about true (complete) precocity or incomplete precocity (pseudoprecocity)?
    a. True precocity occurs because of hormonal stimulation from the pituitary or hypothalamus causing gonadal maturation and fertility.
    b. Pseudoprecocity does not involve development of any secondary sex characteristics.
    c. Incomplete precocity is caused by adrenal or gonadal tumors or dysfunction and results in increased linear growth but no development of secondary sex characteristics.
    d. Incomplete precocity leads to testicular enlargement and ovulation.

37. An adolescent who has tall stature, increased arm span, arachnodactyly, laxity of joints, pectus excavatum, and an abnormal echocardiogram would be suspected of having:
    a. Turner syndrome
    b. Beckwith-Wiedemann syndrome
    c. Marfan syndrome
    d. Klinefelter syndrome

38. Which one of the following is not found in children with growth hormone excess?
    a. Tall stature
    b. Prominent mandible and supraorbital ridge
    c. Enlargement of nose, ears, and jaw
    d. Short stature

39. A pathognomonic skin finding in children with chronic adrenal insufficiency (Addison's disease) is:
    a. Purple striae
    b. Increased pigmentation in the axilla, groin, areola, hand creases, and along surgical scars
    c. Darkened, thickened skin
    d. Increased perspiration and heat intolerance

40. Which of the following findings is not characteristic of children and infants with hyperadrenocorticism?
    a. Advanced skeletal maturation
    b. Moon facies
    c. Weight gain
    d. "Buffalo type" adiposity of face, neck, and trunk

41. Transient neonatal hypoglycemia is:
    a. Most common in AGA infants
    b. Low in premature SGA infants
    c. Most common in LGA infants
    d. Least common in LGA infants

42. Which of the following statements regarding therapy in a child with type 1 diabetes is not true?
    a. Provide normal growth and development with minimal hypo- or hyperglycemic episodes.
    b. Treat the metabolic acidemia initially and then decrease doses and maintain glycemic control with diet and exercise.
    c. Insulin therapy is a life-saving treatment that will need to be continued.
    d. Insulin therapy can mimic normal pancreatic physiology with a combination of rapid-acting analogs and long-acting analog insulins.

43. The preferred name now for insulin-dependent diabetes mellitus (IDDM) is:
    a. Maturity-onset diabetes
    b. Type 1 diabetes
    c. Type 2 diabetes
    d. Insulin resistance syndrome

44. Blood glucose levels of younger children with diabetes are maintained at slightly higher levels than blood glucose levels of older children because:
    a. Children have a greater need for available glucose in the blood system.
    b. Younger children tend to be more active.
    c. Younger children become more irritable than do older children.
    d. Lowering the risk of hypoglycemia in younger children is particularly important to avoid the potential for hypoglycemia with consequent neurologic system damage.

45. Fasting blood glucose goals for children younger than the age of 6 years with diabetes should be:
    a. Between 100 and 180 mg/dL
    b. Between 70 and 120 mg/dL
    c. Between 60 and 80 mg/dL
    d. Slightly over 200 mg/dL

46. Glucagon should be used to treat:
    a. Children with mild hypoglycemia
    b. Children with moderate hypoglycemia
    c. Children with severe hyperglycemia
    d. Children with severe hypoglycemia

47. Which finding is not a sign or symptom of diabetes onset in children?
    a. Alopecia
    b. Polyphagia
    c. Polydipsia
    d. Polyuria

48. Abdominal pain and vomiting are particularly critical to monitor in children with diabetes because these findings may represent the onset of:
    a. Ketoacidosis
    b. Gastrointestinal infection
    c. Hyperglycemia
    d. Autoimmune pancreatitis

49. Which of the following statements is not true about type 2 diabetes?
    a. The patient treatment regimen may include insulin, metformin, 30 minutes of daily exercise, and meal plan to decrease weight by 5–7% of total body weight.
    b. The incidence of type 2 diabetes is decreasing in the Hispanic and African American populations.
    c. Children with type 2 diabetes can present with overweight and acanthosis nigricans.
    d. Three factors influence a child's potential to develop type 2 diabetes—genetic predisposition, autoimmune response, and exposure to viral or chemical agents.

50. Which of the following statements is *not* true about the childhood/adolescent obesity epidemic?
    a. There is only one pharmacologic treatment, orlistat, approved by the FDA for the treatment of obesity.
    b. Prevention is critical in limiting the epidemic with promotion of healthy eating, exercise, and lifestyle changes.
    c. Obesity in children is described as a BMI >30 kg/m².
    d. BMI should be calculated at every well-child examination and plotted on the age- and gender-specific growth charts available from the CDC.

51. Precocious pubertal development is defined as the development of secondary sexual characteristics in boys before the age of _____ years and menses in girls before the age of _____ years.
    a. 10 years; 10 years
    b. 6 years; 8 years

c. 9 years; 9.5 years
d. 6 years; 9 years

52. In boys, lack of secondary sexual characteristics after 17 years suggests:
    a. Anorchia
    b. Abnormal testicular function
    c. True hermaphroditism
    d. Pituitary adenoma

53. The peak incidence for adolescent gynecomastia occurs at age:
    a. 9 to 10 years
    b. 13 to 14 years
    c. 16 to 18 years
    d. >18 years

54. The most common cause of primary amenorrhea is:
    a. Pregnancy
    b. Primary ovarian insufficiency
    c. Secondary ovarian insufficiency
    d. Constitutional or familial

☐ ANSWERS AND RATIONALES

1. C: Congenital thyroid screening is included in the newborn screen done prior to discharge and before day 7 of life by measuring T_4 and thyroid-stimulating hormone (TSH). If the free T_4 is <6.5 µg/dL and the TSH is >20 mIU/L, the infant should be started immediately on thyroid replacement and referred to a pediatric endocrinologist. Any delay in starting thyroid replacement can lead to mental retardation and neurologic consequences.

2. D: In hyperthyroidism, the thyroid-stimulating hormone (TSH) level is decreased; the other answers are consistent with signs of Graves' disease.

3. A: Levothyroxine is the drug of choice for treating hypothyroidism. The other answers are treatment options for hyperthyroidism.

4. C: Constitutional delay is characterized by a bone age that is delayed for chronologic age and a normal growth velocity for bone age. Familial short stature is characterized by slow growth during the first 2–3 years followed by low-normal growth velocity. Endocrine abnormality may be present in a child with dysmorphic features, indicating a genetic cause or skeletal abnormalities, and disproportionate features may indicate skeletal dysplasia or metabolic bone disease.

5. B: Turner syndrome, which occurs in girls, is associated with stature below the third percentile in 99% of affected cases. Down syndrome can affect girls and boys. Klinefelter syndrome is associated with tall stature and hypogonadism. Prader-Willi syndrome is a genetic disorder characterized by hyperphagia and obesity, hypotonia, and reduced mental ability.

6. D: Achondroplasia, or skeletal dysplasia, is an autosomal dominant mutation that results in disproportionate short stature (e.g., shortened limbs, macrocephaly, and bowing of legs). It is not responsive to growth

hormone therapy. Growth delay can be caused by malabsorption of certain nutrients, such as caused by intolerance to gluten in celiac disease. Growth delay associated with Noonan syndrome is related to delayed bone maturation and may respond to growth hormone therapy. Growth delay associated with endocrinopathies can include hypothyroidism, growth hormone deficiency, and other hormone disorders.

7. C: Sexual precocity is idiopathic in 80% of girls. The pediatric nurse practitioner (PNP), however, should refer the child to a pediatric endocrinologist for evaluation of advancing bone age and progressive clinical signs since some children require treatment. Enzyme defects, such as congenital adrenal hyperplasia, may require estrogen replacement during puberty. Systemic central nervous system (CNS) disease may cause signs of precocious puberty as well as neurologic defects, such as visual field deficits. Classic features of long-standing hypothyroidism can be pseudoprecocity, including thelarche; however, there is also absence of pubic hair and delayed linear growth. Treatment is thyroid replacement.

8. D: Precocious puberty is defined as secondary sex characteristics appearing before age 9 in boys and age 8 in girls; the other ages are within normal limits of pubertal development.

9. B: Central precocious puberty (CPP) is suppressed with analogs of long-acting gonadotropin-releasing hormone (GnRH). Follicle-stimulating hormone (FSH) stimulates the ovarian follicles and is not a treatment for CPP.

10. A: Type 1 diabetes is an autoimmune disease in which islet cell antibodies destroy the pancreatic beta cells. The other answers are related to the pathophysiology of type 2 diabetes.

11. A: Signs of type 1 diabetes mellitus include polyuria, polydipsia, polyphagia, and weight loss; these can be easily checked in the office with a urine dipstick or random blood glucose level. Symptoms of hyperthyroidism can include hyperactivity, irritability, heat intolerance, tachycardia, palpitations, weight loss despite increased appetite, hyperreflexia, and hair loss. Symptoms of adrenocortical insufficiency begin very gradually and may include fatigue and muscle weakness, nausea, vomiting and/or diarrhea, orthostatic hypotension, and abdominal discomfort. Nephrotic syndrome may present following an influenza-like episode with periorbital and/or peripheral edema, shortness of breath from pulmonary edema, and dry skin.

12. C: Glycosylated hemoglobin or A1c is a blood test that measures the percentage of glucose that is attached to the hemoglobin cell; once attached, the glucose remains attached for the life of the hemoglobin cell, which is usually not more than 3 months. The normal A1c is between 4% and 6.5%. Because the test measures glycemic control over time, doing the A1c weekly or monthly is not recommended. Measuring

A1c every 6 months may miss signs of deteriorating glycemic control, especially during periods of growth and development such as childhood and adolescence.

13. D: Congenital hearing loss is not related to gestational diabetes; however, the infant of a mother with gestational diabetes is only slightly more at risk for congenital anomalies and is more likely to have transient neonatal hypoglycemia and birth trauma, including shoulder dystocia.

14. B: Intrauterine growth restriction (IUGR) infants have reduced glucose stores in the form of glycogen and body fat and therefore are prone to hypoglycemia; however, infants with IUGR generally have an increased metabolic rate, they do not become acidotic because of hypoglycemia, and hypoglycemia does not make them more prone to sepsis.

15. C: CAH is the most common cause of ambiguous genitalia. Idiopathic, chromosomal defect, and embryologic disorders are less common causes of ambiguous genitalia.

16. A: Hyponatremia (not hypernatremia) is a sign of CAH because there is excessive sodium loss through the kidneys and an inability to maintain serum electrolyte balance. Progressive weight loss, dehydration, and hyperkalemia are symptoms associated with congenital adrenal hyperplasia.

17. D: Families must be counseled about the need for lifelong medication therapy and follow-up. They will also need to understand "stress" dosing (injectable form) for fevers of greater than 101°F, trauma, surgery, and persistent vomiting to prevent metabolic decompensation. CAH is not a self-limiting disease but a long-term, genetic disease affecting the adrenal gland. Genetic counseling should be offered to families of children with CAH to answer questions about the condition, explain choices during future pregnancies, and discuss how to test other family members. Since glucocorticoids are necessary to treat CAH, overweight and bone health are consequences of treatment and should be addressed to prevent long-term health issues.

18. C: Breast buds are the first sign of puberty in girls, and typically, 1½ to 3 years pass from thelarche to menses, so this is within normal pubertal development. A pregnancy test would be a first step for secondary amenorrhea. A buccal smear for chromosomal analysis and luteinizing hormone (LH) and follicle-stimulating hormone (FSH) levels are expensive and unnecessary tests that may increase the anxiety for the family in this setting.

19. A: Primary dysmenorrhea is due to an excessive production of uterine prostaglandins that leads to increased uterine tone and stronger and more frequent menstrual cramping. Pelvic inflammatory disease, endometriosis, and fibroids are associated with secondary dysmenorrhea.

20. B: Anemia is considered to be a complication of dysfunctional uterine bleeding rather than a part of the

differential diagnosis. Pregnancy-related disorders, foreign bodies, and endometriosis should be considered in the differential diagnosis of DUB.

21. D: Rickets is often connected to nutrition. By 11 months of age, babies need a wide variety of foods. Additionally, breastmilk in African American mothers is lower in vitamin D concentrations than is breastmilk from mothers of other ethnicities. Children with trauma may present with a past history of falls or accidents with inconsistent physical findings, such as bruising in various stages of healing. Developmental variations, such as physiologic genu varum, are common in children younger than age 18 months and usually resolve by the age of 3 years. Chromosomal abnormalities, such as hypophosphatasia, can affect bone and tooth development and can present with bowed legs as well as enlarged wrist and ankle joints and abnormal skull shape.

22. D: Excess release of thyroid hormone beyond the newborn period is related to secondary hypothyroidism; the other answers are associated with primary/congenital hypothyroidism.

23. B: There is a higher incidence of congenital hypothyroidism in Hispanic and Native Americans. The other populations do not have a higher incidence of congenital hypothyroidism.

24. B: Symptoms of hypothyroidism are associated with "slower" body functions. Constipation is more likely than frequent stooling. Hoarse cry, coarse features, and lethargy are signs/symptoms of congenital hypothyroidism.

25. A: Thyroid cancer, thyroid nodules, and pituitary tumor are not common in children and teens but are in adults. Most thyroid cancer can be cured with treatment; thyroid nodules and pituitary tumors are unlikely in children and adolescents.

26. C: Weight gain is a more common symptom of hypothyroidism, whereas symptoms of hyperthyroid disease can include an enlarged thyroid, rapid heart rate (tachycardia), widened pulse pressure, a hyperthyroid stare (infrequent blinking) or frank exophthalmos, tremor, sweating, palpitations, smooth moist skin, frequent bowel movements or diarrhea, sleeplessness, attention problems in school, irritability, and weight loss.

27. B: Amenorrhea is common in hypothyroidism, and heat intolerance is more specific for thyroid disease. The restlessness of the 16-year-old and the preteen's problems relate to behavior problems, not hyperthyroidism, and the 6-year-old-girl's symptom is very nonspecific.

28. D: Hashimoto's or chronic autoimmune thyroiditis is the most common cause of goiter/hypothyroidism in childhood (ages 8–15 years; females affected more than males 4:1; increased incidence with type 1 diabetes). Infections and exposure to radiation or trauma are less common in children and teens.

29. C: Nephrogenic diabetes insipidus (DI) is caused by decreased renal responsiveness to ADH. It is not mediated by the central nervous system. Central DI is related to anatomic defects in the brain or damage to the hypothalamus or pituitary. Polydipsia, not oliguria, is a primary presenting symptom.

30. A: Symptoms of diabetes insipidus (DI) in an infant include unexplained fever, rapid onset of vomiting and constipation, clear urine, and poor weight gain. Homocystinuria is a metabolic disorder affecting connective tissue, muscles, the central nervous system, and the cardiovascular system. The primary symptoms of growth hormone deficiency in infants is hypoglycemia, exaggerated jaundice, and micropenis in boys. Hyperglycemia is associated with preterm infants or physiologic stress, including surgery, sepsis, respiratory distress, and hypoxia.

31. C: Constitutional growth delay is considered a normal growth variant with delayed physical maturity but normal final adult height. There is a strong family history in familial short stature, not constitutional growth delay. There is often a familial or genetic variant that a "small" child remains small as an adult. Children with constitutional growth delay start to fall on the growth curve between the ages of 1 and 3 years.

32. A: Infants with growth hormone deficiency may have a normal birthweight or a birthweight <50th percentile, small hands and feet, CNS findings, and a stretched penile length of <2.5 cm (with normal of 4 cm). Congenital hypothyroidism can present with very subtle signs in the first month of life; the infant may have lethargy, poor feeding, and prolonged elevated bilirubin >10 mg/dL for an infant >3 days of age.

33. B: Males with Klinefelter syndrome have additional X genetic material, 47, XXY, causing hypogonadism and sterility often not noticed until puberty. Symptoms include increased height, less muscle mass, youthful appearance, language or reading problems, and small testicles. Adrenal hyperplasia is usually diagnosed with the newborn screening, and the infant presents with electrolyte imbalances and ambiguous genitalia. A teen with Marfan syndrome can be tall and have other distinct physical characteristics, including long, thin arms and legs, loose and flexible joints, and vision and cardiovascular problems (related to the genetic connective tissue disorder). Cerebral gigantism (Sotos syndrome) often presents with excessive physical growth in the first 2 to 3 years of life caused by a rare genetic disorder, and it may be accompanied by cognitive and developmental delays.

34. D: A craving for salt is common in patients with chronic adrenal insufficiency as well as chronic, worsening fatigue and muscle weakness, loss of appetite, and weight loss. The other symptoms are nonspecific and are not related to chronic adrenal insufficiency.

35. D: In utero, the IDM can experience elevated maternal blood glucose and increased insulin production, which stops after delivery, leading to transient neonatal hypoglycemia. This can also cause additional fat

deposits in the infant, leading to large for gestational age (LGA)—not small for gestational age or intrauterine growth restriction. Disorders in bone development are not more common in IDMs.

36. A: True precocity happens when the pituitary gland releases gonadotropins, which stimulate the development of the ovaries in girls and testes in boys, which in turn triggers the female sex hormone estrogen in girls and the male sex hormone testosterone in boys. In pseudoprecocious puberty, the development of secondary sex characteristics is caused by estrogen or testosterone from either the adrenal gland or the gonad, independent of the hypothalamic-pituitary portion of the pubertal axis. Incomplete precocity is considered a normal variant that includes premature thelarche and premature adrenarche without advanced linear growth. Incomplete precocity, or pseudoprecocity, is caused by estrogen and testosterone secreted by tumors in the adrenal glands or gonads; unlike true precocious puberty, the ovaries or testes do not mature.

37. C: Symptoms of Marfan syndrome include tall, thin stature; loose, flexible joints; pectus excavatum or pectus carinatum; and, the most serious, electrocardiogram (ECG) abnormalities caused by prolapse of the valves, aortic aneurysm, and/or aortic dissection. Turner syndrome affects females and is caused by missing or incomplete sex chromosomes. Characteristics include delayed growth, webbed neck, receding lower jaw, low-set ears, drooping eyelids, broad chest with widely spaced nipples, learning disabilities, and lack of physical development through puberty. Beckwith-Wiedemann syndrome is a congenital disorder usually associated with a defect in chromosome 11, causes neonatal hypoglycemia, and can be associated with microglossia and increased tumor development, including Wilms' tumor or adrenal carcinoma. Klinefelter syndrome is associated with tall stature as well as hypotonia and muscle weakness, hypogonadism and infertility, and some degree of reading and learning impairment.

38. D: Short stature is generally associated with growth hormone *deficiency*, whereas growth hormone excess is associated with tall stature, prominent mandible and supraorbital ridge, and enlargement of the nose, ears, and jaw as well as headaches, excessive perspiration, visual impairment, coarse facial features, large hands and feet, menstrual irregularity, and joint pain.

39. B: In Addison's disease, the axilla, groin, areola, hand creases, and surgical scars can have increased bronze skin pigmentation in the extensor surfaces of the skin. Purple striae are common along the sides and lower abdomen due to weight gain in Cushing syndrome or obesity. Darkened, thickened skin (acanthosis nigricans) is associated with increased insulin resistance in type 2 diabetes and/or obesity. Increased perspiration and heat intolerance can be indicative of hyperthyroidism.

40. A: *Hyperadrenocorticism* refers to an increase in the hormone cortisol (Cushing syndrome). Common symptoms include thinning of the skin, weakness, weight gain, bruising, hypertension, diabetes, weak bones (osteoporosis), facial puffiness, and "Buffalo type" adiposity of face, neck, and trunk. Advanced skeletal maturation is associated with precocious puberty.

41. C: Large for gestational age (LGA) infants have increased adipose tissue and are relatively hyperinsulinemic in utero. After delivery and with continued insulin metabolism, the LGA baby is likely to experience hypoglycemia. Appropriate for gestational age (AGA) infants do not commonly experience hypoglycemia unless there is significant birth stress or temperature instability. Premature small for gestational age (SGA) infants can experience hypoglycemia due to a lack of glycogen stores and immature liver function. That transient neonatal hypoglycemia is least common in LGA infants is an untrue statement.

42. B: Patients with type 1 diabetes are insulin-dependent as a result of autoimmune destruction of pancreatic beta cells. Some patients with type 2 diabetes can be managed with diet and exercise.

43. B: A majority of patients with type 1 diabetes are diagnosed before the age of 18 years. Type 1 diabetes can be diagnosed at any age. Type 2 diabetes is now called maturity-onset diabetes and can be managed with diet, exercise, and oral agents; therefore, it is *not* insulin-dependent. Insulin resistance syndrome refers to prediabetes, and early diagnosis and treatment can prevent the onset of type 2 diabetes.

44. D: It is important to avoid hypoglycemia in a younger child whose brain/neurologic system is not fully developed. Younger children have the same need for available glucose in the bloodstream as do older children and adults.

45. A: The target goals are higher in younger children to reduce the risk of hypoglycemia and its effects on developing brains. Children are more likely to have "hypoglycemic unawareness" due to lack of ability to describe symptoms of hypoglycemia. A blood glucose of between 70 and 120 mg/dL is the target for laboratory "normal" blood glucose levels. The other levels given are outside target ranges and can be associated with morbidity.

46. D: Glucagon is an injectable prescription medication used for the treatment of severe hypoglycemia when the child with diabetes is unable to swallow oral carbohydrates, is unconscious, or is experiencing seizures. Mild and moderate hypoglycemia can be treated with a quick-acting carbohydrate, such as glucose tablets, glucose gel, fruit juice, or a regular (sugar-containing) soda or beverage. Glucagon is not a treatment for hyperglycemia; treatment would be a correction dose of rapid-acting insulin analog.

47. A: Alopecia is not associated with diabetes. Signs and symptoms of diabetes include polyuria, polydipsia, polyphagia, and weight loss.

48. A: Diabetic ketoacidosis (DKA) is a medical emergency and can be life-threatening; prompt identification and treatment with insulin, fluids, and treatment of any underlying or concurrent illness are required. Gastrointestinal infection is a common childhood condition involving vomiting and diarrhea, which is managed by maintaining hydration and glucose levels in children with diabetes. Hyperglycemia is diagnosed by elevated blood glucose levels and generally does not involve abdominal pain and vomiting; treatment is a correction dose of insulin. Autoimmune pancreatitis occurs most often in an adult population with initial presentation between the ages of 50 and 60 years.

49. D: The three factors—genetic predisposition, autoimmune response, and viral/chemical exposure—are associated with the development of type 1 diabetes.

50. C: The CDC does not use the term *obese* for children and teens ages 2 to 20 years but uses "at risk for overweight" for those with a BMI between the 85th and 95th percentiles for age and "overweight" for those with a BMI >95th percentile for age.

51. C: The definition of precocious puberty is the development of secondary sex characteristics at an age younger than the accepted lower limits of puberty, namely, before 9.5 years in boys and 9 years in girls.

52. B: Lack of secondary sexual characteristics after the age of 17 years suggests abnormal testicular function, including primary failure due to anorchia, Klinefelter syndrome, radiation, trauma, or tumor. Anorchia is the absence of both testes at birth and is diagnosed before the age of 17 years. True hermaphroditism presents as ambiguous genitalia and is diagnosed in the neonatal period. Pituitary adenoma is one feature of multiple endocrine neoplasia (MEN), an inherited endocrine syndrome that affects 1 in 30,000 persons and that may cause facial tumors.

53. B: Gynecomastia is more common in pubertal males ages 13–14 years with Tanner III for pubic hair and testicular volume between 8 and 10 mL. Children 9 to 10 years are likely to be prepubertal. Children 16 to 18 years and older are generally beyond Tanner III in pubertal development.

54. D: Constitutional or familial primary amenorrhea is delayed pubertal development, including amenorrhea, and is the most common cause of primary amenorrhea. During the initial assessment, it is important to distinguish between a normal variant and any underlying pathology. A pregnancy is the most common cause of secondary amenorrhea. Ovarian insufficiency is considered primary if the ovary fails to function normally in response to appropriate gonadotropin stimulation provided by the hypothalamus and pituitary. Ovarian insufficiency is considered secondary if the hypothalamus and pituitary fail to provide appropriate gonadotropin stimulation.

☐ BIBLIOGRAPHY

Alemzadeh, R., Rising, R., & Lifshitz, F. (2007). In F. Lifshitz (Ed.), *Pediatric endocrinology* (5th ed., Vol. *1*, pp. 1–56). New York, NY: Informa Healthcare USA.

American Diabetes Association. (2014). Standards of medical care in diabetes—2014. *Diabetes Care, 37* (Suppl.), S14–S80.

Ballal, S. A., & McIntosh, P. (2009). Endocrinology. In J. W. Custer & R. E. Rau (Eds.), *The Harriet Lane handbook* (18th ed., pp. 269–300). Philadelphia, PA: Elsevier Mosby.

Blondell, R. D, Foster, M. B., & Dave, K. C. (1999). Disorders of puberty. *American Family Physician, 60*(1), 209–218.

Brock, C. G. D., & Brown, R. S. (Eds.). (2008). *Handbook of clinical pediatric endocrinology*. Malden, MA: Blackwell Publishing.

Buck, M. L. (Ed.). (2008). Levothyroxine use in infants and children with congenital or acquired hypothyroidism. *Pediatric Pharmacotherapy, 14*(10).

Carrillo, A. A., & Bao, Y. (2007). Hormonal dynamic tests and genetic tests used in pediatric endocrinology. In F. Lifshitz (Ed.), *Pediatric endocrinology* (5th ed., Vol. *2*, pp. 737–767). New York, NY: Informa Healthcare USA.

Chase, H. P. (2006). *Understanding diabetes* (11th ed.). Denver, CO: Barbara Davis Center for Childhood Diabetes.

Cooke, D. W., & Plotnick, L. (2008). Type 1 diabetes mellitus in pediatrics. *Pediatrics in Review, 29*(11), 374–385.

Crimmins, N. A., & Dolan, L. M. (2008). Definition, diagnosis, and classification of diabetes in youth. In D. Dabelea & G. J. Klingensmith (Eds.), *Epidemiology of pediatric and adolescent diabetes* (pp. 1–19). New York, NY: Informa Healthcare USA.

Dallas, J. S. (2007). Hyperthyroidism. In F. Lifshitz (Ed.), *Pediatric endocrinology* (5th ed., Vol. *2*, pp. 391–404). New York, NY: Informa Healthcare USA.

Farrag, H. M., & Cowett, R. M. (2007). Hypoglycemia in the newborn. In F. Lifshitz (Ed.), *Pediatric endocrinology* (5th ed., Vol. *2*, pp. 330–358). New York, NY: Informa Healthcare USA.

Fleishman, A., & Gordon, C. (2007). Adolescent menstrual abnormalities. In F. Lifshitz (Ed.), *Pediatric endocrinology* (5th ed., Vol. *2*, pp. 349–363). New York, NY: Informa Healthcare USA.

Freedman, D. S, Mei, Z., Srinvasin, S. R., Berenson, G. S. & Dietz, W. H. (2007). Cardiovascular risk factors and excess adiposity among overweight children and adolescents: The Bogalusa Heart Study. *Journal of Pediatrics, 150*(1),12–17.

Garber, J. R., & Koury, C. B. (2009). Treatment of hyper- and hypothyroidism. *Review of Endocrinology, 3*(4), 20–22.

Gharib, H., & Koury, C. B. (2009). Diagnosis and management of thyroid nodules: An overview. *Review of Endocrinology, 3*(4), 23–25.

Grimberg, A., & De Leon, D. D. (2005). Disorders of growth. In T. Moshang (Ed.), *Pediatric endocrinology:*

The requisites in pediatrics (pp. 127–167). St. Louis, MO: Mosby.

Grimberg, A., & Lifshitz, F. (2008). Worrisome growth. In M. Sperling (Ed.), *Pediatric endocrinology* (3rd ed., pp. 1–50). Philadelphia, PA: Saunders.

Halac, I., & Zimmerman, D. (2004). Evaluating short stature in children. *Pediatric Annals, 33*(3), 170–176.

Henry, J. J. (2004). *Cortisol replacement therapy: An educational booklet for parents and children* (2nd ed.). Gaithersburg, MD: Pediatric Endocrinology Nursing Society.

Henwood, M. J., & Levitt Katz, L. E. (2005). Disorders of the adrenal gland. In T. Moshang (Ed.), *Pediatric endocrinology: The requisites in pediatrics* (pp. 193–213). St. Louis, MO: Mosby.

Huang, S. A. (2007). Hypothyroidism. In F. Lifshitz (Ed.), *Pediatric endocrinology* (5th ed., Vol. *2*, pp. 391–404). New York, NY: Informa Healthcare USA.

Huang, S. A. (2007). Thyromegly. In F. Lifshitz (Ed.), *Pediatric endocrinology* (5th ed., Vol. *2*, pp. 443–453). New York, NY: Informa Healthcare USA.

Hubbard, V. S. (2000). Defining overweight and obesity: What are the issues? *American Journal Clinical Nursing, 72*(5), 1067–1068.

Iglesias, P., & Diez, J. J. (2009). Thyroid dysfunction and kidney disease. *European Journal of Endocrinology, 160,* 503–515.

Jacobson, D., Small, L., & Mazurek Melnyk, B. (2013). Overweight and obesity. In B. Mazurek Melnyk & J. Jenson (Eds.), *A practical guide to child and adolescent mental health screening: Early interventions and health promotion* (2nd ed., Section 16, pp. 319–332). New York, NY: National Association of Pediatric Nurse Practitioners.

Kache, S., & Ferry, R. J., Jr. (2005). Diabetes insipidus. In T. Moshang (Ed.), *Pediatric endocrinology: The requisites in pediatrics* (pp. 257–267). St. Louis, MO: Mosby.

Kappy, M. S., Steelman, J. W., Travers, S. H., & Zeitler, P. S. (2003). Endocrine disorders. In W. W. Hay, Jr., A. R. Hayward, M. J. Levin, & J. M. Sondheimer (Eds.), *Current pediatric diagnosis and treatment* (16th ed., pp. 937–977). New York, NY: Lange Medical/ McGraw-Hill.

Lee, P. A. (2005). Early pubertal development. In T. Moshang (Ed.), *Pediatric endocrinology: The requisites in pediatrics* (pp. 73–86). St. Louis, MO: Mosby.

Lee, P. A., & Houk, C. P. (2007). Puberty and its disorders. In F. Lifshitz (Ed.), *Pediatric endocrinology* (5th ed., Vol. *2*, pp. 273–324). New York, NY: Informa Healthcare USA.

Lee, P. A., & Kulin, H. E. (2005). Normal pubertal development. In T. Moshang (Ed.) *Pediatric endocrinology: The requisites in pediatrics* (pp. 63–72). St. Louis, MO: Mosby.

Loscalzo, M. L. (2008). Turner syndrome. *Pediatrics in Review, 29*(7), 219–226.

Lustig, R. H., & Weiss, R. (2008). In M. Sperling (Ed.), *Pediatric endocrinology* (3rd ed., pp. 788–838). Philadelphia, PA: Saunders.

Lyles, S. P., Silverstein, J. H., & Rosenbloom, A. L. (2007). Practical aspects of diabetes care. In F. Lifshitz (Ed.), *Pediatric endocrinology* (5th ed., Vol. *1*, pp. 125–154). New York, NY: Informa Healthcare USA.

Mahoney, C. P. (1990). Adolescent gynecomastia: Differential diagnosis and management. *Pediatric Clinics of North America, 37*(6), 1389–1404.

Mathiesen, E., & Damm, P. (2014). Gestational diabetes. Diapedia. Retrieved from http://dx.doi.org/10.14496/dia.41040851387.25

Migeon, C. J., & Lanes, R. (2007). Adrenal cortex: Hypo- and hyperfunction. In F. Lifshitz (Ed.), *Pediatric endocrinology* (5th ed., Vol. *2*, pp. 195–229). New York, NY: Informa Healthcare USA.

Miller, W. L., Achermann, J. C., & Fluck, C. E. (2008). The adrenal cortex and its disorders. In M. Sperling (Ed.), *Pediatric endocrinology* (3rd ed., pp. 444–511), Philadelphia, PA: Saunders.

Muglia, L. J., & Majzoub, J. A. (2008). Disorders of the posterior pituitary. In M. Sperling (Ed.), *Pediatric endocrinology* (3rd ed., pp. 335–373). Philadelphia, PA: Saunders.

Muir, A. (2006). Precocious puberty. *Pediatrics in Review, 27*(10), 373–381.

New, M. I., Ghizzoni, L., & Lin-Su, K. (2007). An update of congenital adrenal hyperplasia. In F. Lifshitz (Ed.), *Pediatric endocrinology* (5th ed., Vol. *2*, pp. 227–245). New York, NY: Informa Healthcare USA.

Ogden, C. L., Carroll, M. D., Kit, B. K, & Flegal, K. M. (2014). Prevalence of childhood and adult obesity in the U.S. 2011–2012. *Journal of the American Medical Association, 311*(8), 806–814.

Radovick, S., & MacGillivary, M. H. (Eds.). (2003). *Pediatric endocrinology: A practical guide.* Totowa, NJ: Humana Press.

Raine, J. E., Donaldson, M. D., Gregory, J. W., Savage, M. O., & Hintz, R. L. (Eds.). (2006). *Practical endocrinology and diabetes in children* (2nd ed., pp. 91–108). Malden, MA: Blackwell.

Rogovick, A. L., & Goldman, R. D. (2011). Pharmacologic treatment of pediatric obesity. *Canadian Family Physician, 57*(2) 195–197.

Rosenbloom, A. L., & Connor, E. L. (2007). Hypopituitarism and other disorders of the growth-hormone-insulin-like growth factor-1 axis. In F. Lifshitz (Ed.), *Pediatric endocrinology* (5th ed., Vol. *2*, pp. 65–99). New York, NY: Informa Healthcare USA.

Rosenfeld, R .G., & Cohen, P. (2008). Disorders of growth hormone/insulin-like growth factor secretion and action. In M. Sperling (Ed.), *Pediatric endocrinology* (3rd ed., pp. 254–334). Philadelphia, PA: Saunders.

Rosenfield, R. L., Cooke, D. W., & Radovick, S. (2008). Puberty and its disorders in the female. In M. Sperling (Ed.), *Pediatric endocrinology* (3rd ed., pp. 530–609). Philadelphia, PA: Saunders.

Rossi, W. C., Caplin, N., & Alter, C. A. (2005). Thyroid disorders in children. In T. Moshang (Ed.), *Pediatric endocrinology: The requisites in pediatrics* (pp. 171–190). St. Louis, MO: Mosby.

Sarafoglou, K. (Ed.). (2009). *Pediatric endocrinology and inborn errors of metabolism*. New York, NY: McGraw Medical.

Shomaker, K., Bradford, K., & Key-Solle, M. (2009). The infant with ambiguous genitalia: The pediatrician's role. *Contemporary pediatrics, 26*(4), 40–56.

Thorton, P. S. (2005). Thyroid disorders in children. In T. Moshang (Ed.), *Pediatric endocrinology: The requisites in pediatrics* (pp. 37–59). St. Louis, MO: Mosby.

Treadwell, J. R., Sun, F., & Scholles, K. (2008). Systemic review and meta-analysis of bariatric surgery for pediatric obesity. *Annals of Surgery, 248*(5), 763–776.

U.S. Food and Drug Administration. (2010, April 21). FDA drug safety communication: New boxed warning on severe liver injury with propyithlouracil. Retrieved from http://www.fda.gov/Drugs/DrugSafety/Postmarket DrugSafetyInformationforPatientsandProviders/ucm 209023.htm

Van Vliet, G., & Polack, M. (2007). Thyroid disorders in infancy. In F. Lifshitz (Ed.), *Pediatric endocrinology* (5th ed., Vol. *2*, pp. 391–404). New York, NY: Informa Healthcare USA.

Vivian, E. M. (2006). Type 2 diabetes in children and adolescents—the next epidemic. *Current Medical Research and Opinions, 22*(2), 297–306.

Winter, W. E. (2007). Autoimmune endocrinopathies. In F. Lifshitz (Ed.), *Pediatric endocrinology* (5th ed., Vol. *2*, pp. 595–616). New York, NY: Informa Healthcare USA.

☐ EDUCATIONAL WEBSITES

CARES Foundation—congenital adrenal hyperplasia: http://www.caresfoundation.org

Children with Diabetes—pediatric diabetes: http://www.childrenwithdiabetes.com

American Diabetes Association—all diabetes: http://www.diabetes.org

American Diabetes Association—ADA's training curriculum for schools: http://www.diabetes.org/schooltraining

Intersex Society of North America—*Clinical Guidelines for the Management of Disorders of Sex Development in Childhood*: http://www.dsdguidelines.org/files/clinical.pdf

Human Growth Foundation: http://www.hgfound.org

Hormone Health Network: http://www.hormone.org

Juvenile Diabetes Research Foundation: http://www.jdrf.org

Magic Foundation—all endocrine disorders: http://www.magicfoundation.org

Pediatric Endocrinology Nursing Society: http://www.pens.org

Pituitary Network Association: http://www.pituitary.org

Multisystem and Genetic Disorders

Rita Marie John

CHAPTER 15

☐ INTRODUCTION

Although the disorders in this chapter are more rare, care of the patient needs to be coordinated, comprehensive, continuous, culturally sensitive, and multidisciplinary, with quality and safety involved. The concept of the medical home model in primary care provides the family with comprehensive care that coordinates community agencies and personnel. Although the medical societies do not see that a pediatric nurse practitioner (PNP) can head the medical home, the National Association of Pediatric Nurse Practitioners (NAPNAP) has issued a position statement that clearly states that PNPs can be the head of the medical home. Care concepts revolving around comprehensive, culturally sensitive, compassionate, coordinated care centered around families and children as well as providing transitional care are key to the medical home (National Association of Pediatric Nurse Practitioners, 2009). It is important to coordinate specialty care. Knowledge about each condition and its management is rapidly expanding, and personnel at such centers are most current in this essential practice foundation.

The PNP remains responsible for assisting the child and family with all primary care issues, some of which will be disorder specific. The PNP is a central contact for the child and family for issues of care coordination and community-based interventions, advocacy, assistance with stress management, and promotion of positive adaptation and coping. PNPs working with children who have any of these disorders must become familiar with the issues commonly confronting such children and their families, legislation protecting the rights of individuals who have chronic illness or disability, and support organizations and agencies that can be helpful to caregivers and families.

Several resources are available for children with developmental disabilities. There are University Centers for Excellence in Developmental Disabilities (UCEDD), funded by the Administration on Developmental Disabilities (ADD); Leadership Education in Neurodevelopmental Disabilities (LEND) programs, funded by the Maternal and Child Health Bureau (MCHB); and Intellectual and Developmental Disability Research Centers (IDDRCs). The latter are primarily funded by the Eunice Kennedy Shriver National Institute for Child Health and Development (NICHD). Information about these programs can be found at http://www.aucd.org/template/page.cfm?id=1. The UCEDD has federal partners, including the Administration on Developmental Disabilities, MCHB, National Center on Birth Defects and Developmental Disabilities (NCBDDD) at the Centers for Disease Control and Prevention (CDC), and NICHD.

In addition, collaborating partners include the Association of Maternal Child Health Programs, Corporation for National and Community Service, External Partners Group, National Leadership Consortium on Developmental Disabilities, and National Service Inclusion Project (NSIP). All of these organizations have websites that can be accessed via a search engine. The Alliance of Genetic Support Groups (202-966-5557 and http://www.genetic alliance.org) is a comprehensive resource for conditions with a genetic basis. In addition, the National Association for Rare Disorders can also be a source of information for parents and providers looking to find out more information about rare disorders.

Where possible, information about disorder-specific support organizations is included in the management sections of this chapter. *Exceptional Parent* magazine (416 Main Street, Johnstown, PA 15901, 800-EPARENT or 1-800-372-7368, ext. 203, and http://www.eparent.com) provides a wealth of information for parents of children who have various special healthcare needs. The March of Dimes Birth Defects Foundation (1275 Mamaroneck Avenue, White Plains, NY 10605, 1-888-663-4637 and http://www.marchofdimes.com) provides information about congenital diseases and disorders, and the National Information Center for Children and Youth with Disabilities (NICHCY; 1825 Connecticut Avenue NW, Suite 700, Washington, DC 20009, http://www.nichcy.org) provides information on all disabling conditions.

☐ CONGENITAL DISEASES

Acquired Immune Deficiency Syndrome (AIDS)

- Definition: Advanced stage of illness in individuals infected with the human immunodeficiency virus (HIV); CDC case definition of HIV classifies children according to presence or absence of clinical signs and symptoms and according to status of immune function and clinical findings
- Etiology/Incidence
  1. Each year approximately 6000 HIV-infected women with HIV-1 give birth; preventive strategies reduce the risk of mother-to-child transmission to the infant to 1% to 2%
  2. In the absence of antiretroviral (ARV) therapy, 25% to 30% of nonbreastfeeding infants with HIV-positive mothers will become infected during birth, and if they have prolonged breastfeeding, 50% of infants will become infected (Silberry, 2014)
  3. The predominant mode of transmission remains mother-to-child transmission in utero, intrapartum, or through breastfeeding postnatally
  4. Infants with positive virologic test results at or before 48 hours are considered to have been infected in utero, but infants who have a negative virologic test during the first week and have subsequent positive test are considered to have intrapartum infection
  5. Sexual transmission is an important mode of transmission in adolescence.
  6. Transfusion with blood products: Screening for HIV has virtually eliminated this mode of transmission.
  7. Percutaneous exposure via a needle stick: Greatly reduced due to needleless systems
  8. HIV-infected caretakers who chew their infant's food and then feed it to the child can transmit HIV infection
- Prevention Strategies
  1. HIV screening should be done in all pregnant women; consider repeating an HIV test during the third trimester and this should be done in all women at high risk for HIV. Women who have not been tested during pregnancy should be tested as soon as possible after delivery. If a woman is suspected of having an acute HIV infection, a plasma HIV RNA assay or antigen/antibody combination immunoassay should be done because other tests may not be positive. (Panel on Antiretroviral Therapy and Medical Management of HIV-Infected Children, 2014)
  2. Administration of combination of three ARV drugs from at least two different classes (cARV) prophylaxis during pregnancy and labor has lowered the rate of infection to less than 1% to 2%
     a. Regimes consist of three ARVs during pregnancy and labor
     b. Intravenous zidovudine (AZT) is given to all pregnant women with HIV-1 infection during labor even if they receive the above combination
  3. Elective cesarean delivery at 38 weeks before the onset of labor and before the rupture of membranes for women with a viral load 1000 copies per mL or who have unknown viral load even if they have received three ARVs
  4. Complete avoidance of breastfeeding
- Care of the HIV-1-Exposed Infant
  1. Review history for possible maternal co-infections, including tuberculosis, syphilis, toxoplasmosis, hepatitis B or C, cytomegalovirus, or herpes simplex
  2. Evaluate the infant for signs of co-infection
  3. At baseline, the following must be done:
     a. History and physical
     b. Complete blood count (CBC) with differential, comprehensive metabolic profile include aspartate aminotransferase (AST)/alanine aminotransferase (ALT)
     c. Albumin, total protein, phosphate, calcium
     d. HIV RNA
     e. Drug resistance testing
     f. Lipid panel
     g. Urinalysis (Silberry, 2014)
  4. Measurement of CD4 T-lymphocyte counts can be extended to every 6 to 12 months in children and adolescents who are adherent to therapy, have significantly elevated CD4 levels (above the risk for opportunistic infection risk), have sustained viral suppression, and have a stable clinical status for more than 2 to 3 years. (Panel on Antiretroviral Therapy and Medical Management of HIV-Infected Children, 2014)
- Signs and Symptoms: Median onset for infants with perinatal infection is 12 to 18 months; HIV, however, can be latent for years
  1. Prematurity
  2. Low birth weight
  3. Recurrent serious bacterial or viral infections—especially oral thrush
  4. Failure to thrive
  5. Recurrent fevers

6. Chronic diarrhea
7. Diminished activity
8. Developmental delays
- Differential Diagnosis
  1. Infectious disease or other associated conditions without underlying HIV
  2. Other immune deficiencies of infancy
- Physical Findings in Acute Human Immunodeficiency Viral Infection
  1. General
     a. Falling ratio of head circumference to height and weight due to encephalopathic direct effect on brain growth
     b. Weight loss with failure to thrive (FTT) and pubertal delay
     c. Recurrent, severe, or unusual infections
     d. Fever with fatigue
  2. Lymphoreticular
     a. Lymphadenopathy—>0.5 cm at more than two sites; bilateral at one site
     b. Hepatosplenomegaly
     c. Leukopenia
  3. Head, ears, eyes, nose, and throat (HEENT)
     a. Parotitis, oral ulcers
     b. Central nervous system (CNS) complaints, including headache, meningitis
  4. Cardiac
     a. Cardiomyopathy
     b. Pericardial effusions
     c. Vasculopathy
  5. Gastrointestinal (GI)
     a. GI upset or gastritis
     b. Diarrhea
     c. Hepatitis, pancreatitis
     d. Abdominal pain
  6. Dermatological
     a. Rash, including eczema, seborrhea, urticarial, herpes simplex, tinea corporis
     b. Molluscum, warts
  7. Renal
     a. Proteinuria
     b. Renal tubular acidosis
     c. Renal failure
     d. Hypertension
  8. Infections
     a. Unusual or opportunistic infections
     b. New sexually transmitted disease
- Diagnostic Tests/Findings
  1. Detection of HIV in a neonate
     a. All infants and toddlers should have direct HIV viral assays done—HIV DNA polymerase chain reaction and HIV RNA assays
     b. For HIV-exposed infants, the recommended times for testing are 14–21 days, 1–2 months, and 4–6 months.
     c. Viral testing should be done in any known HIV-exposed infant as well as in infants at high risk for HIV infection
     d. Repeat viral testing should occur 2–4 weeks after the cessation of ARV therapy
     e. A positive test for direct HIV viral assays should be repeated as soon as possible
     f. To definitely exclude any HIV testing, two test results are needed, but their timing is also important:
        (1) Two negative tests after 6 months
        (2) One negative direct HIV viral assay test after 1 month with a second one after 4 months
     g. Nucleic acid amplification tests (NATs) must be used in infants and toddlers due to the maternal transfer of antibodies that would be detected using the newer tests discussed in the Care of the HIV-1-Exposed Infant section. Therefore, there are different types of NAT tests—HIV DNA tests, RNA polymerase chain reaction assays (PCR tests), as well as related RNA quantitative or qualitative assays
        (1) HIV DNA tests: HIV DNA PCR is 99.8% specific at birth and 100% specific at 1, 3, and 6 months. However, the sensitivity is only 55% at birth but increases to 90% by 2–4 weeks and 100% by age 3–6 months. This explains why two tests are needed (Branson et al., 2014)
  2. Detection of HIV for adolescents and children ≥24 months (Panel on Antiretroviral Therapy and Medical Management of HIV-Infected Children, 2014)
     a. The two-step process previously recommended is no longer acceptable (Branson et al., 2014). This involved using saliva or blood screening using an enzyme-linked immunoassay (EIA). EIA tests could not be used in acute infection and missed early HIV infection. The Western blot test, which followed an EIA, is no longer recommended. This was first recommended in 1989 and now there are improved fourth-generation tests able to detect the early rise of p24 antigen that occurs after initial infection with HIV and before HIV antibody is produced. It can reduce the window period that occurs after the initial infection of HIV but before detectable antibodies are produced. These HIV tests detect the HIV p24 antigen and both anti-HIV IgM and IgG antibodies
     b. As shown in **Figure 15-1**, a test negative for HIV-1 and HIV-2 antibody test and p24 antigen requires no follow-up
     c. A positive fourth-generation test must be followed with a U.S. Food and Drug Administration (FDA)-approved immunoassay test that differentiates HIV-1 antibodies from HIV-2 antibodies
     d. A specimen that is positive on the initial fourth-generation test but HIV-1 negative or indeterminate on the HIV-1/HIV-2 antibody differential immunoassay should be repeated with an HIV-1 NAT test
        (1) An indeterminate HIV-1/HIV-2 antibody differentiation but a reactive HIV-1 NAT result indicates HIV-1 infection

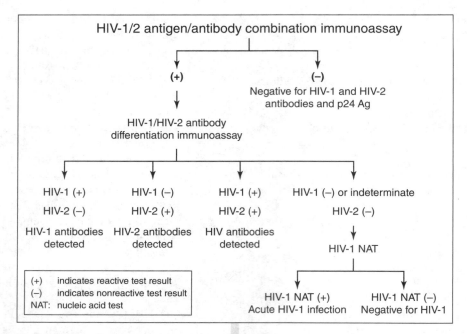

Figure 15-1 HIV-1/2 antigen/antibody combination immunoassay.

Source: Centers for Disease Control and Prevention and Association of Public Health Laboratories. Laboratory Testing for the Diagnosis of HIV Infection: Updated Recommendations. Available at http://stacks.cdc.gov/view/cdc/23447. Published June 27, 2014.

(2) A negative HIV-1 NAT result in the presences of a nonreactive or indeterminate HIV-1/HIV-2 antibody differentiation assay is indicative of a false positive on the initial immunoassay

- Management/Treatment
1. Risk reduction through prevention of maternal infection, ensuring clean blood and tissue supplies, prevention of sexually transmitted diseases (STDs) and needle sharing
2. Reduction of risk of perinatal HIV—through treatment of pregnant mother and perinatal chemoprophylaxis of mother and infant
3. At birth, history, physical, and risk assessment, continue or start ARV prophylaxis
4. If mother's HIV-1 serostatus is unknown at the time of labor or birth, do a rapid HIV-1 antibody test on mother or newborn with consent
5. Treatment with zidovudine to *all* HIV-exposed newborns as soon as possible, usually within 6 to 12 hours, younger than 12 months regardless of symptoms, immunologic, or virologic measures
6. At 12 to 18 months, enzyme immunoassay for antibody to HIV-1
7. Pneumocystis carinii pneumonia prophylaxis in infants should start at 6 weeks regardless of CD5 cell count or percentages
8. Standard immunizations are given
9. Tests done at baseline include monitoring of CD4+ lymphocyte count and percentage, CBC, differential, platelet count
10. Antiretroviral therapy in consultation with HIV management specialists
11. Immunize and tuberculosis (TB) screening according to guidelines

12. Treatment of infections and other associated conditions—consult an infectious disease (ID) specialist
13. Early intervention for developmental delay
14. Maximum supportive care for child and family
15. CDC National Prevention Information Network
    P.O. Box 6003
    Rockville, MD 20849-6003
    1-800-458-5231
    http://www.cdcnpin.org

Chlamydia Trachomatis

- Definition: There are three species that cause human infection: *Chlamydia trachomatis*, *Chlamydophila pneumoniae*, and *Chlamydophila psittaci*. Chlamydiaceae divides into two genera, *Chlamydophila* and *Chlamydia*; *Chlamydophila* includes *C. pneumoniae*, *C. psittaci*, and nonhuman pathogens; *Chlamydia* includes *C. trachomatis* and nonhuman pathogens. The organism is an obligate intracellular replicating bacterium that has an infectious elementary body. The elementary body attaches to the cell membrane and enters the cells using a phagosome. The elementary body is reorganized into a metabolically active reticulocyte body, which replicates by binary fission and secondary differentiation. Then it is released out of the cell as an elementary body again and reinfects new cells. The life cycle is 48–72 hours, which is much longer than most bacteria, whose life cycle is 20 minutes. There is no long-lasting immunity
- Etiology/Incidence
1. Chlamydia causes neonatal conjunctivitis, trachoma, pneumonia in young infants, genital tract infections,

trachoma, and lymphogranuloma venereum (American Academy of Pediatrics [AAP], 2012)

2. *C. trachomatis* is divided into three biovars, two of which cause human infection—trachoma and lymphogranuloma venereum (LVG). There are 18 serovars of the biovars that cause human infection

3. *C. trachomatis* (biovar trachoma, serotypes D, Da, E, G, G, H, I, Ia, J, and K) is the most common sexually transmitted bacterial infection in the United States, with an incubation of at least 1 week. *C. trachomatis* (biovar trachoma, serotypes A, B, Ba, and C) causes ocular disease and is a major cause of blindness outside of the United States. The ocular disease found in Africa, Asia, Middle East, Central America, South America, and Australia is most common in preschool children

4. 25% to 50% of perinatally infected infants develop conjunctivitis (Siqueira, 2014)

5. Transmission occurs from cervical maternal infection to infant during vaginal delivery 50% of the time

6. Prevalence among sexually active women about 5%; among adolescents may be as high as 20%

7. *Chlamydia trachomatis* is the most prevalent sexually transmitted disease in the United States, with highest rate from 14 to 24 years

8. Incidence of neonatal pneumonia if mother is infected is approximately 5% to 30%

- Signs and Symptoms: *Chlamydia trachomatis* in the neonate
  1. Neonatal conjunctivitis—mild to severe
     a. Typically develops 5 to 14 days after birth but can develop as late as 5 weeks
     b. Lasts for longer than 2 weeks
     c. Conjunctival edema and injection
     d. Watery to mucopurulent eye discharge
     e. Pseudomembrane with bloody discharge if prolonged
     f. Routine prophylactic ophthalmic drops of silver nitrate, erythromycin, and tetracycline used to prevent *Neisseria gonorrhoeae* is not effective against *C. trachomatis*
  2. Neonatal pneumonia
     a. 3 to 19 weeks of age with an incubation period of 7 to 21 days
     b. Preceding signs include rhinorrhea, congestion, and conjunctivitis
     c. Tachypnea with persistent "staccato" cough with congestion
     d. Rales and rarely wheezing
     e. Preterm infants can have apnea
  3. Genitourinary tract manifestations
     a. Includes urethritis, cervicitis, endometritis, perihepatitis (Fitz-Hugh-Curtis syndrome, and Reiter syndrome)
- Differential Diagnosis
  1. A different infectious agent, *Staphylococcus aureus*, *Haemophilus influenzae*, streptococcus, herpes simplex, enteric bacteria

  2. Chemical reaction to silver nitrate
  3. Bronchitis/pneumonia—respiratory syncytial virus, other viral or bacterial infections
- Physical Findings
  1. Neonatal conjunctivitis
     a. Injected conjunctiva with exudate within first weeks of life
     b. Pseudomembrane
     c. Friable conjunctiva and eyelid swelling
  2. Neonatal pneumonia
     a. Afebrile
     b. Tachypnea
     c. Rales, but rarely wheezes
- Diagnostic Tests/Findings
  1. Chest radiograph shows hyperinflation with bilateral interstitial or patchy infiltrates but usually there is no lobar consolidations or pleural effusion
  2. Peripheral eosinophilia (>400 cells μ/L)
  3. Pneumonia: Use of a serum acute microimmunofluorescent (MIF) titer for IgM-specific microimmunofluorescent of 1:32 or greater. CF titers >1:64 and MIF titers >1:256 are strongly suggestive of LGV
  4. Gold standard is culture and is approved by FDA for use at all sites/culture; the specimen must contain epithelial cells since *Chlamydia* are intracellular; highly specific (98% to 100%) and sensitive (AAP, 2012)
  5. Nucleic acid amplification tests (NAAT) tests are highly sensitive and specific (>95%) and have a rapid turnover; have potential for false-positive results and not approved for use in extragenital sites, including conjunctivitis
  6. Enzyme immunoassays (EIAs) have a specificity and sensitivity of 60% to 70%
     a. Perinatally acquired vaginal and rectal infection can be present for up to 18 months; after this, sexual abuse needs to be considered
     b. Lower genital tract infection is generally asymptomatic
- Management/Treatment: Topical therapy is ineffective; infants younger than 6 months, oral erythromycin suspension, 50 mg/kg/day for 14 days; approximately 20% of infants need second course of treatment; erythromycin is associated with increased risk of pyloric stenosis

Gonococcal Infection

- Definition: Infections caused by acquisition of *Neisseria gonorrhoeae* (GC) that occurs only in humans
- Etiology/Incidence
  1. Maternal transmission to neonate from contact with vaginal secretions during birth
  2. Second most common sexually transmitted infection with 15- to 19- and 20- to 24-year-old women highest rates of gonorrhea in 2007
  3. Screen for chlamydia if positive for GC
- Signs and Symptoms
  1. Infections in newborn infant usually involve the eye
     a. Ophthalmic; injected
     b. Swollen conjunctiva with exudate

2. Other types of infection include scalp abscess, disseminated disease with bacteremia, arthritis, or meningitis
   a. Fever
   b. Irritability
   c. Rapid respiration
   d. Rapid heart rate
- Differential Diagnosis
  1. Conjunctivitis
     a. Chemical reaction to silver nitrate
     b. Infections due to chlamydia, *Staphylococcus aureus*, *Haemophilus influenzae*, streptococcus, herpes simplex, or enteric bacteria
  2. Bronchitis/pneumonia—respiratory syncytial virus (RSV), other viral, bacterial causes
  3. Skin, oropharyngeal, arthritic, vaginal, urethral, rectal, systemic infection
  4. Other causative organisms
  5. Allergy
- Physical Findings
  1. Gonococcal ophthalmia neonatorum—conjunctivitis, appearing 2 to 5 days after birth, occasionally up to 25 days
     a. Thin, clear discharge from eye that becomes thick, mucoid, sometimes bloody
     b. Edema of lids, conjunctiva
     c. Untreated, may progress to edema and ulceration of cornea, globe perforation and blindness, and/or may become systemic infection
  2. Other—scalp abscesses, disseminated infection with signs of sepsis, meningitis, or pain, and decrease in motion if septic arthritis
- Diagnostic Tests/Findings
  1. Gram stain at initial evaluation—microscopic identification of Gram-negative intracellular diplococci in smears of exudate followed by laboratory-based testing
  2. Culture is preferred—swab from orifice or blood, synovial fluid from affected joint or cerebrospinal fluid specimen
  3. Verify initial positive test (NAAT tests are not approved for prepubertal children)
- Management/Treatment: Follow current CDC guidelines
  1. Ophthalmia neonatorum prophylaxis—silver nitrate 1% aqueous; erythromycin ophthalmic ointment 0.5%; tetracycline ophthalmic ointment 1%
  2. Hospitalize infected neonates and evaluate for disseminated disease
     a. Ceftriaxone 25 to 50 mg/kg IV or IM in a single dose, not to exceed 125 mg for GC conjunctivitis without dissemination. Hospitalization is advised while child is being evaluated for dissemination
     b. Cefotaxime is recommended for infants with hyperbilirubinemia
  3. Neonatal disseminated infection
     a. Ceftriaxone 25 to 50 mg/kg/day IV or IM in a single daily dose for 7 days, with a duration of 10 to 14 days, if meningitis is documented OR
     b. Cefotaxime 25 mg/kg IV or IM every 12 hours for 7 days, with a duration of 10 to 14 days, if meningitis is documented

Congenital Syphilis

- Definition: An infection caused by *Treponema pallidum* that can be acquired in adolescents and congenitally in infants; congenital infection occurs by transplacental transmission of *T. pallidum*, a spirochete; facilitates infection with HIV
- Etiology/Incidence
  1. Rates of congenital syphilis in United States have doubled since 2000. In 2000, the rate was 2.1 per 100,000 and is presently 5.3 per 1000 (Patton, Su, Nelson, & Weinstock, 2014). However, the rates are higher due to men having sex with men rather than among females (0.9 per 100,000). Racial and ethnic disparity continues with the rate 13.2 times higher among black women as compared to white women and 2.7 times higher among Hispanic than among white women. The rate is the western United States was the highest in 2014, and for the first time, the south did not have the highest rate (Patton et al., 2014)
  2. *Treponema pallidum*—mother with history of syphilis whose treatment is not documented as complete with full follow-up
  3. Transmission is more common when a mother has primary and secondary infection rather than latent infection. If the mother has early, untreated syphilis, there is a 40% risk of spontaneous abortion. The World Health Organization (WHO) estimated that of the 1 million pregnancies affected by syphilis, 460,000 result in stillbirth, hydrops fetalis abortion, or perinatal death; low-birth-weight or preterm infants occur in 270,000, and 270,000 will have congenital syphilis
  4. Maternal risk factors are lack of prenatal care and cocaine abuse
  5. Can be contracted at any stage of pregnancy
- Signs and Symptoms
  1. 60% of infants with congenital infection have no symptoms in the 1st week of life, but will develop symptoms if not immediately treated; initial presentation up to 2 years of age. The presentation at birth of congenital syphilis is stillbirth, hydrops fetalis, preterm delivery, or asymptomatic
  2. Early congenital syphilis—liver, hematologic, mucous membrane, musculoskeletal, CNS, eye, renal, GI
     a. Low birth weight/prematurity
     b. Rhinitis (snuffles), mucous patches
     c. Jaundice with elevated liver enzymes
     d. Lymphadenopathy with Coombs-negative hemolytic anemia, thrombocytopenia
     e. Osteochondritis, which causes resistance to movement (pseudoparalysis of Parrot)
     f. Rash similar to secondary syphilis with desquamation of hands/feet
     g. CNS abnormalities

3. Late congenital syphilis
   a. Signs and symptoms of syphilis in children between 2 and 5 years include central nervous system abnormalities, bone, joint, teeth, eye, and skin issues
   b. Signs and symptoms of syphilis in children between 5 and 20 years include interstitial keratitis, Hutchinson teeth, anterior bowing of the skins, Clutton joints (symmetrical joint swelling), saddle nose, frontal bossing, mulberry molars (molars with enamel growths), rhagades (fissures or cracks in the skin at the mouth angle or nose angle) (Eckerle, Howard, & John, 2013)
- Differential Diagnosis
  1. Any of the TORCH (*Toxoplasma*, others, rubella, cytomegalovirus [CMV], herpes) congenital conditions
  2. Rash stage—pityriasis rosea, scabies, tinea
- Physical Findings
  1. May be asymptomatic at birth
  2. Nonimmune hydrops
  3. Hepatomegaly
  4. Splenomegaly
  5. Lymphadenopathy
  6. Rhinitis (snuffles)
  7. Pseudoparalysis of Parrot
- Diagnostic Tests/Findings
  1. Tests for syphilis: After the newborn period, reverse screening is generally done with treponemal tests first, then confirming with nontreponemal tests. The nontreponemal tests are used to monitor effectiveness of treatment (AAP, 2012)
     a. Direct visualization of spirochete by dark field microscopy; direct fluorescent antibody test for *Treponema pallidum*: definitive diagnosis
     b. Nontreponemal tests—Venereal Disease Research Laboratory microscopic slide test (VDRL); rapid plasma reagin (RPR)
     c. Treponemal test—fluorescent treponemal antibody absorbed; microhemagglutination assay for antibody to *Treponema pallidum* (TP-PA or FTA-ABS). These remain positive for life and are not diagnostic of a new infection. These tests correlate poorly with disease activity and should not be used to monitor effectiveness of therapy
  2. If the mother has a reactive nontreponemal and treponemal test, the infant's cord blood results should be evaluated with a quantitative nontreponemal serological test (RPR or VDRL) since umbilical cord blood could be contaminated with mother's blood and lead to a false positive; a treponemal test is not necessary
  3. Elevated liver function tests (LFTs); positive VDRL in cerebrospinal fluid (CSF)
  4. Coombs-negative hemolytic anemia, thrombocytopenia
  5. Radiographic changes ("moth eaten" metaphysis)
- Management/Treatment
  1. Prenatal screen all pregnant women; treat all infected individuals, especially sexually active women and partners

  2. Treat infants with proven or highly probable disease and an abnormal physical examination that is consistent with congenital syphilis, a serum quantitative nontreponemal serologic titer that is fourfold higher than the mother's titer, or has a positive dark field or fluorescent antibody test of body fluid with:
     a. Aqueous crystalline penicillin G 100,000–150,000 units/kg/day, administered as 50,000 units/kg/dose IV every 12 hours during the first 7 days of life or every 8 hours if the infant is older than 1 week of age for a total of 10 days OR
     b. Procaine penicillin G 50,000 units/kg/dose IM in a single daily dose for 10 days
     c. Follow up to determine appropriately falling titers of the serologic testing (nontreponemal test) every 2 to 3 months until there is a decrease fourfold in test or the test becomes nonreactive
  3. For children with reactive serologic tests for syphilis identified after 1 month, the provider should review maternal serology to determine whether the child has congenital or acquired syphilis; treatment consists of:
     a. Aqueous crystalline penicillin G 200,000 to 300,000 units/kg/day IV, administered as 50,000 units/kg every 4 to 6 hours for 10 days
     b. Follow up as above for infected neonates

Herpes

- Definition: Group of infectious diseases caused by the herpes simplex virus (HSV) type 1 or 2; HSV-1 is associated with infections of EENT and central nervous system, and HSV-2 is associated with anogenital infections; establishes viral latency in sensory ganglia following primary infection. The clinical presentation of herpes in the newborn period includes: (1) disseminated disease involving multiple organ systems but predominantly liver and lungs (25%), (2) localized CNS disease (30%), and (3) skin, eyes, and/or mouth disease (45%) (Pinninti & Kimberlin, 2013)
- Etiology/Incidence
  1. More than 80 herpesvirus, 8 infect humans—HSV-1, HSV-2, varicella-zoster virus (VZV), human herpesvirus (HHV-6 and HHV-7), Epstein-Barr virus, cytomegalovirus (CMV), and Kaposi's sarcoma–associated herpesvirus (HHV-8)
  2. Transmitted through exposure to mucous membranes or skin with active lesion through direct contact of virus with host mucous membrane or abraded skin. The transmission can occur at three different times: (1) in utero (5%); (2) during peripartum period (85%); or (3) postnatal (10%). In utero infections present with cutaneous, ophthalmologic, and CNS disease
  3. HSV can be transmitted to neonatals with an incidence of 1:32,000 live births, with 1500 cases in United States annually (Pinninti & Kimberlin, 2013). Neonatal herpes is a severe infection with high morbidity and mortality even in the face of antiviral treatment

- Signs and Symptoms
  1. Congenital in utero infection
     a. Often die in utero
     b. If survive to term, vesicular lesions, chorioretinitis, microphthalmia, microcephaly, with abnormal CNS
  2. Neonatal skin-eye-mouth (SEM) disease
     a. Usually presents in first 2 weeks of life
     b. Cutaneous lesions generally located on scalp, mouth, nose, and eye with the baby contracted from the mother's genitals
  3. Neonatal CNS disease
     a. Infant in 2nd to 3rd week of life
     b. Neurologic signs—lethargy, irritability, poor feeding, temperature instability, seizures, apneic episodes
     c. Permanent neurologic disability in 40% of survivors, but mortality is 4%
  4. Neonatal disseminated disease
     a. Mortality rate of 29% (Pinninti & Kimerlin, 2013)
     b. Acutely ill infant during 1st week of life
     c. Multisystem involvement—shock, disseminated intravascular coagulation, and multiorgan failure with liver and lungs most
     d. Unresponsive to antibiotic therapy
- Differential Diagnosis
  1. Bacterial sepsis such as group B streptococcus and viral infections—enterovirus, varicella, influenza A/B, parainfluenza, and adenovirus
  2. Langerhans cell histiocytosis and incontinentia pigmenti can present with vesicles
- Physical Findings
  1. Neonatal skin-eye-mouth (SEM) disease
     a. Vesicles with erythematous base, clear or cloudy fluid, sometimes appearing pustular, limited to skin, eyes, and mouth
     b. Transient fever, malaise (low acuity)
  2. Neonatal CNS disease
     a. Herpetic skin lesions in 60% of cases
     b. Cranial nerve abnormalities
     c. Seizures
  3. Neonatal disseminated disease
     a. Septic picture—seizures, lethargy
     b. Fever, tachypnea, labored breathing with onset of HSV pneumonitis
     c. Hepatomegaly
- Diagnostic Tests/Findings
  1. Virus isolation from skin, mucous membranes, urine, blood, stool, or CSF
  2. Detection of fluorescent antibodies (especially when skin lesions are active)
  3. Polymerase chain reaction (PCR)—helpful in CNS infection where the specificities range from 71% to 100% and sensitivities range from 75% to 100% (Pinninti & Kimberlin, 2014)
  4. Serology rarely useful in acute HSV infection
  5. Increased CSF protein and pleocytosis

  6. Pulmonary radiograph reveals bilateral, patchy infiltrates from 3 to 10 days of neonatal disseminated disease
  7. Abnormal liver function test results
- Management/Treatment
  1. Infant with known or suspected herpes
     a. Acyclovir 20 mg/kg body weight IV every 8 hours for 21 days for disseminated and CNS disease (60 mg/kg per day)
     b. Acyclovir 20 mg/kg IV every 8 for 14 days for SEM (60 mg/kg per day)
  2. Infants with ocular involvement
     a. 1% trifluridine, or
     b. 0.1% iododeoxyuridine, or
     c. 3% vidarabine for ocular HSV or for neonatal HSV with SEM involvement

Cytomegalovirus (CMV)

- Definition: Congenital infection with cytomegalovirus, a member of the herpesvirus family, can be symptomatic (10%) or asymptomatic (90%); CMV affects 1 out of 750 babies; asymptomatic infections are the most common, but some congenitally infected infants who are asymptomatic at birth can have hearing loss or learning disability later in life. CMV establishes lifelong latency in the monocyte and granulocyte
- Etiology/Incidence
  1. Most common intrauterine infection, affecting 0.6% to 0.7% of newborns (Swanson & Schleiss, 2013). No seasonality to this infection. CMV may be acquired in infancy via intrapartum or postnatal routes. Breast milk may transmit the infection and low-birth-weight premature infants are at increased risk via this route
  2. Prevalence varies with age, socioeconomic status, ethnicity, and nationality, with increasing prevalence with age, coming from a developing nation, low socioeconomic group, and being African American
  3. Risk of severe disease is greater if exposed to gestational primary infection; however, congenital infection can result from reactivation of latent CMV infection
  4. Preterm infants are at greater risk of symptomatic infection
  5. Vertical transmission to infant
     a. In utero via placenta
     b. At birth through passage
     c. Postnatal infection by ingestion of CMV-positive human milk
- Signs and Symptoms
  1. Symptomatic infection at birth
     a. Intrauterine growth restriction
     b. Developmental delay
     c. Jaundice, hepatosplenomegaly
     d. Purpura, generalized petechiae, thrombocytopenia
     e. Bone abnormalities

f. Periventricular calcifications, seizures, sensorineural hearing loss, microcephaly

g. Retinitis and pneumonitis

2. Asymptomatic infection at birth

   a. Sensorineural hearing loss is most common sequela (AAP, 2012) with 21% of all hearing loss at birth secondary to CMV and 25% of all hearing loss at 4 years secondary to CMV

   b. Intellectual consequences with greater risk of school failure

- Differential Diagnosis

1. Congenital toxoplasmosis

2. Rubella

3. Herpes

- Physical Findings: Classic congenital CMV manifestations are noted above

- Diagnostic Tests/Findings

1. Isolation of CMV from infant urine, pharynx, or peripheral blood leukocytes within first 3 weeks of life

2. Other tests with variable efficacy

   a. CMV-specific IGM is used beyond the neonatal period by looking for a fourfold antibody titer increase in paired serum specimen of the IgM serum antibody.

   b. PCR testing of neonatal blood and cerebrospinal fluid

   c. CMV antigenemia

- Management/Treatment

1. Primary prevention in women of child-bearing age and younger, since both initial infection and reactivation during pregnancy can cause fetal infection

   a. Of all the congenital infections, only 22% of mothers knew about this infection; more education regarding this infection is needed among all women

2. Congenitally affected infants

   a. Treatment with IV ganciclovir 6 mg/kg for 6 weeks for infants with symptomatic disease or CNS involvement at birth. Must monitor CBC for neutropenia, which occurs in about 60% of patients. Treatment with human granulocyte colony-stimulating factor can be used to restore neutrophil count and monitoring for renal function with dosage adjustment as needed. Valganciclovir can also be used at 16 mg/kg/dose every 12 hours with the same toxicity profile as ganciclovir

   b. Diagnostic studies in suspected CMV infection should include liver function tests, CBC, bilirubin, chest x-ray, and audiologic screening

   c. In asymptomatic infections, no antivirals are recommended, but careful series measures of head circumference, careful physical exams, audiologic evaluations are needed (AAP, 2012; Swanson & Schleiss, 2013)

   d. Refer to developmental disabilities center for interdisciplinary management

3. Asymptomatic infants with congenital CMV

   a. Refer to audiology for periodic sensorineural hearing evaluation

   b. Screen frequently for growth retardation and emerging developmental delays

   c. Refer to ophthalmology—emerging chorioretinitis

   d. Refer to dentistry—defective tooth enamel

4. Neonatal acquisition—often presents as afebrile pneumonia after 8-week incubation period; test suspect infants

5. Seek specialist consultation regarding use of ganciclovir

Congenital Rubella Syndrome (CRS)

- Definition: Rubella is a *Rubivirus* in the Togaviridae family. The disease is mild in most adults; however, it can cause multisystem involvement in the fetus when associated with maternal infection during the first 12 weeks of gestation (McLean, Fiebelkorn, Temte, & Wallace, 2013). The risk for congenital infection is highest during the first 12 weeks and congenital defects are rare over 20 weeks. Subclinical disease in the mother can cause congenital malformations in the fetus. The incubation period ranges from 12 to 23 days after exposure, with an average of 18.

- Etiology/Incidence

1. Maternal to fetal transmission of rubella virus

2. From 2005 to 2011, a total of 11 rubella cases were reported each year (McLean et al., 2013) with only 6 cases of CRS reported between 2013 and 2014 (Seetoo et al., 2013)

- Signs and Symptoms

1. Early manifestation of rubella

   a. Ophthalmologic—cataracts, pigmentary retinopathy, microphthalmos, congenital glaucoma

   b. Neurologic—behavior disorders, meningoencephalitis, mental retardation

   c. Cardiac—patent ductus, peripheral pulmonary artery stenosis

   d. Auditory—deafness

   e. Growth—failure to thrive, related to heart defects

   f. To confirm diagnosis must have a symptom from one of each of the two following categories:

      (1) Cataracts, congenital glaucoma, congenital heart disease (most commonly patent ductus arteriosus or peripheral pulmonary artery stenosis), loss of hearing, pigmentary retinopathy

      (2) Purpura, hepatosplenomegaly, jaundice, microcephaly, developmental delay, meningoencephalitis, radiolucent bone disease

2. Delayed manifestation of congenital rubella syndrome

   a. Can be delayed from 2 to 4 years

   b. Diabetes mellitus

   c. Progressive encephalopathy resembling subacute sclerosing panencephalitis

   d. Higher than expected incidence of autism

- Differential Diagnosis
  1. Congenital CMV
  2. Syphilis
  3. Toxoplasmosis
- Physical Findings
  1. Growth restriction
  2. Meningoencephalitis
  3. Hepatosplenomegaly
  4. Thrombocytopenia
  5. Blueberry muffin lesions (dermal erythropoiesis)
  6. Cataracts, retinopathy, glaucoma, cataracts
  7. Petechial or purpuric rash
  8. Sensorineural hearing impairment
  9. Microphthalmia
  10. Radiolucent bones
- Diagnostic Tests/Findings
  1. Reliable evidence of acute rubella infection
     a. Positive viral culture for rubella
     b. Detection of rubella virus by polymerase chain reaction
     c. Presence of rubella-specific IgM antibody
     d. Demonstration of a significant rise in IgG antibody from paired acute- and convalescent-phase sera
     e. Serology is most common
- Management/Treatment
  1. Isolate infants with CRS from pregnant/potentially pregnant women for 1 full year
  2. Two-thirds of infants with CRS show no symptoms at birth; if maternal infection known or suspected, obtain cultures to determine whether infant is shedding virus
  3. Early intervention for developmental stimulation
  4. Refer to cardiology, ophthalmology, audiology for evaluation
  5. Psychosocial support to child and family
  6. Ensure appropriate school placement and supports
  7. Rubella is a reportable disease

Hepatitis B

- Definition: Hepatitis B is a Hepadnaviridae virus that primarily affects the liver that can cause an acute hepatitis with recovery, an acute hepatitis with liver failure, or chronic hepatitis that can lead to cirrhosis, primary carcinoma of the liver, or liver failure. Untreated perinatal transmission results in lifelong chronic infection in over 90% of newborns. Infection in children ages 1 year to 5 years results in a 25% to 50% chronic disease rate. Chronic infection leads to cirrhosis (scarring) or hepatocellular carcinoma (Eckerle et al., 2013)
- Etiology/Incidence
  1. Person-to-person transmission of hepatitis B virus via close personal contact, saliva and other secretions, blood and blood products through wound exudates, or sexual contact with infected individuals; perinatal vertical transmission from infected/carrier mother to infant

  2. Infants born to mothers positive for hepatitis B surface antigen (HBsAg) and hepatitis B "e" antigen (HBeAg) have a 70% to 90% chance of acquiring perinatal HBV if infant does not receive postexposure prophylaxis. The perinatal transmission risk is about 10% if the mother only is positive for HBsAg; around 90% of infected infants eventually become chronically infected with HBV
  3. 24% of chronic infections are from perinatal transmission
  4. HBV is transmitted through infected body fluids
- Signs and Symptoms
  1. Long incubation period 60 to 150 days, average of 90 days
  2. Malaise, anorexia, nausea, vomiting
  3. Right upper quadrant abdominal pain, fever, headache
  4. Myalgia, arthralgia, and arthritis
  5. Skin rash
  6. Dark urine, begins 1 to 2 days before the onset of jaundice
- Differential Diagnosis
  1. Hepatitis A, hepatitis C, hepatitis D, hepatitis E
  2. Cystic fibrosis, Wilson's disease, metabolic liver disease
  3. Infectious causes such as CMV, toxoplasmosis, enterovirus, Epstein-Barr virus
- Physical Findings
  1. Neonatal infection usually results in "healthy" chronic carrier state
  2. Later, progression to liver disease with:
     a. Liver enlargement, tenderness
     b. Jaundice
     c. Arthralgia or arthritis
     d. Rash or urticaria
- Diagnostic Tests/Findings
  1. Presence of surface antigen HBsAg, HBeAg antigen antibodies to either of these or HBcAg (core antigen)
  2. Aminotransferase elevation—peaks at about 1 month
  3. Bilirubin elevation
  4. Elevated white blood cells (WBCs); elevated serum α-fetoprotein concentration
- Management/Treatment
  1. Chronic infection with hepatitis B occurs if there is an absence of IgM anti-HBc or the persistence of HBsAg for 6 months
  2. To try to avoid perinatal transmission—HBIG 0.5 mL 1 vaccination in first 12 hours of life; the second dose must be given at 1 to 2 months with third dose at 6 months; the infant should have testing for HBsAg and anti-HBs at 9 to 18 months to measure success of vaccination with HBIG at birth
  3. Prevention of hepatitis B is by universally vaccinating all children so that they cannot become carriers of hepatitis B
  4. The drugs to treat hepatitis B have been approved by the FDA and include interferon ≥1 year, lamivudine

≥3 years, and adefovir ≥12 years, telbivudine ≥16 years, and entecavir ≥16 years. Treatment of chronic hepatitis B should be referred to a healthcare provider with an expertise in treating chronic hepatitis B (AAP, 2012)

5. Chronic infection with hepatitis B is being treated in adults with liver failure and chronic hepatitis C; there are two classes of agent interferons (interferon-a2b and peginterferon-a2a) or long-term use of nucleosides/nucleotide analogs (lamivudine, adefovir, entecavir, tenofovir, and telbivudine) being used as monotherapy or in combination

Toxoplasmosis

- Definition: *Toxoplasma* is an obligate intracellular protozoan. Infection with protozoan *Toxoplasma gondii* occurs after consumption of undercooked meat or ingestion of the oocyte of *T. gondii* from unwashed fruits and vegetables. It can also be transmitted by the definitive host: domestic or feral cats. The cat excretes oocytes in soil and cat litter; changing litter can transmit it
- Etiology/Incidence
  1. Primary infection is a self-limited illness that in 10% to 20% of immunocompetent hosts will have isolated occipital or cervical adenopathy
  2. *T. gondii* has the highest rate of transmission to the fetus between 10 and 24 weeks of gestation and will lead to the greatest burden of disease in the fetus during this time (Barry, Weatherhead, Hotez, & Woc-Colburn, 2013)
  3. 85% of women of child-bearing age are susceptible to infection
  4. Estimated 400 to 4000 cases per year in the United States or 1 to 10 per 10,000 live births (AAP, 2012)
  5. Asymptomatic infection occurs in the neonate, and these infants will develop signs and symptoms of the disease
  6. The incubation of acquired infection is on average 7 days, with a range of 4 to 21 days
- Signs and Symptoms
  1. An acute infection during pregnancy results in the classic triad—chorioretinitis, intracranial calcification, and hydrocephalus; in the newborn this triad occurs in less than 10%
  2. Asymptomatic at birth in 70% to 90%
  3. Nonspecific manifestations of symptomatic congenital infection
     a. Microcephaly
     b. Seizures
     c. Maculopapular rash
     d. Hepatosplenomegaly
     e. Jaundice
     f. Thrombocytopenia
  4. Later manifestations of congenital infection
     a. Blindness, epilepsy, psychomotor retardation, mental retardation can occur as late as 2nd or 3rd decade

     b. Blindness is the result of chorioretinitis, which damages the retina. Acute infection can manifest as blurred vision, eye pain, floaters, scotoma, and photophobia with initially and later chorioretinitis resulting in unilateral vision loss
  5. In childhood, the acquisition of *T. gondii* infections may be asymptomatic or may be nonspecific. Cervical lymphadenopathy is the most common sign with malaise, fever, sore throat, arthralgia, and myalgia being nonspecific for this disease. Mononucleosis-like illness can occur with rash and hepatomegaly
- Differential Diagnosis
  1. Cytomegalovirus
  2. Syphilis
  3. Rubella
  4. Hemolytic disease of the newborn
- Physical Findings
  1. Severe
     a. Microcephaly or hydrocephalus with or without intracranial calcification
     b. Retinal lesions on fundoscopic examination
     c. Splenomegaly, hepatomegaly
     d. Lymphadenopathy
     e. Jaundice
     f. Growth failure
  2. Subclinical (later signs)—retinal lesions on fundoscopic examination
- Diagnostic Tests/Findings
  1. Prenatal—fetal blood or tissue analysis; ultrasonography for bilateral, symmetrical ventriculomegaly
  2. The testing can be direct or indirect method
     a. Indirect methods: Organism-specific serology immunoglobulin IgA, IgM, and IgG are useful to identify pregnant women at risk of acquiring the infection during pregnancy. IgG test is positive 1–2 months postinfection. A positive *gondii*-specific test can be sent to PAMF-TSF (available at http://www .pamf.org/serology) for confirmatory testing. Enzyme immunoassays are most sensitive for IgM and can be detected 2 weeks postinfection and become undetectable within 6 to 9 month in most people
     b. Direct methods: Looking at the fluids and tissues via microscope and evaluating the DNA PCR of bronchoalveolar lavage fluids or other tissue
  3. In utero testing by polymerase chain reaction (PCR) assay (detection of genomic material in amniotic fluid can be used with sensitivity of 94% and specificity of 100%), or immunoperoxidase staining can be done with any body fluid for confirmatory diagnosis
  4. Visual detection of tachyzoites in newborn CSF, ventricular fluid, blood, bone marrow, brain or placental tissue, or detection 1 to 6 weeks
  5. Intracerebral calcifications with or without hydrocephalus
- Management/Treatment
  1. Prevention is best—pregnant women should not eat raw or undercooked meat; they should wash fruits

and vegetables prior to eating and should wear gloves while gardening, avoid changing cat litter

2. For symptomatic and asymptomatic congenital infection—pyrimethamine combined with sulfadiazine supplemented with folic acid for 1 year is the initial therapy (AAP, 2012) in conjunction with ID consult

3. Maternal infection—spiramycin treatment can be used in pregnant women to prevent transmission to the fetus but will not work if the fetus is already infected. This is an investigational drug and can be obtained following advice of PAMF-TSl and with authorization of FDA

   a. Maternal treatment with pyrimethoamine and sulfadiazine if there is fetal infection confirmed after 18 weeks or the mother acquires the infection during the third trimester

❏ FETAL ALCOHOL SYNDROME (FAS) AND FETAL ALCOHOL SPECTRUM DISORDERS (FASD)

- Definition: An umbrella term for a set of disorders that result from the consumption of alcohol during pregnancy; FASD occurs three times more often than FAS. Prenatal alcohol exposure (PAE) causes a wide range of features that are characterized by minor facial dysmorphic features, growth deficiency, and central nervous systems symptoms (Dorrie, Föcker, Freunscht, & Hebebrand, 2014)
- Etiology/Incidence
  1. An estimated 1000 to 6000 infants will be born with FAS, with a worldwide estimate of FASD of 1 in 100
  2. Dose that causes damage is unknown, but occurs even at low levels of consumption; cell adhesion molecules are inhibiting, affecting neuronal migration
  3. Alcohol raises acetaldehyde levels and causes apoptotic damage from excess glutamate activity due to gamma amino butyric acid (GABA) withdrawal; this causes apoptotic neurodegeneration reaction, deleting neurons from developing sites in the CNS
  4. The finding that PAE of one drink per week has an association with aggressive behavior at 6–7 years suggests that there is no safe amount of PAE (Dorrie et al., 2014)
- Signs and Symptoms
  1. History of drinking during pregnancy
  2. Infant alcohol withdrawal symptoms (irritability, hyperactivity, jitteriness) and alcohol odor to amniotic fluid if alcohol abuse during last days of pregnancy
  3. There needs to be a CNS abnormality showing at least one of three types of deficits or abnormalities—structural, neurologic, and functional
  4. Fetal alcohol spectrum disorders—diagnostic features must include facial features, growth retardation, structural and/or functional CNS dysfunction, and

a history of prenatal alcohol exposure (see Signs and Symptoms for more information)

   a. Fetal alcohol syndrome (FAS)—full-blown syndrome involving every diagnostic feature as above
   b. Partial fetal alcohol syndrome (pFAS)—some but not all of the facial features are present, CNS dysfunction as in FAS
   c. Alcohol-related neurodevelopmental disorder (ARND)—CNS abnormalities without facial abnormalities with confirmed PAE
   d. Alcohol-related birth defects (ARBD)—various birth defects without CNS disease with confirmed PAE
   e. Static encephalopathy/alcohol exposed (SE/AE)—significant structural defects. Neurologic defects, but no growth or facial features
   f. Neurodevelopmental disorder (alcohol exposed)—confirmed PAE with cognitive and behaviors problems, but no CNS damage. Behavior effects include problems with math, memory or attention difficulties, poor school performance, and poor impulse control (Dorrie et al., 2014)

- Differential Diagnosis: Other deletion syndrome, Williams syndrome, Dubowitz syndrome, fetal Dilantin (phenytoin) syndrome, Down syndrome
- Physical Findings: Will vary
  1. Diagnostic facial features include a thin upper lip, short palpebral fissures, and flattened philtrum
     a. Other facial features include widely spaced eyes with narrow lids and epicanthal folds; short, upturned, or beaklike nose with broad nasal bridge; thin upper lip with vermilion border; micrognathia and dental malocclusion
  2. Growth retardation, which can be prenatal or postnatal growth deficit
  3. Structural and/or functional CNS dysfunction includes intellectual disability, psychiatric conditions (attention deficit hyperactivity disorder [ADHD], conduct disorders, oppositional defiant disorders, anxiety disorders, adjustment disorders, sleep disorders, and depression), language disorder, microcephaly, motor disorder, and memory disorder
  4. Other congenital defects, including congenital heart defects, cleft palate, limb deficiencies
  5. Hip subluxation or dislocation
  6. Seizure disorder
  7. Ophthalmologic disorders—myopia/strabismus
  8. Hearing impairment
- Diagnostic Tests/Findings
  1. IQ usually in 60 to 80 range, stable throughout life
  2. History of maternal alcohol abuse during pregnancy
- Management/Treatment
  1. Prevention is key; ensure pregnant women know risk of alcohol intake on fetal development
  2. No known treatment to reverse primary defects
  3. Needs appropriate educational plan with needed support to reduce negative impact
  4. Screen for vision, hearing, neurologic disorders

5. Refer to http://www.cdc.gov/ncbddd/fas/default.htm
6. For information on FASD: National Organization on Fetal Alcohol Syndrome http://www.nofas.org/

☐ GENETIC SYNDROMES

Trisomy 18 (Edwards Syndrome)

- Definition: Autosomal chromosomal disorder with karyotype 47 XY or XX 1 18, trisomy of chromosome 18; associated with severe mental retardation and other congenital defects associated with advanced maternal age; less than 5% survive beyond 1st year of life
- Etiology/Incidence
  1. Nondisjunction during meiotic division resulting in trisomy of chromosome 18
  2. 1 in 5000 live births
  3. 10% of cases are mosaic
  4. If there is only a partial duplication of chromosome 18, they will have a milder presentation
- Signs and Symptoms
  1. Growth retardation
  2. Faces—low-set ears with prominent occiput and micrognathia
  3. Musculoskeletal—rocker-bottom feet and overlapping fingers (second over third, and fifth over fourth)
  4. Cardiac—congenital heart defects
  5. Neurologic—severe global developmental delays, CNS defects with hypertonia
  6. Feeding problems
- Differential Diagnosis: Trisomy 13; other rare chromosomal aberrations
- Physical Findings
  1. Retardation of growth with severe failure to thrive (FTT)
  2. Microcephaly, low-set ears, prominent occiput, micrognathia
  3. Heart murmur
  4. Clenched hands with overriding fingers and crossed thumb
- Diagnostic Tests/Findings
  1. Karyotype
     a. Fluorescent in situ hybridization (FISH) analysis
     b. Results usually available within 48 hours
  2. Maternal serum quadruple screen include α-fetoprotein, human chorionic gonadotropin, unconjugated estriol, and inhibin A; this test has 11% greater detection rate than the triple screen, with a 5% screen positive rate
  3. Echocardiogram to detect congenital cardiac defects
  4. Chorionic villus sampling or amniocentesis with subsequent pregnancies
- Management/Treatment
  1. Genetic counseling
  2. Psychosocial support to parents and family
  3. Refer to cardiology
  4. Support nutritional needs; may require gastric feedings

5. Prophylactic antibiotics to prevent subacute bacterial endocarditis (SBE) if cardiac effects present
6. Enroll in early intervention program for habilitative therapies
7. Assist family with management of special needs child—may require in-home nursing
8. Support Organization for Trisomy 18, 13, and Related Disorders (SOFT) http://www.trisomy.org/

Down Syndrome (DS) (Trisomy 21)

- Definition: Down syndrome, or trisomy 21, is the most common inherited genetic syndrome associated with a variable degree of mental impairment and karyotype 47 XY or XX 1 21
- Etiology/Incidence
  1. Three different genetic alterations
     a. In 95%, Down syndrome is result of a random non-disjunction (trisomy 21)
     b. Less commonly, it occurs as mosaicism where some cells are affected and others are normal
     c. Balanced translocation, often involves chromosomes 21 and 14
  2. 1 in 691 live births (Hobson-Rohrer & Samson-Fang, 2013)
  3. Affects males and females equally
  4. Risk factors include advanced maternal age, previous child with Down syndrome or another chromosomal abnormality, parental balanced translocation, parents with chromosomal problems
- Signs and Symptoms
  1. Mental retardation, mild to severe
  2. Typical phenotypic signs at birth
     a. Head—midface hypoplasia; small brachycephalic head with epicanthal folds, flat nasal bridge, upward-slanting palpebral fissures, Brushfield spots, small mouth
     b. Ears—small ears
     c. Neck—excessive skin at the nape of the neck
     d. Hands and feet—simian crease and short fifth finger with clinodactyly; a wide space, often with a deep fissure between the first and second toes; lymphedema, brachydactyly (shortened digits)
     e. Neurologic—mental impairment is variable, ranging from mild (IQ: 50–70), to moderate (IQ: 35–50), and only occasionally severe (IQ: 20–35)
     f. Cardiac—increased risk of congenital heart defects (50%)
     g. GI—Hirschsprung disease (1%); gastrointestinal atresias (12%)
     h. Musculoskeletal—hypotonia; hyperflexability; wide gap between first and second toes, acquired hip dislocation (6%)
     i. Skin—dry, single transverse palmar crease
- Differential Diagnosis: Other genetic or chromosomal syndromes

- Physical Findings
  1. Phenotype as above
  2. Hearing loss (75%); otitis media (50–70%)
  3. Obstructive sleep apnea (50–75%)
  4. Signs of congenital heart disease—50%; endocardial cushion defect most common (45%) with ventricular septal defects (35%) second
  5. Signs of hypothyroidism and other endocrine problems—15%; by adulthood 60% will develop hypothyroidism (Hobson-Rohrer & Samson-Fang, 2013)
  6. Signs of anomaly of GI tract 5%; celiac disease 15% (Davidson, 2008)
  7. Ligamentous laxity—100%
  8. Hematological—leukemia (<1%)
  9. Eye—eye disease (60%), including cataracts (15%), and severe refractive errors (50%)
  10. Obesity—50% by early childhood
  11. Musculoskeletal—ankle pronation and pes planus
  12. Premature aging
- Diagnostic Tests/Findings
  1. Pre- or postnatal chromosome analysis reveals 47,XY or 47,XX,+21 karyotype
  2. CBC with differential to identify those with leukemia; 10- to 15-fold increased risk
  3. Symptoms of atlantoaxial instability (neck pain, decreased range of motion of the neck, gait disturbance, bowel or bladder dysfunction, hyperreflexia, or paresthesias)—routine radiographs for atlantoaxial instability are no longer recommended (Hobson-Rohrer & Samson-Fang, 2013)
  4. Ophthalmologic evaluations every 2 years between 3 and 5 years of age, and then yearly after this (50% risk of refractive errors between 3 and 5 years)
- Management/Treatment
  1. For complete guidelines by age for patients with Down syndrome, see http://pediatrics.aappublications.org/content/128/2/393.full.pdf+html
  2. Primary prevention via education re: risk factors; secondary prevention via prenatal diagnosis
  3. Monitor for growth and family support every well visit
  4. Annual screening TSH, hemoglobin; hearing screen if normal screening at 6 months
  5. Initial evaluation by cardiology to rule out congenital heart defect even if no murmurs are heard
  6. Screen for celiac disease if symptomatic; screen for symptoms at every visit
  7. Early intervention by physical therapy (PT), occupational therapy (OT), speech therapists; special education; review individualized education program
  8. Genetic counseling for parents and older siblings
  9. Periodic full history and physical with sensory and developmental evaluations
  10. Nutritional support
  11. Observe for signs of autism and refer if suspicious of autism spectrum disorder (ASD)
  12. Prompt referral for associated conditions; regular ophthalmology evaluation
  13. Parental education around increased risk of infections; encouragement of self-help skills; care of dry skin; avoidance of contact sports and trampolines; to call provider if changes in gait, use of hands, bowel or bladder dysfunction, or new onset of weakness due to risk of atlantoaxial instability; discuss cervical spine protection during anesthesia; awareness of delayed dentition and psychosocial changes during puberty (Bull & American Academy of Pediatrics, 2011)
  14. Patient advocate and guide family during transition to adult care
  15. Referral to appropriate websites for education and support
     a. National Down Syndrome Society: http://www.ndss.org/
     b. National Association for Down Syndrome: http://www.nads.org/
     c. National Down Syndrome Congress: http://www.ndsccenter.org/

Fragile X Syndrome (FXS)

- Definition: Fragile X syndrome is associated with a range of intellectual impairments, from learning problems to autism and anxiety. The disorder is linked to a fragile site on the long arm of the X chromosome at band q27.2. The amount of repeats of the CGG in a normal individual ranges from 5 to 40, but 30 repeats is the most common. This leads to gene silencing, which in turn causes decreased or absent levels of fragile X mental retardation protein (FMRP). Full mutation range occurs when there are more than 200 CGG repeats in the coding of the protein or by a point mutation or deletion in the fragile X mental retardation gene. Premutation occurs when the CGG repeat number is between 55 and 100, they are unstable meiotically, and they produce FMRP that may be in lower amounts than normal. The severity of cognitive impairment depends on the degree of the FMR1 methylation and gene silencing rather than the number of CGG repeats. Different FMRP levels have different clinical presentations since the methylation may differ
- Etiology/Incidence
  1. Genetic anomaly, labeled FMRI, on X chromosome at Xq27.3, the same position as the fragile site
  2. Males are more severely affected than females since they only have one X chromosome; if a male has a methylated full mutation, he will have mild to moderate intellectual disability; females with the full mutation typically have learning disabilities, but about 15% have intellectual disabilities
  3. If the individual has premutation, he or she can have mild cognitive and/or behavioral deficits, primary ovarian insufficiency, and, in older adult premutation carriers, especially males, a fragile X–associated tremor/ataxia syndrome (FXTAS). A small number of female carriers of a permutation have some of the physical features of fragile X—prominent ears or

hypermobile finger joints as well as emotional problems, including anxiety, depression, obsessional thoughts, or schizotypy. Males with a permutation have problems with executive functions, social deficits, attention problems, and obsessive-compulsive behavior

4. Affected individuals—1:4000 males; 1:8000 females
5. Premutation—1 in 813 males and 1:259 in females (Hersh, Saul, & Committee on Genetics, 2011)
   a. Testing for carriage should be done if:
      (1) Family history of mental retardation, developmental disabilities, or autism
      (2) Infertile women with increased FSH at younger than 40 years
      (3) Egg and sperm donors
6. Approximately 20% of males asymptomatic, but can transmit gene, resulting in symptomatic offspring
7. Most common inherited cause of mental retardation (MR)
   a. Children with developmental delay, mental retardation, or autism spectrum should undergo molecular testing for fragile X (Hersh et al., 2011)

- Signs and Symptoms
  1. Eye: Strabismus with refractive errors may be present. Occasionally nystagmus and ptosis are found
  2. Face: Long, narrow face, prominent jaw, with high arched palate, dental crowding, and malocclusion
  3. ENT: Protuberant ears by late childhood, chronic otitis media
  4. GI: Gastroesophageal reflux
  5. GU: Macro-orchidism occurs in more than 80% of adolescents and is less common in childhood
  6. Skin findings: Soft velvet skin, joint hypermobility, pes planus, scoliosis, and clubfoot
  7. Neuro: Seizures occur in 13% to 18% of affected males and 5% of females with the full mutation; macrocephaly, speech delay, echolalia, perseverative speech
  8. Musculoskeletal: Poor gross motor coordination
  9. Behavior phenotype of FXS
     a. Poor eye contact with excessive shyness and anxiety with hand flapping and biting
     b. Tactile defensives
     c. Attentional deficit with hyperactivity, hyperarousal to sensory stimuli, and ASD

- Differential Diagnosis
  1. Autism, Asperger syndrome, or pervasive developmental disorder
  2. Mental retardation with nonspecific etiology
  3. Klinefelter syndrome, Sotos syndrome
  4. Attention deficit hyperactivity disorder

- Physical Findings
  1. Macrocephaly
  2. Prominent forehead with long, thin face and prominent jaw, especially in adolescence
  3. Macro-orchidism in adolescent males; may be seen as early as age 5
  4. Protuberant, large ears, long or wide
  5. Soft, smooth skin
  6. Heart murmur or apical midsystolic click
  7. Serous otitis media
  8. Strabismus—40%
  9. Joint laxity (especially fingers), hip subluxation, occasionally clubfoot

- Diagnostic Tests/Findings
  1. DNA analysis from whole blood in approved laboratory to confirm diagnosis
  2. Prenatal testing from chorionic villus or amniocentesis sample

- Management/Treatment
  1. Treatment of the behavioral problems with the appropriate psychotropic medication and counseling
  2. Psychosocial support to parents, child, and family
  3. Genetic counseling—no spontaneous mutations have been found for fragile X syndrome; all family members should undergo genetic testing to identify transmitting males, carrier females, and affected individuals
  4. Regular well-child examination with attention to:
     a. Cardiac auscultation—if click or murmur heard, obtain echocardiogram, consider referral to cardiologist for possible mitral valve prolapse
     b. Otoscopic evaluation—serous otitis media
     c. Ophthalmologic evaluation—strabismus (40%), myopia
     d. Developmental evaluation—mild to severe delays (usually moderate)
     e. Anticipatory guidance
  5. Enroll in early intervention as soon as delays are recognized; speech-language therapy and sensory/motor integration therapy thought to be most helpful
  6. Ensure appropriate educational placement with necessary supports
  7. National Fragile X Foundation: https://fragilex.org/

Turner Syndrome (TS) (XO Karyotype)

- Definition: Chromosomal anomaly resulting from multiple karyotypes, including 45,X, 45,X/46,XX mosaicism, and a structurally abnormal X, leading to developmental, cardiac, reproductive, genetic, and psychosocial issues. To make the diagnosis, the female must have the characteristic features of TS with the complete or partial absence of the second X sex chromosome with or without mosaicism of the cell line. If the patient does not have the clinical features of TS but does have the 45,X cell populations, she does not have TS. Typically, the 45,X monosomy presents with the most severe phenotype (Milbrant & Thomas, 2013)
- Etiology/Incidence
  1. Nondisjunction during meiotic division, usually maternal; more than half have a mosaic chromosomal complement (45,XO/46,XX)
  2. TS is present in one of 2500 live-born females; many affected embryos do not survive to term (Milbrant & Thomas, 2013

- Signs and Symptoms
  1. Female with unexplained growth failure or pubertal delay
  2. Constellation of any of the following findings
     a. Edema of the hands or feet (particularly in newborn)
     b. Nuchal folds (webbed neck)
     c. Left-sided cardiac anomalies, especially coarctation of aorta or hypoplastic left heart
     d. Low hairline and high-arched palate
     e. Low-set ears with small mandible; chronic otitis media
     f. Short statures with growth velocity less than the 10th percentile for age
     g. Marked elevated FSH
     h. Cubitus valgus
     i. Nail hypoplasia
     j. Multiple pigmented nevi
     k. Short fourth metacarpal (Bondy, 2007)
     l. Intrauterine growth restriction (IUGR)
  3. Lack of development of secondary sexual characteristics
- Differential Diagnosis
  1. Congenital lymphedema without Turner karyotype
  2. Coarctation of aorta without Turner karyotype
- Physical Findings
  1. Signs and symptoms listed above plus:
  2. Neonatal—lymphedema (usually resolved by age 2 years)
  3. Widely spaced, often inverted nipples with "shield"-shaped chest
  4. Hypertension and aortic murmur
  5. Ear deformities
  6. Strabismus, amblyopia, ptosis
  7. Scoliosis (10%)
  8. Defective dentition
- Diagnostic Tests/Findings
  1. All Turner syndrome patients
     a. Cytogenetic testing for karyotype
     b. Orthopedic evaluation for hip dislocation, scoliosis, and kyphosis
     c. Evaluation for hearing loss; adult risk of sensorineural loss is 60%
     d. Cardiac echocardiogram or MRI for:
        (1) Coarctation of aorta (20%)
        (2) Bicuspid aortic valve (50%)
     e. Annually from age 4 onward, T_4, TSH due to high rate of autoimmune thyroid disease
     f. Abdominal and pelvic ultrasound to detect gonadal dysgenesis and renal anomalies, which are found in 30% to 50% of females, with a horseshoe kidney being the most common
     g. Plasma gonadotropin studies to detect low levels of normal female hormones
- Management/Treatment
  1. Refer to endocrinology
     a. To increase adult height, growth hormone therapy
     b. Hormone (estrogen) replacement therapy beginning about 12 to 13 years of age
     c. Monitor for hypothyroidism
  2. Genetic counseling
  3. Psychosocial support
  4. Assistance in school if there are learning disabilities; intelligence in normal
  5. Referral to cardiology for cardiac anomaly diagnosis and treatment
  6. Referral to ophthalmology—strabismus and hyperopia (farsightedness) each occur in 25% to 35% of these children (Bondy, 2007)
  7. Referral to ENT if recurrent otitis due to abnormal relationship between the Eustachian tube and middle ear since the cranial base is different
  8. Referral to orthodontist due to narrowed maxilla and wide, micrognathic mandible as well as pediatric dentist
  9. Referral to orthopedics, urology if scoliosis, renal anomalies
  10. Screen for celiac disease, which runs from 4% to 6% in patients with Turner syndrome
  11. Turner's Syndrome Society of the United States: http://www.turnersyndrome.org/
  12. Information on Turner's syndrome: http://turners.nichd.nih.gov/

Klinefelter Syndrome (XXY Karyotype)

- Definition: Klinefelter syndrome is the most common sex chromosome disorder in males with 47,XXY karyotype or a variant with an estimated frequency of 1:660 male newborns (Groth, Skakkebaek, Host, Gravhold, & Bojesen, 2013); the extra X chromosome can come from either parent; linked to advanced maternal age; men with mosaicism are less affected and tend to go undiagnosed until later in life
- Etiology/Incidence
  1. Maternal meiotic nondisjunction resulting in contribution of two X chromosomes to maternal zygote (ovum); when ovum is fertilized by sperm containing one Y chromosome, resulting embryo has Klinefelter karyotype
  2. Most common numerical chromosomal aberration is double X and a Y
  3. Most common cause of hypogonadism and infertility in men
- Signs and Symptoms
  1. Classic description: Cardinal feature is small testicles (>95%) with infertility (95–99%), increased gonadotropin levels (>95%), gynecomastia (38–75%), learning difficulties (>75%)
     a. Tall eunuchoid body proportion in males, especially at adolescence and beyond
     b. Slow, incomplete pubertal development with sparse facial and pubic hair, small testicles and infertility

c. Increased risk of mediastinal cancers (~500-fold); breast cancer (~50-fold increase)

d. Cleft palate (18%), mitral valve prolapse (~55%)

e. Metabolic syndrome with abdominal adiposity, type 2 diabetes

f. Behavioral and psychiatric disorders (shy, immature, anxious, aggressive, antisocial)

g. Osteoporosis

2. More common

a. Learning disabilities in reading and spelling with syntax problems

b. Speech and language dysfunction and impairment in executive function

c. Infertility

d. Low testosterone such as erectile dysfunction and poor libido

e. Harder testicles with a volume of 10 mL regardless of penile size, body proportions, or level of androgenization

- Differential Diagnosis
  1. Marfan syndrome
  2. Sotos syndrome
  3. Trisomy 8p
- Physical Findings
  1. Tall for age, with disproportionate lower limb length
  2. Gynecomastia
  3. Small, firm testes
  4. Cryptorchidism
  5. Small phallus
  6. Hypospadias
  7. Less pubic and facial hair
- Diagnostic Tests/Findings
  1. Chromosome analysis yields 47,XXY karyotype or mosaic
  2. Sex hormone: Testosterone, estrogen, LH, FSH, sex hormone-binding globulin (SHBG)
  3. Fasting glucose, lipids, and HbA1c
  4. Thyroid screen, hemoglobin, hematocrit
  5. Bone densitometry and vitamin D status (Groth et al., 2013)
- Management/Treatment
  1. Early intervention for learning disorders
  2. Counseling/therapy for behavioral disorders and encourage exercise. Check regarding well-being, sexual activity, libido
  3. Psychosocial support for family
  4. Genetic counseling
  5. Refer to endocrinology for consideration of testosterone therapy at age 11 or 12; echocardiograph if; referral to plastic surgery for management of gynecomastia; psychologist referral if self-esteem issues or if psychiatric problems
  6. Screen for breast cancer (4%)
  7. Reduction mammoplasty for severe gynecomastia
  8. Questions regarding physical activity, sexual function
  9. American Association for Klinefelter Syndrome Information and Support: http://www.aaksis.org/
  10. Klinefelter's Syndrome Assistance and Resource (UK): http://www.ksa-uk.co.uk/

Tay-Sachs Disease

- Definition: Inborn error of metabolism, which causes a deficiency of hexosaminidase A. This lysosomal storage disease, classified as a sphingolipidosis, results in the accumulation of G_{m2} ganglioside in the lysosomes of various tissues, which results in progressive neurologic degenerative disease and death. Unlike cerebral palsy, it is progressive and marked by an exaggerated startle response, failure to thrive, loss of normal milestones, spasticity, and developmental regression (Krishnamoorthy, Eichler, Rapalino, & Frosch, 2014)

- Etiology/Incidence
  1. Autosomal recessive single gene disorder; deficiency of hexosaminidase A (hex A), which is necessary for breakdown of ganglioside G_{m2}; as glycoside accumulates in neurons, axons degenerate and demyelination occurs
  2. Ashkenazi Jewish population (80%), some Pennsylvania Dutch, Louisiana Cajun, French Canadian; carrier rate may be as high 1:52 of Irish Americans
  3. Autosomal recessive transmission of the *HEXA* gene, located on chromosome 15

- Signs and Symptoms
  1. Normal development until age 3 to 6 months, then progressive deterioration
  2. Earliest symptom is irritability and increased reaction to sound with emerging spasticity
  3. Hypotonia with development delay, then deterioration
  4. Vision starts to deteriorate by age 6 months, with blindness as early as 1 year; cherry-red spot of the macula is due to degeneration of the ganglion cells
  5. Macrocephalic due to accumulation of the cerebral G_{m2}
  6. Frequent upper respiratory infections
  7. Seizure activity as early as 6 months

- Differential Diagnosis
  1. Sandhoff disease
  2. Krabbe disease
  3. Niemann-Pick disease
  4. Farber lipogranulomatosis
  5. Gaucher disease
  6. Beals syndrome (congenital contractural arachnodactyly)
  7. Homocystinuria
  8. Metachromatic leukodystrophy
  9. Peroxysomal disorders
  10. Mitochondrial disorders

- Diagnostic Tests/Findings
  1. Gene testing for known mutations
  2. Serum enzymatic assay yields deficiency of hexosaminidase A
  3. MRI shows changes in the ventral thalamus, white matter hypomyelination, enlarged caudate nucleus, later progression to cerebral atrophy

- Management/Treatment
  1. Genetic counseling
  2. Primary prevention via carrier screening
  3. Secondary prevention via prenatal diagnosis and elective termination of pregnancy
  4. No known treatment for underlying metabolic deficiency
  5. Supportive/comfort care for child; assist to obtain home nursing services as disease progresses and care burden increases
  6. Psychosocial support for parents and family
  7. Referral to pain management and palliative care
  8. The National Tay-Sachs and Allied Diseases Association: http://www.ntsad.org/

Marfan Syndrome

- Definition: Inherited disorder of connective tissue; affects the skeletal, cardiovascular, and ocular systems
- Etiology/Incidence
  1. Autosomal dominant inheritance of defective fibrillin gene (*FBN1* mapped to chromosome 15 [15q21.1]); 15% sporadic mutation
  2. Incidence is 1:5000
- Signs and Symptoms
  1. The Ghent diagnostic criteria for Marfan syndrome was revised and includes any one of the following:
     a. Aortic root ≥2 z score and ectopia lentis
     b. Aortic root ≥2 z score and *FBN1* mutation
     c. Aortic root ≥2 z score and systemic score ≥7
     d. Ectopia lentis and *FBN1* mutation known to be associated with Marfan syndrome
     e. Positive family history of Marfan syndrome and ectopia lentis
     f. Positive family history of Marfan syndrome and systemic score ≥7
     g. Positive family history of Marfan syndrome and aortic root ≥3 z score in those <20 years of age or ≥2 z score in an adult (>20 years of age)
     h. The systemic scores include the following: Wrist and thumb sign (3), wrist or thumb sign (1), pectus carinatum (2), pectus excavatum or chest asymmetry (1), hind foot deformity (e.g., valgus) (2), pes planus (1), pneumothorax (2), dural ectasia (2), protrusio acetabulae (2), reduced upper-to-lower body segment ratio and increased arm-span-to-height ratio (1), scoliosis or thoracolumbar kyphosis (1), reduced elbow extension (1), craniofacial features: three of the following—dolichocephaly, downward-slanting palpebral fissures, enophthalmos, retrognathia, and malar hypoplasia (1), skin striae (1), myopia (1), or mitral valve prolapse (1) (Tinkle, Saal, & AAP Committee on Genetics 2013)
     i. A potential Marfan syndrome diagnosis includes an *FBN1* mutation with aortic root with a z score <3 in those <20 years of age

- Differential Diagnosis
  1. Mitral valve prolapse syndrome
  2. Loeys-Dietz syndrome
  3. Homocystinuria
  4. Vascular type of Ehlers-Danlos syndrome
  5. Stickler syndrome
  6. Fragile X
  7. Familial thoracic aortic aneurysm
  8. Congenital contractual arachnodactyly
- Diagnostic Tests/Findings
  1. Genetic testing to evaluate for the defects in *FBN1*
  2. Positive family history of Marfan syndrome
  3. Cardiac evaluation (echocardiogram to evaluate for mitral valve prolapse; signs of dilatation of aortic root, or dissecting aortic aneurysm)
  4. Ocular evaluation—slit-lamp examination for ectopic lentis
  5. Skeletal evaluation—scoliosis screening; trunk/extremities ratio
  6. Urine screening for amino acids at birth to evaluate for homocystinuria
- Management/Treatment
  1. Refer to cardiology for periodic echocardiogram to detect dissecting aortic aneurysm, mitral valve prolapse in severe cases; surgical graft repair of the ascending aorta and aortic valve has been successful
  2. Propranolol to reduce effect of ventricular ejection on ascending aorta
  3. Refer to ophthalmology for treatment of myopia, lens subluxation, cataracts, glaucoma, and retinal detachment
  4. Refer to endocrinology for hormonal treatment to curtail height, valuable psychological effect; prevention of scoliosis and kyphosis; prevention of secondary problems of feet
  5. Psychosocial support for patient and family
  6. Genetic counseling
  7. Ensure mainstream or inclusive school placement with any necessary supports, with attention to physical activity limitations if cardiovascular involvement
  8. Avoidance of wind instruments, sky diving, scuba diving, mountaineering in patients with emphysematous lung disease
  9. National Marfan Foundation (NMF): http://www.marfan.org

Mucopolysaccharidosis (MPS)

- Definition: Rare group of lysosomal storage disorders of glycosaminoglycan (GAG) catabolism. This type of disorder leads to an accumulation of partially degraded GAG, resulting from a deficiency of a specific lysosomal enzyme, that leads to GAG fragments, causes progressive cellular damage in multiple organ systems, and eventually causes organ failure. Most of the MPS disorders are autosomal recessive with the exception of MPS II, which is an X-linked recessive disorder affecting males. Early diagnosis and treatment improve the outcome. Today there are enzymes replacements for MPS I, II, and VI (Muenzer, 2011)

- Etiology/Incidence
  1. MPS I is due to the deficiency of lysosomal enzyme α-L-iduronidase; the patient accumulates glycosaminoglycan within lysosomes and there is multiorgan dysfunction and damage as a result (Hurler-Scheie syndrome)
  2. MPS II, or Hunter syndrome, is a deficiency of iduronate-2-sulphatase, and MPS III A–D is Sanfilippo syndrome, with each subtype having a deficiency of different enzymes
  3. MPS IV A, B, is Morquio syndrome, and MPS V (Scheie syndrome) has actually been reclassified as MPS I. MPS VI is Maroteauz-Lamy syndrome, and MPS VII is Sly syndrome
  4. MPS VIII is no longer used since it was s single case report that was classified as MPS II. Finally, MPS IX is a deficiency of hyaluronan
  5. There are different presentations within each type, ranging from mild and occurring later to severe

- Signs and Symptoms
  1. Attenuated MPS I can go undiagnosed for years and there is no cognitive impairment
  2. Severe MPS I may not be diagnosed until after 12 month to 18 months. The skeletal changes seen in MPS I are referred to as dysostosis multiplex and result in profound loss of joint motion, restricted mobility and growth
  3. Progressive cognitive impairment with progressive neurodegenerative disorder in severe MPS I; early development is normal and delay is more obvious by 1 to 2 years of age
  4. Over time, coarse facial features with enlarged tongue, full lips, flat nasal bridge become more obvious
  5. Communicating hydrocephalus develops over months
  6. Onset of language skills is delayed
  7. Behavior tends to be placid rather than hyperactive or aggressive as seen in MPS II or III
  8. Recurrent upper respiratory tract infections with otitis
  9. Snoring and coarse breathing occur due to adenoidal and tonsillar enlargement
  10. Recurrent inguinal hernia
  11. Restrictive lung disease with sleep apnea and asthma
  12. Vision loss due to corneal clouding, and sensorineural hearing impairments
  13. Progressive skeletal and joint disease leading to dysostosis multiplex, scoliosis, kyphosis, and hip dislocation
  14. Short stature

- Differential Diagnosis: Other progressive neuropathies and inborn errors of metabolism, particularly other mucopolysaccharidoses and thyroid deficiency

- Physical Findings
  1. Orthopedic—skeletal abnormalities, including spinal anomalies/gibbus formation, joint stiffness, short stature, atlantoaxial instability
  2. Neurologic—macrocephaly, hydrocephalus, scaphocephaly, severe to mild cognitive impairment
  3. Eyes—clouded corneas, retinal degeneration
  4. HEENT—deafness, tonsillar hypertrophy
  5. Cardiac—congestive heart failure, valvular disease, angina, hypertension
  6. GI—hepatosplenomegaly, inguinal/umbilical hernia

- Diagnostic Tests/Findings
  1. Prenatal diagnosis with amniocentesis or chorionic villus sampling and enzyme analysis
  2. Enzyme activity assay based on cultured leucocytes, plasma, serum, or cultured fibroblasts is the gold standard for diagnosis
  3. Measurement of urinary GAG levels can be helpful if the results are positive and suggest an MPS disorder. However, there is a high false-negative rate, and a negative urinary GAG analysis does not rule out an MPS disorder

- Management/Treatment
  1. Multidisciplinary team including genetic counselor
  2. Hematopoietic stem cell transplant can preserve intellectual capacity, but not the corneal clouding, cardiac valvular deformities, and skeletal abnormalities. It does not reverse cognitive damage
  3. Enzyme replacement therapy (ERT) with recombinant human enzyme is approved for MPS I, II, and IVA. Laronidase (Aldurazyme) treats MPS type I (Hurler and Hurler-Scheie forms), whereas idursulfase (Elaprase) treats MPS type II. In February 2014, elosulfase alfa was approved to treat MPS IVA (Morquio A syndrome) but does not improve the neurocognitive effects because it does not cross the blood–brain barrier. The benefits of ERT include joint mobility improvements, walking ability, pulmonary function improvement, and decrease in hepatosplenomegaly (Muenzer, 2011)
  4. Psychosocial support and anticipatory guidance
  5. Early intervention; appropriate school placement with supports as needed
  6. MRI of brain and spine
  7. Annual audiology tests and ophthalmologic exams
  8. Pulmonary function tests and sleep studies
  9. Cardiology and orthopedics evaluation
  10. Bone marrow transplantation in selected cases, especially if a human leukocyte antigen (HLA)-matched sibling donor is available
  11. Refer to audiology and ophthalmology for evaluation and treatment as indicated
  12. National MPS Society: http://www.mpssociety.org/

Prader-Willi Syndrome (PWS)

- Definition: Prader-Willi is caused by a failure of expression of the paternally acquired imprinted region on chromosome 15q11-q13 that results in a recognizable set of signs and symptoms that affect the neurologic and endocrine systems. It is characterized by voracious, uncontrollable appetite and obesity

- Etiology/Incidence
  1. It equally affects both sexes and has equal worldwide incidence
  2. 1:15,000 to 1:25,000 incidence (Committee on Genetics, 2011)
- Signs and Symptoms
  1. In infancy, the child has hypotonia, failure to thrive, and early feeding problems. Later, hyperphagia (voracious appetite) develops with characteristic behavioral problems and global developmental delay
  2. Behavioral problems include temper tantrums and obsessive-compulsive disorders, including skin picking, stubbornness, perseverant speech, psychosis
  3. Sleep apnea with hypoventilation, excessive daytime sleepiness and early-morning walking
  4. Hypernasal speech with a weak or squeaky cry during infancy
  5. Temperature instability with high pain threshold
- Differential Diagnosis: Other neurologic and musculoskeletal disorders with early hypotonia (including cerebral palsy) and developmental delay
- Physical Findings
  1. Growth—short stature, failure to thrive in infancy, obesity
  2. Face—dolichocephaly, narrow bitemporal diameter, almond-shaped up-slanting palpebral fissures, strabismus, nystagmus, myopia, hyperopia, thin upper lip, small mouth with downturned corners, and viscous saliva
  3. Genitourinary (GU)—small genitalia, cryptorchidism
  4. Skin—hypopigmented, blond to brown hair, frontal hair upsweep
  5. Orthopedics—osteoporosis, kyphosis, small hands and feet, clinodactyly, narrow hands with straight ulnar border, scoliosis
  6. Neurologic—poor fine and gross motor skills, mild to moderate mental retardation, in the neonatal period there is a poor suck and swallow with feeding problems (Committee on Genetics, 2011)
- Diagnostic Tests/Findings
  1. FISH study to look at the PWS region—there are four things that can be seen: (1) In 70%, the paternally inherited chromosome 15 has microdeletions of 3-4 megabases of genetic material in the PWS region; (2) in around 20%, the child acquired two copies from the mother and none from the father: (3) in around 5%, there is a defect in the process of imprinting in when the father passes on the region he received from his mother; and (4) a balanced translocation that moves the imprinting center away from the correct region
  2. Orthopedics, dental, endocrine, ophthalmology, dietician evaluations
  3. Growth hormone deficiency frequent, but not universal
  4. Thyroid screening with TSH every 2–3 years

- Management/Treatment
  1. Behavioral therapy for control of eating and other problem behaviors
  2. Genetic counseling
  3. Early intervention and appropriate school placement with supports
  4. Psychosocial support for child and family
  5. Refer to endocrinology for evaluation and management of growth hormone deficiency
  6. Education of parents regarding need for follow-up with specialists, dietary management, the high pain tolerance, increased risk of febrile seizures (5–10%); high rates of obstructive sleep apnea, behavioral management skills, family adjustment, family planning methods as the child ages.
  7. Prader-Willi Syndrome Association: http://www.pwsausa.org/

☐ MULTISYSTEM DISORDERS

Cerebral Palsy (CP)

- Definition: A group of static disorders that affect development of motor control, posture, and balance due to a static injury to the developing fetal brain or to the infant brain. There are a range of symptoms in the child with CP. The motor disorders are often accompanied with disorders of sensation, cognition, perception, behavior, or communication with or without seizure disorder (Liptak, Murray, & Council on Children with Disabilities, 2011). Although the manifestations can change over time, the brain lesion is static; the damage that occurs to the brain is permanent, but the outcome can improve due to the plasticity of the CNS and the ability of the child to improve. The classification of the four types of CP is based on the changes in muscle tone, anatomic region of involvement, and severity of the problem—spastic (diplegia, quadriplegia, hemiplegia), dyskinetic (choreoathetoid, dystonic), hypotonic, and mixed
- Etiology/Incidence
  1. Prevalence is 3.6 per 1000 live births (Liptak et al., 2011)
  2. The etiology can be a CNS insult in the prenatal, perinatal, postnatal periods or a result of prematurity
  3. Prenatal causes include brain malformation, in utero stroke, congenital cytomegalovirus infection
  4. Perinatal causes include hypoxic ischemic encephalopathy, viral encephalitis, and meningitis
  5. Postnatal causes include accidental head trauma, anoxic insult, and child abuse
  6. High association with prematurity and very low birth weight
  7. In most preterm infants, there is usually no single factor identified as the cause, but there may be multiple risk factors
  8. There are several disorders that mimic CP, but they are progressive. These diseases include mitochondrial

disorders, leukodystrophies, lysosomal storage disease, and ataxia telangiectasia

- Signs and Symptoms
  1. The essential findings include delayed motor milestones, abnormal muscle tone, hyperreflexia, absence of regression, or evidence of a different diagnosis
  2. There may be transient abnormalities in tone and reflexes that interfere with motor progress and can be outgrown
  3. The infant may show hand preference before age 12 months, palmar thumb at 8 months, scissoring of the legs when held up under the arms, or hyperreflexia. They should not show a diurnal variation in symptoms
  4. Vision impairment (50%)
  5. Hearing impairment (10%)
  6. Seizures (30%)
  7. Cognitive impairment (50%)
  8. High risk of dental disease
  9. Higher risk of sleep disorders (23%)
- Differential Diagnosis
  1. Neurodegenerative disorders such as Duchenne muscular dystrophy
  2. Metabolic disorders, lysosomal storage diseases, ataxia telangiectasia, leukodystrophy
  3. Transient toe walking
  4. Familial spastic paraplegia
  5. Genetic disorders such as Miller-Dieker or Rett syndrome
  6. Mitochondrial disorders
  7. Spinal cord tumor/syrinx
  8. Brain tumor
  9. Hydrocephalus, dystonias
- Physical Findings
  1. Abnormal muscle tone (hypo- or hypertonia) with developmental delay
  2. Muscle weakness
  3. Loss of selective control/or persistent infant reflexes
  4. Retained primitive reflexes or pathologic reflexes
  5. Hyperactive tendon and heightened stretch reflexes; positive Babinski
  6. Restricted joint range of motion
  7. Hip click or clunk on Barlow maneuver or Ortolani test
  8. Movement-related muscle spasms with spasticity
  9. Low weight for height
  10. Neuromuscular scoliosis
  11. Visual and hearing problems
  12. Swallowing and feeding difficulty with failure to thrive
  13. Respiratory problems, including aspiration pneumonia, infections
  14. Incontinence
- Diagnostic Tests/Findings
  1. Developmental evaluation—delays in gross motor, fine motor, speech, according to type of CP and presence of mental retardation
  2. Brain MRI is recommended if there has been no perinatal imaging showing the signs of CP—90% will show

changes, including in utero strokes, major and minor brain malformations, and white matter loss, including periventricular leukomalacia (low-birth-weight infants)

- Management/Treatment
  1. Coordinate interdisciplinary management to promote optimum health and function
  2. Enroll in early intervention services—speech, OT, PT services
  3. Identify and treat associated conditions (e.g., seizures, visual impairment, hearing impairment, gastroesophageal reflux) and make appropriate referrals
  4. Prevent secondary conditions (e.g., failure to thrive, skin breakdown, dental caries)
  5. Functional therapies to build on strengths and promote compensation for physical impairments
     a. Adaptive seating
     b. Bracing
     c. Wheeled mobility
  6. Parent/family support for positive coping and stress relief—Office of Developmental Disabilities can provide respite care
  7. Spasticity relief
     a. Enteral medication—lioresal, diazepam, dantrium sodium, tizanidine hydrochloride
     b. Botulinum toxin IM to major affected muscles, or nerve block injections
     c. Intrathecal lioresal
     d. Selective dorsal root rhizotomy
  8. Support growth and nutrition, gastrostomy if needed, medication for reflux
  9. Ensure appropriate education with supportive services and therapies
  10. Oromotor therapy, including chewing, swallowing, and speech therapy
  11. Seizure prevention
  12. Orthopedist referral for corrective casting, muscle release and lengthening, split tendon transfers, osteotomies, and arthrodeses
  13. Osteoporosis can develop especially with the use of anticonvulsants, so supplements of calcium and vitamin D are needed
  14. Transitional care to adult provider when ready
  15. United Cerebral Palsy: http://www.ucp.org
  16. Support group for kids: http://www.hemikids.org
  17. National Institute for Neurological Disorders and Stroke: http://www.ninds.nih.gov/disorders/cerebral_palsy/cerebral_palsy.htm

Spina Bifida

- Definition: Congenital abnormality of the CNS or the spine resulting from failure of neural tube to close during early embryonic development; risk factors for neural tube defect include maternal folic acid deficiency, maternal use of valproic acid or carbamazepine, or maternal diabetes

- Etiology/Incidence
  1. Multifactorial inheritance pattern; environmental contribution not well understood, although addition of folic acid to dietary intake reduces occurrence probability by one-half
  2. Spina bifida occulta—incidence up to 10% of population
  3. Myelomeningocele—1:1000; decreasing, probably due to folic acid supplementation and prenatal diagnosis with selective termination (not proven)
- Signs and Symptoms
  1. Neurologic—can have hydrocephalus, Chiari malformation and hydromyelia, tethered cord
  2. Orthopedics—hip dislocation, knee contractures, spinal deformities such as kyphosis, scoliosis, fractures
  3. Urological—urinary "dribbling," unable to achieve urinary continence, frequent urinary tract infections, ureteral reflux with renal damage
  4. GI—chronic constipation, difficulty with bowel continence
  5. Motor developmental delays, especially lower extremity–related gross motor delays
  6. Latex allergies
  7. Intelligence in normal range, but with learning disorders, often with attention deficit hyperactivity disorder (ADHD)
- Differential Diagnosis: Syndromes of which spina bifida is associated, e.g., Meckel-Gruber syndrome
- Physical Findings
  1. Spina bifida occulta—usually benign; may have sacral dimple, hairy patch at base of spine, uneven gluteal folds
  2. Arnold-Chiari Type II CNS malformation (nearly 100%)—associated with progressive hydrocephalus, difficulty swallowing, hypoventilation, apnea
  3. Meningocele or myelomeningocele—signs at birth include lesion at some point along thoraco-lumbar-sacral spine, often with a cystlike structure protruding; neural elements may be apparently absent or may be easily visualized within the sac
  4. Widely spaced cranial sutures, bulging fontanel, macrocephaly (with hydrocephalus)
  5. Lack of typical lower extremity function, sometimes with orthopedic deformity (clubfoot, dislocated or subluxed hip, tibial torsion)
  6. Abnormal deep tendon reflexes in lower extremities
  7. Abnormal neonatal reflexes in lower extremities
  8. Decreased or absent anal wink
  9. Atrophied lower extremity/hip muscles
  10. Scoliosis, kyphosis
  11. Obesity in older children and adolescents (>50%)
  12. Neurogenic bowel and bladder
  13. Latex sensitivity (>40%)
- Diagnostic Tests/Findings
  1. Prenatal diagnosis possible by maternal serum screening for elevated α-fetoprotein, followed by ultrasound diagnostics for spinal anomaly and head "lemon sign"
  2. Postnatal diagnosis made on clinical basis
  3. Hydrocephalus after birth, increasing head circumference out of proportion to other growth parameters
- Management/Treatment
  1. Infants diagnosed prenatally should be referred to tertiary center with appropriate supports for birth (possible planned C-section) and immediate neonatal intensive care
  2. Refer to multidisciplinary treatment center for specialty management—assistance from orthopedist, urologist, neurosurgeon, developmental pediatrician, orthotist, physical and occupational therapists, nutritionist, advanced practice nurse, and social worker
  3. Enroll infant in early intervention program as soon as medically stable
  4. Monitor for urinary tract infections; expect less common organisms; monitor for shunt malfunction if presence of shunted hydrocephalus; baseline head CT scan; follow up if increased intracranial pressure suspected; refer to neurosurgeon for evaluation of suspected shunt malfunction or tethered cord
  5. Monitor for development of orthopedic problems, especially scoliosis and unilateral hip subluxation or dislocation; baseline and follow-up radiographic studies
  6. Monitor for skin breakdown
  7. Nutritional and behavioral intervention to prevent obesity
  8. Test for latex sensitivity (skin or RAST); latex precautions
  9. Anticipatory guidance for development, safety
  10. Psychosocial support to family and child
  11. Assistance finding least restrictive school placement and other community supports—restrict from heavy-contact sports only; otherwise full inclusion should be encouraged
  12. Genetic counseling
  13. All women of childbearing age should consume 0.8 mg folic acid daily to help prevent neural tube defects
  14. Referral to Spina Bifida Association of America (SBAA): http://www.sbaa.org/

Sudden Infant Death Syndrome (SIDS)

- Definition: The death of infants who are younger than 1 year without a physiologic cause despite a complete examination of the case, including an autopsy, examination of scene of death, and a review of the child's medical history and record (Task Force on Sudden Infant Death Syndrome, 2011). Other causes of death in infancy include ill-defined and unknown cause of mortality due to lack of thorough investigation, and accidental suffocation and strangulation in bed. The latter is due to suffocation by soft bedding, overlaying by parents, entrapment between the wall and another object, and strangulation
- Etiology/Incidence
  1. Unknown cause but felt that some deaths attributed to SIDS were related to co-sleeping

2. 2000 SIDS deaths per year with rates among non-Hispanic blacks and American Indian/Alaska Natives twice as high as among white infants (Mathews & MacDorman, 2013)
3. Peak incidence 2 to 4 months; uncommon before 2 weeks and after 6 months

- Signs and Symptoms: Infant unexpectedly found lifeless after a period of sleep
- Differential Diagnosis
  1. Meningitis
  2. Intracranial hemorrhage
  3. Myocarditis
  4. Accidental trauma
  5. Child abuse
  6. Metabolic disorder like medium-chain acyl-CoA dehydrogenase (MCAD) deficiency
- Physical Findings
  1. Full cardiorespiratory arrest
  2. Unresponsive to resuscitation
- Diagnostic Tests/Findings: Diagnosis of exclusion, with autopsy and investigation, failure to find adequate cause of death
- Management/Treatment
  1. Risk reduction
     a. Encourage prenatal care to ensure patient education
     b. Supine sleeping position, not side-lying position
     c. Avoid maternal and passive smoking
     d. Separate sleeping place for infants; do not allow sleeping on beds due to risk of entrapment and strangulation
     e. Avoid soft bedding, sheets, or blankets
     f. Maintain comfortable room temperature
     g. Avoid overheating, no heavy blankets, overbundling
     h. Consider offering a clean pacifier at nap and bedtime, but do not force it
     i. Avoid commercial devices to reduce risk of SIDS
     j. Avoid positional plagiocephaly by encouraging the mother to turn the baby's head from side to side, encouraging observed awake tummy time, and avoid excessive time in car seat carriers
     k. No bumper pads on crib slats
     l. Offer a pacifier at bedtime, but do not hang them around the infant's neck
     m. Encourage breastfeeding and avoid pacifier use in breastfed infants until 3–4 weeks of age
     n. No cardiorespiratory monitors to reduce the risk of SIDS (Task Force on Sudden Infant Death, 2011)
  2. After infant's death
     a. Maximum support to family, others
     b. Provide factual information
     c. Assist with necessary tasks
     d. Assist nursing mother with abrupt cessation of breastfeeding
  3. National SIDS Resource Center: http://www.sidscenter.org

QUESTIONS

Select the best answer.

1. Which of the following is a characteristic physical sign of fragile X syndrome in adolescent males?
   a. Small, posteriorly rotated ears
   b. Macro-orchidism
   c. Hypertonia
   d. Double hair whirl

2. Which of the following physical stigmata are common in newborns with Down syndrome?
   a. Microcephaly, flattened philtrum, downward-slanting eyes
   b. Hypotonia, large-appearing tongue and small mouth, upward slant to eyes
   c. Lymphadenopathy, coarctation of the aorta, webbed neck
   d. Funnel or pigeon-breasted chest, arachnodactyly, Brushfield spots

3. A 2-month-old infant, with a history of sacral myelomeningocele repair, has an increase in head circumference from the 75th to the 95th percentile. What is the most appropriate *first* action?
   a. Order a stat head CT scan
   b. Refer to neurosurgery for management
   c. Recheck it at the next well-child visit
   d. Recheck and replot the child's head circumference

4. A 2-week-old presents with mucopurulent eye discharge with injection and edema of the conjunctiva. The 15-year-old mother had no prenatal care. What is the most likely organism?
   a. *Staphylococcus aureus*
   b. Gonococcus
   c. *C. pneumoniae*
   d. *C. trachomatis*

5. A newborn presents with a large VSD, rocker-bottom feet, overlapping second and third fingers, and fourth and fifth fingers with hypotonia. What is the most likely diagnosis?
   a. Fragile X syndrome
   b. Down syndrome
   c. Edwards syndrome
   d. Klinefelter syndrome

6. Which of the following problems is common in a child with Hurler syndrome?
   a. Developmental delay from birth
   b. Obstructive sleep apnea
   c. Ectopic lentis
   d. Congenital heart disease

7. What is an expected finding in young infants with cerebral palsy (CP)?
   a. Voracious appetite and weight gain
   b. Hepatosplenomegaly
   c. Hypotonia in the first weeks of life
   d. Unusually severe reactions to their first immunizations

8. A mother with a newborn asks about co-sleeping. Based on the latest guidelines, what would be the most appropriate response?
   a. Do not co-sleep because you can roll over on your baby
   b. Tell me more about beliefs around co-sleeping
   c. Babies need to sleep on their back in the same room as their mother
   d. Never co-sleep with your baby

9. A mother with Marfan syndrome comes with her 5-year-old for a checkup. The child has myopia and a positive wrist and thumb sign. She reports that she was told by her last healthcare provider not to worry about this child. What is the next best step?
   a. Raise the issue of a genetic referral.
   b. Reassure her.
   c. Follow the child for further signs of Marfan syndrome.
   d. Refer to ophthalmology.

10. Which of the following is appropriate advice for the mother of a newborn?
    a. The child should sleep on her back.
    b. The child should sleep on her back or side.
    c. The child should be allowed to sleep in a car seat at night.
    d. The child can sleep on her comforter.

11. A 5-year-old female presents for a school physical with a complaint of hyperactivity, a mild developmental delay, aversion of gaze, hand mannerisms, and long, thin face with a slightly dysmorphic ear. What is the most likely diagnosis?
    a. Fragile X
    b. Turner syndrome
    c. Fetal alcohol syndrome
    d. Williams syndrome

12. A child has a negative HIV-1 and HIV-2 antibody test and a p24 antigen test that is negative. What is the next step?
    a. Do an HIV DNA PCR.
    b. Do two HIV DNA PCRs.
    c. Do RNA polymerase chain reaction assays (PCR tests).
    d. No further follow-up is needed.

13. A newborn presents with cataracts, congenital glaucoma, congenital heart disease, hepatosplenomegaly, thrombocytopenia, blueberry muffin rash, and growth retardation. What is the most likely diagnosis?
    a. Cytomegalovirus
    b. Toxoplasmosis
    c. Rubella syndrome
    d. Syphilis

14. A well-appearing, well-dressed 11-month-old has a long philtrum, midface hypoplasia, microcephaly, developmental delay, and myopia. The mother denies drinking alcohol during the pregnancy. What is the next best step?

a. Refer the mother and child to child protective services.
b. Refer the child to early intervention.
c. Refer the child to cardiology.
d. Refer the mother to Alcoholics Anonymous.

15. An 18-month-old child exposed to HIV in utero had negative HIV DNA at 2 weeks and 8 weeks. What is indicated at the 18-month visit?
    a. No further testing is needed.
    b. HIV DNA should be repeated.
    c. Enzyme immunoassay for antibody to HIV-1 should be performed.
    d. CBC with differential and immunoglobulins is needed.

16. A newborn fails his newborn hearing test. Because the mother is an adolescent and there is evidence of the presence of intrauterine growth restriction, jaundice, and mild hepatomegaly, you suspect cytomegalovirus (CMV). What is the best way to establish the diagnosis of congenital CMV?
    a. CMV-specific IgM
    b. Isolation of CMV from infant urine, pharynx, or peripheral blood leukocytes within first 3 weeks of life
    c. Enzyme-linked immunosorbent assays (ELISA)
    d. CMV antigenemia

17. A baby is born to a mother with chronic hepatitis B. What is the best treatment approach?
    a. Administer interferon within 24 hours.
    b. Administer hepatitis B vaccine within 24 hours.
    c. Administer interferon and nucleotide in combination daily.
    d. Administer HBIG and hepatitis B vaccine within 12 hours.

18. A 2-year-old female has lymphedema of the hands and feet, with low posterior hairline, cubitus valgus, and a history of intrauterine growth restriction. Which of the following defects is the most common among the children with these signs?
    a. Supravalvular aortic valve stenosis
    b. Mitral valve prolapse
    c. Dissecting aortic arch
    d. Coarctation of the aorta

19. Joshua is the 9-month-old son of parents of Louisiana-French descent. The child stopped rolling over. Mother reports he is increasingly irritable. Which of the following physical exam findings is most consistent with Tay-Sachs disease?
    a. Cardiomyopathy
    b. Retinal detachment
    c. "Cherry-red" spot on retina
    d. Hyporeflexia

20. What is the hallmark of Prader-Willi syndrome in infancy?
    a. Failure to thrive
    b. 100% detection rate with chromosome analysis for a 15q deletion

c. Emergence of spasticity during toddler years

d. Voracious appetite and development of obesity

21. A 15-day-old infant with respiratory distress arrives in the ED. The exam reveals mild cyanosis, hepatosplenomegaly, and features consistent with Down syndrome. Which of the following is the most likely diagnosis?
    a. Complete AV canal (endocardial cushion defect)
    b. Patent ductus arteriosus
    c. Atrial septal defect
    d. Ventricular septal defect

22. A newborn presents with lymphadenopathy, a decrease in the ability to move the left leg, Coombs-negative hemolytic anemia, hepatomegaly, and snuffles. What is the most likely diagnosis?
    a. Congenital herpes infections
    b. Congenital cytomegalovirus (CMV) infection
    c. Congenital syphilis
    d. Congenital gonococcal infection

23. To which of the following substances is a child with spina bifida likely to be allergic?
    a. Eggs
    b. Pollens
    c. Latex
    d. Dust mite feces

24. What is the preferred treatment of choice for syphilis?
    a. Erythromycin
    b. Penicillin
    c. Cefotaxime
    d. Zithromax

25. Which of the following is consistent with neonatal disseminated herpes disease?
    a. Hyperactive newborn with apparent spasticity
    b. Multiple papules scattered over the body
    c. Fever, grouped vesicles on the skin
    d. Purpuric rash over the body

26. A 2-month-old child presents after an episode of sepsis for a follow-up visit. He has gained 2 pounds since birth and has a decrease in head circumference from the 50th to the 25th percentile. In addition, he has inguinal and axillary adenopathy of 1 cm and has hepatomegaly. Which of the following is included in the infectious disease differential?
    a. Herpes simplex type 2 infection
    b. Human immunodeficiency virus infection
    c. Chlamydia infection
    d. Congenital gonorrhea

27. Which of the following is the most helpful in confirming a diagnosis of *Chlamydia pneumoniae* in a 1-month-old child with a cough?
    a. Chest x-ray showing lobar consolidation
    b. Decrease serum immunoglobulins
    c. Lymphocytosis
    d. Mother with no prenatal care

28. A social worker brings a child in prior to placement with a chief complaint of copious vaginal discharge. A culture is positive for *Chlamydia*. From the social perspective, what is the next best step?
    a. Reassure the social worker that this is a prenatal transmission.
    b. Tell the social worker the result and allow her to decide the next step.
    c. Tell the social worker the result and inform her of the likelihood of sexual abuse.
    d. Call the foster family with the result.

29. Which of the following is a nontreponemal test for syphilis?
    a. Venereal Disease Research Laboratory (VDRL) microscopic slide test
    b. Fluorescent treponemal antibody absorbed (FTA-ABS)
    c. *Treponema pallidum* particle agglutination (TP-PA)
    d. TORCH titer

30. Which anticipatory guidance would be helpful in decreasing the risk of toxoplasmosis?
    a. When camping, treat water from streams with iodine.
    b. Do not go barefoot in high-risk areas.
    c. Wash hands after changing cat litter.
    d. Avoid handling contaminated diapers.

31. What would you expect to find in a child with congenital toxoplasmosis?
    a. Jaundice
    b. Microcephaly
    c. Cerebral calcifications
    d. Congenital heart disease

32. What congenital infection can present with snuffles, lymphadenopathy, pseudoparalysis of Parrot, CNS abnormalities, and low birth weight?
    a. Cytomegalovirus
    b. Rubella
    c. Toxoplasmosis
    d. Syphilis

33. A child presents with chorioretinitis, intracranial calcification, and hydrocephalus. What is the most likely diagnosis?
    a. Congenital toxoplasmosis
    b. Congenital syphilis
    c. Fetal alcohol syndrome
    d. Edwards syndrome

34. Which of the following screenings is done annually after 1 year of age in a child with Down syndrome?
    a. Cervical spine
    b. Urinalysis
    c. Celiac screening
    d. Thyroid screening

35. A 6-year-old child has increased reflexes, toe walking, and a clumsy gait. Which of the following diagnostic tests would be helpful in making a diagnosis of cerebral palsy?
    a. Skull x-ray
    b. Computerized tomography of the head

c. Magnetic resonance imaging of the head

d. Magnetic resonance imaging of the lumbosacral spine

36. What hormone must be replaced in adolescents with Klinefelter syndrome?

a. Thyroid hormone

b. Growth hormone

c. Estrogen

d. Testosterone

37. A 9-month-old child of Jewish parents presents with increasing irritability and noise sensitivity. What is the next best step?

a. Encourage the mother to decrease environmental stimuli.

b. Refer to a pediatric neurologist.

c. Refer for further developmental screening.

d. Reevaluate at the 12-month examination.

38. A newborn presents with microcephaly, low-set ears, prominent occiput, micrognathia, heart murmur, and clenched hands with overriding fingers and crossed thumb. What is best diagnostic test?

a. Karyotype

b. Amino acid urine screen

c. Newborn screening

d. Methylation test

39. A 2.5-year-old child presents with a macrocephaly, developmental delay, coarse facial features, large tongue, kyphosis, hip dislocation, tonsillar and adenoidal hypertrophy, and hepatomegaly. She is receiving early intervention services without improvement. What is the next best step?

a. Referral to genetics for further evaluation

b. Follow up in 3 months

c. Reassure the parents

d. Follow up in 6 months

☐ ANSWERS AND RATIONALES

1. B: Macro-orchidism occurs in patients with fragile X in adolescence rather than during infancy and early childhood. A double hair whirl is not significant for fragile X. Hypotonia rather than hypertonia is found in fragile X. Large, not small, ears are characteristic of fragile X.

2. B: Microcephaly, flattened philtrum, and downward-slanting eyes are related to fetal alcohol spectrum disorder, and hypotonia, large-appearing tongue and small mouth, and upward slant to eyes points to Turner syndrome. Funnel or pigeon-breasted chest, arachnodactyly, and Brushfield spots represent a combination of syndromes, with the first two signs being signs of Marfan syndrome and Brushfield spots found in Down syndrome.

3. D: Although the child with a sacral myelomeningocele is at risk for hydrocephalus, careful reexamination of the head circumference should be done before ordering a stat head CT or a neurosurgical evaluation. It

would be more appropriate to start with a head ultrasound if the head circumference is abnormal to avoid exposure to radiation. "Image gently" is a warning to all providers to avoid radiation to avoid increasing a child's risk of cancer due to exposure to radiation.

4. D: This question is designed to review the fact that *Chlamydia trachomatis* is the number one cause of sexually transmitted disease in adolescents. In this case, due to lack of prenatal care, the adolescent did not receive a screen for chlamydia and therefore was at risk for passing this on to the newborn. *C. pneumoniae* is an organism that affects the respiratory tract in school-aged children and adolescents. *S. aureus* and *N. gonorrhoeae* are possible pathogens but less likely than *Chlamydia*.

5. C: The description gives the classic signs of Edwards syndrome, or trisomy 18. In Down syndrome, overlapping fingers and rocker-bottom feet are not found, and although hypotonia is common, the rest of the features are not pathognomonic. In Klinefelter syndrome, there is micropenis in early childhood, and later features include small testicles with gynecomastia. In fragile X, large ears and long face with significant developmental delay are characteristic.

6. B: The newborn with Hurler syndrome may not show any specific signs in infancy. The development of obstructive sleep apnea is very common in this disease due to tonsillar hypertrophy resulting from accumulation of partially degraded glycosaminoglycan (GAG). In severe mucopolysaccharidosis, the diagnosis is usually not made until the 2nd year of life. Developmental delays from birth can be seen with several genetic disorders and neuromuscular disease such as spinal muscular atrophy, type 1. Congenital heart disease (CHD) is common with a variety of genetic disorder and congenital infections. Gene deletions are chromosome 22 may be involved in isolated CHD.

7. C: The finding of hypotonia is a common presentation in young infants with CP. The finding of hepatosplenomegaly points to a metabolic disorder or neonatal infections. A voracious appetite may be present, but weight gain may be slow due to increased calorie needs. There is no association with immunization reactions and a static disorder like CP.

8. B: You need to explore this issue with the parent so that she can partner with you in deciding that this may not be the best idea. Although co-sleeping can lead to infant death due to rollover accidents, as PNPs we need to understand that this practice is steeped in tradition. It would be important to work with the family's cultural beliefs.

9. A: Exploration of the issues of a genetic referral would be important to help this mother to decide what she wants to do. While the child may need an ophthalmology evaluation due to myopia and possible Marfan syndrome, she needs to have other evaluations, including cardiology referral. It would be better to

start with the referral that would give the mother a broader view of the problem. False reassurance is not helpful.

10. A: The new American Academy of Pediatricians (AAP) guidelines published in 2011 were clear that side-lying positioning, comforters or soft bedding, as well as car seats were not appropriate for babies to sleep. The only answer that is completely correct is that the child should sleep on her back.

11. A: The symptoms and signs of fragile X are outlined in this question. Turner syndrome presents with delay in the onset of puberty, short stature, webbed neck, and coarctation of the aorta. Children with Williams syndrome have supravalvular aortic stenosis, cheerful affect, typical "elfin" faces, and developmental delay. The facial characteristics of fetal alcohol syndrome include a thin upper lip, short palpebral fissures and flattened philtrum, CNS dysfunction, and growth retardation.

12. D: This child needs no further follow-up and does not need any further tests.

13. C: Rubella syndrome is most likely to present with eye findings, blueberry muffin rash, growth retardation, and hepatosplenomegaly. Syphilis is characterized by lymphadenopathy, bone lesions, and snuffles.

14. B: No matter what the reason, a child with a developmental delay needs a referral to early intervention to help improve developmental outcomes. Although the child may benefit from a referral to neurology, there is no cardiac signs of disease, and the child does not need to go to cardiology. The presenting signs and symptoms can go with other genetic disorders, and it would be important to consider referral to genetics.

15. B: An HIV DNA should be done to confirm after 4 months that the child does not have HIV.

16. B: The isolation of CMV from the infant's body secretions is the best way to confirm the diagnosis of CMV. CMV-specific IgM or CMV antigenemia are typically used after the newborn period. ELISA is not available for testing for CMV.

17. D: The best treatment approach is to use both hepatitis-B-specific immunoglobin and hepatitis B vaccine. Interferon is used in the treatment and is used in combination with a nucleotide. Hepatitis B vaccine is needed, but the baby needs a booster to help fight the infection.

18. D: Coarctation of the aorta is the most common cardiac defect seen in this Turner's syndrome. A dissecting aortic arch and a mitral valve prolapse would be characteristic of Marfan syndrome. Children with Williams syndrome have supravalvular aortic stenosis.

19. C: A cherry-red spot on the retina is the hallmark of Tay-Sachs disease in a child with developmental regression. Cardiomyopathy can be found in Duchenne muscular dystrophy as well as mucopolysaccharidosis. Hyperreflexia would be more common in children with increased tone.

20. A: Although a voracious appetite with obesity is the hallmark of children with Prader-Willi syndrome, in infancy these children have hypotonia and feeding difficulties with failure to thrive. The detection rate for the deletion is not 100%.

21. A: The following congenital cardiac lesions are acyanotic—patent ductus arteriosus, atrial septal defect, and ventricular septal defect. This patient is cyanotic.

22. C: Congenital syphilis presents with snuffles, lymphadenopathy, Coombs-negative hemolytic anemia, and pseudoparalysis of Parrot. CMV is usually an asymptomatic infection, and when it is symptomatic in the newborn, the presentation would include intrauterine growth restriction, developmental delay, jaundice, hepatosplenomegaly, purpura, generalized petechiae, thrombocytopenia, and bone abnormalities. Congenital gonococcal infection would usually present with a severe conjunctivitis as the presenting complaint.

23. C: Latex is the most common allergy in patients with spinal bifida as a result of the high number of medical procedures and exposure to latex in a hospital setting. It is important to recognize that children with latex allergy may be allergic to foods, including avocado, kiwi, banana, chestnut (high risk) and apple, carrot, celery, melons, papaya, potato, and tomato (medium risk). There are other fruits that carry a low risk of crossover, and therefore the latex–fruit allergic association does exist.

24. B: Penicillin is the drug of choice for syphilis.

25. C: Grouped vesicles is the hallmark of herpes simplex. Papular lesions are not usually due to herpes simplex virus, and a purpuric rash would point to meningococcemia.

26. B: Human immunodeficiency virus can present with lymphadenopathy, poor weight gain, decreased head circumference, and serious bacterial infections.

27. D: A chest x-ray of a child will show hyperinflation rather than lobar infiltrates. The child with chlamydia will have elevated immunoglobulins and peripheral eosinophilia. The lack of prenatal care is a risk factor for chlamydia pneumonitis.

28. C: The child with an active chlamydia infection after age 18 months is a victim of childhood sexual assault. This infection needs to be treated, but the social worker needs to be aware of the implication of a positive result.

29. A: There are nontreponemal tests such as Venereal Disease Research Laboratory (VDRL) microscopic slide test and rapid plasma reagin (RPR), which are initial screening tests. Usually, a nontreponemal test is performed first, and if it is reactive, then a treponemal test is done. The fluorescent treponemal antibody absorbed is the treponemal test most used to confirm a positive RPR. The FTA-ABS remains positive and becomes reactive earlier. Since it remains positive after treatment, the test does not indicate current disease

state or the need for treatment. The other treponemal test used to confirm a nontreponemal test is a *Treponema pallidum* particle agglutination (TP-PA).

30. C: Transmission of toxoplasmosis occurs through handling of cat feces. Pregnant women should avoid contact with cat litter, and others should wash hands thoroughly when handling cat litter.

31. B: Newborns with congenital toxoplasmosis will have cerebral calcifications.

32. D: The classic presentation of congenitally acquired syphilis includes low birth weight/prematurity; rhinitis (snuffles); mucous patches; jaundice with elevated liver enzymes; lymphadenopathy with Coombs-negative hemolytic anemia; osteochondritis, which causes resistance to movement (pseudoparalysis of Parrot); CNS abnormalities; and a rash similar to secondary syphilis with desquamation of hands and feet (AAP, 2012). The presentation of toxoplasmosis includes microcephaly, seizures, maculopapular rash, hepatosplenomegaly, and jaundice.

33. C: Chorioretinitis, intracranial calcification, and hydrocephalus are the classic triad of congenital toxoplasmosis and are found in less than 10%. The physical findings of fetal alcohol syndrome involve classic facial features, growth retardation, and CNS abnormality.

34. D: Children with Down syndrome are at greater risk for thyroid disease and leukemia. The guidelines from the American Academy of Pediatrics (2011) recommend a thyroid screening yearly by objective laboratory testing at birth, at 6 months, and yearly thereafter. Atlantoaxial dislocation can be screened for at 3 years of age. Celiac disease can be found in up to 5% to 12% of patients affected by Down syndrome.

35. C: MRI of the brain is the most helpful in children with suspected cerebral palsy, and about 90% will show some abnormalities, including major and minor brain malformation, strokes, and white matter loss.

36. D: Males with Klinefelter syndrome need testosterone as a result of inadequate virilization. The thyroid is not usually affected.

37. B: Tay-Sachs disease is seen in families of Ashkenazi Jewish descent and is characterized by degenerative CNS signs and hyperreaction to noise. A consultation with the pediatric neurologist is indicated because of the possibility of Tay-Sachs disease.

38. A: Individuals with Edwards syndrome have trisomy of chromosome 18, which can be evaluated with a karyotype. A newborn screening screens for biochemical, hemoglobin, thyroid, and metabolic disorders. Amino acid screening specifically evaluates for amino acid deficiencies or excesses but would not be helpful in this case. In doing methylation tests, there is polymerase chain reaction (PCR) amplification of individual DNA fragments. These tests are done to rule out such genetic disorders as Prader-Willi syndrome and Angelman syndrome.

39. A: This child has many of the signs of Hurler's syndrome. Given the lack of progress in early intervention and the physical assessment findings, a referral to genetics would be the best approach in this child.

☐ BIBLIOGRAPHY

American Academy of Pediatrics. (2012). *Red book: 2012 report of the committee on infectious diseases* (28th ed.). Elk Grove Village, IL: Author.

Barry, M. A., Weatherhead, J. E., Hotez, P., & Woc-Colburn, L. (2013). Childhood parasitic infections endemic to the United States. *Pediatric Clinics of North America, 60,* 471–485.

Bondy, C., for the Turner Syndrome Consensus Study Group. (2007). Clinical Practice Guidelines: Care of girls and women with Turner syndrome: A guideline of the Turner Syndrome Study Group. *Journal of Clinical Endocrinology and Metabolism, 92*(1), 10–25.

Boss, R. D., Holmes, K. W., Althaus, J., Rushton, C., McNee, H., & McNee, T. (2013). Trisomy 18 and complex congenital heart disease; seeking the threshold benefit. *Pediatrics, 132,* 161–165.

Branson, B. M., Owen, S. M., Wesolowski, L. G., Bennett, B., Werner, B. G., Wroblewski, K. E., & Pentella, M. A. (2014, June 27). *Laboratory Testing for the Diagnosis of HIV Infections: Updated Recommendations.* Retrieved from http://www.cdc.gov/hiv/pdf/HIVtestingAlgorithm Recommendation-Final.pdf

Bull, M., & American Academy of Pediatrics. (2011). Health supervision for children with Down syndrome. *Pediatrics, 128*(2), 393–406. Retrieved from http://aappolicy.aappublications.org

Committee on Genetics. (2011). Health supervision for children with Prader-Willi syndrome. *Pediatrics, 127,* 195–204.

Davidson, M. (2008) Primary care for children and adolescents with Down syndrome. *Pediatric Clinics of North America. 55*(5), 1099–1111.

Dorrie, N., Föcker, M., Freunscht, I., & Hebebrand, J. (2014). Fetal alcohol disorders. *European Child & Adolescent Psychiatry, 23*(10), 863–875. doi:10.1007/s00787-014-0571-6

Eckerle, J. K., Howard, C., & John, C. C. (2013). Infections in internationally adopted children. *Pediatric Clinics of North America, 60,* 487–505.

Groth, K. A., Skakkebaek, A., Host, C., Gravholt, C. H., & Boiesen, A. (2013). Clinical review: Klinefelter syndrome—a clinical update. *Journal of Clinical Endocrinology and Metabolism, 98*(1), 20–30. doi:10.1210/jc.2012-2382

Hersh, J. H., Saul, R. A., & Committee on Genetics. (2011). Health supervision for children with fragile X syndrome. *Pediatrics, 127,* 994–1006.

Hobson-Rohrer, W. L., & Samson-Fang, L. (2013). Down syndrome. *Pediatrics in Review, 34,* 573. doi:10.1542/pir.34-12-573

Krishnamoorthy, K. S., Eichler, F., Rapalino, O., &. Frosch, M. P. (2014). Case 14-2014: An 11-month-old girl with developmental delay. *New England Journal of Medicine, 370*, 1830–1841. doi:10.1056/NEJMcpc1305987

Liptak, G., Murphy, N., & Council on Children with Disabilities. (2011). Providing a primary care medical home for children and youth with cerebral palsy. *Pediatrics, 128*, e1321–1329.

Mathews, T. J., & MacDorman, M. F. (2013). Infant mortality statistics from the 2009 period linked birth/infant death data set. *National Vital Statistics Reports, 61*(8).

McLean, H. Q., Fiebelkorn, A. P., Temte, J. L., & Wallace, G. S. (2013, June 14). Prevention of measles, rubella, congenital rubella syndrome, and mumps, 2013: summary recommendations of the Advisory Committee on Immunization Practices (ACIP) recommendations and reports. *Morbidity and Mortality Weekly Reports, 62*(RR04),1–34.

Milbrant, T., & Thomas, E. (2013). Turner's syndrome. *Pediatrics in Review, 34*, 420–423. doi:10.1542/pir.34-9-420

Muenzer, J. (2011). Overview of mucopolysaccharidoses. *Rheumatology, 50*, V4–V12.

National Association of Pediatric Nurse Practitioners. (2009). NAPNAP position statement on pediatric health care/medical home: Key issues on delivery, reimbursement, and leadership. *Journal of Pediatric Health Care, 23*, 23a–24a.

Panel on Antiretroviral Therapy and Medical Management of HIV-Infected Children. (2014). *Guidelines for the Use of Antiretroviral Agents in Pediatric HIV Infection.* Retrieved from https://aidsinfo.nih.gov/contentfiles/lvguidelines/PediatricGuidelines.pdf

Panel on Opportunistic Infections in HIV-Exposed and HIV-Infected Children. (2013). Guidelines for the prevention and treatment of opportunistic infections in HIV-exposed and HIV-infected children. Washington, DC: U.S. Department of Health and Human Services. Retrieved from http://www.guideline.gov/content.aspx?id=47539

Panel on Opportunistic Infections in HIV-Infected Adults and Adolescents. (2015). Guidelines for the Prevention and Treatment of Opportunistic Infections in HIV-Infected Adults and Adolescents. Retrieved from https://aidsinfo.nih.gov/contentfiles/lvguidelines/adult_oi.pdf

Panel on Treatment of HIV-Infected Pregnant Women and Prevention of Perinatal Transmission. (2014). *Recommendations for Use of Antiretroviral drugs in Pregnancy HIV-1-Infected Women for Maternal Health and Interventions to Reduce Perinatal HIV Transmission in the United States.* Retrieved from https://aidsinfo.nih.gov/contentfiles/lvguidelines/PerinatalGL.pdf

Patton, M. E., Su, J. R., Nelson, R., & Weinstock, H. (2014, May 9). Primary and secondary syphilis—United States, 2005–2013. *Morbidity and Mortality Weekly Report, 63*(18), 402–406.

Pinninti, S. G., & Kimberlin, D. W. (2013). Neonatal herpes simplex virus infections. *Pediatric Clinics of North America, 60*,351–366.

Sakzewski, L., Ziviani, J., & Boyd R. N. (2014). Efficacy of upper limb therapies for unilateral cerebral palsy: A meta-analysis. *Pediatrics, 133*, e175–204.

Seetoo, K., Carlos, M. P., Blythe, D., Trivedi, L., Myers, R,. England, T., Agee, C. . . . Grant, Y. (2013, March 29). Three cases of congenital rubella syndrome in the postelimination era—Maryland, Alabama, and Illinois, 2012. *Morbidity and Mortality Weekly Report, 62*(12), 226–229.

Silberry, G. K. (2014). Preventing and managing HIV infection in infants, children, and adolescents in the United States. *Pediatrics in Review, 35*, 268–286.

Siqueira, L. M. (2014). Chlamydia in children and adolescents. *Pediatrics in Review, 35*, 145–157.

Smith, D., Martin, M., Lansky, A., Mermin, J., & Choopanya, K. (2013, June 14). Update to interim guidance for pre-exposure prophylaxis (PrEP) for the prevention of HIV infection: PrEP for injecting drug users. *Morbidity and Mortality Weekly Report, 62*(23), 463–466.

Swanson, E., & Schleiss, M. (2013). Congenital cytomegalovirus infection: New prospects for prevention and therapy. *Pediatrics Clinics of North America, 60*, 335–350.

Task Force on Sudden Infant Death Syndrome. (2011). SIDS and other sleep-related infant deaths: Expansion of recommendations for a safe infant sleeping environment. *Pediatrics, 128*, 1030–1039.

Tinkle, B., Saal., H. M., & American Academy of Pediatrics, Committee on Genetics. (2013). Health supervision for the child with Marfan syndrome. *Pediatrics, 132*, e1059–1072.

Advanced Practice, Role Development, Current Trends, and Health Policy

Janet S. Selway

CHAPTER 16

☐ INTRODUCTION

Advanced practice registered nurses (APRNs) must remain informed regarding role development, current issues and trends related to their practice, and changes in healthcare policy, as each has an impact on the evolving practice environment. In July, 2008, the National Council of State Boards of Nursing (NCSBN) APRN Committee, and the Advanced Practice Nursing Consensus Work Group completed a regulatory model for the future regulation of Advanced Practice Nursing. This document delineates the definition of an APRN based on seven characteristics.

☐ ADVANCED PRACTICE NURSING

1. Definition of Advanced Practice Registered Nurse (APRN): According to the Consensus Model for APRN Regulation (APRN Consensus),

    The definition of an APRN is a nurse:

    a. who has completed an accredited graduate-level education program preparing him/her for one of the four recognized APRN roles;

    b. who has passed a national certification examination that measures APRN, role and population-focused competencies and who maintains continued competence as evidenced by recertification in the role and population through the national certification program;

    c. who has acquired advanced clinical knowledge and skills preparing him/her to provide direct care to patients, as well as a component of indirect care; however, the defining factor for all APRNs is that a significant component

of the education and practice focuses on direct care of individuals;

    d. whose practice builds on the competencies of registered nurses (RNs) by demonstrating a greater depth and breadth of knowledge, a greater synthesis of data, increased complexity of skills and interventions, and greater role autonomy;

    e. who is educationally prepared to assume responsibility and accountability for health promotion and/or maintenance as well as the assessment, diagnosis, and management of patient problems, which includes the use and prescription of pharmacologic and non-pharmacologic interventions;

    f. who has clinical experience of sufficient depth and breadth to reflect the intended license; and

    g. who has obtained a license to practice as an APRN in one of the four APRN roles: certified registered nurse anesthetist (CRNA), certified nurse-midwife (CNM), clinical nurse specialist (CNS), or certified nurse practitioner. (p. 6) Reproduced from National Council of State Boards of Nursing, 2008.

2. APRNs are educated in one of the four roles and in at least one of six population foci: family/individual across the life span, adult-gerontology, pediatrics, neonatal, women's health/gender-related, or psych/mental health.

3. Many nurses with advanced graduate nursing preparation practice in roles and specialties that do not focus on direct care to individuals, and, therefore, their practice does not require regulatory recognition beyond the Registered Nurse license granted by state boards of

nursing. These other advanced, graduate nursing roles are not APRN roles (APRN Consensus, 2008).

4. The National Association of Pediatric Nurse Practitioners (NAPNAP) (formerly known as the National Association of Pediatric Nurse Associates and Practitioners) endorsed the July 2008 Consensus Model for APRN Regulation. According to the Consensus Model, a nurse practitioner should have education in the role of nurse practitioner and one or more population foci, including pediatrics as a distinct population focus.

5. In 2013, NAPNAP released its position statement on the Doctorate of Nursing Practice (DNP), endorsing the DNP as the appropriate credential and level of education for advanced practice nursing. This document replaced the NAPNAP 2008 position statement on the DNP.

Role Development

- First NP program established in 1964 prepared pediatric nurse practitioners (PNPs) through collaborative efforts of Loretta C. Ford, EdD, RN, and Henry K. Silver, MD, at the University of Colorado
  1. PNP role development provided a model for other emerging nurse practitioner (NP) specialties
  2. Original support of PNP role as "physician extender" to improve access concerns due to shortage of primary care providers
  3. Most early PNP education occurred within certificate and/or continuing education programs; e.g., Colorado program included 4 months didactic study followed by 18 months clinical practicum training
  4. Early research focused on quality of care, cost-effectiveness, productivity, clinical decision-making skills, and role satisfaction of the PNP
  5. National Association of Pediatric Nurse Practitioners organized in 1973 to establish PNP practice guidelines
  6. Early resistance to NP role as too much of a "medical model" from mainstream graduate nursing education, contrasted with the "nursing model" of Clinical Nurse Specialist (CNS) role development
  7. From 1980 to 1989 more physicians resulted in less need for nurse practitioners (NPs)
  8. From 1990 to 1998 increased emphasis on primary care resulted in decreased need for specialty care; NP seen as viable, cost-effective member of healthcare delivery team
  9. The role of the PNP continues to expand, and now involves secondary and tertiary care. PNPs now practice in a variety of settings

Advanced Practice Trends and Issues

1. Consensus Model for Regulation of Advanced Practice Nursing endorsed by 48 nursing entities in 2008. The model defines the APRN as an "independent practitioner" and says APRNs should be licensed with no regulatory requirements for collaboration, direction or supervision.

2. Robert Wood Johnson Foundation (RWJF) Institute of Medicine (IOM) report *The Future of Nursing: Leading Change, Advancing Health* was published in 2010. The purpose of this 2-year initiative of the RWJF and the IOM was to establish a report that would provide an action-oriented blueprint for the future of nursing. The Consensus Model for Regulation of Advanced Practice Nursing is Appendix D of the *Future of Nursing* report. The four major messages of this landmark report are:
   a. Nurses should practice to the full extent of their education and training.
   b. Nurses should achieve higher levels of education and training through an improved education system that promotes seamless academic progression.
   c. Nurses should be full partners, with physicians and other healthcare professionals, in redesigning health care in the United States.
   d. Effective workforce planning and policy require better data collection and an improved information infrastructure.

- Standards and Scope of Practice
  1. Standards of practice
     a. Described by the American Nurses Association (American Nurses Association [ANA], 2010) as authoritative statements by which to measure quality of practice, service, or education
     b. Establishes minimum levels of acceptable performance
     c. Provides consumer with means to measure quality of care received
     d. Both generic and specific specialty standards exist
     e. Specialty groups have also developed standards, including National Association of Pediatric Nurse Practitioners (NAPNAP) and Association for Women's Health, Obstetric, and Neonatal Nurses (AWHONN) (formerly NAACOG)
     f. PNP-relevant standards of practice
        (1) American Nurses Association Maternal-Child Health (MCH) Standards—first published in 1983
        (2) NAPNAP Standards—first published in 1987, most recently updated 2004
        (3) AWHONN Standards
     g. Can be used to provide legal expectations of practice, but were not designed to define standards of practice for clinical or legal purposes
  2. Scope of practice
     a. Based on what is legally allowable in each state under its Nurse Practice Act
     b. Provides guidelines vs. specific mandates for nursing practice
     c. Is not mandated
     d. Varies widely from state to state and over time
     e. Often based on legal requirements within state and national standards

f. NAPNAP first published Scope of Practice for PNPs in 1983 with updated statements published in 1990, 2000, and 2004

g. *Chart Overview of Nurse Practitioner Scopes of Practice in the United States* (Christian, Dower, & O'Neill, 2007)

3. Prescriptive authority

   a. Physician signature on prescriptions written by NP is *not* required in any state

   b. Controlled substance prescriptions must include the NP's name and Drug Enforcement Administration (DEA) number

   c. As of 1998, all states have approved and/or implemented some degree of prescriptive authority

   d. Required pharmacology education within graduate program and continuing education to maintain authority—specific requirements vary by state

   e. Scope of prescriptive authority varies by state; full scope includes ability to obtain federal DEA registration number

   f. The APRN Consensus Model says that all APRNs should have prescriptive authority

4. NAPNAP Position Statement on Nurse Practitioner Prescriptive Privileges, 2010, https://www.napnap.org/napnap-position-statements-0. NAPNAP advocates for:

   a. Full prescriptive authority as appropriate

   b. NP authority to prescribe all medical devices, i.e., durable medical equipment

   c. NP prescriber name displayed on prescription pads, dispenser bottle labels

   d. Implementation of e-prescribing

   e. Diagnosis, treatment, prescriptive authority clearly stated in state Nurse Practice Act

   f. Provider-inclusive language in all legislation affecting health care of children

   g. All NPs obtain National Provider Identification (NPI) number, DEA number, and state controlled substances license

   h. Routine continuing education in pharmacology

5. Nurse practice acts

   a. Authorizes Boards of Nursing in each state to establish statutory authority for licensure of registered nurse (RN)

   b. Authority includes use of title, authorization for scope of practice, and disciplinary grounds

   c. Evolves from statutory law, which, after interpretation, becomes regulatory language

6. Clinical practice guidelines or protocols

   a. Definition: "Systematically developed statements to assist practitioner and patient about appropriate care for specific clinical outcomes" (Institute of Medicine [IOM], 1990)

   b. Need/requirements for guidelines/protocol development

      (1) The PNP uses a framework for clinical practice that incorporates both scientific and theoretical bases

(2) The scope of healthcare services and standards of practice provided by PNPs are affected by state Nurse Practice Acts, licensure and regulatory mechanisms, work setting privileges, and/or credentialing and collaborative agreements where necessary (NAPNAP, 2004)

(3) Variable requirements depending on individual state Nurse Practice Act and standards of practice

(4) Protocol requirements may be met with recognized reference books and published clinical guidelines

c. Examples of pediatric-related practice guidelines for preventive care

   (1) Bright Futures (Maternal and Child Health Bureau [MCHB])

   (2) Guidelines for Adolescent Preventive Services (American medical Association [AMA])

   (3) Guide to Clinical Preventive Services

d. Examples of pediatric-related practice guidelines for illness management

   (1) Asthma (National Institutes of health [NIH], American Academy of Pediatrics [AAP])

   (2) Hearing screening (NIH, AAP)

   (3) HIV (Agency for Healthcare Research and Quality [AHRQ], formerly Agency for Health Care Policy and Research [AHCPR])

   (4) Otitis media with effusion (AHRQ)

   (5) Pain (AHRQ)

   (6) Sickle cell disease (AHRQ)

Regulation of Advanced Nursing Practice

1. APRN regulatory model

   a. The Consensus Model for Future Regulation of APRN Practice (APRN Joint Dialogue Group Report, 2008) describes the APRN regulatory model as including four essential components: licensure, accreditation, certification, and education (LACE)

   b. "LACE" is proposed as a communication network including the organizations that represent the four components of APRN regulation: licensure, accreditation, certification, and education. Past tension between certification bodies, state Boards of Nursing, and nursing education accrediting organizations regarding role and responsibility for credentialing is being addressed by the development of a mechanism called LACE that enhances the communication and transparency among APRN licensure, accreditation, certification, and education bodies

2. Credentialing—regulatory mechanism(s) to ensure accountability for competent practice

   a. Mandates accountability/responsibility for competent practice

   b. Validation of required education, licensure, and certification

   c. Necessary to assure public of safe health care provided by qualified individuals
   d. Necessary to ensure compliance with federal and state laws related to nursing practice
   e. Acknowledges APRN advanced scope of practice
   f. Should provide appropriate avenues for public or individual practice complaints
   g. Allows profession to be accountable to public and its members by enforcing professional standards for practice
3. Clinical privileges
   a. In 1983, possibility of hospital staff membership opened to nonphysician providers by Joint Commission on Accreditation of Health Care Organizations (JCAHO; now The Joint Commission)
   b. Current issue for APRN practice
4. Licensure: Defined in the APRN Consensus Model as "the granting of authority to practice" (APRN Consensus Workgroup & the NCSBN APRN Advisory Committee, 2008, p. 7). Licensure occurs at the role and population focus level, not at the specialty level
   a. Licensure is also defined as "the process by which boards of nursing grant permission to an individual to engage in nursing practice after determining that the applicant has attained the competency necessary to perform a unique scope of practice" (National Council of State Boards of Nursing [NCSBN], 2015)
   b. "The licensing title Advanced Practice Registered Nurse is the title to be used for the subset of nurses prepared with advanced, graduate-level nursing knowledge to provide direct patient care in four roles: certified registered nurse anesthetist, certified nurse-midwife, clinical nurse specialist, and certified nurse practitioner" (Reproduced from National Council of State Boards of Nursing, 2008; APRN Joint Dialogue Group Report, 2008, p. 9)
   c. An interstate compact is a formal agreement between two or more states to remedy a problem of mutual concern
   d. Multistate Nurse Licensure Compact—since 1998, 24 states have passed legislation to recognize nursing RN licensure among participating states
   e. The APRN Compact, drafted by the APRN Compact Working Group, was first adopted in 2002 but has yet to be implemented (National Council of State Boards of Nursing, n.d.)
   f. The 2014 iteration of the APRN Compact mirrors the APRN Consensus Model. Goal is adoption by NCSBN Delegate Assembly and consideration by state legislatures by January 2016
5. Accreditation: The APRN Consensus Model defines accreditation as "the formal review and approval by a recognized agency of educational degree or certification programs in nursing or nursing-related programs" (APRN Joint Dialogue Group Report, 2008, p. 7)
   a. The U.S. Department of Education (n.d.-a) defines accreditation as "the recognition that an institution maintains standards requisite for its graduates to gain admission to other reputable institutions of higher learning or to achieve credentials for professional practice" (U.S. Department of Education, n.d.-a).
   b. All APRN education programs must undergo a preapproval, preaccreditation, or accreditation process prior to admitting students. Two accrediting agencies offer, and one is developing, accrediting services that include evaluation of master's or higher degree nurse practitioner programs:
      (1) The Commission of Collegiate Nursing Education (CCNE) is an autonomous arm of the American Association of Colleges of Nursing (AACN). CCNE evaluates baccalaureate and graduate nursing programs, including programs offering distance education. CCNE accreditation is based on compliance with CCNE accreditation standards. The National Task Force Criteria for Evaluation of Nurse Practitioner Programs (NTF Criteria) are incorporated into CCNE accrediting standards.
      (2) The Accreditation Commission on Education in Nursing (ACEN) was formerly the National League for Nursing Accreditation Commission (NLNAC), a subsidiary of the National League for Nursing (NLN). As of 2013, ACEN is an autonomous accreditation agency and offers accrediting services to all types of nursing education programs.
      (3) The National League for Nursing Commission for Nursing Education Accreditation (NLN CNEA) was initiated in 2013. The NLN CNEA, a new autonomous accrediting arm of the NLN, is undergoing development and anticipates offering accrediting services by 2016 to all types of nursing education programs. http://www.nln.org/accreditation-services/faqs
      (4) The NLN endorsed the National Task Force Criteria for Evaluation of Nurse Practitioner Programs
6. Certification
   a. Definition—"The formal recognition of the knowledge, skills, and experience demonstrated by the achievement of standards identified by the profession" (Reproduced from National Council of State Boards of Nursing, 2008; APRN Joint Dialogue Group Report, 2008, p. 7)
   b. Purpose—to assure the public that an individual has mastered a body of knowledge and acquired skills in a particular specialty
   c. May be required for state licensure and reimbursement
   d. Required for Medicare reimbursement
   e. Required for APRN practice in most states
   f. NP credentialing currently available through National Commission for Certifying Agencies (NCCA)-recognized certifying agencies (Institute for Credentialing Excellence, 2015)

g. Certifying Agencies for Nurse Practitioners (entry level):
   (1) Pediatric Nursing Certification Board (PNCB)—formerly NCBPNPN
       800 South Frederick Avenue, Suite 104
       Gaithersburg, MD 20877-4250
       301-330-2921 and 1-888-641-2767
   PNCB offers NP certification examinations for:
       (a) Certified Pediatric Nurse Practitioner-Primary Care (CPNP-PC)
       (b) Certified Pediatric Nurse Practitioner-Acute Care (CPNP-AC)
   (2) American Nurses Credentialing Center (ANCC)
       600 Maryland Avenue, SW Suite 100 West
       Washington, DC 20024-2572
       1-800-284-2378
   ANCC offers NP certification examinations for:
       (a) Pediatric NP (PNP-BC)
       (b) Family NP (FNP-BC)
       (c) Adult-Gerontology Primary Care NP (AGPCNP-BC)
       (d) Adult-Gerontology Acute Care NP (AGACNP-BC)
       (e) Psychiatric Mental Health NP –Family (PMHNP-BC)
   (3) American Academy of Nurse Practitioners Certification Program (AANPCP)
       Capitol Station, LBJ Building
       P.O. Box 12926
       Austin, TX 78711-2926
       1-855-822-6727
   AANPCP offers NP certification examinations for:
       (a) Adult-Gerontology (Primary Care) AGNP-C and
       (b) Family Nurse Practitioner FNP-C
   (4) National Certification Corporation for the Obstetric, Gynecologic, and Neonatal Specialties (NCC)
       676 North Michigan Avenue
       Suite 3600
       Chicago, IL 60611-0082
   NCC offers NP certification examination for:
       (a) Neonatal Nurse Practitioner (NNP)
       (b) Women's Health Nurse Practitioner (WHNP)
   (5) Oncology Nursing Certification Corporation
       125 Enterprise Drive
       Pittsburgh, PA 15275
       412-859-6104 and 1-877-769-ONCC
   ONCC offers one NP certification examination for:
       (a) Advanced Oncology Certified Nurse Practitioner (AOCNP)
   (6) American Association of Critical-Care Nurses Certification Corporation (AACNCC)
       101 Columbia
       Aliso Viejo, CA 92656-4101
       1-800-899-AACN

AACNCC offers one NP certification examination as a renewal option only for
       (a) Acute Care NP-Adult-Gerontology (ACNP-AG)

7. Education is defined as "the formal preparation of APRNs in graduate degree-granting or postgraduate certificate programs" (Reproduced from National Council of State Boards of Nursing, 2008; APRN Joint Dialogue Group Report, 2008, p. 7)
   a. *Criteria for Evaluation of Nurse Practitioner Programs*, 4th Edition
      (1) Released August 2012 by a multiorganizational task force, the National Task Force on Quality Nurse Practitioner Education (NTF). This is the fourth release of the NTF Criteria, which is recognized as the national standard for nurse practitioner educational programs
      (2) The NTF 2012 was co-facilitated by the National Organization of Nurse Practitioner Faculties (NONPF) and the American Association of Colleges of Nursing (AACN)
      (3) Additional NTF members in 2012 included five NP certification bodies (AANPCP, AACNCC, ANCC, NCC, and PNCB), two accrediting agencies (CCNE and NLNAC), and several NP specialty national associations
      (4) Friends of the NTF who regularly participated in discussions included the National Council of State Boards of Nursing and the Division of Nursing within the Bureau of Health Professions/Health Resources and Services Administration
   b. Selected key recommendations for APRN education from APRN Consensus Model:
      (1) Formal education in an accredited graduate or postgraduate certificate (master's or doctoral) program in a university.
      (2) Broad-based APRN education: *Population focus*, rather than *specialty*, is the term now used to describe nurse practitioner tracks. *Population focus* best describes the broad area of practice for which competencies exist to supplement core role preparation. *Specialty* is a more narrow focus of practice that may include added emphasis of education after the initial broad-based education of role and population focus.
      (3) At minimum, all APRN education must include the APRN core: three separate graduate-level courses in advanced pharmacology, advanced physiology/pathophysiology, and advanced health assessment.
      (4) APRNs must be prepared at a minimum in one role and one population focus. Additional content specific to role and population should be integrated throughout the other role and population clinical and didactic content.
      (5) The graduate should be prepared to assume responsibility for clinical decision making,

i.e., assessment, diagnosis and management of patient problems, health promotion/health maintenance.

c. APRN entry level:
(1) American Association of Colleges of Nursing (2004) publishes position statement: The practice doctorate should be the DNP degree and should be the entry level for advanced nursing practice, including the four APRN roles: nurse practitioner, nurse-midwife, nurse anesthetist, and clinical nurse specialist. The DNP is not a degree limited to the four APRN roles.
(2) In 2012, NAPNAP endorsed the DNP as the appropriate credential and level of education for APRNs, noting that master's-prepared PNPs have and will continue to have a significant role in the improvement of the health and welfare of children.

☐ PRACTICE ISSUES

1. Interprofessional Collaborative Practice
   a. *Core Competencies for Interprofessional Collaborative Practice: Report of an Expert Panel* published in 2011 (http://www.aacn.nche.edu/education-resources/ipecreport.pdf)
   b. Definition of interprofessional collaboration: Interprofessional collaborative practice, when multiple health workers from different professional backgrounds work together with patients, families, carers, and communities to deliver the highest quality of care (Reprinted from Framework for action on interprofessional education and collaborative practice, © World Health Organization 2010.)
   c. Expert Panel report sponsors:
      (1) American Association of Colleges of Nursing
      (2) American Association of Colleges of Osteopathic Medicine
      (3) American Association of Colleges of Pharmacy
      (4) American Dental Education Association
      (5) Association of American Medical Colleges
      (6) Association of Schools of Public Health
   d. Four general core competency domain statements for interprofessional collaborative practice:
      (1) Values and Ethics: "Work with individuals of other professions to maintain a climate of mutual respect and shared values" (p. 19)
      (2) Roles/Responsibilities: "Use the knowledge of one's own role and those of other professions to appropriately assess and address the healthcare needs of the patients and populations served" (p. 21)
      (3) Interprofessional communication: "Communicate with patients, families, communities, and other health professionals in a responsive and responsible manner that supports a team approach to the maintenance of health and the treatment of disease" (p. 23)
      (4) Teams and Teamwork: "Apply relationship-building values and the principles of team dynamics to perform effectively in different team roles to plan and deliver patient-/population-centered care that is safe, timely, efficient, effective, and equitable" (p. 25). Reproduced from Interprofessional Education Collaborative Expert Panel. (2011). Core competencies for interprofessional collaborative practice: Report of an expert panel. Washington, D.C.: Interprofessional Education Collaborative.

2. Case management
   a. Definitions
      (1) "Case management is a collaborative process of assessment, planning, facilitation, care coordination, evaluation and advocacy for options and services to meet an individual's and family's comprehensive health needs through communication and available resources to promote quality cost effective outcomes" Reprinted with permission, the Case Management Society of America, 6301 Ranch Drive, Little Rock, AR 72223, www.cmsa.org.
      (2) Nursing Case Management is a collaborative method of assisting patients and families in accessing health care services. Coordinating care is a key feature with the goal of meeting individuals' health care needs in a participatory way. Important concepts include avoiding duplication and fragmented care, ensuring high quality clinical outcomes, and maintaining cost effective health care. Nurse case management includes: assessment, planning, implementation, evaluation, and interaction. (Llewellyn & Leonard, 2009, p. 12)
   b. Case management is not a profession unto itself but a practice that encompasses many disciplines. The goal of case management is to formulate a plan that enables the patient to move smoothly through the healthcare system
   c. Components of the role and function of the case manager, according to the Case Management Society of America's Standards of Practice:
      (1) Assessment of health and psychosocial needs, including health literacy, and development of a case management plan collaboratively with all stakeholders
      (2) Planning with all stakeholders to maximize healthcare responses, quality and cost-effective outcomes
      (3) Facilitating communication and coordination among stakeholders, involving the patient in the decision-making process in order to minimize service fragmentation
      (4) Educating the patient and all stakeholders on treatment options, community resources, insurance benefits, and psychosocial concerns so that timely and informed decisions can be made

(5) Empowering the patient to problem solve by exploring care options and alternative plans, when necessary, to achieve desired outcome

(6) Encouraging the appropriate use of healthcare services and striving to improve the quality of care and maintain cost-effectiveness on a case-by-case basis

(7) Assisting the client in safe transitions of care to the next most appropriate level

(8) Striving to promote patient self-advocacy and self-determination

(9) Advocating for both the patient and stakeholders, to facilitate positive outcomes. However, if a conflict arises, the patient must be the priority (CMSA, 2014)

3. Quality improvement (QI)
   a. National Quality Forum (NQF) is a not-for-profit, nonpartisan membership-based organization that works to catalyze improvements in health care
   b. National Committee for Quality Assurance
   c. The Healthcare Effectiveness Data and Information Set (HEDIS) is a tool used by more than 90% of America's health plans to measure performance on important dimensions of care and service. Altogether, HEDIS consists of 81 measures across 5 domains of care
   d. Quality improvement (QI) consists of systematic and continuous actions that lead to measurable improvement in healthcare services and the health status of targeted patient groups
   e. Quality in health care is defined by the Institute of Medicine as a direct correlation between the level of improved health services and the desired health outcomes of individuals and populations
   f. Performance measurement is the regular collection of data to assess whether the correct processes are being performed and desired results are being achieved
   g. "Meaningful Use"—the American Recovery and Reinvestment Act authorizes the Centers for Medicare and Medicaid Services (CMS) to provide a reimbursement incentive for physician and hospital providers who are successful in becoming "meaningful users" of an electronic health record (EHR). These incentive payments began in 2011 and gradually phase down. By 2015, providers are expected to have adopted and be actively utilizing an EHR in compliance with the "meaningful use" definition, or they will be subject to financial penalties under Medicare (Centers for Medicare and Medicaid Services, 2015)
   h. Patient-centered medical home (sometimes known as a primary care medical home) is defined as "an approach to providing comprehensive primary care … that facilitates partnerships between individual patients, and their personal physicians, and when appropriate, the patient's family"
   i. Alternative terms—total quality management (TQM); continuous quality improvement (CQI); QI

differs from quality assurance (QA) in being a continuous rather than an episodic process
   j. Systematic, organized structures, processes, and expected outcomes focus on defining excellence and ensuring accountability for quality of care
   k. QI provides framework for ongoing evaluation of practice through identification of norms, criteria, and standards that measure program effectiveness and minimize liability
   l. QI mechanisms and strategies
      (1) Peer review
         (a) Recognize and reward nursing practice
         (b) Leads to higher standards of practice
         (c) Discourages practice beyond scope of legal authority
         (d) Improves quality of care
         (e) Provides for accountability and responsibility
      (2) Other methods of evaluation
         (a) Audit—retrospective measurement of quality
         (b) Interviews and questionnaires
         (c) Patient satisfaction surveys or interviews

4. Risk management
   a. Systems and activities designed to recognize and intervene to decrease risk of injury to patients and subsequent claims against healthcare providers; based on assumption that many injuries to patients are preventable
   b. Evaluates sources of legal liability in practice such as:
      (1) Patients
      (2) Procedures
      (3) Quality of record keeping
   c. Areas of liability risk
      (1) Practitioner–client relationship
      (2) Communication and informed consent
      (3) Clinical expertise
      (4) Self-evaluation by professionals of need to stay current
      (5) Documentation
      (6) Consultation and referral
      (7) Policies, procedures, and protocols
      (8) Supervision of others
   d. Includes educational activities that decrease risk in identified areas

5. Malpractice
   a. Professional misconduct, unreasonable lack of skill; infidelity in professional or fiduciary duties; illegal, immoral conduct resulting in patient harm
   b. Alleged professional failure to render services with degree of care, diligence, and precaution that another member of same profession in similar circumstances would render to prevent patient injury
   c. Malpractice insurance
      (1) Does not protect APRN from charges of practicing medicine without a license if APRN is practicing outside legal scope of practice for that state

(2) National Practitioner Data Bank collects information on adverse actions against healthcare practitioners, including nurses

(3) Types of coverage

    (a) Occurrence coverage—covers malpractice event that occurred during policy period, regardless of date of discovery or when claim filed

    (b) Claims made coverage—covers only claims filed during policy coverage period, regardless of when event occurred; optional tail coverage contract extends the coverage of a claims made policy into the future to cover all claims filed after the basic claims made coverage period

6. Negligence—failure of individual to do what a reasonable person would do that results in injury to another

7. Reimbursement: Whether working independently, sharing a joint practice with a physician, or practicing within a hospital or managed care system, APRNs must be reimbursed appropriately. Standards that determine private pay insurance mechanisms are often modeled after federal policies such as Medicaid and Medicare. However, even when the federal government establishes mandates that encourage direct payment of nonphysician healthcare providers, barriers to reimbursement are often encountered in state-level rules and regulations. National survey data indicate that just over one-fourth of all major managed care organizations in the United States refuse to credential nurse practitioners as primary care providers.

a. Medicaid

    (1) Authorized in 1965 as Title XIX of Social Security Act

    (2) Federal/state matching program with federal oversight

    (3) Financed through federal and state taxes, with between 50% and 83% of total Medicaid costs covered by federal government

    (4) The Affordable Care Act of 2010 created a national Medicaid minimum eligibility level of 133% of the federal poverty level (FPL) ($32,252.50 for a family of four in 2015) for nearly all Americans younger than age 65 years. This expansion went into effect January 1, 2014. States had the option of expanding this coverage with federal support any time before January 14, 2014

    (5) Other nonfinancial eligibility criteria include federal and state requirements regarding residency, immigration status, and documentation of U.S. citizenship

    (6) State Medicaid programs are required by federal government to cover certain categories such as:

        (a) Recipients of Aid to Families with Dependent Children (AFDC)—states set own eligibility requirements for AFDC

        (b) People older than 65, blind, or totally disabled who are eligible for cash assistance under federal Supplemental Security Income (SSI) program

        (c) Pregnant women (for pregnancy-related services only) and children under 6 years with family incomes up to 133% of federal poverty level

        (d) Medicaid and the Children's Health Insurance Program (CHIP) provide health coverage to half of all low-income children in the United States (>43 million children). Minimum eligibility guidelines are set by the federal government; states can choose to expand coverage. All states have done so. The average CHIP income eligibility level for children is 241% of the federal poverty level

        (e) All children from birth to age 6 years with family incomes up to 133% of FPL and children ages 6–18 years with family incomes up to 100% of FPL are eligible for Medicaid

        (f) Other eligible children include infants born to women covered by Medicaid (known as "deemed newborns"), certain children in foster care or an adoption assistance program, and certain children with disabilities

        (g) All children enrolled in Medicaid are entitled to Early, Periodic Screening, Diagnosis, and Treatment (EPSDT). CHIP also ensures a comprehensive set of benefits for children, but states have flexibility to design the benefit package

    (7) States can apply to CMS for waivers to populations beyond what can traditionally be covered under the state plan

    (8) States can choose to cover "medically needy"

    (9) Coverage required for certain services

        (a) Hospital and physician services

        (b) Laboratory and radiographic services

        (c) Nursing home and home healthcare services

        (d) Prenatal and preventive services

        (e) Medically necessary transportation

    (10) States can add services to list and can place certain limitations on federally mandated services

    (11) Although Medicaid recipients cannot be billed for services, states can impose nominal copayments or deductibles for certain services

b. Medicare

    (1) Federally mandated program established in 1965, provides health insurance for aged and disabled individuals, and people of all ages with end-stage renal disease

    (2) Medicare eligibility

        (a) Eligibility covers hospital service, physician services, and other medical services

(b) Income level does not impact eligibility

(c) Those 65 years of age and older who are eligible for Social Security are automatically enrolled whether or not they are retired—persons are eligible for Social Security when they (or their spouses) have paid into Social Security system through employment for 40 quarters or more

(d) Those who have paid into system for fewer than 40 quarters can enroll in Medicare Part A by paying monthly premium

(e) Those who are younger than age 65 and are totally and permanently disabled may enroll in Medicare Part A after receiving Social Security disability benefits for 24 months

(f) Those with chronic renal disease requiring dialysis or transplant may also be eligible for Part A without a 2-year waiting period

(g) Services covered include some hospitalization costs; some skilled nursing facility costs, although custodial care is not covered; home health care—100% for skilled care, 80% of approved amount for medical equipment; and hospice care—100% for most services

(h) Payment for hospitalization is based on projected costs of caring for patient with given problem—each Medicare patient admitted to a hospital is classified according to a diagnosis-related group (DRG); the hospital is then paid a predetermined amount for each patient admitted with the given DRG, if hospital costs are above payment rate, the hospital must absorb loss; if costs are below payment rate, hospital allowed to keep a percentage of excess

(3) "Original Medicare" is Part A and Part B: Medicare Part A covers:

(a) Hospital care

(b) Skilled nursing facility care

(c) Nursing home care (but not if only custodial care)

(d) Hospice

(e) Home health services

(4) Medicare Part B—Supplementary Medical Insurance (SMI)

(a) Monthly premium is charged

(b) Some low-income people are eligible to have monthly premium paid by Medicaid

(c) Financed by general federal revenues and by Part B monthly premiums

(d) Covers all medically necessary services—80% of an approved amount after annual deductible; includes physician services, physical, occupational, and speech therapy; medical equipment and diagnostic tests; and

some preventive care such as Pap tests, mammograms, hepatitis B, pneumococcal and influenza vaccines can be included in medical expenses

(5) Medicare Part C (Medicare Advantage)

(a) Medicare Advantage, also called Part C, includes both Part A and Part B Medicare (Original Medicare)

(b) Part C coverage is provided by private insurance plans approved by Medicare

(c) Medicare Advantage plans cover all Part A and Part B services and may offer extra coverage

(d) Medicare pays a fixed amount each month for a person's care to the Medicare Advantage plan.

(e) Medicare Advantage plans usually include a prescription drug benefit

(6) Medicare Part D—prescription drug benefit

(a) Medicare Prescription Drug Plan may be added to Part C Medicare Advantage or may be added to Original Medicare or other types of Medicare plans

(b) Each Medicare drug plan has a formulary

(c) Part D costs vary according to various plans and drugs used

c. APRN—Medicaid/Medicare coverage

(1) Omnibus Budget Reconciliation Act (OBRA) 1989—mandated Medicaid reimbursement for certified pediatric and family nurse practitioners began July 1, 1990; providers required to practice within the scope of state law and do not have to be under supervision or associated with a physician or other provider

(a) Level of payment determined by states—reimbursement rates range from 70% to 100% of fee-for-service physician Medicaid rate

(b) Pediatric and family nurse practitioners may bill Medicaid directly after attaining provider number from state Medicaid agency

(c) States can elect to pass laws allowing them to extend Medicaid payment to other types of NPs not identified in federal statutes

(2) Legislation provides direct Medicare reimbursement for APRNs in all geographic locations

(a) APRN reimbursement at 85% of physician fee schedule when billing independently using APRN billing number; direct physician supervision not required

(b) When APRN is employed by physician, the physician practice may receive 100% of customary physician charge, according to "Incident to" rules (Centers for Medicare and Medicaid Services, 2013)

(c) Nurse practitioners who have their own billing number and provide shared visits with physicians in hospitals may bill for services at 100% as long as the physician has also seen the patient the same day in a "face-to-face" encounter. Billing will take place under the physician billing number (American Association of Nurse Practitioners, 2013)

(d) In order to bill Medicare, a nurse practitioner must meet the following conditions:

   i. Be a registered professional nurse who is authorized by the state in which the services are furnished to practice as a nurse practitioner in accordance with state law; and

   ii. Be certified as a nurse practitioner by a recognized national certifying body that has established standards for nurse practitioners; and

   iii. Possess a master's degree in nursing

(e) National certifying bodies for nurse practitioners that fulfill Medicare billing requirements include:

   i. AANPCP

   ii. ANCC

   iii. NCC

   iv. PNCB

   v. ONCC

   vi. AACNCC

   vii. Hospice and Palliative Certification Corporation (formerly the National Board on Certification of Hospice and Palliative Nurses). This is a specialty certification for APRNs who have already earned a master's, postgraduate, or doctoral degree from an APRN program that is CCNE or ACEN accredited.

(f) NP covered services are limited to services an NP is legally authorized to perform under the state law in which the NP practices and must meet training, education, and experience requirements prescribed by the Secretary of Health and Human Services

(3) NP services covered under Part B if service would be considered physician's services if furnished by MD or Doctor of Osteopathy (DO); if NP is legally authorized to perform services in the state in which they are performed; if services are performed in collaboration with MD/DO (collaboration specified as a process whereby NP works with physician to deliver health care within scope of NP expertise with medical direction and appropriate supervision as provided for in jointly developed guidelines or other mechanisms defined by federal regulations and law of the state in which services are performed); and services are otherwise precluded from coverage because of one of the statutory exclusions

(4) "Incident to" refers to services provided as an integral, yet incidental, part of the physician's personal, professional services in the course of diagnosis or treatment of injury or illness—these services must occur under direct personal supervision of a physician, and the APRN must be an employee of the physician group; services must occur during the course of treatment where the physician performs an initial service and subsequent services in a manner that reflects the physician's active participation and management of the course of treatment—direct personal supervision does not mean that the physician must be in the same room as the APRN; however, the physician must be present in the office suite and available for assistance and direction while the APRN provides patient care

(5) When APRN performs "incident to" service in physician's office, billing must be submitted to Medicare by employing physician, under the physician's name, provider number, and CPT code—payment is made at full physician rate and is paid to physician or physician practice

(6) When APRN provides service in skilled nursing facility, or nursing facility located in urban area as defined by law, Medicare payment can be obtained—Medicare reimbursement is also available for APRN services in skilled nursing facilities (SNFs) in nonrural areas on a reasonable charge basis; this amount may not exceed physician fee schedule amount for service and payment is made to the APRN's employer

(7) Centers for Medicare and Medicaid Services (CMS)

   (a) Formerly Health Care Financing and Administration (HCFA)

   (b) Oversight of several federal programs, including Medicare, Medicaid, State Children's Health Insurance Program (SCHIP), Health Insurance Portability and Accountability Act (HIPAA), and Clinical Laboratory Improvement Amendments (CLIA)

   (c) Website: http://cms.hhs.gov

d. Other third-party payers

(1) Private insurer reimbursement is contract specific per state insurance commission

(2) Civilian Health and Medical Program of the United States (CHAMPUS)

   (a) Federal health plan for military personnel, including surviving dependents, families, and retirees

   (b) APRN reimbursement for services

(3) Federal Employees Health Benefit Program (FEHBP)

(a) One of largest employer-sponsored group health insurance programs

(b) APRN recognized as designated healthcare provider

e. Methods of payment for advanced practice nurses

(1) Fee-for-service model

(a) Unit of payment by visit or procedure

(b) Can occur with utilization review in which case payer has right to authorize or deny payment of expensive medical interventions such as hospital admission, extra hospital days, and surgery

(2) Episodic model

(a) One sum is paid for all services delivered during a given illness

(b) DRG fee payment

(3) Capitation model, PPO, and HMO are covered in section on Managed Care in this chapter

❑ PROFESSIONAL ORGANIZATIONS

1. Purpose and benefits
   a. Establish practice standards
   b. Collective voice to promote nursing and quality of care
   c. Monitor and influence policy and legislative initiatives
   d. Position papers on practice issues
   e. Disseminate information
2. Examples
   a. American Nurses Association (ANA)
   b. National Association of Pediatric Nurse Practitioners (NAPNAP)
   c. Gerontological Advanced Practice Nurses Association (GAPNA)
   d. National Organization of Nurse Practitioner Faculties (NONPF)
   e. American Association of Nurse Practitioners (AANP)
   f. Nurse Practitioner Associates for Continuing Education (NPACE)
   g. National Association of School Nurses
   h. Association for Women's Health, Obstetrics, and Neonatal Nurses (AWHONN)
   i. National Association of Nurse Practitioners in Women's Health (NPWH)
- Research in Advanced Practice: Practice-based research is essential to the ongoing development of advanced practice nursing.
1. Major trend is outcome studies
2. Sources of federal funding
   a. Agency for Healthcare Research and Quality (AHRQ)
      (1) Formerly the Agency for Health Care Policy and Research (AHCPR)
      (2) http://www.ahrq.gov/

b. National Institutes of Health (NIH)
   (1) Includes the National Institute for Nursing Research (NINR)
   (2) http://www.nih.gov/
c. Maternal and Child Health Bureau (MCHB)
   (1) Functions within Health Resources and Services Administration (HRSA)
   (2) http://www.mchb.hrsa.gov/
3. Sources of research findings
   a. Conferences
   b. Scholarly publications
   c. Distribution of summaries of research studies
4. Use of research in practice setting
   a. Use evidence-based practice routinely
   b. Translate clinical evidence into practice settings and with practice issues
   c. Develop research-based clinical pathways
   d. Track clinical outcomes and variances
   e. Demonstrate quality and cost-effectiveness of care
   f. Give structure to demonstration projects
   g. Persuade lawmakers of NP value and contributions in today's healthcare system
   h. Improve quality and patient outcomes
5. Benefit of research for patients
   a. Provides thorough understanding of patient situation
   b. Provides more accurate assessment of situations
   c. Increases effectiveness of interventions
   d. Increases provider sensitivity to patient situations
   e. Assists providers to more accurately determine need for and effectiveness of interventions
6. Barriers to research utilization
   a. Time and cost of conducting research studies
   b. Resistance to change in work setting
   c. Lack of rewards for using research findings
   d. Lack of understanding or uncertainty regarding research outcomes
7. Strategies to overcome barriers to research utilization
   a. Creation of organizational culture that values and uses research
   b. Creation of environment where questions are encouraged, critical thinking is appreciated, and nursing care is evaluated
   c. Support for research through time allocation and financial commitment

❑ HEALTH POLICY

- Policy Influences
1. Healthy People 2020—10-year program (HealthyPeople.gov. (n.d.). *Health People 2020 Framework.* retrieved from https://www.healthypeople.gov/sites/default/files/HP2020Framework.pdf)
2. Vision—a society in which all people live long, healthy lives
3. Mission
   a. Identify nationwide health improvement priorities

b. Increase public awareness and understanding of the determinants of health, disease, and disability and the opportunities for progress

c. Provide measurable objectives and goals that are applicable at the national, state, and local levels

d. Engage multiple sectors to take actions to strengthen policies and improve practices that are driven by the best available evidence and knowledge

e. Identify critical research, evaluation, and data collection needs

4. Healthy People 2020 overarching goals:

a. Attain high-quality, longer lives free of preventable disease, disability, injury, and premature death

b. Achieve health equity, eliminate disparities, and improve the health of all groups

c. Create social and physical environments that promote good health for all

d. Promote quality of life, healthy development, and healthy behaviors across all life stages

5. Healthy People 2020—Foundation Measures Category and Measures of Progress:

a. General Health Status

(1) Life expectancy

(2) Healthy life expectancy

(3) Physical and mental unhealthy days

(4) Self-assessed health status

(5) Limitation of activity

(6) Chronic disease prevalence

(7) International comparisons

b. Disparities and Inequity

(1) Race/ethnicity

(2) Gender

(3) Socioeconomic status

(4) Lesbian, gay, bisexual, transgender status

(5) Geography

c. Social Determinants of Health

(1) Social and economic factors

(2) Natural and built environments

(3) Policies and programs

d. Health-Related Quality of Life and Well-Being

(1) Well-being/satisfaction

(2) Physical, mental, and social health-related quality of life

(3) Participation in common activities

6. Healthy People 2020—Leading Health Indicators (LHIs): There are 26 LHIs organized under 12 topics, available at: https://www.healthypeople.gov/sites/default/files/HP2020_brochure_with_LHI_508_FNL.pdf

a. Topic 1, Access to Health Services

(1) LHIs 1 and 2: Health insurance; have a primary care provider

b. Topic 2, Clinical Preventive Services

(1) LHIs 3, 4, 5, and 6: Colorectal cancer screening, hypertension control, diabetic with HbA1c >9%; child immunizations

c. Topic 3, Environmental Quality

(1) LHIs 7 and 8: Air quality index >100; child age 3–11 years exposed to secondhand smoke

d. Topic 4, Injury and Violence

(1) LHIs 9 and 10: Fatal injuries, homicide

e. Topic 5, Maternal, Infant, and Child Health

(1) LHIs 11 and 12: Infant deaths; preterm births

f. Topic 6, Mental Health

(1) LHIs 13 and 14: Suicides; adolescents who experience major depressive episodes

g. Topic 7, Nutrition, Physical Activity, and Obesity

(1) LHIs 15, 16, 17, and 18: Adults who meet federal physical activity guidelines; adults who are obese; children and adolescents who are obese; total vegetable intake for persons age ≥2 years

h. Topic 8, Oral Health

(1) LHI 19: Persons age ≥2 years who used oral health system in last 12 months

i. Topic 9, Reproductive and Sexual Health

(1) LHIs 20 and 21: Sexually active females ages 15–44 years who received reproductive health services in past 12 months; persons living with HIV who know their serostatus

j. Topic 10, Social Determinants

(1) LHI 22: Students who graduate with a diploma 4 years after starting 9th grade

k. Topic 11, Substance Abuse

(1) LHIs 23 and 24: Adolescents using alcohol or any illicit drugs during the past 30 days; adults engaging in binge drinking during the past 30 days

l. Topic 12, Tobacco

(1) LHIs 25 and 26: Adults who are current cigarette smokers; adolescents who smoked cigarettes in the past 30 days

7. Healthy People 2010—Summary of Progress (selected pediatric LHIs)

a. Healthy People 2010 consisted of 969 specific objectives in 28 focus areas

b. Evaluation of Healthy People 2010 Leading Health Indicators include:

(1) Longevity at birth increased 1.2% over the decade

(2) Percentage of women receiving prenatal care improved but only achieved 15% of the 2010 targeted change

(3) Avoidance of unnecessary hospitalization for pediatric asthma declined by 21.7%

(4) Exposure of children age <6 years to tobacco smoke reduced by 69%, exceeding the targeted change

(5) Childhood immunizations met the 2010 target

(6) Overweight in children ages 6–12 years increased by 58.75%, moving considerably far away from the 2010 target

(7) Students in grades 9–12 who reported never having sexual intercourse increased by 4.4%, moving one-third of distance to target

(8) Students in grades 9–12 who reported using a condom at last intercourse increased by 6%, moving halfway toward the 2010 target

(9) Percentage of adolescents reporting not using alcohol or illicit drugs in the last 30 days increased by 2.7%

(10) Percentage of adolescents using tobacco declined by 42.5%

- Utilization of Health Policy
  1. Shifting trend toward primary care and early preventive measures; supports need for APRN
  2. Four major policy and regulation initiatives impacting APRN practice:
     a. Consensus Model for APRN Regulation: Licensure, Accreditation, Certification and Education (APRN Joint Dialogue Group, 2008)
     b. The Doctor of Nursing Practice movement
     c. *The Future of Nursing* RWJF/IOM report (2010)
     d. Patient Protection and Affordable Care Act
  3. Triple Aim of health care: The Institute for Healthcare Improvement (IHI) developed the Triple Aim as a statement of purpose for fundamentally new health systems that contribute to the overall health of populations while reducing costs
     a. Better care
     b. Better health
     c. Lower healthcare cost
- Types of Healthcare Delivery Systems
  1. Primary health care
     a. Definition: Primary care is the provision of integrated, accessible healthcare services by clinicians who are accountable for addressing a large majority of personal healthcare needs, developing a sustained partnership with patients, and practicing in the context of family and community
     b. Activities and/or functions define boundaries of primary care, such as curing or alleviating common illnesses and disabilities
     c. Entry point to a system that includes access to secondary and tertiary care
     d. Attributes include care that is accessible, comprehensive, coordinated, continuous, and accountable
     e. Strategy for organizing healthcare system as a whole; gives priority and allocates resources to community-based rather than hospital-based care
     f. Categories of primary care providers (PCPs) and nature of care
        (1) Medical specialties—family medicine, general internal medicine, general pediatrics, obstetrics and gynecology
        (2) Other experts have included NP and physician assistants (PAs) as primary care providers (PCPs)
     g. Many definitions stress self-responsibility for health
  2. Managed care
     a. Definition: A network that is integrated and combines financing and delivery of healthcare services to covered individuals
        (1) Network connects consumers, sponsors, providers, and third-party payers

(2) Initial managed care organization was Kaiser Health Plan (California) established in 1930s

b. Objectives
   (1) Manage use and price of healthcare delivery system
   (2) Control type, level, and frequency of treatment
   (3) Restrict level of reimbursement for services
c. Type of health insurance plan designed to control costs while ensuring quality care is provided
d. Obligation to manage is shared among providers, consumers, and payers
   (1) Providers no longer dictate price of care delivery; must assume more financial risk for population assigned to them for care
   (2) Consumers have fewer choices of coverage, providers, and greater financial responsibility
   (3) Payers manage healthcare dollars through benefit design, selective contracting, and shifting financial risk to providers
e. Types of managed care plans
   (1) Health maintenance organizations (HMOs)
      (a) Most common type
      (b) Over 70 million Americans are enrolled in an HMO (National Conference of State Legislators, 2013)
      (c) Offer preestablished benefit package—including preventive, inpatient, and outpatient care
      (d) HMO contracts with providers to provide care to enrollees
      (e) Providers at financial risk, resulting in incentive to provide high-quality, cost-effective care
      (f) Enrollees select a primary care provider (PCP) who manages total care by authorizing specialty visits, hospitalization, and other services
      (g) PCP may be MD, APRN, or PA provider; serving as "gate keeper" and expert in an individual's care
   (2) Preferred provider organizations (PPOs)
      (a) Compromised managed care option that is alternative between indemnity and HMO insurance
      (b) Uses financial incentives to influence consumer and provider behaviors
      (c) Refers to variety of arrangements between insurers, providers, and third-party payers rather than standard plan
      (d) Often owned by large insurance companies such as Prudential, Travelers, and Aetna
      (e) Available primarily to employed commercial population
   (3) Point of service plans (POS)
      (a) Consumers decide whether to use a provider network or seek care outside the network

(b) If variation of HMO plan, PCP coordinates care for enrollees; if variation of PPO plan, enrollees may choose lower cost options outside of provider network

(c) Most rapidly growing type of managed care

   (4) Integrated delivery systems

(a) Vertical integration of services across levels of care into seamless system with improved access for enrollees

(b) Capitated payment—financial risk shifts from payer to provider; unit of value is cost per member per month (PMPM); providers receive age- and sex-adjusted budget to cover services to maintain wellness of specific target population

(c) Emphasis on provision of appropriate but not unlimited care with financial benefit of keeping population healthy through systematic preventive services

   (5) Accountable care organizations (ACOs)

(a) Groups of doctors, hospitals, and other healthcare providers, who come together voluntarily to give coordinated high-quality care to their Medicare patients

(b) The goal of coordinated care is to ensure that patients, especially the chronically ill, get the right care at the right time, while avoiding unnecessary duplication of services and preventing medical errors

(c) When an ACO succeeds both in delivering high-quality care and spending healthcare dollars more wisely, it will share in the savings it achieves for the Medicare program (Centers for Medicare and Medicaid Services, 2015)

  f. Reimbursement under managed care

   (1) Providers accept financial risk for care provided to specific population of enrollees

   (2) Capitated payment

(a) Provider receives payment in advance

(b) Payment level reflects expected utilization by enrolled population for which provider is responsible

   (3) Provider must control volume and cost

   (4) Efficiency usually rewarded through bonus payments for operating within budget and meeting goals for quality and efficiency

  g. Monitoring, evaluation, and accreditation in managed care

   (1) Health Plan Employer Data and Information Set (HEDIS)—provides quality measures and compares with benchmark standards and goals

   (2) National Committee for Quality Assurance (NCQA)

(a) Major accreditation body for health plans, provider organizations such as ACOs, and health plan contracting organizations

  h. Challenges and opportunities of managed care for APRNs

   (1) Need for balance between quality of care and costs inherent in diagnosis/management per client visit

(a) Education programs must incorporate managed care content into curriculum

(b) APRN must combine strong clinical and financial skills to determine cost of providing care to target population

   (2) APRN strategies for success within evolving managed care environment

(a) Determine strategies to increase efficiency without sacrificing quality of client–provider interactions; e.g., group well-child visits

(b) Lobby for APRN inclusion on provider panels

(c) Maintain partnerships with APRN education programs for collaborative study and documentation of APRN effectiveness

- Health Insurance Portability and Accountability Act of 1996 (HIPPA)

1. Health insurance reform—addresses preexisting conditions and provides portability of health insurance when an employee changes jobs or loses a job

2. Administrative simplification required by Centers for Medicare and Medicaid Services :

  a. Electronic transactions and code set standards

  b. Privacy requirements

  c. Security requirements

  d. National identifier requirements

3. CMS responsible for oversight and compliance with administrative simplification mandates except for privacy provisions, which are overseen by the Office of Civil Rights (OCR)

4. Target dates for implementation and compliance with administrative simplification

  a. Administrative simplification provisions required Department of Health and Human Services to adopt national standards for electronic healthcare transactions and code sets, unique health identifiers and security

  b. Final Privacy Rule published in December 2000 and modified in August 2002. Set national standards for the protection of individually identifiable health information by the three types of covered entities

  c. Final Security Rule was published in 2003. Sets national standards for protecting the confidentiality, integrity, and availability of electronic protected health information

5. "Covered entities"

  a. Health plans

  b. Healthcare clearinghouses

  c. Healthcare providers who conduct any electronic transitions of health-related information

6. Website information
   a. Department of Health and Human Services page: http://www.hhs.gov/ocr/privacy/hipaa/administrative/index.html
   b. OCR page: http://www.hhs.gov/ocr/privacy/index.html

☐ QUESTIONS

Select the best answer.

1. Which of the following is congruent with the APRN Consensus Model?
   a. APRN licensure occurs at the level of role and population foci.
   b. APRN education programs must be doctoral level.
   c. National certification by a recognized APRN certifying body is optional.
   d. Accreditation by the U.S. Department of Education is the minimum requirement for APRN programs.

2. Which of the following objectives from Healthy People 2010 has not made progress toward achieving its targeted goal?
   a. Reduce exposure of children age ≤6 years to tobacco smoke
   b. Reduce percentage of adolescents using tobacco
   c. Increase childhood immunization rates
   d. Reduce number of children ages 6 to 12 years who are overweight

3. The nurse practitioner role was initially established to:
   a. Reduce the nursing shortage and improve access to care
   b. Improve working conditions of nurses while improving access to care
   c. Improve access to care and partially solve physician shortage
   d. Improve nursing's image through expansion of the role

4. Early NP-related research focused on:
   a. The response of policymakers to the nursing shortage
   b. The effectiveness of the NP as a primary caregiver
   c. An effort to demonstrate quality and cost-effectiveness of NPs
   d. The role of the NP as a physician extender

5. Standards of practice are:
   a. Authoritative statements used to measure quality
   b. Used to measure outcome but are not authoritative
   c. Designed for legal purposes
   d. Not designed for legal purposes and cannot be used to measure quality

6. Quality improvement activities include:
   a. Patient satisfaction surveys only
   b. Peer review, patient satisfaction surveys, chart audits
   c. Defining four practice domains
   d. Systems to decrease risk of injury to patients

7. Most risk management programs are based on the assumption that:
   a. Many injuries to patients are preventable.
   b. Most legal liability is a result of poor documentation.
   c. Most injuries to patients are not preventable.
   d. Malpractice insurance is generally unnecessary.

8. What is regarded as the national standard for nurse practitioner education?
   a. APRN Consensus Model
   b. *Criteria for Evaluation of Nurse Practitioner Programs*, 4th Edition
   c. IOM *Future of Nursing* report
   d. AACN Essentials of Master's Education

9. Standards of practice may be used to:
   a. Establish minimal levels of performance
   b. Establish reimbursement schemes for APRNs
   c. Mandate nursing practice across the nation
   d. Mandate nursing practice in certain states

10. Scope of practice:
    a. Is identical across the states
    b. Is determined by the federal government
    c. Is mandated by the federal government
    d. Varies from state to state

11. Medicaid provides health insurance coverage to:
    a. Certain categories of people whose personal income falls below a certain percentage of the federal poverty level
    b. Anyone whose personal income falls below the federal poverty level
    c. Newborns, pregnant women, and those older than 65 years whose personal income falls below the federal poverty level
    d. Those who are elderly

12. Which children do *not* meet the federal minimum financial eligibility criteria for Medicaid?
    a. Infants born to women who already receive Medicaid ("deemed newborns")
    b. Ages up to 6 years and family income <133% of federal poverty level
    c. Ages 6 to 18 years and family income <100% of federal poverty level
    d. Ages 6 to 18 years and family income >133% of federal poverty level

13. Medicare reimbursement for services:
    a. Is not dependent on the patient's income level
    b. Depends on the patient's income level
    c. Is not available to APRNs under any circumstances
    d. Is only available to APRNs who are in collaborative practice with a physician

14. Medicare Part A covers:
    a. Hospital, skilled nursing facility, and hospice care
    b. All medically necessary services
    c. Skilled nursing facility (SNF) care only
    d. Hospice care only

15. Medicare Part B covers:
    a. All medically necessary services
    b. Inpatient hospital care

c. Outpatient physician services only

d. Skilled nursing facility and hospice care

16. In order to bill Medicare, a nurse practitioner must meet which conditions?

a. Have a DNP and state authorization to practice

b. Have a PhD and be nationally certified

c. State authorization to practice and nationally certified

d. Have a master's in nursing; national certification optional

17. The term "incident to" refers to:

a. The occasions when an APRN practices independently but occasionally consults with a physician

b. The notion that the physician must be present in the office suite and immediately available to provide assistance in order for the APRN to bill for services rendered

c. The notion that a physician must examine the patient along with the APRN if Medicare is to be billed for services rendered

d. Medicaid only and is not pertinent to Medicare billing

18. "Incident to" billing is specific only to:

a. Medicare and Medicaid

b. Medicaid

c. Medicare

d. Private insurance companies

19. Which certifying bodies certify pediatric nurse practitioners?

a. ANCC and PNCB

b. NAPNAP and AANPPC

c. PNCB and NAPNAP

d. NCC and PNCB

20. Legal authority for APRN practice is granted by:

a. Federal law

b. Regulations from the Department of Health and Human Services

c. State law and regulations

d. The Board of Medicine in most states

21. Malpractice insurance:

a. Protects APRNs from charges of practicing medicine without a license when they are practicing outside the legal scope of practice

b. Does not protect APRNs from charges of practicing medicine without a license when they are practicing outside the legal scope of practice

c. Does not pay for legal defense if the APRN is practicing beyond the legal scope of practice

d. Is important but should not be purchased if the facility in which the APRN is employed carries good coverage

22. Which of the following is one of the four general core competency domains of interprofessional collaborative practice according to the Interprofessional Education Collaborative Expert Panel?

a. Working with individuals of other professions to maintain a climate of mutual respect and shared values

b. Maintaining a silo perspective so all benefit from expert knowledge

c. Understanding that hierarchical team-based care is the best care and therefore teams should be led by physicians

d. Accepting that the patient is the most important member of the interprofessional team

23. Certification is:

a. A procedure through which the government appraises and grants a certificate to the APRN

b. Granted by the individual states

c. Governed by each state's Board of Nursing

d. The formal recognition of the knowledge, skills, and experience demonstrated by the achievement of standards identified by the profession

24. Licensure:

a. Is a federal process that is used to standardize healthcare facilities

b. Is the granting of authority to practice

c. Cannot be used to prohibit anyone from practicing a given profession

d. Is a federal process that is used to standardize education programs

25. The APRN Consensus Model is:

a. A mandate from the NCSBN that defines advanced practice nursing

b. A proposed regulatory model for advanced practice nursing

c. A proposal for federal legislation for advanced practice nursing

d. Approved only by the American Nurses Association

26. Which of the following is *not* one of the four major recommendations of the Robert Wood Johnson Foundation Institute of Medicine report *The Future of Nursing: Leading Change, Advancing Health*?

a. Nurses should practice to a limited extent of their education and training as defined by Boards of Medicine.

b. Nurses should achieve higher levels of education and training through an improved education system that promotes seamless academic progression.

c. Nurses should be full partners, with physicians and other healthcare professionals, in redesigning health care in the United States.

d. Effective workforce planning and policymaking require better data collection and an improved information infrastructure.

27. Which of the following is *not* congruent with U.S. prescribing laws and nurse practitioners?

a. Physician signature on prescriptions written by NP is required in all states.

b. Controlled substance prescriptions must include the NP's name and DEA number.

c. As of 1998, all states have approved and/or implemented some degree of prescriptive authority for nurse practitioners.

d. Pharmacology education within graduate programs and continuing education is required to maintain authority—specific requirements vary by state.

☐ ANSWERS AND RATIONALES

1. A: According to the APRN Consensus Model, APRN licensure must occur at the level of role and population foci. APRN education is at the minimum master's level. APRNs should be nationally certified, and APRN programs should be accredited by a nursing accrediting agency.

2. D: Overweight status in children ages 6 to 12 years increased by 58.75%.

3. C: The first nurse practitioner (NP) role was pediatric nurse practitioner (PNP). Original support of PNP role was as a "physician extender" to improve access concerns due to shortage of primary care providers.

4. C: Early research focused on quality of care, cost-effectiveness, productivity, clinical decision-making skills, and role satisfaction of the PNP.

5. A: Standards of practice were described by the American Nurses Association as authoritative statements by which to measure quality of practice, service, or education.

6. B: Quality improvement (QI) consists of systematic and continuous actions, such as peer review, patient satisfaction surveys, and chart audits, that lead to measurable improvement in healthcare services and the health status of targeted patient groups.

7. A: Risk management consists of systems and activities designed to recognize and intervene to decrease risk of injury to patients and subsequent claims against healthcare providers and is based on the assumption that many injuries to patients are preventable.

8. B: The National Task Force on Quality Nurse Practitioner Education published the fourth edition of *Criteria for Evaluation of Nurse Practitioner Programs* in 2012, and it is recognized as the national standard for nurse practitioner education.

9. A: Standards of practice establish minimum levels of acceptable performance.

10. D: Scope of practice is based on what is legally allowable in each state according to a state's Nurse Practice Act and varies widely for APRNs across states.

11. A: States set individual eligibility criteria for Medicaid within federal minimum standards. The Affordable Care Act of 2010 (PPACA) created a national minimum Medicaid eligibility criteria of 133% of the federal poverty level.

12. D: Income >133% of federal poverty level exceeds the federal government minimum financial eligibility criteria for Medicaid. States may choose to expand coverage, and all states have done so.

13. A: Income level does not impact Medicare eligibility.

14. A: Medicare Part A covers hospital care, SNF care, nursing home care (but not if only custodial care), hospice, and home health services.

15. A: Medicare Part B covers all medically necessary services—80% of an approved amount after annual deductible. All medically necessary services include physician services; physical, occupational, and speech therapy; medical equipment and diagnostic tests. Some preventive care such as Pap tests, mammograms, and hepatitis B, pneumococcal, and influenza vaccines can be included in medical expenses.

16. C: To bill Medicare, an NP must possess a master's degree in nursing (minimum), have state authorization to practice in state in which services are furnished, and be nationally certified by a certifying body recognized by the Centers for Medicare and Medicaid Services.

17. B: "Incident to" means that the physician must be present in the office suite and available for assistance and direction while the APRN provides patient care. When an APRN performs "incident to" service in a physician's office, billing must be submitted to Medicare by employing the physician, under the physician's name, provider number, and CPT code—payment is made at full physician rate and is paid to physician or physician practice.

18. C: "Incident to" rules apply only to Medicare billing.

19. A: American Nurses Credentialing Center (ANCC) and Pediatric Nursing Certification Board (PNCB) offer certification exams for pediatric nurse practitioners. National Association of Pediatric Nurse Practitioners (NAPNAP) is a professional association, not a certifying body. National Certification Corporation (NCC) offers certification exams for neonatal and women's health NPs.

20. C: Scope of practice of APRN is based on what is legally allowable in each state under its Nurse Practice Act.

21. B: Does not protect an APRN from charges of practicing medicine without a license if the APRN is practicing outside legal scope of practice for that state.

22. A: Working with individuals of other professions describes the Values/Ethics general core competency for interprofessional collaborative practice. Maintaining a silo perspective means maintaining a limited worldview of one discipline's perspective. Implementing hierarchical team-based care supports a silo perspective. Although the patient is the most important member of the interprofessional team, this is not one of the four competencies described in the IPEC Expert Panel report.

23. D: The correct answer is how the APRN Consensus Model describes certification.

24. B: The correct answer is how the APRN Consensus Model defines licensure.

25. B: The Consensus Model for Future Regulation of APRN Practice (2008) describes the APRN regulatory model as including four essential components: licensure, accreditation, certification, and education (LACE).

26. A: The incorrect answers are three of the four key recommendations of the IOM *Future of Nursing* report. The correct fourth message is: "Nurses should work to the full extent of their education and training."

27. A: The incorrect answers are true. Physician signature on prescriptions written by NPs is *not* required in any state.

❐ BIBLIOGRAPHY

American Association of Colleges of Nursing. (2004). *AACN position statement on the practice doctorate in nursing*. Retrieved from http://www.aacn.nche.edu /DNP/DNPPositionStatement.htm

American Association of Nurse Practitioners. (2013). Medicare update. Retrieved from http://www.aanp.org /legislation-regulation/federal-legislation/medicare /68-articles/326-medicare-update

American Nurses Association. (2010). *Nursing: Scope and standards of practice* (2nd ed.). Silver Spring, Maryland: American Nurses Association.

American Nurses Association, National Association of Pediatric Nurse Practitioners, & Society of Pediatric Nurses. (2008). *Pediatric nursing: Scope and standards of practice*. Silver Spring, Maryland: American Nurses Association.

APRN Consensus Work Group & the National Council of State Boards of Nursing (NCSBN) APRN Advisory Committee (2008). *Consensus Model for APRN Regulation: Licensure, Accreditation, Certification & Education*. Chicago, Illinois: NCSBN

APRN Joint Dialogue Group Report. (2008). *Consensus model for PRN regulation: Licensure, accreditation, certification, and education*. Retrieved from http://www .aacn.nche.edu/education-resources/APRNReport.pdf

Case Management Society of America (CMSA). (2014). *What is a case manager?* Available at: http://www.cmsa.org/Home /CMSA/WhatisaCaseManager/tabid/224/Default.aspx

Centers for Medicare and Medicaid Services. (2013). *HIPAA general information*. Available at: https://www.cms .gov/Regulations-and-Guidance/HIPAA-Administrative -Simplification/HIPAAGenInfo/index.html

Centers for Medicare and Medicaid Services. (2015). *Electronic medical record*. Available at http://www.cms.gov /Regulations-and-Guidance/Legislation/EHRIncentive Programs/Downloads/FAQs_Apr_2014.pdf

Christian, S., Dower, C., & O'Neill, E. O. (2007). *Chart overview of nurse practitioner scopes of practice in the United States*. San Francisco: UCSF Center for the Health Professions. Retrieved from http://www.health.state.mn.us /healthreform/workforce/npcomparison.pdf

Hansen-Turton, T., Ware, J., Bond, L., Doria, N., & Cunningham, P. (2013). Are managed care organizations in the United States impeding the delivery of primary care by nurse practitioners? A 2012 update on managed care organization credentialing and reimbursement practices. *Population Health Management, 16*(5), 306–309.

Institute for Credentialing Excellence. (2015). NCAA accreditation. Retrieved from http://www.credentialing excellence.org/ncca

Llewellyn, A., & Leonard, M. (2009). *Nursing case management review and resource manual* (3rd ed.). Silver Spring, MD: American Nurses Credentialing Center.

National Association of Pediatric Nurse Practitioners. (2010). NAPNAP position statement on nurse practitioner prescriptive privileges. *Journal of Pediatric Health Care, 24*(6), 21A–22A.

National Association of Pediatric Nurse Practitioners. (2013). NAPNAP position on the doctorate of nursing practice (DNP). *Journal of Pediatric Health Care, 27*(1), 78–79.

National Conference of State Legislatures. (2013). *Managed car, market reports, and the states*. Retrieved from http://www.ncsl.org/research/health/managed-care -and-the-states.aspx

National Council of State Boards of Nursing. (n.d.) *Licensure*. Available at https://www.ncsbn.org/licensure.htm

National Council of State Boards of Nursing. (n.d.) *Licensure compacts*. Retrieved from https://www.ncsbn.org /compacts.htm

National Task Force on Quality NP Education. (2012). *Criteria for evaluation of nurse practitioner programs*. National Organization of Nurse Practitioner Faculties. Retrieved from http://www.aacn.nche.edu/education-resources/evalcriteria2012.pdf

Nurse Practitioner Roundtable. (2008, June). *Nurse practitioner DNP education certification and titling: A unified statement*. Washington, DC. Retrieved from http://www .pncb.org/ptistore/resource/content/forms/DNP_Unified _Statement.pdf

Sondik, E. J., Huang, D. T., Klein, R. J., & Satcher, D. (2010). Progress toward the Healthy People 2010 goals and objectives. *Annual Review in Public Health, 31*, 271–281.

Stiefel, M., & Nolan, K. (2012). *A guide to measuring the Triple Aim: Population health, experience of care, and per capita cost*. IHI Innovation Series white paper. Cambridge, MA: Institute for Healthcare Improvement. Retrieved from http://www.ihi.org/resources/Pages /IHIWhitePapers/AGuidetoMeasuringTripleAim.aspx

Stokowski, L. A. (2015). APRN prescribing law: A state-by-state summary. Medscape Multispecialty. Retrieved from http://www.medscape.com/viewarticle/440315

U.S. Department of Education. (n.d.-a). FAQs about accreditation. Retrieved from http://ope.ed.gov/accreditation/FAQAccr.aspx

U.S. Department of Health and Human Services. (n.d.-b). HIPAA Administrative Simplification statute and rules. Retrieved from http://www.hhs.gov/ocr/privacy/hipaa /administrative/index.html

World Health Organization (WHO). 2010. *Framework for Action on Interprofessional Education & Collaborative Practice*. Geneva, Switzerland: WHO. Retrieved from: http://whqlibdoc.who.int/hq/2010/WHO_HRH_ HPN_10.3_eng.pdf?ua=1

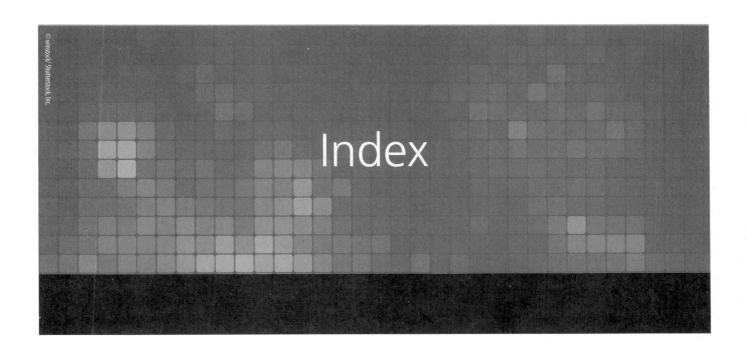

Index